Integrative Psychiatry and Brain Health

Integrative Medicine Library

Published and Forthcoming Volumes

SERIES EDITOR

Andrew Weil, MD

Donald I. Abrams and Andrew Weil: *Integrative Oncology, 2nd edition*
Robert Bonakdar and Andrew W. Sukiennik: *Integrative Pain Management*
Timothy P. Culbert and Karen Olness: *Integrative Pediatrics*
Stephen DeVries and James Dalen: *Integrative Cardiology*
Randy Horwitz and Daniel Muller: *Integrative Rheumatology, Allergy, and Immunology*
Mary Jo Kreitzer and Mary Koithan: *Integrative Nursing*
Gerard Mullin: *Integrative Gastroenterology*
Robert Norman, Philip D. Shenefelt, and Reena N. Rupani: *Integrative Dermatology*
Myles D. Spar and George E. Munoz: *Integrative Men's Health*
Victoria Maizes and Tieraona Low Dog: *Integrative Women's Health, 2nd edition*
Aly Cohen, Frederick S. vom Saal, and Andrew Weil: *Integrative Environmental Medicine*
Richard Carmona and Mark Liponis: *Integrative Preventive Medicine*
Mikhael Kogan: *Integrative Geriatric Medicine*
Daniel A. Monti and Andrew B. Newberg: *Integrative Psychiatry and Brain Health, 2nd edition*
Barbara Bartlik, Geovanni Espinosa, and Janet Mindes: *Integrative Sexual Health*
Shahla Modir and George Munoz: *Integrative Addiction and Recovery*

Integrative Psychiatry and Brain Health

Second Edition

EDITED BY

Daniel A. Monti, MD, MBA
Director
Marcus Institute of Integrative Health
The Ellen and Ron Caplan Chair
Department of Integrative Medicine and Nutritional Sciences
Sidney Kimmel Medical College of Thomas Jefferson University
Philadelphia, PA

Andrew B. Newberg, MD
Director of Research
Marcus Institute of Integrative Health
Department of Integrative Medicine and Nutritional Sciences
Professor of Emergency Medicine and Radiology
Sidney Kimmel Medical College of Thomas Jefferson University
Philadelphia, PA

SERIES EDITOR

Andrew Weil, MD
Founder and Director
Arizona Center for Integrative Medicine
University of Arizona
Tucson, AZ

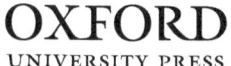

OXFORD
UNIVERSITY PRESS

Oxford University Press is a department of the University of Oxford. It furthers
the University's objective of excellence in research, scholarship, and education
by publishing worldwide. Oxford is a registered trade mark of Oxford University
Press in the UK and certain other countries.

Published in the United States of America by Oxford University Press
198 Madison Avenue, New York, NY 10016, United States of America.

© Oxford University Press 2018

First Edition published in 2010
Second Edition published in 2018

All rights reserved. No part of this publication may be reproduced, stored in
a retrieval system, or transmitted, in any form or by any means, without the
prior permission in writing of Oxford University Press, or as expressly permitted
by law, by license, or under terms agreed with the appropriate reproduction
rights organization. Inquiries concerning reproduction outside the scope of the
above should be sent to the Rights Department, Oxford University Press, at the
address above.

You must not circulate this work in any other form
and you must impose this same condition on any acquirer.

Library of Congress Cataloging-in-Publication Data
Names: Monti, Daniel A., editor. | Newberg, Andrew B., 1966– editor.
Title: Integrative psychiatry and brain health / edited by Daniel A. Monti, Andrew B. Newberg.
Other titles: Integrative psychiatry (Monti) | Weil integrative medicine library.
Description: Second edition. | New York, NY : Oxford University Press, [2018] |
Series: Weil integrative medicine library |
Preceeded by: Integrative psychiatry / edited by Daniel A. Monti,
Bernard D. Beitman. 2010. | Includes bibliographical references and index.
Identifiers: LCCN 2017036634 | ISBN 9780190690557 (pbk.)
Subjects: | MESH: Mental Disorders—therapy | Brain—physiology |
Complementary Therapies | Integrative Medicine—methods
Classification: LCC RC480.5 | NLM WM 400 | DDC 616.89/14—dc23
LC record available at https://lccn.loc.gov/2017036634

This material is not intended to be, and should not be considered, a substitute for medical or other
professional advice. Treatment for the conditions described in this material is highly dependent on
the individual circumstances. And, while this material is designed to offer accurate information with
respect to the subject matter covered and to be current as of the time it was written, research and
knowledge about medical and health issues is constantly evolving and dose schedules for medications
are being revised continually, with new side effects recognized and accounted for regularly. Readers
must therefore always check the product information and clinical procedures with the most up-to-
date published product information and data sheets provided by the manufacturers and the most
recent codes of conduct and safety regulation. The publisher and the authors make no representations
or warranties to readers, express or implied, as to the accuracy or completeness of this material.
Without limiting the foregoing, the publisher and the authors make no representations or warranties
as to the accuracy or efficacy of the drug dosages mentioned in the material. The authors and the
publisher do not accept, and expressly disclaim, any responsibility for any liability, loss or risk that
may be claimed or incurred as a consequence of the use and/ or application of any of the contents of
this material.

3 5 7 9 8 6 4 2
Printed by Webcom, Inc., Canada

CONTENTS

Foreword to the Second Edition   vii
Acknowledgments   ix
About the Editors   x
Contributors   xi

Section 1   Lifestyle Effects on Brain Health

1. Diet, Gut, and Brain: A New Horizon   3
   Anthony J. Bazzan and Daniel A. Monti

2. Key Nutrients for Normal Brain Health   19
   Rashna K. Staid

3. Effects of Exercise on Mental Health   50
   Stephen Olex and Krista Olex

4. The Neurobiology of Meditation and Stress Reduction   97
   Andrew B. Newberg and David B. Yaden

5. The Interaction of Religion and Health   118
   David B. Yaden and Andrew B. Newberg

6. Behavioral Strategies for Happiness and Satisfaction   157
   Cathy Greenberg and Relly Nadler

Section 2   Healing Systems: Theory and Evidence

7. Botanicals of Interest to Psychiatrists   177
   Daniel A. Monti and Andrew B. Newberg

8. Acupuncture and Chinese Medicine   205
   Jingduan Yang and Daniel A. Monti

9. The Role of Chiropractic in Mind–Body Health   238
   George Zabrecky

10. Homeopathy and Psychiatry 258
   Bernardo A. Merizalde

11. Hypnosis and Biofeedback as Prototypes of Mind–Body Medicine 287
    Marie Stoner

12. Mindfulness-Based Interventions for Psychiatric Disorders 312
    Aleeze Moss and Diane Reibel

13. Neuromodulation in Psychiatric Disorders 329
    Christina Herring

Section 3 Integrative Psychiatry in Practice

14. Functional Neuroimaging: A Transformative Tool for Integrative Psychiatry 347
    Abass Alavi and Andrew B. Newberg

15. Commonly Encountered Sleep Disorders 382
    Karl Doghramji

16. Cognitive Interventions: Brain Training and Rehabilitation 404
    Thomas Swirsky-Sacchetti and Robert L. Rider

17. Integrative Approaches to Cognitive Decline 431
    Thomas J. Kelly IV and Mijail Serruya

18. Integrative Approaches to Depression 472
    Nancy Wintering and Andrew B. Newberg

19. Integrative Treatment of Anxiety 498
    Birgit Rakel

20. Integrative Treatment of Emotional Traumas 530
    Anna Tobia

21. Addictions: Evidence for Integrative Treatment 555
    Mary F. Morrison, Karen Lin, and Susan Gersh

Index 575

FOREWORD TO THE SECOND EDITION

ANDREW WEIL, MD
Series Editor

Integrative Psychiatry was first published in 2010. Since then, interest in the field has grown among both patients and providers, driven largely by concerns about overmedication.

More people than ever take psychiatric medications. Many mental health professionals say they are tired of being pill pushers. Many patients find the drugs problematical, not as effective as promised and often causing adverse effects and dependence. All of us should be troubled by the vast numbers of children and adolescents on them, because we do not know what are the effects on the developing brain of long-term use of psychiatric drugs. I am particularly uneasy about the casual dispensing of antipsychotic agents—drugs intended for management of schizophrenia—now given as first-line interventions along with SSRI antidepressants to boost the often disappointing efficacy of those products.

And since 2010, the evidence base for nonpharmacological management of mental and emotional disorders has grown substantially. Cognitive Behavioral Therapy (CBT) and mindfulness practice, for example, appear to be as effective as medication in treating mild to moderate depression. We are learning more about lifestyle influences on mental health, particularly dietary habits. A surprising and exciting recent discovery is the complex interaction of the gut microbiome and brain. The first chapter of this updated edition is devoted to the subject.

Drs. Monti and Newberg have made the second edition of *Integrative Psychiatry* a most useful handbook for putting this new model into practice. It advances the field by presenting evidence-based approaches for managing the most common psychiatric disorders and will greatly benefit both patients and practitioners.

ACKNOWLEDGMENTS

We would like to express our gratitude to Andrew Weil, MD, for the opportunity to contribute to this important *Integrative Medicine* textbook series. Andy has been a teacher and friend, and we share a common mission of expanding the horizons of health and wellness care. In addition, we would like to thank our editors, Andrea Knobloch and Tiffany Lu, at Oxford University Press for all of their help in making this book a reality. We also would like to thank our students, Huiqing Xu and Jacqueline Muscella, for their help with formatting the manuscript. Finally, we are deeply appreciative to our colleagues for the superb chapters they contributed with the common goal of providing the most up-to-date and comprehensive book on integrative psychiatry and brain health.

ABOUT THE EDITORS

Daniel A. Monti, MD, MBA, is founding Director of the Marcus Institute of Integrative Health and founding Chair of the Department of Integrative Medicine and Nutritional Sciences, the first medical school department in the nation devoted to the field of Integrative Medicine, at the Sidney Kimmel Medical College of Thomas Jefferson University. He also is Professor in the departments of Psychiatry and Emergency Medicine. Dr. Monti's extensive research has focused on assessing promising mind-body interventions, understanding brain mechanisms of stress and emotional regulation, and testing natural molecules for therapeutic efficacy in nervous system diseases and cancer. He is author of dozens of scholarly papers and one popular press book, and editor of three textbooks.

Andrew B. Newberg, MD, is currently the Director of Research at the Marcus Institute of Integrative Health and the Department of Integrative Medicine and Nutritional Sciences at the Sidney Kimmel Medical College of Thomas Jefferson University. He is also a Professor in the Departments of Emergency Medicine and Radiology. Dr. Newberg has actively pursued a number of neuroimaging research projects which have included the study of aging and dementia, epilepsy, and other neurological and psychiatric disorders. He has also studied the more general mind/body relationship including understanding the physiological correlates of acupuncture, meditation, and other types of integrative therapies. He has published over 200 peer reviewed articles and chapters as well as two best-selling books.

CONTRIBUTORS

Abass Alavi, MD, MD (Hon), PhD (Hon), DSc (Hon)
Professor of Radiology
Hospital of the University of Pennsylvania
Associate Director, Center for the Study of Aging
University of Pennsylvania
Philadelphia, PA

Anthony J. Bazzan, MD, FACN, ABIHM
Assistant Professor
Associate Director, Marcus Institute of Integrative Health
Thomas Jefferson University
Philadelphia, PA

Karl Doghramji, MD
Professor of Psychiatry, Neurology, and Medicine
Medical Director, Jefferson Sleep Disorders Center
Program Director, Fellowship in Sleep Medicine
Thomas Jefferson University
Philadelphia, PA

Susan Gersh, MD
Professor of Clinical Medicine, Internal Medicine
Lewis Katz School of Medicine
Temple University
Philadelphia, PA

Cathy Greenberg, PhD, PCC
Executive Coach and Founder, The Fearless Leaders Group
Faculty, College of Executive Coaching
Arroyo Grande, CA

Christina Herring, MD
Associate Professor of Psychiatry
Marcus Institute of Integrative Health
Thomas Jefferson University
Philadelphia, PA

Thomas J. Kelly IV, BA
Department of Neurology
Thomas Jefferson University
Philadelphia, PA

Karen Lin, MD, MPH
Associate Professor of Clinical
 Medicine, Internal Medicine
Director, Acupuncture Program at
 Temple General Internal Medicine
Lewis Katz School of Medicine
Temple University
Philadelphia, PA

Bernardo A. Merizalde, MD
Clinical Assistant Professor
Marcus Institute of Integrative Health
Thomas Jefferson University
Philadelphia, PA

Daniel A. Monti, MD, MBA
Director
Marcus Institute of Integrative Health
The Ellen and Ron Caplan Chair
Department of Integrative Medicine
 and Nutritional Sciences
Sidney Kimmel Medical College of
 Thomas Jefferson University
Philadelphia, PA

Mary F. Morrison, MD, MS
Vice Chairperson for Research and
 Professor of Psychiatry
Lewis Katz School of Medicine
Temple University
Philadelphia, PA

Aleeze Moss, PhD
Associate Director
Myrna Brind Center for Mindfulness
Marcus Institute of Integrative Health
Thomas Jefferson University
Philadelphia, PA

Relly Nadler, PsyD, MCC
President/CEO, True North Leadership
Co-Founder/Chief Executive Coach;
 Vital Signs, Vital Skills
Santa Barbara, CA

Andrew B. Newberg, MD
Director of Research
Marcus Institute of Integrative Health
Department of Integrative Medicine
 and Nutritional Sciences
Professor of Emergency Medicine and
 Radiology
Sidney Kimmel Medical College of
 Thomas Jefferson University
Philadelphia, PA

Krista Olex, PsyD
Clinical Psychology
Behavioral Health Consulting
Washington, DC

Stephen Olex, MD
Integrative Cardiology
Marcus Institute of Integrative Health
Thomas Jefferson University
Villanova, PA

Birgit Rakel, MD
Assistant Professor
Director, Integrative Women's Health
 Program
Marcus Institute of Integrative Health
Thomas Jefferson University
Philadelphia, PA

Diane Reibel, PhD
Director
Myrna Brind Center for Mindfulness
Marcus Institute of Integrative Health
Thomas Jefferson University
Philadelphia, PA

Robert L. Rider, PhD
Diversified Psychological Resources
Philadelphia, PA

Mijail Serruya, MD, PhD
Assistant Professor
Department of Neurology
Co-Medical Director, Comprehensive Concussion Center
Thomas Jefferson University
Philadelphia, PA

Rashna K. Staid, MD, ABIHM, FACP
Clinical Instructor and Co-Director of Executive Medicine Program
Marcus Institute of Integrative Health
Thomas Jefferson University
Philadelphia, PA

Marie Stoner, MEd
Director of Programming/Co-Founder, Activate Brain & Body, Inc.
Consultant, Marcus Institute of Integrative Health
Thomas Jefferson University
Philadelphia, PA

Thomas Swirsky-Sacchetti, PhD, ABPP-CN
Diversified Psychological Resources
Consultant, Marcus Institute of Integrative Health
Thomas Jefferson University
Philadelphia, PA

Anna Tobia, PhD
Clinical Psychologist
Marcus Institute of Integrative Health
Thomas Jefferson University
Philadelphia, PA

Nancy Wintering, MSW, LCSW, CCRP
Research Program Manager
Marcus Institute of Integrative Health
Thomas Jefferson University
Philadelphia, PA

David B. Yaden, MA
PhD Candidate
University of Pennsylvania
Philadelphia, PA

Jingduan Yang, MD, FAPA
Founder and President
American Institute for Clinical Acupuncture
Philadelphia, PA
Faculty, Fellowship in Integrative Medicine
Center for Integrative Medicine
University of Arizona
Tuscon, AZ

George Zabrecky, DC, MD
Founder and Director
Life Extension Center
Villanova, PA
Research Assistant Professor
Marcus Institute of Integrative Health
Thomas Jefferson University
Philadelphia, PA

Integrative Psychiatry and Brain Health

SECTION 1

Lifestyle Effects on Brain Health

1

Diet, Gut, and Brain: A New Horizon

ANTHONY J. BAZZAN AND DANIEL A. MONTI

> **Key Points**
>
> - There is growing data that dietary factors have profound effects on inflammation, the gut microbiome, intestinal permeability, and the blood–brain barrier, all of which impact brain health.
> - The Western diet is deleterious for both physical and cognitive/emotional health.
> - Recent research advances elucidate that understanding the harmful physiological effects of certain dietary behaviors is as important as knowing the role of critical nutrients for optimal brain health.

Introduction

Many Americans consume what is commonly referred to as the Western diet (WD), which broadly includes fried foods, sugars, red meat, refined grains, high-fat dairy products, as well as other processed and fast foods. This dietary approach is known to promote obesity, metabolic syndrome, cardiovascular disease, cancer, and many other health problems (Manzel et al., 2014; Stott-Miller, Neuhouser, & Stanford, 2013; Tantamango-Bartley, Jaceldo-Siegl, Fan, & Fraser, 2013).

A recent study (Akbaraly et al., 2013) shows that those who consume a predominantly WD are at increased risk for premature death and those who do survive to old age are less likely to remain in good health. The study included nearly 3,800 men and 1,600 women, with an average age of 51, who were followed for nearly 25 years. Other data suggests that diet has direct correlates with emotional state. For example, a prospective study of diet quality and mental health in adolescents showed that a healthier diet (i.e., more vegetables, fruits, and whole grains) was associated with less anxiety and depression (Jacka, Kremer, Taylor, Berk, & Stansfeld, 2011).

Western Diet, Inflammation, and Mood

One frequently discussed mechanism for the deleterious effects of the WD is inflammation. Western-type foods and body fat are independent risk factors for inflammation. Hence, certain foods themselves may induce inflammation (Tantamango-Bartley et al., 2013), and the increased body fat that results from these foods are a source of inflammation. For example, consumption of unhealthy fats increases inflammatory factors, and adipocytes are known to release inflammatory substances including interleukin (IL-) 1, IL-6, and tumor necrosis factor (TNF).

Inflammation, in turn, can negatively affect mood. Inflammatory markers are associated with depressed mood (Harrison et al., 2009), and antidepressants can have an anti-inflammatory affect (Hashioka, McGeer, Monji, & Kanba, 2009). Acute inflammation is known to cause a negative mood state, mediated by cytokine activation (Wright, Strike, Brydon, & Steptoe, 2005). In addition, the mood changes caused by inflammation have been observed to do so through alterations of subgenual cingulate activity and mesolimbic connectivity (Harrison et al., 2009).

Of note, many non-WD diet foods, such as those associated with a Mediterranean-type diet, are associated with decreased inflammation. For example, omega-3 fatty acids have been shown to have anti-inflammatory and immune-enhancing properties (Mori & Beilin, 2004), as is the case with many plant foods (Recio, Andujar, & Rios, 2012) and dietary fiber (Ma et al., 2012).

The Gut Microbiome

An important recent development in the understanding of a key source of inflammation is the functioning of the gut microbiome. The gut microbiota has diverse and essential roles in metabolism of nutrients, in development of the immune system, and as resistance to pathogen colonization via interactions with gut-associated lymphoid tissue. Perturbations of the gut microbiota, referred to as gut dysbiosis, are commonly described in diseases involving inflammation, including inflammatory bowel disease, infection, colorectal cancer, and food allergies. Importantly, the inflamed microenvironment in the gut is particularly conducive to proliferation of *Enterobacteriaceae*, while families of potentially healthful bacteria succumb to environmental changes caused by inflammation (Zeng, Inohara, & Nuñez, 2017).

Diet has a pivotal role in determining the composition of the gut microbiota. For example, the abundance of oligosaccharides in human breast milk favors the proliferation of helpful bacteria equipped with carbohydrate-processing enzymes, such as Bifidobacterium, in comparison to formula-fed infants who have higher levels of *Clostridium* spp. (Fallani et al., 2010; Marcobal et al., 2010). Mice fed on a WD with high sugar and fat display a reduction in Bacteroidetes but an overgrowth of Firmicutes (Daniel et al., 2014), an unfavorable ratio that is discussed in further detail later. A vegetarian diet in humans is associated with lower intestinal pH and increased short-chain fatty acids (SCFAs) that might have an inhibitive effect on the growth of *Escherichia coli* and other members of Enterobacteriaceae (Zimmer et al., 2012). Consumption of a diet high in milk-derived saturated fat, but not plant-derived polyunsaturated fat, changes the conditions for microbial balance in a way that was shown to be associated with a proinflammatory immune response and increased incidence of colitis in genetically susceptible mice (Devkota, 2012). Hence food may have a profound role in shaping the composition of the gut microbiota. In the inflamed gut, collateral damage of the mucosal epithelium due to inflammatory response and increased shedding of dead epithelial cells contributes to an environment for unfavorable proliferation of unhealthful and pathogenic microbiota (Zimmer et al., 2012).

The human gut microbiome has been thought to contain at least 10 times more cells than the human body, or about 1% to 3% of total body mass (MacDougall, 2012). However, some suggest the new ratio of bacteria to human cells is closer to 1:1 (3.8×10^T to 3.0×10^T for total number of bacteria and human cells, respectively; Sender, Fuchs, & Milo, 2016).

The human gut harbors 10^{11} to 10^{12} per gram colonic content (>10^{14} total bacteria). More important than absolute cell numbers is that total bacterial genes outnumber human genes by about 150:1, and more than 10,000 different species are resident in the human. The human genome has 23,000 genes whereas the human microbiome has over 1 million genes. Hence, we walk around with approximately 1,023,000 genes with the majority of those genes not us but the microbiome within us, the implications of which are massive.

So the realization comes that the gene expression of our 23,000 chromosomes means whether we build a healthy or a sick body comes not so much from our family history as from the bacterial mass we host in our guts. That mass is highly dependent on environmental factors and principally our diets.

As sobering as this is, it is also great news when it comes to strategies to prevent or reverse chronic diseases.

The intestinal microbiota functions like an organ with metabolic activity that rivals the liver. It is important for immune and gastrointestinal maturation, normal central nervous system development, colonization resistance, immune system modulation, and metabolic maturation. For example, the microbiota has important effects on both multiple immune mechanisms. Innate mechanisms, such as epithelial production of protective mucin layers maintaining spatial segregation in the intestine, as well as epithelial cell secretion of a broad range of antimicrobial peptides, all work in tandem to protect and balance physiological processes in the gut and body. Further, adaptive mechanisms such as specific microbial species within the gut stimulate induction of regulatory T cells while others induce effector T cells (Elson & Alexander, 2015). Hence, there is ongoing communication between the microbiota and immune system, underscoring the potential importance of the composition of the microorganisms themselves. Changes in the mucosal barrier from infection or other means can induce effector T cells that are reactive to the intestinal microbiota. These cells can persist as memory cells for extended periods of time and can become pathogenic effector cells when they reencounter the antigen. Brain and body health is associated with a diverse gut microbiota that functions to maintain the balance between T effector and T regulatory cells in the intestine. Whether dysbiosis can be reversed in patients who have immunologically mediated diseases, and subsequently restore health, is an important clinical and research question.

As we consider the gut microbiota and its effects on human health, the following categorizations are noted:

- **Microbiome** (Who is there?): The composite of commensal, symbiotic, and pathogenic microbial species that are living in the gut. There are numerous emerging technologies and techniques to assess the microenvironment of the gut.
- **Metagenomics** (What language do they speak?): Genomic analysis of microbial DNA that is extracted directly from communities in environmental samples. This technology—genomics on a large scale—enables a survey of the different microorganisms present in a specific environment, for example the human gut.
- **Metascriptomics** (What are they talking about?): A branch of transcriptomics that studies and correlates the transcriptomes of a group of interacting organisms or species. This technique enables us to identify the actively transcribed ribosomal and messenger ribonucleic acid (RNA) from a community.

In terms of the microbiome itself, the two largest phyla are Firmicutes and Bacteroidetes (Box 1.1). The altered relationship of the Firmicutes/Bacteroidetes ratio has been associated with a number of pathological conditions. For example, obesity has been associated with an increased abundance of Firmicutes and/or a decrease in Bacteroidetes (Hildebrandt et al., 2009). This ratio is also related to disruption of metabolic homeostasis (e.g., type 2 diabetes mellitus and non-alcoholic fatty liver disease) and elevated markers of inflammation such as IL-6 (Milner & Beck, 2012).

The short-term consumption of a diet entirely of animal or plant products alters the gut microbial gene expression rapidly (David et al., 2014). This is an important observation suggesting that dietary interventions may be potentially the most powerful factor affecting the gut microbiome. Likewise, metagenomic and metabolomic studies show that in obesity some microbiota show a more efficient intestinal absorption of calories and increased lipid deposition (Hildebrandt et al., 2009).

Animal-based diet consumption leads to increased bile-tolerant microbiota (i.e., *Alistipes* spp., *Bilophila* spp., *Bacteroidetes* spp.) and decreased dietary plant polysaccharide fermenters (i.e., *Firmicutes, Roseburia* spp.,

---

Box 1.1 Two Largest Phyla: Firmicutes and Bacteroidetes

Examples of Firmicutes

- *Anaerotruncus colihominis* spp.
- *Butyrivibrio crossotus* spp.
- *Clostridium* spp.
- *Coprococcus eutactus* spp.
- *Faecalibacterium prausnitzii* spp.
- *Lactobacillus* spp.
- *Pseudoflavonifractor* spp.
- *Roseburia* spp.
- *Ruminococcus* spp.
- *Veillonella* spp.

Examples of Bacteroidetes

- *Bacteroides–Prevotella* spp.
- *B. vulgatus* spp.
- *Prevotella* spp.
- *Barnesiella* spp.
- *Odoribacter* spp.

Eubacterium rectale spp., *Ruminococcus bromii* spp.) while at the same time increased presence of *Bilophila wadsworthia*, a gram-negative anaerobe that is associated with gut inflammatory conditions including acute appendicitis and inflammatory bowel disease (David, et al. 2014; Finegold, Summanen, Hunt Gerardo, & Baron, 1992). This latter relationship was discovered as a result of administration of high-dose intravenous antibiotics.

The Diet and Microbiota Interact with Gut Regulators

Multiple studies have shown that gut microbiota have effects on gut permeability (Cani et al., 2007; Lam et al., 2012; Maffeis et al., 2016; Mokkala et al., 2016; Pendyala, Walker, & Holt, 2012; Tulstrup et al., 2015), and WD significantly alters the distribution of bacteria in the gastrointestinal tract. The intestinal barrier consists of specialized, semipermeable cell layers united by tight junction proteins. This barrier serves to regulate nutrient and water entry and prevents the entry of undesired compounds (Turner, 2009). It protects us from the outside world, more so than the skin or lungs. In effect it determines who is coming in, who is not coming in, and the regulation of everything the gut comes into contact with.

The intestinal barrier has important structures between adjacent cells in the gut: tight junctions, gap junctions, and desmosomes. Tight junctions are watertight doors when they are working properly. Zonulin, a protein from prehaptoglobin (HP)2, has the ability to open these doors, presumably for the purpose of sampling the outside to train the immune system (Fasano, 2012). Hence, zonulin is a physiologic modulator of intercellular tight junctions and is the only protein currently described in trafficking of macromolecules for tolerance/immune response balance.

Gluten can activate zonulin and open the doors, as can several microbiota. Celiac disease is a great model for understanding the activity of these doors. Gluten is composed of a mixture of two main proteins, gliadins and glutenins. Glutenin forms a meshwork of fibers in which globular gliadins are embedded. This leads to a number of inflammatory processes across several organ systems. Both types of proteins can result in significant symptoms in patients with celiac disease.

Tight junctions are extremely complex structures and have numerous redundancies and back-up systems. If the zonulin pathway is deregulated in genetically susceptible individuals, disorders can occur. We have known for a long time that in order to develop many of the common illnesses of today, a combination of genes and environmental exposures (diet, stress, toxins, pollutants, etc.) is needed. However, it is increasingly apparent that the rest of the puzzle includes the microbiome, gut permeability, and dysregulation of immune response, and they are all interrelated.

Zonulin as a Potential Marker of Gut–Brain Dysfunction

The genes for zonulin are on chromosome 16. It is interesting to note that there is tremendous overlap in the diseases known to have a genetic link on chromosome 16 and those for which zonulin has emerged as a biomarker, including autoimmune diseases, cancers, and diseases of the nervous system.

The composition of tight junctions involves occludin and zonula occludens (ZO) proteins such as ZO-1, ZO-2, and ZO-3. Zonulin binding to the cell surface results in rearrangement of the cell cytoskeleton, loss of occludin-ZO1 protein–protein interaction, and increased membrane permeability (Drago et al., 2006). This provides an explanation for the connection of seemingly disparate diseases and a common pathway of altered intestinal permeability. ZO proteins may be affected by diet. For example, in rodents, WD foods decrease levels of tight junction protein ZO-1 and transepithelial resistance in the proximal colon, both markers of gut barrier dysfunction (Lam et al., 2012). A compromised gut barrier makes the intestinal tract vulnerable to gram-negative lipopolysaccharides (LPS), which promotes endotoxemia and systemic inflammation (Cani et al., 2007, 2008).

In a study focused on detecting schizophrenia-related changes of plasma proteins, the genetic relationship between acute phase proteins and schizophrenia disease was assessed by testing HP α1/HP α2 (i.e., zonulin) polymorphism and two single nucleotide polymorphisms of HP, rs2070937 and rs5473, for associations with schizophrenia. The authors found that four proteins in the family of positive acute phase proteins were all upregulated in patients. There were significant associations between schizophrenia and polymorphisms related to the HP gene. Schizophrenia is accompanied by both an altered expression of HP and a different genotype distribution of the HP gene. Thus the HP gene is associated with schizophrenia (Wan et al., 2007). Similar results were previously reported by Maes et al. (2001), who examined HP phenotypic and genotypic frequencies in 98 northwestern Italian schizophrenic patients compared with healthy controls. The frequency of the HP gene was significantly higher in schizophrenic patients compared to controls.

The Role of Vitamin D in the Gut–Brain Connection

Vitamin D_3 induces the expression of occludin, ZO-1, ZO-2, and vinculin, and vitamin D_3 treatment promotes the translocation of ZO-1 to the plasma membrane (Pálmer et al., 2001). Chronic infection with intracellular bacteria dysregulates vitamin D metabolism by causing vitamin D receptor dysfunction within phagocytes (Waterhouse, Perez, & Albert, 2009). This underscores an increasing importance of vitamin D levels in patients who present with a myriad of issues that may be associated with intestinal permeability problems.

Another observation in regard to the gut–brain connection is that vitamin D levels have inversely correlated with depression in observational studies, increasing risk by 14% to 60% (Jorde, Sneve, Figenschau, Svartberg, & Waterloo, 2008). There also is data that vitamin D can have a positive treatment effect on depression. In a randomized trial of 441 obese patients with low vitamin D levels, high-dose supplementation was associated with improved depression outcomes at one year (Jorde et al., 2008). A case series of depressed adolescents showed significant improvement of depressive symptoms with vitamin D supplementation in combination with psychotherapy (Högberg, 2012).

Gut, Microbiome, and Cognition

Changes in the gut microbiome may contribute to changes in cognition. It has been shown that supplementation with multispecies microorganisms can influence brain function, including induction of hippocampal synaptic plasticity and production of brain-derived neurotrophic factor, in animal models. In addition, spectroscopy analysis revealed regional-specific changes in brain metabolites in response to microorganism supplementation, which indicates changes in several pathways contributing to modulation of neural signaling (O'Hagan et al., 2017).

A recent human study using brain relaxometry and cognitive testing showed that changes in waist circumference were associated with brain iron deposition in the striatum, amygdala, and hippocampus in parallel to visual-spatial constructional ability and circulating beta amyloid Aβ42 levels. These changes were linked to shifts in gut microbiome; hence, changes in the gut metagenome were associated longitudinally with cognitive function and brain iron deposition (Blasco, 2017). In addition, gut metagenome changes were associated with bacterial generation of siderophores (iron-reducing compounds), suggestive of more virulent microorganisms (Heesemann et al., 1993). This study also extends previous work in animal models on the gut microbiota and obesity. The obese microbiota differs from the lean microbiota and may produce more SCFAs and, hence, extract more energy from a given diet than the lean microbiota. The relative proportion of Bacteroidetes was lower and Firmicutes was higher in obese than lean individuals, which also has been observed in diet-related cognitive impairment (Hildebrandt et al., 2009).

In a recent study prebiotics were shown to have anxiolytic and antidepressant-like effects and reverse the impact of chronic stress in mice (Burokas et al., 2017). These combined findings suggest that more research is warranted to further explore the potential for therapeutic targeting of the gut microbiota for cognitive health.

The blood–brain barrier (BBB) itself may be affected by dietary factors and the microbiome. The BBB is the regulator for the entry of blood-derived nutrients and compounds required for healthy brain function. It is the protector from the entry of potentially harmful blood-derived toxins. It is composed mainly of endothelial cells, pericytes, and glial cells that together provide the scaffolding that encompasses microvascular networks within the central nervous system.

The gut microbiome influences cognitive function via the gut–brain axis and BBB integrity, which is negatively affected by the WD, particular high-fat and high-sugar diets that increase Firmicutes and decrease Bacteroidales (Braniste et al., 2014). Recent evidence links the gut microbiome with dietary- and metabolic-associated hippocampal impairment. In one study, rats on a WD for 90 days exhibited a leaky BBB in the hippocampus and reduced mRNA expression of the tight junction proteins claudin-5 and claudin-12 (Kanoski, Zhang, Zheng, & Davidson, 2010). The hippocampus in humans is located in the temporal lobes and is part of the limbic system. It is responsible for processing of long-term memory and emotional responses, storage of long-term memories, and memory of the location of objects or people. Others have observed cognitive impairment.

Western Diet Effects on the Brain

SCFAs, such as acetate, propionate, and butyrate, are produced in the gut by microbiota fermentation of indigestible carbohydrates, such as resistant starch and non-starch polysaccharides from whole grains, vegetables, and fruits (MacFarlane & MacFarlane, 2011). These acids nourish the cells of the gastrointestinal tract. They are indispensable for the health of the cells, the gut, and therefore the individual. Most SCFAs in portal circulation are metabolized by the liver. SCFAs produced in the distal colon bypass portal circulation and reach the brain through general circulation (MacFabe, 2012).

The production of SCFAs is significantly reduced in humans within days following a change from a plant-based diet to an animal-based diet high in saturated fat and low in complex carbohydrates (David et al., 2014). SCFAs have a neuroprotective effect. Sodium butyrate promotes cell proliferation and differentiation in the dentate gyrus resulting in brain-derived neurotrophic factor and glia-derived neurotrophic factor. An example of the potential clinical significance is that sodium butyrate improves memory performance in the novel object recognition task (Intlekofer et al., 2013; Stefanko et al., 2009). Butyrate has anti-inflammatory actions in the gut and brain by preventing the induction of TNFa by LPS via the suppression of nuclear factor kB (Segain et al., 2000). Recently butyrate has been shown to stabilize hypoxia-inducible factor, critical for maintaining gut barrier integrity and protecting against the influx of toxins (Kelly et al., 2015).

Animal models consistently show that chronic consumption of a WD elevates levels of neuroinflammatory markers, with associated impaired cognition (Camer et al., 2015; Hsu et al., 2015; Ledreux et al., 2016; Puig et al., 2012). Gut microbiota can directly stimulate the production of IL-1b and TNFa, which impair hippocampal-dependent memories in rodents (Hein et al., 2010; Heumann et al., 1994; Rachal Pugh et al., 2001). Along with cognitive impairments, rats fed a WD have increased neuro-inflammation in both the hippocampus and the cortex (Camer et al., 2015; Herculano et al., 2013; Hsu et al., 2015; Ledreux et al., 2016; Pistell et al., 2010; Puig et al., 2012). WD consumption elevates levels of inflammatory endotoxins such as LPS, and increased levels of microbiome-derived LPS in circulation stimulate inflammatory pathways (Amar et al., 2008; Bruce-Keller et al., 2009; Cani et al., 2007). There is data to suggest this research may be generalizable to humans, with reports implicating an association between circulating inflammatory factors and cognitive decline in humans (Sellbom & Gunstad, 2012; Sweat et al., 2008).

The bacterial species *Akkermania muciniphila* is reduced by the diet species that is negatively associated with inflammation (Bruce-Keller et al., 2015; Schneeberger et al., 2015), while anti-inflammatory *Lactobacilli* are reduced by WDs. In addition, supplementation with *Lactobacillus helveticus* prevents spatial memory impairment in WD-fed mice lacking the anti-inflammatory cytokine IL-10 (Lecomte et al., 2015; Ohland et al., 2013).

Insulin is released in response to brain cues and circulating glucose. Insulin crosses the BBB via a saturable transporter, and insulin receptors are present in neurons primarily localized to synapses. WD-induced peripheral insulin resistance has been associated with impaired cognitive function and reduced synaptic plasticity in rat models (Pavlik et al., 2013; Stranahan et al., 2008). In humans, increased circulating insulin and insulin resistance also is associated with an increased risk for developing dementia including Alzheimer's disease (Arvanitakis et al., 2004; Luchsinger et al., 2004; Rönnemaa et al., 2008).

Conclusion

Consumption of a WD that is high in saturated fat and added sugars may negatively impact cognitive function, particularly processes that rely on the integrity of the hippocampus. Reviewed mechanisms that link the WD with cognitive dysfunction include dysbiosis, reduced SCFA production, altered gut barrier and BBB integrity, neuro-inflammation, and insulin receptor resistance. Currently available data suggest that the gut microbiome influences cognitive function via a gut–brain axis and that WD factors significantly alter the proportions of commensal bacteria in the gastrointestinal tract. We underscore data linking gut bacteria to altered intestinal permeability and BBB integrity, thus making the brain more vulnerable to the influx of harmful substances from the gastrointestinal tract and, eventually, circulation. The WD also increases production of endotoxin by commensal bacteria, which in turn can promote brain inflammation leading to emotional and cognitive dysfunction. There is limited but growing evidence that specific probiotics or prebiotics may positively impact the deleterious effects of WD consumption, particularly neuropsychological outcomes.

Together the current evidence supports the notion that some disease processes can be modified if the damaging interplay between genes and environment is prevented by avoiding environmental triggers and that health may be retrieved or enhanced by reestablishing the intestinal barrier and lowering systemic inflammation. Also, the WD is more critical in causing dysbiosis than an overweight or obese body mass index (Davis, Yadav, Barrow, & Robertson, 2017). It is then clear that dietary factors are emerging as crucial factors, and clinicians should consider diet as a potential risk factor as well as a potential therapy in the overall evaluation of brain heath. More human studies exploring gut–brain axis pathways are needed to facilitate the development of therapies that target the microbiome, such as probiotics, prebiotics, antibiotics, or microbiota transfer to treat neurobiological and cognitive dysfunction.

REFERENCES

Akbaraly, T., Sabia, S., Hagger-Johnson, G., Tabak, A. G., Shipley, M. J., Jokela, M., et al. (2013). Does overall diet in midlife predict future aging phenotypes? A cohort study. *American Journal of Medicine, 126*(5), 411–419.

Amar, J., Burcelin, R., Ruidavets, J. B., Cani, P. D., Fauvel, J., Alessi, M. C., Chamontin, B., & Ferriéres, J. (2008). Energy intake is associated with endotoxemia in apparently healthy men. *American Journal of Clinical Nutrition, 87*(5), 1219–1223.

Arvanitakis, Z., Wilson, R. S., Bienias, J. L., Evans, D. A., & Bennett, D. A. (2004). Diabetes mellitus and risk of Alzheimer disease and decline in cognitive function. *Archives of Neurology, 61*(5), 661–666.

Blasco, G., Moreno-Navarrete, J. M., Rivero, M., Pérez-Brocal, V., Garre-Olmo, J., Puig, J., et al. (2017). The Gut Metagenome Changes in Parallel to Waist Circumference, Brain Iron Deposition, and Cognitive Function. *Journal of Clinical Endocrinology and Metabolism, 102*(8), 2962–2973.

Braniste, V., Al-Asmakh, M., Kowal, C., Anuar, F., Abbaspour, A., Tóth, M., et al. (2014). The gut microbiota influences blood-brain barrier permeability in mice. *Science Translational Medicine, 6*(263), 263ra158. doi:10.1126/scitranslmed.3009759

Bruce-Keller, A. J., Keller, J. N., & Morrison, C. D. (2009). Obesity and vulnerability of the CNS. *Biochimica et Biophysica Acta, 1792*(5), 395–400.

Burokas, A., Arboleya, S., Moloney, R. D., Peterson, V. L., Murphy, K., Clarke, G., et al. (2017). Targeting the microbiota-gut–brain axis: Prebiotics have anxiolytic and antidepressant-like effects and reverse the impact of chronic stress in mice. *Biological Psychiatry, 82*(7), 472–487.

Cani, P. D., Amar, J., Iglesias, M. A., Poggi, M., Knauf, C., Bastelica, D., et al. (2007). Metabolic endotoxemia initiates obesity and insulin resistance. *Diabetes, 56*, 1761–1772.

Daniel, H., Gholami, A. M., Berry, D., Desmarchelier, C., Hahne, H., Loh, G., et al. (2014). High-fat diet alters gut microbiota physiology in mice. *The ISME Journal, 8*(2), 295–308. doi:10.1038/ismej.2013.155

David, L. A., Maurice, C. F., Carmody, R. N., Gootenberg, D. B., Button, J. E., Wolfe, B., et al. (2014) Diet rapidly and reproducibly alters the human gut microbiome. *Nature, 505*, 559–563.

Davis, S. C., Yadav, J. S., Barrow, S. D., & Robertson, B. K. (2017). Gut microbiome diversity influenced more by the Westernized dietary regime than the body mass index as assessed using effect size statistic. *Microbiology Open,* doi:10.1002/mbo3.476

Devkota, S. (2012). Dietary-fat-induced taurocholic acid promotes pathobiont expansion and colitis in Il10$^{-/-}$ mice. *Nature, 487*, 104–108.

Drago, S., El Asmar, R., Di Pierro, M., Clemente, M. G., Sapone, A. T. A., Thakar, M., et al. (2006). Gliadin, zonulin and gut permeability: Effects on celiac and non-celiac intestinal mucosa and intestinal cell lines. *Scandinavian Journal of Gastroenterology, 41*(4), 408–419.

Elson, C., & Alexander, K. (2015). Host-microbiota interactions in the intestine. *Digestive Diseases, 33*(2), 131–136.

Fallani, M., Young, D., Scott, J., Norin, E., Amarri, S., Adam, R. et al. (2010). Intestinal microbiota of 6-week-old infants across Europe: Geographic influence beyond delivery mode, breast-feeding, and anti-biotics. *Journal of Pediatric Gastroenterology & Nutrition, 51*, 77–84.

Fasano, A. (2012). Zonulin, regulation of tight junctions, and autoimmune diseases. *Annals of the New York Academy of Sciences, 1258*(1), 25–33.

Finegold, S., Summanen, P., Hunt Gerardo, S., & Baron, E. (1992). Clinical importance of Bilophila wadsworthia. *European Journal of Clinical Microbiology & Infectious Diseases, 11*, 1058–1063.

Harrison, N. A., Brydon, L., Walker, C., Gray, M. A., Steptoe, A., & Critchley, H. D. (2009). Inflammation causes mood changes through alterations of subgenual cingulate activity and mesolimbic connectivity. *Biological Psychiatry.66*(5), 407–414.

Hashioka, S., McGeer, P. L., Monji, A., & Kanba, S. (2009). Anti-inflammatory effects of antidepressants: Possibilities for preventives against Alzheimer's disease. *Central Nervous System Agents in Medicinal Chemistry, 9*(1), 12–19.

Heesemann, J., Hantke, K., Vocke, T., Saken, E., Rakin, A., Stojiljkovic, I., & Berner, R. (1993). Virulence of Yersinia enterocolitica is closely associated with siderophore production, expression of an iron-repressible outer membrane polypeptide of 65,000 Da and pesticin sensitivity. *Molecular Microbiology, 8*, 397–408.

Hein, A. M., Stasko, M. R., Matousek, S. B., Scott-McKean, J. J., Maier, S. F., Olschowka, J. A., Costa, A. C., & O'Banion, M. K. (2010). Sustained hippocampal IL-1beta overexpression impairs contextual and spatial memory in transgenic mice. *Brain, Behavior, and Immunity, 24*(2), 243–253.

Hildebrandt, M. A., Hoffmann, C., Sherrill-Mix, S. A., Keilbaugh, S. A., Hamady, M., Chen, Y.-Y., et al. (2009). High-fat diet determines the composition of the murine gut microbiome independently of obesity. *Gastroenterology, 137*(5), 1716–1724.

Högberg, G. (2012). Depressed adolescents in a case-series were low in vitamin D and depression was ameliorated by vitamin D supplementation. *Acta Paediatrica, 101*(7), 779–783.

Intlekofer, K. A., Berchtold, N. C., Malvaez, M., Carlos, A. J., McQuown, S. C., Cunningham, M. J., Wood, M. A., & Cotman, C. W. (2013). Exercise and sodium butyrate transform a subthreshold learning event into long-term memory via a brain-derived neurotrophic factor-dependent mechanism. *Neuropsychopharmacology, 38*(10), 2027–2034.

Jacka, F. N., Kremer, P. J., Taylor, S., Berk, M. & Stansfeld, S. A. (2011). A prospective study of diet quality and mental health in adolescents. *PloS One, 6*(9), e24805. doi:10.1371/journal.pone.0024805

Jorde, R., Sneve, M., Figenschau, Y., Svartberg, J., & Waterloo, K. (2008). Effects of vitamin D supplementation on symptoms of depression in overweight and obese subjects: Randomized double blind trial. *Journal of Internal Medicine, 264*(6), 599–609.

Kanoski, S. E., Zhang, Y., Zheng, W., & Davidson, T. L. (2010). The effects of a high-energy diet on hippocampal function and blood-brain barrier integrity in the rat. *Journal of Alzheimer's Disease, 21*(1), 207–219. doi:10.3233/JAD-2010-091414

Kelly, C. J., Zheng, L., Campbell, E. L., Saeedi, B., Scholz, C. C., Bayless, A. J., et al. (2015). Crosstalk between Microbiota-Derived Short-Chain Fatty Acids and Intestinal Epithelial HIF Augments Tissue Barrier Function. *Cell Host & Microbe, 17*(5), 662–671.

Lam, Y. Y., Ha, C. W., Campbell, C. R., Mitchell, A. J., Dinudom, A., Oscarsson, J., et al. (2012). Increased gut permeability and microbiota change associate with mesenteric fat inflammation and metabolic dysfunction in diet-induced obese mice. *PloS One, 7*(3), e34233. doi:10.1371/journal.pone.0034233

Lecomte, X., Gagnaire, V., Briard-Bion, V., Jardin, J., Lortal, S., Dary, A., & Genay, M. (2014). The naturally competent strain Streptococcus thermophilus LMD-9 as a new tool to anchor heterologous proteins on the cell surface. *Microbial Cell Factories, 13*, 82. doi:10.1186/1475-2859-13-82

Ledreux, A., Wang, X., Schultzberg, M., Granholm, A. C., & Freeman, L. R. (2016). Detrimental effects of a high fat/high cholesterol diet on memory and hippocampal markers in aged rats. *Behaviorial Brain Research, 312*, 294–304.

Luchsinger, J. A., Tang, M. X., Shea, S., & Mayeux, R. (2004). Hyperinsulinemia and risk of Alzheimer disease. *Neurology, 63*(7), 1187–1192.

Ma, Y., Griffith, J. A., Chasan-Taber, L., Olendzki, B. C., Jackson, E., Stanek, E. J. III, et al. (2006). Association between dietary fiber and serum C-reactive protein1,2,3. *The American Journal of Clinical Nutrition, 83*, 760–766.

MacDougall, R. (2012). NIH Human Microbiomes Project defines normal bacterial makeup of body. Bethesda, MD: National Institutes of Health.

Macfabe, D. F. (2012). Short-chain fatty acid fermentation products of the gut microbiome: implications in autism spectrum disorders. *Microbial Ecology in Health and Disease*, doi:10.3402/mehd.v23i0.19260

Macfarlane, G. T., & Macfarlane, S. (2011). Fermentation in the human large intestine: its physiologic consequences and the potential contribution of prebiotics. *Journal of Clinical Gastroenterology, 45*(Suppl), S120–S127.

Maes, M., Delanghe, J., Bocchio Chiavetto, L., Bignotti, S., Tura, G.-B., Pioli, R., et al. (2001). Haptoglobin polymorphism and schizophrenia: Genetic variation on chromosome 16. *Psychiatry Research, 104*, 1–9.

Maffeis, C., Martina, A., Corradi, M., Quarella, S., Nori, N., Torriani, S., et al. (2016). Association between intestinal permeability and faecal microbiota composition in Italian children with beta cell autoimmunity at risk for type 1 diabetes. *Diabetes/Metabolism Research and Reviews, 32*(7), 700–709.

Manzel, A., Muller, D. N., Hafler, D. A., Erdman, S. E., Linker, R. A., & Kleinewietfeld, M. (2014). Role of "Western diet" in inflammatory autoimmune diseases. *Current Allergy and Asthma Reports, 14*(1), 404. doi:10.1007/s11882-013-0404-6

Marcobal, A., Barboza, M., Froehlich, J. W., Block, D. E., German, J. B., Lebrilla, C. B., & Mill, D. A. (2010). Consumption of human milk oligosaccharides by gut-related microbes. *Journal of Agricultural and Food Chemistry, 58*, 5334–5340.

Milner, J. J., & Beck, M. A. (2012). The impact of obesity on the immune response to infection. *Proceedings of the Nutrition Society, 71*, 298–306.

Mokkala, K., Röytiö, H., Munukka, E., Pietilä, S., Ekblad, U., Rönnemaa, T., et al. (2016). Microbiota richness and composition and dietary intake of overweight pregnant women are related to serum zonulin concentration, a marker for intestinal permeability. *Journal of Nutrition, 146*(9), 1694–1700.

Mori, T. A., & Beilin, L. J. (2004). Omega-3 fatty acids and inflammation. *Current Atherosclerosis Report, 6*(6), 461–467.

O'Hagan, C., Li, J. V., Marchesi, J. R., Plummer, S., Garaiova, I., & Good, M. A. (2017). Long-term multi-species Lactobacillus and Bifidobacterium dietary supplement enhances memory and changes regional brain metabolites in middle-aged rats. *Neurobiology of Learning and Memory, 144*, 36–47.

Ohland, C. L., Kish, L., Bell, H., Thiesen, A., Hotte, N., Pankiv, E., & Madsen, K. L. (2013). Effects of Lactobacillus helveticus on murine behavior are dependent on diet and genotype and correlate with alterations in the gut microbiome. *Psychoneuroendocrinology, 38*(9), 1738–1747.

Pálmer, H. G., González-Sancho, J. M., Espada, J., Berciano, M. T., Quintanilla, M., Cano, A., et al. (2001). Vitamin D_3 promotes the differentiation of colon carcinoma cells by the induction of E-cadherin and the inhibition of β-catenin signaling. *Journal of Cell Biology, 154*(2), 369–387.

Pavlik, V., Massman, P., Barber, R., & Doody, R. (2013). Differences in the association of peripheral insulin and cognitive function in non-diabetic Alzheimer's disease cases and normal controls. *Journal of Alzheimers Disease, 34*(2), 449–456.

Pendyala, S., Walker, J. M., & Holt, P. R. (2012). A high-fat diet is associated with endotoxemia that originates from the gut. *Gastroenterology, 142*(5), 1100–1101.e2. doi:10.1053/j.gastro

Puig, K. L., Floden, A. M., Adhikari, R., Golovko, M. Y., & Combs, C. K. (2012). Amyloid precursor protein and proinflammatory changes are regulated in brain and adipose tissue in a murine model of high fat diet-induced obesity. *PLoS One, 7*(1), e30378. doi:10.1371/journal.pone.0030378

Rachal Pugh, C., Fleshner, M., Watkins, L. R., Maier, S. F., & Rudy, J. W. (2001). The immune system and memory consolidation: a role for the cytokine IL-1beta. *Neuroscience and Biobehavioral Reviews, 25*(1), 29–41.

Recio, M. C., Andujar, I., & Rios, J. L. (2012). Anti-inflammatory agents from plants: Progress and potential. *Current Medicinal Chemistry, 19*(14), 2088–2103.

Rönnemaa, E., Zethelius, B., Sundelöf, J., Sundström, J., Degerman-Gunnarsson, M., Berne, C., Lannfelt, L., & Kilander, L. (2008). Impaired insulin secretion increases the risk of Alzheimer disease. *Neurology, 71*(14), 1065–1071.

Segain, J. P., Raingeard de la Blétière, D., Bourreille, A., Leray, V., Gervois, N., Rosales, C., Ferrier, L., Bonnet, C., Blottière, H. M., & Galmiche, J. P. (2000). Butyrate inhibits inflammatory responses through NFkappaB inhibition: implications for Crohn's disease. *Gut, 47*(3), 397–403.

Sellbom, K. S., & Gunstad, J. (2012). Cognitive function and decline in obesity. *Journal of Alzheimers Disease, 30*(Suppl 2), S89–95.

Sender, R., Fuchs, S., & Milo, R. (2016) Are we really vastly outnumbered? Revisiting the ratio of bacterial to host cells in humans. *Cell, 164*, 337–340. doi:10.1016/j.cell

Stefanko, D. P., Barrett, R. M., Ly, A. R., Reolon, G. K., & Wood, M. A. (2009). Modulation of long-term memory for object recognition via HDAC inhibition. *Proceedings of the National Academy of Sciences U S A, 106*(23), 9447–9452.

Stott-Miller, M., Neuhouser, M. L., & Stanford, J. L. (2013). Consumption of deep-fried foods and risk of prostate cancer. *Prostate, 73*(9), 960–969.

Stranahan, A. M., Norman, E. D., Lee, K., Cutler, R. G., Telljohann, R. S., Egan, J. M., & Mattson, M. P. (2008). Diet-induced insulin resistance impairs hippocampal synaptic plasticity and cognition in middle-aged rats. *Hippocampus, 18*(11), 1085–1088.

Sweat, V., Starr, V., Bruehl, H., Arentoft, A., Tirsi, A., Javier, E., & Convit, A. (2008). C-reactive protein is linked to lower cognitive performance in overweight and obese women. *Inflammation, 31*(3), 198–207.

Tantamango-Bartley, Y., Jaceldo-Siegl, K., Fan, J., & Fraser, G. (2013). Vegetarian diets and the incidence of cancer in a low-risk population. *Cancer Epidemiology Biomarkers & Prevention, 22*(2), 286–294.

Tulstrup, M. V., Christensen, E. G., Carvalho, V., Linninge, C., Ahrne, S., Højberg, O., et al. (2015). Permeability and gut microbial composition in Wistar rats dependent on antibiotic class. *PLoS One, 10*(12), e0144854.

Turner, J. R. (2009). Intestinal mucosal barrier function in health and disease. *Nature Reviews Immunology, 2009*(11), 799–809. doi:10.1038/nri2653

Wan, C., La, Y., Zhu, H., Yang, Y., Jiang, L., Chen, Y., et al. (2007). Abnormal changes of plasma acute phase proteins in schizophrenia and the relation between schizophrenia and haptoglobin (Hp) gene. *Amino Acids, 32*, 101–108.

Waterhouse, J. C., Perez, T. H., & Albert, P. J. (2009). Reversing bacteria-induced vitamin D receptor dysfunction is key to autoimmune disease. *Annals of the New York Academy of Science, 1173*, 757–765.

Wright, C. E., Strike, P. C., Brydon, L., & Steptoe, A. (2005). Acute inflammation and negative mood: Mediation by cytokine activation. *Brain, Behavior and Immunity, 19*(4), 345–350.

Zeng, M., Inohara, N., & Nuñez, G. (2017). Mechanisms of inflammation-driven bacterial dysbiosis in the gut. *Mucosal Immunology, 10*(1), 18–26.

Zimmer, J., Lange, B., Sauer, H., Klosterhalfen, S., Enck, P., Frick, J.-S., et al. (2012). A vegan or vegetarian diet substantially alters the human colonic faecal microbiota. *European Journal of Clinical Nutrition, 66*, 53–60.

2

Key Nutrients for Normal Brain Health

RASHNA K. STAID

> **Key Points**
>
> - The Standard American Diet has been replete in high-energy foods with little nutritional value along with an inadequate intake of foods that contain essential nutrients.
> - There has been a sharp increase in psychiatric diseases but relatively little attention to improving poor nutritional patterns that affect mental health conditions.
> - Long-term nutrient deprivation results in neuroinflammation, which contributes to causing mental illnesses such as depression, anxiety disorder, schizophrenia, and others.
> - There is a growing body of research to substantiate the benefits of supplementing many nutrients including omega-3 fatty acids, vitamin D, the B complex vitamins, vitamin E, and the minerals magnesium, iron, zinc, choline, calcium, and selenium to help prevent and treat many mental illnesses.
> - It is not just one single nutrient that is important to optimizing brain health but all the nutrients working in concert in a healthy, well-balanced meal that helps to optimize brain function and prevent disease.

Introduction

Over the last 100 years the Standard American Diet (SAD) has been replete in high-energy foods with little nutritional value along with an inadequate intake of foods that contain essential nutrients (Parletta, Milte, & Meyer, 2013). Poor eating habits include undereating, overeating, and not having enough of the healthy foods we need each day. In fact, it is not surprising that the top sources of calories among Americans include grain-based desserts, refined breads, chicken and chicken mix dishes, sweetened soft drinks, pizza, and alcoholic beverages (US Department of Agriculture & US Department of Health and Human Services, 2010). Most, if not all, of these foods are very high in calories and low in nutrient density. Moreover, these combinations of foods are leading to chronic disease. Statistics show that more than one-third (78.6 million) of US adults are obese and at high risk of developing chronic diseases, like unipolar and bipolar depression, anxiety, attention deficit hyperactivity disorder (ADHD), and schizophrenia (Jacka, Maes, Pasco, Williams, & Berk, 2012; Parletta et al., 2013). The World Health Organization estimates that one in four to one in six people in most countries, and approximately 50% of Americans, will meet the criteria for mental disorder over their lifetime (Parletta et al., 2013). Despite the prevalence of mental illness, there has been relatively little attention to improving poor dietary patterns and subsequently affecting mental health conditions. Just consider how major depression, which is one of the worldwide leading causes of years of healthy life lost as a result of disability (Jacka, Mykletun, & Berk, 2012; Sanchez-Villegas & Martínez-González, 2013), could be prevented in millions of people who suffer from the disease (Jacka, Cherbuin, Anstey, & Butterworth, 2015; Sanchez-Villegas & Martínez-González, 2013) by improving diet and essential nutrients intakes.

When comparing the average diet from over 100 years ago we can see where society went wrong. There has been a significant sacrifice in food quality for convenience. Previously, the American diet was rich in whole foods that were low in sugar, high in omega-3 fatty acids, and high in animal fats, but now those foods have been replaced with processed foods that are high in sugar or refined carbohydrates, omega-6 fatty acids, shelf-stable fats, and even new ingredients like artificial dyes and preservatives, not to mention the plastic petroleum products that Americans store and cook their food in. Thus, unfortunately, as people in society became better fed, they ate more calories than ever before in history but were more nutrient deprived than ever. People are subsequently starving on a cellular level (Collective Evolution, 2015). The fundamental problem of long-term nutrient deprivation is that it causes neuroinflammation because nutrient deprivation is associated with an upregulated inflammatory response, characterized by increased levels of proinflammatory cytokines and other acute phase proteins (Milaneschi et al., 2011).

Over time this chronic inflammation may be the underlying mechanism causing and sustaining mental illnesses such as unipolar (Berk et al., 2013; Howren, Lamkin, & Suls, 2009) and bipolar depression (Leboyer et al., 2012), schizophrenia (Metcalf et al., 2016), anxiety disorders, posttraumatic stress disorder (Michopoulos, Powers, Gillespie, Ressler, & Jovanovic, 2016), and many other neuropsychiatric conditions (Flinkkilä, Keski-Rahkonen, Marttunen, & Raevuori, 2016; Michopoulos et al., 2016). So in order to effectively treat an underlying cause of psychiatric disease we need a shift in the usual paradigm and to consider prescribing healthy, nutrient-dense foods and supplements before reflexively prescribing medication. This is just what Hippocrates taught in approximately 400 BCE when he was quoted as saying, "Leave your drugs in the chemist's pot if you can heal the patient with food."

A well-researched healthy diet, such as the Mediterranean-style diet, consisting of healthy fats, fresh fruits and vegetables, fish, legumes, nuts, seeds, whole-grain cereals, and some wine intake, is broken down into essential nutrients such as monounsaturated fats, polyphenols, vitamins, omega-3 fatty acids, minerals, and amino acids. These critically important and essential nutrients in turn increase neuronal survival, neurotransmission, membrane fluidity, and cell membrane integrity, while simultaneously reducing oxidative damage, cell death, and neuroinflammation in a person's brain, leading to a healthier brain that is more resistant to dysfunction and disease (Parletta et al., 2013).

The Nutrients

OMEGA-3 FATTY ACIDS

Omega-3 fatty acids are essential nutrients to the body. Limited storage of the omega-3 fatty acids in adipose tissue suggests that a continued dietary supply is necessary to maintain sufficient levels in the brain tissue (Arterburn, Hall, & Oken, 2006). Three main fatty acids make up the omega-3 fatty acids. Docosahexaenoic acid (DHA) and eicosapentaenoic acid (EPA) are marine derived and are in high levels in fish such as wild salmon, arctic char, mackerel, sardines, black cod, and anchovies (Hobson & Underhill, 2016). The third main omega-3 fatty acid is α-linoleic acid (ALA), which is found in high levels in plant sources such as flaxseed, walnut, linseed, canola, and soy (McNamara & Strawn, 2013). Omega-3 fatty acids, also known as n-3 fatty acids, were named based on the position of the hydrocarbon chains with a methyl group at one end (called the omega position) and a carboxyl group at the other end (Natural Medicines Professional Database, 2016a).

These fatty acids have numerous significant benefits on the brain's overall structure and function. One most notable example is that DHA accounts for 30% to 40% of the fatty acids found in gray matter of the cortex. It has been shown that these higher levels of omega-3 fatty acids correlate to larger brain volumes (Pottala et al., 2014). The omega-3 fatty acids EPA and DHA are also important for signal transmission in the brain (McNamara & Strawn, 2013; Patrick & Ames, 2015). Omega-3s are also critical in reducing inflammation that can negatively impact the brain by causing chronic diseases (Simopoulos, 2002) like unipolar and bipolar depression, schizophrenia, and ADHD (McNamara & Strawn, 2013). Finally, omega-3 fatty acids have been found to help lower the risk of dementia (Samieri et al., 2008; Witte et al., 2014), while enhancing memory, focus, and attention in the very young to the very old (Witte et al., 2014).

Not all omega-3 fatty acids are equivalent for brain health. In humans, the marine-derived EPA and DHA have significant beneficial effects over the omega-3 fatty acid α-linoleic acid. This is because α-linoleic acid is easily oxidized and thus cannot be interconverted into EPA and DHA, the form required by the body (Arterburn et al., 2006). In addition, the SAD is relatively high in omega-6 fatty acids, which results in excess arachidoinic acid (AA) production that has a proinflammatory effect on the brain. Recent evidence shows that the average American's omega-6/omega-3 ratio today, eating the SAD, is roughly 15–20:1. This is significantly different from the omega-6/omega-3 ratio of roughly 2–4:1 in the diet approximately 150 years ago, and the omega-6/omega-3 ratio of 0.8:1 in Paleolithic times (Simopoulos, 2008). The rapid rise in the omega-6/omega-3 ratio appears to have innumerable negative consequences on the body. Consider from an evolutionary standpoint, the modern diet's fatty acid composition has changed drastically within only one to two generations, while human's physiology has not had enough time to adapt to these profound changes. This is made even worse by the fact that not only are people consuming more omega-6 fatty acids, but this consumption is further hindering the conversion of the omega-3 fatty acid α-linoleic to the required EPA and DHA because both alpha-linoleic acid and linoleic acid compete for the same enzymes in the body to be converted into their respective active forms (α-linoleic acid into EPA and DHA versus linoleic acid into AA). In fact studies have shown this conversion of α-linoleic acid to EPA and DHA is extremely inefficient. For example in men the fractional conversion of alpha-linoleic to EPA is between 0.3% and 8%, while the conversion of α-linoleic to DHA is less than 4% and often undetectable. Women appear to have slightly more efficient conversion rates, so up to 21% of α-linoleic acid is converted to EPA, and up to 9% of α-linoleic acid is converted to DHA (Arterburn et al., 2006).

THE EPA AND DHA-SEROTONIN CONNECTION

It is well known that serotonin is a critical neurotransmitter in the brain. It is concentrated in discrete regions known to regulate social cognition and decision-making. Serotonin regulates executive function, impulsivity, sensory gating, and social behavior. Thus dysfunction in the serotonin pathways can lead to diseases such as ADHD, bipolar disorder, schizophrenia, depression, and impulsive behavior (Patrick & Ames, 2015). Patrick and Ames also describe a proposed mechanism of how omega-3 fatty acids regulate serotonin pathways. They explain how high EPA levels allow presynaptic membranes to release the neurotransmitter serotonin across the synaptic space and high DHA levels allow the neurotransmitter serotonin to bind to the postsynaptic receptor, thus improving signal transmission. The opposite holds true with low EPA and DHA levels, where less neurotransmitter is released from the presynaptic terminal, with a low EPA level (Patrick & Ames, 2015). This model helps to explain the critical role of omega-3 fatty acids EPA and DHA in overall brain health and function, as well as how to reduce the incidence of neuropsychiatric symptoms and diseases.

RESEARCHED EFFECTS OF OMEGA-3 FATTY ACID SUPPLEMENTATION ON PSYCHIATRIC ILLNESSES

There is a substantial amount of literature on the effects omega-3 fatty acid supplementation and psychiatric illnesses over the past 10-plus years. It has been found that omega-3 fatty acids EPA and DHA may be beneficial to patients as primary prevention and secondary prevention, as well as augmenting current medication-based psychiatric treatment. In addition it has been found that a low red blood cell DHA and EPA levels can act as a risk biomarker or risk factor associated with psychopathology (McNamara & Strawn, 2013).

Primary and Early Secondary Prevention

As the well-known saying goes, "an ounce of prevention equals a pound of cure," and this important way of thinking can reduce suffering and costs in the rising epidemic of psychiatric diseases present today, which is expected to grow in the foreseeable future. Thus treating patients who are "high risk" or just showing early signs of developing psychiatric symptoms and disorders can stem this growing epidemic. In addition, safer and efficacious therapies, such as omega-3 supplementation of DHA and EPA, may be the ideal therapy for both primary and early secondary prevention in patients meeting these high-risk criteria (McNamara & Strawn, 2013). Preliminary intervention trials have found omega-3 fatty acid monotherapy can significantly reduce the severity of symptoms in patients with psychotic disorders, major depressive disorder (MDD), and bipolar disorder.

A proof of concept study by Amminger et al. (2010) evaluated subjects who were at high risk for developing a psychotic disorder because they were found to have subclinical psychotic symptoms or psychotic proneness and thus were at higher risk of developing a full-blown psychotic disorder A double-blind randomized trial treated subjects at high risk for developing psychosis with either long-chain omega-3 fatty acids or placebo for 12 weeks and then those subjects were observed for an additional 40 weeks. By the end of the 12 months, only 4.9% of the patients treated with long-chain fatty acids versus 27.5% of the patient who received placebo transitioned to the threshold of psychosis. The authors concluded that long-chain omega-3 fatty acids were efficacious for preventing and delaying psychosis transition in high risk patients. They also felt that this was a well-tolerated and safe primary prevention option that warrants further studies (Amminger et al., 2010).

Another study conducted by Nemets, Nemets, Apter, Bracha, and Belmaker, (2006) looked at early secondary prevention of long-chain omega-3 fatty acid treatment in childhood depression. This study was a double-blind, placebo-controlled pilot study of children early in the course of depression who received omega-3 fatty acids monotherapy versus placebo for 16 weeks. The study found that the subjects that were treated with omega-3 fatty acid supplementation exhibited a significant reduction in depression symptom severity relative to subjects who were treated with placebo at eight weeks and again at 16 weeks. In fact, 70% subjects treated with omega-3 fatty acids had a greater than 50% reduction in symptoms, and none of the subjects treated with placebo had a reduction in symptoms severity. In addition, 40% of the subjects treated with omega-3 fatty acids and none of the subjects treated with placebo exhibited symptomatic remission (McNamara & Strawn, 2013; Nemets et al., 2006).

A third study showed that omega-3 fatty acids may also be used in early secondary prevention as monotherapy to treat bipolar symptoms. In a systematic review, Turnbull Cullen-Drill, and Smaldone (2008) reviewed 99 studies and found that subjects who were treated with an omega-3 fatty acid demonstrated statistically significant improvement in bipolar symptoms. Again, the authors felt that the benign side effect profile made using omega-3 fatty acids an important consideration in the treatment of bipolar disease symptoms.

Adjuvant Therapy with Omega-3 Fatty Acids

Millions of people are already receiving conventional antidepressant medication for their psychiatric disorders but unfortunately are still symptomatic.

Omega-3 fatty acids appear to have a role in augmenting the therapeutic benefit of conventional antidepressant, mood stabilizer, and antipsychotic medication therapy. In a double-blind, placebo-controlled trial, Gertsik, Poland, Bresee, and Rapaport (2012) evaluated whether omega-3 fatty acid supplementation could actually augment the benefits of citalopram treatment in patients with MDD. This study compared citalopram 20 mg plus an omega-3 fatty acid capsule against citalopram 20 mg plus an olive oil placebo capsule. Participants were monitored by a psychiatrist every two weeks for two months. At the end of the study, the authors found that omega-3 fatty acid augmentation of citalopram treatment produced significantly greater reduction in depressions scores as compared to citalopram alone (Gertsik et al., 2012).

Omega-3 fatty acids also seem to be beneficial in augmenting mood stabilizer medication in bipolar disorder patients. A double-blind, placebo-controlled trial conducted by Stoll et al. (1999) evaluated patients with bipolar disorder who were on their usual treatment and randomized half the subjects to treatment with omega-3 fatty acids versus a placebo of olive oil. After four months of treatment, they too found that the subjects who were treated with omega-3 fatty acids had a significantly longer period of remission then the placebo group. The subjects also seemed to perform better in nearly every outcome measure than patients treated with the placebo (Stoll et al., 1999).

Finally, a double-blind, placebo-controlled trial conducted by Berger et al. (2007) found that supplementation with ethyl-eicosapentaenoic acid does improve antipsychotic efficacy and tolerability during the first-episode psychosis in schizophrenic patients. In addition, the supplementation permitted a 20% reduction in second-generation antipsychotic doses (McNamara & Strawn, 2013).

OMEGA-3 FATTY ACIDS RECOMMENDED DOSING AND POTENTIAL SIDE EFFECTS

Dosing

Currently the US Food and Drug Administration (FDA) has not approved omega-3 fatty acids for treatment of any psychiatric disorder. However, omega-3 fatty acid supplementation is readily available over-the-counter. In adults the recommended dose based on review of numerous studies evaluating the benefits of omega-3 fatty acids and psychiatric illnesses would be approximately 2 to 3 g daily of combined EPA and DHA in the triglyceride form. In order to both properly store and reduce some of the gastrointestinal symptoms, it is recommended that omega-3 fatty acids capsules be kept in the freezer and taken with cold water and a meal. It is also best to avoid hot beverages for 10 to 15 minutes.

Potential Side Effects

It is well established that omega-3 fatty acid supplementation may cause mild gastrointestinal disease disturbances including nausea, diarrhea, gastroesophageal reflux, eructation, and less commonly emesis (McNamara & Strawn, 2013). In addition, omega-3 fatty acids may have possible drug interactions with warfarin therapy, increasing a patient's bleeding time. Thus patients should be educated and cautioned about being monitored for side effects (Buckley, Goff, & Knapp, 2004). Taking aspirin therapy and high doses of omega-3 fatty acids (> 3 g/daily) has been associated with increased bruising and bleeding times. However, trials that have studied chronic high dose omega-3 fatty acids alone or in combination with aspirin do not show any increased risk for clinically significant bleeding times (Harris, 2007; McNamara & Strawn, 2013).

Cautions

Fish oils containing omega-3 fatty acids have the potential threat of contamination with methyl mercury, PCBs, and other environmental pollutants. Most fish oil supplements today are highly purified and do not exceed the FDA limits to be considered contaminated. However, when buying over-the-counter omega-3 fatty acids it is important to stay with brands that had good manufacturing practices. Several organizations do test the quality of products to make sure the product contains ingredients listed on the label and that they do not contain harmful levels of contaminants. The organizations that offer this quality testing include: US Pharmacopeia, ConsumerLab.com, and NSF International (National Institutes of Health, 2011).

Vitamins

Vitamins are a group of organic compounds that are essential for normal physiological functioning and are for the most part not synthesized by the body. Humans require adequate amount of all 13 vitamins that include the four fat-soluble vitamins (A, D, E, K) and the nine water-soluble vitamins, including vitamin C and the eight B vitamins: thiamine (B1), riboflavin (B2), niacin (B3), pantothenic acid (B5), vitamin B6, biotin (B7), folate (B9), and vitamin B12.

Unfortunately, today we see significant vitamin insufficiencies and deficiencies, resulting in chronic lifestyle diseases (Kennedy, 2016).

VITAMIN D—THE SUNSHINE VITAMIN

Unlike all the other vitamins that cannot be synthesized by the body, vitamin D can be, but most people should not rely on making vitamin D de-novo in the body. Vitamin D is synthesized into its active form 1,25-hydroxyvitamin D_3 in a multistep process. It starts when sunlight (with a specific UVB spectrum of 290–315 nm) comes in contact with the skin and converts 7-dehydrocholesterol to vitamin D_3. Then vitamin D_3 is transferred by plasma to the liver and converted into 25-hydroxyvitamin D_3 (calcidiol), which is then changed by the liver into 1,25-hydroxyvitamin D_3 (calcitriol), the active form of vitamin D_3, which exerts its biological effects on receptors throughout the body (Holick & Chen, 2008).

The process of converting 7-hydroxycholesterol in the skin to the dietary equivalent vitamin D_3 in adequate supply for the body's optimal performance is unfortunately limited by many factors (e.g., age, skin color, latitude, seasonal change, obesity, etc.), and thus it is recommended that people take an additional vitamin D_3 supplement instead of relying on sun exposure (Holick & Chen, 2008). A study conducted by Brot et al. (2001) found that in Denmark (latitude 54°–58° N) no cutaneous vitamin D was made for six to seven months of the year. There was also a two-month time lag before the increase in number of hours of sunshine raised the 25-OH vitamin D concentration. The study also found that the usual amount of sun exposure elderly people have to their hands, face, and arms for 10 to 15 minutes during peak summer sun time hours (from 11 AM to 2 PM) was insufficient to adequately raise 25-OH vitamin D levels. In addition, this does not even take into account that most women today, as opposed to when the study was conducted in the early part of the 1990s, protect their skin more from the damaging rays of the sun by wearing sunblock, which further decreases vitamin D production in the skin (Brot et al., 2001).

The Vitamin D Receptor

The vitamin D receptor also plays a major role in ensuring that we get adequate response from the activated form of vitamin D. Currently, there have been over 900 vitamin D receptors identified throughout the body. The vitamin D level and the receptors play a critical role in many diseases from psychiatric diseases including schizophrenia, depression, anxiety, and seasonal affective disorder to diseases that affect the immune system, lung diseases, cardiovascular diseases, metabolic diseases, cancers, autoimmune diseases, and well-known diseases affecting the bones and muscles such as osteoporosis and muscle weakness (Holick & Chen, 2008).

More recently we have discovered that there are single nucleotide polymorphisms (SNPs) or genetic variations that can cause the vitamin D receptor not to function properly. This increases the vitamin D requirements to initiate the appropriate response from the receptor. In fact, a study looked at the vitamin D receptor gene variant FokI polymorphism (RS 2228570) and found that the GG gene variant was associated with a significantly higher prevalence of depression in both men and women than any other vitamin D receptor variant (Lang et al., 2013). Thus evaluating patients' genetic variations or SNPs may also be an integral part of ensuring their optimal vitamin D levels.

The Vitamin D-Serotonin Connection

Similarly to EPA and DHA, vitamin D has been found to play a critical role in the serotonin pathway. Vitamin D receptors have been found to be co-factors for the tryptophan hydroxylase-2 enzyme (TPH2). Thus when high levels of vitamin D are present there is an increased conversion of tryptophan, which has crossed the blood–brain barrier, into serotonin by the TPH2 enzyme. Conversely, low levels of vitamin D decrease the conversion of tryptophan, which has crossed the blood–brain barrier, into serotonin because the enzyme does not work as efficiently without adequately high levels of the vitamin D cofactor (Patrick & Ames, 2015).

Researched Effects of Vitamin D3 Supplementation on Mood and Psychiatric Illnesses

Vitamin D has had a substantial amount of literature supporting its effectiveness for psychiatric and mood disorders over the past 20-plus years. Beneficial effects have been found even in healthy subjects during the winter, in depressed patients, in children with bipolar spectrum disorder (BSD), and even in adolescent women with premenstrual syndrome–related mood disorders (PMS).

Primary Prevention to Enhance Mood
In a double-blinded, placebo-controlled study, Lansdowne and Provost (1998) looked at how vitamin D_3 can enhance mood in healthy subjects during the winter. They treated 44 healthy subjects with 400 IU, 800 IU, or placebo for

five days. They looked at positive and negative affect schedules that were self-reported prior to administering the vitamin D supplementation and just after. The researchers found that vitamin D_3 significantly enhanced the positive affect of the subjects and that there was also some evidence of a reduction in the negative affect symptoms. Therefore, vitamin D_3 supplementation can even benefit patients who are considered "healthy" (Lansdowne & Provost, 1998).

Therapeutic Benefits with Vitamin D Supplementation

Vitamin D receptors are expressed in key brain regions that may potentially play a crucial role in mood regulation, so it is not surprising that vitamin D_3 supplementation has also been found to be beneficial for the treatment of mania in children with BSD. In an open label study, Sikoglu et al. (2015) looked at 16 children with BSD who had mania on their screening visits with a positive Young Mania Rating Scale (YMRS) ≥ 8 and compared them to typically developing children. They treated all the subjects with vitamin D_3 2000 IU daily for eight weeks and found that the subjects with BSD had a significant improvement in mania symptoms scores (YMRS), which correlated with an improved 25-OH vitamin D level. No other interventions were made during this eight-week course of therapy. Based on the positive findings in the pilot study, the authors concluded that more research is warranted and to possibly consider using higher doses of vitamin D3 supplementation in these children (Sikoglu et al., 2015).

Another double-blinded, randomized, placebo-controlled trial looked at how vitamin D supplementation effected 150 adolescent girls with PMS who were diagnosed with severe hypovitaminosis D (a 25-OH vitamin $D_3 \leq 10$ng/ml). The adolescent girls were either randomly assigned to four months treatment with vitamin D or a placebo. Symptom severity scores were measured at baseline and each month during the trial. The study results showed significant improvement in all five symptom categories including anxiety, irritability, crying easily, sadness, and disturbed relationship. The authors concluded that vitamin D is a safe, effective, and convenient method for improving the quality of life in young women with severe hypovitaminosis D and concomitant mood disorders associated with PMS (Tartagni et al., 2016).

Correlation Study between Depression and Hypovitaminosis D

Despite the belief that vitamin D is beneficial in depression, there is scarce epidemiologic evidence that higher 25-OH vitamin D levels protect against depression. A Finnish study by Jääskeläinen et al. (2015) examined the relationship of serum 25-hydroxy vitamin D with the prevalence of depressive and anxiety disorders. The authors studied the Health 2000 survey results of 5,371 individuals and found 354 diagnosed with depressive disorder and 222 with anxiety disorder. Serum 25-OH vitamin D concentrations were determined from frozen samples. The study found higher serum 25-vitamin D concentrations were associated with the lower prevalence of depressive disorder especially among men, younger people, divorced people, and those who had an unhealthy lifestyle or suffered from a metabolic syndrome. The serum concentrations of 25-OH vitamin D_3 that appeared to give people protection was a level of at least 50 nmol/l. The authors concluded that a larger scale prospective study is needed to confirm these findings.

Vitamin D_3 Recommended Dosing and Potential Side Effects

Dosing

The dosing of vitamin D3 has been a very controversial topic. The Institute of Medicine ([IOM], 2011) in 2010 came up with recommendations for vitamin D therapy based upon its review of the evidence that vitamin D supplementation was beneficial for bone health; there was insufficient evidence to support vitamin D supplementation for any other health condition. Unfortunately, the 2010 IOM report does not take into account the growing evidence in the literature that supports optimizing vitamin D levels for both the prevention and the treatment of diseases that affect people's mental health. After a review of the literature, it appears that most studies seem to support targeting a serum level of 25-OH vitamin D between 50 and 75 nmol per liter. However, most people who live in the Northern latitudes have grossly inadequate baseline 25-OH vitamin D levels. Thus it is proposed that a loading dose of vitamin D3 should be administered to optimize the 25-OH vitamin D3 level. A proposed calculation to determine appropriate loading dose by Van Groningen et al. (2010) is loading dose of vitamin D3 (IU) = 40 × (target serum 25-OHD3 − serum 25-OHD3) × body weight(kg) or Δ25-OHD3 = 0.025 × (dose per kg body weight; see also Balvers et al., 2015). Thereafter, maintenance supplementation should be administered to sustain the optimized level. Given the half-life of vitamin D3 is between three and six weeks, it is recommended that maintenance vitamin D3 be supplemented on a daily, weekly, or at most monthly basis (Balvers et al., 2015; Rolland et al., 2013). Maintenance dosing of vitamin D3 does vary based on age, skin type, UV exposure, obesity, malabsorption problems, and so on (Balvers et al., 2015). However, most individuals over the age of 18, once circulating 25-OH vitamin D levels are optimized, can be maintained on an average vitamin D3 intake of 400 to 800 IUs to a maximum level of 4000 IUs as per recommended by the IOM (Balvers et al., 2015). However, as clinicians, we have all faced situations where patients require significantly higher doses of vitamin D3 supplementation to maintain even sufficient 25-OH vitamin D levels, thus each individual should be assessed and treated in accordance to his or her needs based on a 25-OH vitamin D level that should be checked at least in three months after starting supplementation and then periodically thereafter to ensure levels are optimally maintained.

Potential Side Effects

The safety of vitamin D supplementation has always been a concern because it is a fat-soluble vitamin that is stored in the body and can potentially lead to vitamin D intoxication resulting in hypercalcemia. The adverse effects of hypercalcemia may result in vomiting, pain, fever, anorexia, and weight loss. There has only been anecdotal evidence that extremely high doses of vitamin D of at least 1250 μg per day (50,000 IU) can cause these classical signs of toxicity (Balvers et al., 2015; Hathcock, Shao, Vieth, & Heaney, 2007). However, there seems to be consensus that prolonged intakes of vitamin D3 at 250 μg per day (10,000 IUs per day) does not cause adverse effects (Balvers et al., 2015; Hathcock et al., 2007; Vieth, 1999) because at this level there is no change in circulating calcium levels (Balvers et al., 2015; Vieth, 1999). In fact the IOM converted this to a safety factor by 2.5 times, and thus it recommends the safe upper limit of intake for adults of vitamin D_3 100 μg per day (4000 IUs per day; Balvers et al., 2015). Vitamin D has also been suggested to increase the risk of kidney stones; however, a large prospective analysis of 193,551 participants in the Health Professionals Follow-up Study and Nurses' Health Study I and II did not detect an increased risk of forming kidney stones (Ferraro, Taylor, Gambaro, & Curhan, 2016).

THE B VITAMINS

B vitamins play critical roles in the body. They act as coenzymes in a substantial portion of enzymatic processes that underpin every aspect of cellular and physiological function. The B vitamins are not grouped on the basis of the chemical structure similarity but rather with regard to their water solubility and their interrelated cellular coenzyme functions (Kennedy, 2016). There are two main roles of the B vitamins include catabolic and anabolic metabolism (Kennedy, 2016). In catabolic metabolism, the B vitamins assist in generating the body's energy (ATP) within cells' mitochondria. They are also critical in the construction and transformation of many bioactive molecules including nitric oxide, neurotransmitters, methylation (of DNA, RNA, proteins, and lipids), synthesizing endogenous antioxidants, making substrates for the citric acid cycle, and finally assisting in DNA and RNA synthesis. Therefore it is not hard to imagine that deficiencies in these critical B vitamins can cause significant health problems.

The Homocysteine Hypothesis

B vitamins are essential nutrients for maintaining health in the body, and maintaining optimal levels is critically important to preventing a host of diseases. This has led researchers to find associations between certain B vitamins and increased levels of homocysteine, a potentially toxic amino acid formed in the methionine cycle, which causes cardiovascular disease and Alzheimer's disease, as well as several other forms of mental illness. Thus the homocysteine hypothesis, which has been repeatedly studied, looks at how mild to moderate increases in homocysteine levels are due to insufficiencies in several key vitamins required to recycle homocysteine (Kennedy, 2016; Mech & Farah, 2016). In particular the B vitamins believed to be important in maintaining low levels of homocysteine are folate, vitamin B12, and vitamin B6. However, despite this robust hypothesis, therapy with these vitamins, alone or in combination, has not adequately improved the treatment of psychiatric diseases that are associated with elevated homocysteine levels (Parletta et al., 2013). One explanation for this was eloquently discussed in a review paper by Kennedy et al. (2016) suggesting that most studies have focused on the effects of one to three of the B vitamins (folate, B12, and B6). However, the paper points out, the potential effects and roles of the other five B vitamins have been almost entirely ignored, despite the fact that the entire palette of B vitamins work intricately in concert (Kennedy, 2016). Therefore, the entire B complex should be replenished when trying to optimize benefits of therapy.

Brain-Specific Symptoms in B Vitamin Deficiencies

- Vitamin B1 deficiency can cause irritability, emotional disturbances, confusion, disturbed sleep, and memory loss (Kennedy, 2016; Kerns, Arundel, & Chawla, 2015). Frank deficiency can lead to Wernicke-Korsakoff syndrome, which is characterized by neurodegeneration within the medial thalamus and cerebellum, ataxia, abnormal motor function and eye movement, amnesia, apathy, and confabulation (Kennedy, 2016; Zempleni, 2007).
- Vitamin B2 deficiency may result in symptoms of fatigue, personality change, and brain dysfunction (Kennedy, 2016; Zempleni, 2007).

- Vitamin B3 (niacin) deficiency may result in depression, anxiety, vertigo, memory loss, paranoia, psychotic symptoms, and aggression, also known as Pellagrous insanity (Kennedy, 2016; Zempleni, 2007).
- Vitamin B5 (pantothenic acid) deficiency results in encephalopathy, behavior change, and demyelination (Kennedy, 2016; Zempleni, Suttie, Gregory, & Stover, 2013).
- Vitamin B6 (pyridoxine) deficiency results in irritability, impaired alertness, depression, cognitive decline, dementia, autonomic dysfunction, and convulsions (Kennedy, 2016; Zempleni et al., 2013).
- Vitamin B7 (biotin) deficiency results in depression, lethargy, hallucinations, and seizures (Kennedy, 2016; Zempleni, 2007).
- Vitamins B9 (folate) and vitamin B_{12} deficiency results in affective disorder, behavior changes, psychosis, cognitive impairment/decline, and dementia (including Alzheimer's and vascular diseases; Kennedy, 2016; Reynolds, 2006).

The Genetic Factor: MTHFR

Adequate neurotransmitters production is critical to avoiding imbalances in the brain that lead to diseases such as depression, anxiety, ADHD, and so on. In order to synthesize these monoamine neurotransmitters such as norepinephrine, serotonin, and dopamine, B vitamins must be metabolized to their active coenzyme form in the body (Mech & Farah, 2016). However, this does not always occur sufficiently if there are genetic variations or SNPs exist that impair methyl group donation by reduced or metabolized B vitamins, thus resulting in a deficiency in these critical coenzymes, a rise in homocysteine, and a reduction in monoamine production (Mech & Farah, 2016). The most common of these polymorphisms are the methylenetetrahydrofolate reductase (MTHFR) variants. It is possible that previous studies that failed to show significant benefit of treatment with high-dose folate may have failed because they did not supplement with the methylated or activated form of the vitamin, to compensate for the possible genetic variation found in the subjects.

Mech and Farah (2016) looked at 330 adults with MDD who were positive for either MTHFR C677T or A1298C polymorphisms. In the study 160 subjects were treated with placebo and 170 were treated with a reduced or methylated B vitamin for eight weeks. The Montgomery-Asberg Depression Rating Scale (MADRS) and plasma homocysteine levels were used to evaluate patients at both zero weeks and eight weeks. The results showed the patients who are in the active treatment group improved on average to a 12-point reduction on the MADRS by eight weeks, and 42% achieved full remission ($p < 0.001$). Additionally, in the active treatment group 131 (82.4%) showed a reduction in homocysteine, while patients on placebo demonstrated a small elevation in homocysteine levels. There were no side effects that were significantly different between the groups. The authors concluded that these results support the homocysteine theory of depression and the safety and therapeutic benefit of reduced B vitamins as monotherapy for MDD, particularly in patients with MTHFR variations (Mech & Farah, 2016).

B Vitamin Recommended Dosing and Potential Side Effects

Dosing

Although large-scale studies are lacking, there is considerable evidence that insufficiencies/deficiencies in B vitamins contribute to many psychiatric symptoms and disorders including depression, anxiety, ADHD, and so on. Optimal dosing of B vitamins can be based on direct serum levels of the vitamins, indirectly with markers such as homocysteine or methylmalonic acid, or with nutrient panels that measure white blood cell intracellular levels. However, caution needs to be used in interpreting normal serum levels; for example vitamin B12 deficiency with subclinical disease has been found despite normal serum levels of vitamin B_{12} in about 50% of patients (Oh & Brown, 2003). Additional testing of genetic variations or SNPs such as MTHFR, methionine synthetase reductase (MTRR), cystathionine beta synthetase (CBS), methionine synthetase (MTR), transcobolamine 1 (TCN1), and transcobolamine 2 (TCN2; Matteini et al., 2010) are also starting to help direct therapeutic treatment with certain B vitamins, since theses genetic variations may lead to upregulation or downregulation of a specific enzymatic process altering the requirement of the vitamin cofactor. However, if routine testing is not readily available or too expensive, it is recommended that a vitamin B complex 100 tablet be taken daily; this will contain approximately 100 mg of each of the major B vitamins (Rakel, 2012).

Precautions

B vitamins are water soluble, so any excessive intake should be excreted in the urine, and thus they are considered safe at any level or at least considerably higher than the US Recommended Daily Allowance (RDA) except for three notable exceptions:

- Folic acid: High levels of folic acid can mask the symptoms of vitamin B12 deficiency and result in a hidden accumulation of permanent damage including cognitive impairment (Kennedy, 2016; Morris, Jacques, Rosenberg, & Selhub, 2007) and neuropathy (Bell, 2010). There also may be a potential detrimental effect of consuming high doses of folic acid that can interfere with normal folate metabolism and immune function. In addition, high folate levels may interfere with the effects of anti-folate medications prescribed for several conditions including rheumatoid arthritis, psoriasis, cancer, bacterial infections, and malaria. There is also concern of a biphasic effect with regard to cancer, conferring protection at lower concentrations but increasing carcinogenesis at higher concentrations. Currently, there is no consensus as to optimal blood folate levels or levels that may cause harm (Kennedy, 2016).

- Niacin: High levels of niacin can cause nausea, vomiting, diarrhea, and in rare cases liver damage with extended uses of niacin in amounts greater than 1 g per day. The recommended maximum intake of niacin is 35 mg per day, based on the fact that greater than 100 mg per day causes temporary flushing (Kennedy, 2016).
- Vitamin B6 (pyridoxine): The upper limit of B6 is set at 100 mg/day, which is approximately 75 times the US RDA. This level was set based on case reports of reversible sensory neuropathy following doses of greater than 1000 mg taken for extended periods. However, it is important to note that several clinical trials of subjects consuming up to 750 mg/day of vitamin B6 for a number of years have not demonstrated any neuropathic side effects (Kennedy, 2016).

VITAMIN E

Vitamin E is a family of eight naturally occurring compounds: four tocopherols and four tocotrienols (T3s). From a nutritional and physiological perspective, alpha-tocopherol is the most important form of the vitamin (Gumpricht & Rockway, 2014). Recent data supports using T3s because they have been found to transverse into the brain, are potent antioxidants, and have neuroprotective effects (Gumpricht & Rockway, 2014).

Benefits of Vitamin E—The Research

Vitamin E has been found to have numerous benefits that help improve or protect brain health. The most well-known benefits of vitamin E is that it protects cell membranes from damage by free radicals because vitamin E is a hydrophobic molecule that acts as an antioxidant to protect the polyunsaturated fatty acids (PUFAs) found in biological membranes (i.e., brain tissue) against oxidative damage (Gumpricht & Rockway, 2014; Muñoz, Solé, & Coma, 2005; Niki & Traber, 2012). This protective effect also may explain the protective role vitamin E plays in reducing the brain amyloid beta peptide that accumulates in in patients suffering from Alzheimer's disease (Muñoz et al., 2005). Additionally, low levels of vitamin E indicate fewer antioxidant defenses against lipid peroxidation, which can increase depression (German et al., 2011; Rubio-López, Morales-Suárez-Varela, Pico, Livianos-Aldana, & Llopis-González, 2016).

Tocotrienols

Recent research now suggests that α-tocopherol is not the only beneficial form of vitamin E for brain health, since recent literature points to T3 forms of vitamin E exerting significant benefits in the brain, protecting it against ischemia (Aggarwal & Nesaretnam, 2012), and inflammation (Jiang, 2012). This appears to be a hot area for research, and more studies will help us understand the T3s' potentially important role in human health.

Vitamin E Recommended Dosing and Potential Side Effects

Dosing
Unfortunately to date there are no significant human studies to suggest optimal vitamin E dosing to protect brain health and prevent or treat psychiatric disease states. Additionally, most of the research thus far centers on dosing α-tocopherol and basically neglects to look at the other forms of vitamin E. However, what has been studied is the optimization of α-tocopherol vitamin E supplementation as a key essential lipophilic chain-breaking antioxidant that protects human lipoproteins, PUFAs, cellular, and intracellular membranes from oxidative damage (Raederstorff, Wyss, Calder, Weber, & Eggersdorfer, 2015). According to the literature, the dose of vitamin E supplementation should be based on the amount of PUFAs in the diet (Valk & Hornstra, 2000). The higher the PUFA level in the diet, the higher the dose of vitamin E is required to be effective protection. A proposed calculation to determine an individual's optimal intake of vitamin E is a basal level of 4–5 mg/d of RRR-α-tocopherol plus 0.5mg of RRR-α-tocopherol/g of PUFA in the diet, which comes out to be an average vitamin E (α-tocopherol level) of 12 to 20 mg for the typical range of PUFA intake (Raederstorff et al., 2015). In adults

older than 18, the tolerable upper limit of dosing for supplementary alpha-tocopherol recommended by the IOM is 1,000 mg daily (equivalent to 1,500 IU), and this limit is not altered during pregnancy or breastfeeding (Natural Medicines Professional Database, 2016d).

Potential Side Effects
Vitamin E in high doses can potentially cause nausea, diarrhea, stomach cramps, fatigue, weakness, headache, blurred vision, rash, and bruising and bleeding (Natural Medicines Professional Database, 2016b,c).

The Minerals

MAGNESIUM

About 100 years ago the beneficial effects of $MgSO_4$ given hypodermically to patients with agitated depression was published, and since then magnesium has been used in patients regularly for multiple conditions. It is one of the most essential minerals in the human body, connected with brain biochemistry and the fluidity of neuronal membrane (Serefko et al., 2013). It is effective treatment for both psychiatric and neurological symptoms, some of which include hyperexcitability, agitation, headaches, irritability, fits, fatigue, confusion, hallucinations, anxiety, insomnia, nervousness, PMS, and depression (Serefko et al., 2013). It appears to be related to many of the aforementioned symptoms due to its many roles. Magnesium functions as a coenzyme and plays an important role in the metabolism of carbohydrates, proteins, and fats to produce ATP and in the synthesis of nucleic acids (DNA and RNA; Kaplan, Crawford, Field, & Simpson, 2007). It actively transports ions (such as potassium and calcium) across cell membranes and for cell signaling (Kaplan et al., 2007). It is essential for greater than 300 biochemical reactions in the body, including maintenance of normal nerve function (Kaplan et al., 2007). Finally, magnesium insufficiency leads to neuronal damage that can cause depression (Rubio-López et al., 2016).

Benefits of Magnesium—The Research

Clinical studies have found magnesium treatment and/or supplementation to be effective in the treatment of depression and agitation. One possible mechanism of action is inadequate brain magnesium appears to reduce serotonin levels, and since antidepressants have been shown to have the action of raising brain magnesium, it is understandable that magnesium is effective therapy (Eby & Eby, 2010). In fact it has also been found that cotreatment of magnesium salts and antidepressants (i.e., fluoxetine, imipramine, and bupropion) result in the synergistic antidepressant-like effects (Cardoso et al., 2009; Serefko et al., 2013). Thus it makes sense that treatment will be found beneficial for nearly all depressives patients as it has been found in postpartum and MDD, reducing depressive symptoms in chronic fatigue syndrome, reducing depressive symptoms in women with PMS, patients with both depression and paresthesia (Serefko et al., 2013), and in treatment-resistant depressive disorder (Eby & Eby, 2010).

Magnesium Recommended Dosing and Potential Side Effects

Dosing

As a prevention strategy for depression symptoms, a recommended daily intake of 600 to 800 mg of magnesium salt should be taken daily, with the exception of the ineffective salt form of magnesium oxide (Serefko et al., 2013). Magnesium oxide should not be used to replete the magnesium insufficiency or deficiency because of his poor bioavailability. Other magnesium salts such as magnesium citrate, magnesium glycinate, magnesium maleate, magnesium glutamate, and magnesium aspartate all have a much higher bioavailability (Belkouch et al., 2016; Firoz & Graber, 2001). Additionally, it is best to avoid compositions of magnesium glutamate or aspartate in depressive individuals since these forms can potentially worsen symptoms of depression, since excesses of glutamate and aspartate in the brain are neurotoxic (Mark et al., 2001; Serefko et al., 2013).

Potential Side Effects

One possible problem with long-term administration of magnesium is the development of tolerance to the antidepressant effect, but there has been conflicting evidence of this phenomena in rats versus mouse studies (Serefko et al., 2013). The adverse effect that occurs most frequently occurs after intake of a high dose of magnesium is diarrhea. Some forms of magnesium, like magnesium glycinate, are less likely to cause diarrhea than the other salt forms. Diarrhea can also be avoided by giving magnesium preparation by parenteral or topical routes (Serefko et al., 2013).

IRON

Iron deficiency is the most prevalent single nutrient deficiency worldwide (Kim & Wessling-Resnick, 2014). Both too little and too much iron can be a cause for diseases. Iron is an essential cofactor in the production of ATP for brain energy, and it plays an essential role in hemoglobin, ensuring sufficient oxygen for oxidative brain metabolism (Kaplan et al., 2007). In addition, iron functions in the enzyme systems involved in the production of neurotransmitters such as serotonin, norepinephrine, and epinephrine, while concurrently enhancing their binding to proteins receptors in the frontal cortex (Kaplan et al., 2007).

Benefits of Iron—The Research

Iron insufficiency and deficiency affect people of all ages, but inadequate levels are most critical during developmental years. In young children iron deficiency appears to cause irreversible problems in terms of behavior and developmental milestones, and deficiency causes developmental delays (Kim & Wessling-Resnick, 2014; Lozoff et al., 2003). Iron deficiency is also associated with cognitive alterations in adolescents (Bruner, Joffe, Duggan, Casella, & Brandt, 1996; Kim & Wessling-Resnick, 2014). Finally, children with iron deficiency have been found to have increased anxiety and/or depression with social and attentional problems, while iron supplementation has improved symptoms of anxiety and depression (Kim & Wessling-Resnick, 2014). In adults, iron supplementation has also been found to be beneficial in reversing symptoms of postpartum depression in mothers who also had an low iron stores (Sheikh, Hantoushzadeh, Shariat, Farahani, & Ebrahiminasab, 2017).

However, as stated previously, too much iron can also have deleterious effects on the brain. It appears there is a J-curve relationship, which explains why iron levels need to be maintained in a healthy range in order to prevent disease. For instance, excess iron in the brain is implicated in the development and pathogenesis of neurodegenerative disorders like Alzheimer's, Parkinson's disease, and Huntington's disease as well as causing anxiety-like behavior and mood (Kim & Wessling-Resnick, 2014).

Iron Recommended Dosing and Potential Side Effects

Dosing

Safe and effective iron supplementation should be based on several factors including: age, sex, menstruation status, kidney function, genetic factors, type of diet, other medications/supplements a person is using, as well as the individual's blood parameters including hemoglobin, hematocrit, and iron profile (serum iron, TIBC, and ferritin levels). Thus, if needed, it is better to dose iron supplements to normalize the patient's blood parameters that are based on the individual's given age and sex and treatment goal(s). Currently, most laboratories report a large normal range of ferritin for males 12 to 300 ng/mL and females 12 to 150 ng/mL. However, the lower end of that range is suboptimal, and thus the ferritin level should be at least 60 ng/mL (Rakel, 2012). Recommended daily dose of iron for adults with iron deficiency is 100 to 200 mg of elemental iron. Iron sulfate is the most commonly used form of iron, but other preparations are available (Longo & Camaschella, 2015). Iron bisglycinate may be preferred since it seems to have a more tolerable side effect profile with reduced constipation side effects.

Potential Side Effects
The adverse effects to iron supplementation are mainly gastrointestinal (Natural Medicines Professional Database, 2016c).

ZINC

Zinc is the most abundant intracellular trace element and has numerous roles from protein synthesis to structure and regulation of gene expression (Kaplan et al., 2007). It has also been found to be a cofactor for over 200 different enzymes, present in over 300 metalloenzymes involved in all aspects of metabolism (Kaplan et al., 2007). In the brain, zinc is also found in neurons and glial cells. In fact, there are certain zinc-enriched regions (e.g., hippocampus) that are very responsive to dietary zinc deprivation that can cause brain dysfunctions, such as learning impairment (Kaplan et al., 2007).

Benefits of Zinc—The Research

Zinc supplementation has been found to be beneficial in several different types of studies that have looked at zinc and depression. First, an 80-person observational study found that patients with minor depression had serum zinc levels that were approximately 93% that of controls, whereas patients with major depression had serum zinc levels that were 88% of controls ($p < 0.001$; Cope & Levenson, 2010; Maes et al., 1994). A second small pilot study looked at the treatment of zinc and improvement in depression symptoms in 15 women and found that when women were given a MVI containing 7mg of zinc for 10 weeks they had an increased serum zinc level, which was associated with a significant decrease in anger/hostility and depression/dejection scores compared to women given the same MVI without zinc (Cope & Levenson, 2010; Sawada

& Yokoi, 2010). Finally, a third study looked to see if zinc enhanced therapy in treatment-resistant patients. The 12-week, double-blind, placebo-controlled study looked at patients that were previously refractory to the antidepressant drug imipramine. The study randomized them into two groups, one group receiving zinc 25 mg with the drug therapy daily and the other group receiving a placebo and drug therapy daily. The results showed the group receiving the zinc supplements significantly improved depression inventory scores and had improved outcomes compared to patients receiving drug therapy and placebo (Cope & Levenson, 2010; Siwek et al., 2009).

Zinc Recommended Dosing and Potential Side Effects

Dosing

For mood disorder specifically, 7 to 25 mg daily of zinc has been shown to be beneficial in adult patients (Natural Medicines Professional Database, 2016c; Sawada & Yokoi, 2010; Siwek et al., 2009). One must use caution with treatment of zinc because it can inhibit copper absorption, leading to a deficiency (Rakel, 2012).

Potential Side Effects

Zinc is a relatively safe mineral with few if any reported side effects. However, according to reports from the California Poison Control System, zinc ingestion was cited as a common cause of adverse events, including increased heart rate (45%), agitation (30%), vomiting (30%), and nausea (15%; Dennehy, Tsourounis, & Horn, 2005; Natural Medicines Professional Database, 2016d).

OTHER NOTABLE MINERALS FOR BRAIN HEALTH

- Choline is important for the structural integrity of cell membranes, for cell signaling, as it is the precursor to acetylcholine, and for nerve impulse transmission. It is also a major source of methyl groups for methylation reactions (Kaplan et al., 2007; Zeisel, 2000).
- Selenium is an essential trace mineral and is part of the antioxidant enzymes that protect cells from effects of free radicals (Kaplan et al., 2007).
- Calcium is a very important intracellular messenger and cofactor for enzymes. It also has the critical role in the release of neurotransmitters and other chemical signaling between cells (Kaplan et al., 2007).

NUTRIENT SYNERGIES

It is not just one single nutrient or food that is important to optimizing brain health but all the nutrients working in concert that helps to optimize brain function and prevent disease. Thus it takes a healthy, balanced meal to provide the variety of nutrients we need. So it is not surprising that these nutrients work synergistically together to benefit the body. A study by Jerneren et al. (2015) evaluated if B vitamin supplementation had an effect on brain atrophy rates in patients with differing plasma omega-3 fatty acid levels. The study found that there was a significant benefit in reducing brain atrophy only in subjects that had a high serum level omega-3 fatty acids that were supplemented with B vitamins (Jerneren et al., 2015). Another example of nutrient synergies is in the proposed mechanism by Patrick and Ames in 2015, where they proposed that vitamin D is an important cofactor to the enzyme TPH2 in the presynaptic neuron and omega-3 fatty acids EPA and DHA are important for the release of serotonin across the synaptic space. Accordingly, people who are deficient in vitamin D, and/or omega-3 fatty acids EPA or DHA, would have reduced serotonin production and transmission, while people who have high levels of vitamin D and omega-3 fatty acids EPA and DHA have normal serotonin production and cell signaling (Patrick & Ames, 2015). Both of these are good examples of how we must look for synergies of nutrients to better understand brain nutrient needs.

Conclusion and Future Directions

The SAD is nutrient poor, and this has been shown to negatively impact brain health/function. Optimally, eating a diet rich in organic whole foods including vegetables, fruits, nuts, legumes, health fats/oils, and grass-fed lean proteins would give our brains the synergist nutrients they need to perform and age well. However, since eating a well-balanced, whole-food, organic diet is not always feasible, it makes sense to try and understand which key nutrients may be supplemented in patients at high risk for disease. Studies over the past 20 years have started to show how omega-3 fatty acids, vitamins D, the B complex, vitamin E, and minerals including magnesium, iron and zinc, choline, selenium, and calcium are critical brain nutrients in preventing disease. However, thus far the research is far from conclusive or robust to understand the dynamic intricacies of which nutrients are important for treating specific brain dysfunctions. This is even more complicated since an individual's genetic variations (SNPs) may alter a person's need for a particular nutrient. More research is needed to understand what Hippocrates innately believed and or observed approximately 2400 years ago, "Let food be thy medicine and medicine be thy food."

REFERENCES

Aggarwal, B., & Nesaretnam, K. (2012). Vitamin E tocotrienols: life beyond tocopherols. *Genes and Nutrition, 7*(1), 1. doi:10.1007/s12263-011-0234-x.

Amminger, G. P., Schäfer, M. R., Papageorgiou, K., Klier, C. M., Cotton, S. M., Harrigan, S. M., et al. (2010). Long-chain ω-3 fatty acids for indicated prevention of psychotic disorders. *Archives of General Psychiatry, 67*(2), 146. doi.org/10.1001/archgenpsychiatry.2009.192

Arterburn, L. M., Hall, E. B., & Oken, H. (2006). Distribution, interconversion, and dose response of n-3 fatty acids in humans. *The American Journal of Clinical Nutrition, 83*(6 Suppl.), 1467S–1476S. Retrieved from http://www.ncbi.nlm.nih.gov/pubmed/16841856

Balvers, M. G. J., Brouwer-Brolsma, E. M., Endenburg, S., de Groot, L. C. P. G. M., Kok, F. J., & Gunnewiek, J. K. (2015). Recommended intakes of vitamin D to optimise health, associated circulating 25-hydroxyvitamin D concentrations, and dosing regimens to treat deficiency: Workshop report and overview of current literature. *Journal of Nutritional Science, 4*, e23. doi.org/10.1017/jns.2015.10

Belkouch, M., Hachem, M., Elgot, A., Van, A. Lo, Picq, M., Guichardant, M., et al. (2016). The pleiotropic effects of omega-3 docosahexaenoic acid on the hallmarks of Alzheimer's disease. *The Journal of Nutritional Biochemistry, 38*, 1–11. doi.org/10.1016/j.jnutbio.2016.03.002

Bell, D. S. H. (2010). Metformin-induced vitamin B12 deficiency presenting as a peripheral neuropathy. *The Southern Medical Journal, 103*(3), 265–267. doi.org/10.1097/SMJ.0b013e3181ce0e4d

Berk, M., Williams, L. J., Jacka, F. N., O'Neil, A., Pasco, J. A., Moylan, S., et al. (2013). So depression is an inflammatory disease, but where does the inflammation come from? *BMC Medicine, 11*, 200. doi.org/10.1186/1741-7015-11-200

Brot, C., Vestergaard, P., Kolthoff, N., Gram, J., Hermann, A. P., Sørensen, O. H., et al. (2001). Vitamin D status and its adequacy in healthy Danish perimenopausal women: Relationships to dietary intake, sun exposure and serum parathyroid hormone. *British Journal of Nutrition, 86*(Suppl. 1), S97. doi.org/10.1079/BJN2001345

Bruner, A. B., Joffe, A., Duggan, A. K., Casella, J. F., & Brandt, J. (1996). Randomised study of cognitive effects of iron supplementation in non-anaemic iron-deficient adolescent girls. *The Lancet, 348*, 992–996.

Buckley, M. S., Goff, A. D., & Knapp, W. E. (2004). Fish oil interaction with warfarin. *Annals of Pharmacotherapy, 38*(1), 50–52. doi.org/10.1345/aph.1D007

Cardoso, C. C., Lobato, K. R., Binfaré, R. W., Ferreira, P. K., Rosa, A. O., Santos, A. R., & Rodrigues, A. L. (2009). Evidence for the involvement of the monoaminergic system in the antidepressant-like effect of magnesium. *Progress in Neuropsychopharmacology and Biological Psychiatry, 33*(2), 235–242.

Collective Evolution. (2015). The real food guide: How we ate 100 years ago. Retrieved from http://www.collective-evolution.com/2015/02/27/the-real-food-guide-how-we-ate-100-years-ago/

Cope, E. C., & Levenson, C. W. (2010). Role of zinc in the development and treatment of mood disorders. *Current Opinion in Clinical Nutrition and Metabolic Care, 13*(6), 685–689. doi.org/10.1097/MCO.0b013e32833df61a

Dennehy, C. E., Tsourounis, C., & Horn, A. J. (2005). Dietary supplement-related adverse events reported to the California Poison Control System. *American Journal of Health-System Pharmacy, 62*, 1476–1482. doi.org/10.2146/ajhp040412

Eby, G. A., & Eby, K. L. (2010). Magnesium for treatment-resistant depression: A review and hypothesis. *Medical Hypotheses, 74*(4), 649–660. doi.org/10.1016/j.mehy.2009.10.051

Ferraro, P. M., Taylor, E. N., Gambaro, G., & Curhan, G. C. (2016). Vitamin D intake and the risk of incident kidney stones. *The Journal of Urology, 197*(2), 405–410. doi.org/10.1016/j.juro.2016.08.084

Firoz, M., & Graber, M. (2001). Bioavailability of US commercial magnesium preparations. *Magnesium Research, 14*(4), 257–262.

Flinkkilä, E., Keski-Rahkonen, A., Marttunen, M., & Raevuori, A. (2016). Prenatal inflammation, infections and mental disorders. *Psychopathology, 49*(5), 317–333. doi.org/10.1159/000448054

German, L., Kahana, C., Rosenfeld, V., Zabrowsky, I., Wiezer, Z., Fraser, D., & Shahar, D. R. (2011). Depressive symptoms are associated with food insufficiency and nutritional deficiencies in poor community-dwelling elderly people. *The Journal of Nutrition, Health & Aging, 15*(1), 3–8. Retrieved from http://www.ncbi.nlm.nih.gov/pubmed/21267514

Gertsik, L., Poland, R. E., Bresee, C., & Rapaport, M. H. (2012). Omega-3 fatty acid augmentation of citalopram treatment for patients with major depressive disorder. *Journal of Clinical Psychopharmacology, 32*(1), 61–64. doi.org/10.1097/JCP.0b013e31823f3b5f

Gumpricht, E., & Rockway, S. (2014). Can ω-3 fatty acids and tocotrienol-rich vitamin E reduce symptoms of neurodevelopmental disorders? *Nutrition, 30*(7), 733–738. doi.org/10.1016/j.nut.2013.11.001

Harris, W. S. (2007). Expert opinion: Omega-3 fatty acids and bleeding—cause for concern? *American Journal Cardiology, 99*(Suppl.), 44C–46C. doi.org/10.1016/j.amjcard.2006.11.021

Hathcock, J. N., Shao, A., Vieth, R., & Heaney, R. (2007). Risk assessment for vitamin D. *The American Journal of Clinical Nutrition, 85*(1), 6–18. Retrieved from http://ajcn.nutrition.org/cgi/content/long/85/1/6

Hobson, K., & Underhill, A. (2016). 13 best fish: High in omega-3s. Retrieved from http://health.usnews.com/wellness/slideshows/13-best-fish-high-in-omega-3sand-environment-friendly

Holick, M. F., & Chen, T. C. (2008). Vitamin D deficiency: A worldwide problem with health consequences. *The American Journal of Clinical Nutrition, 87*(4), 1080S–1086S. Retrieved from http://www.ncbi.nlm.nih.gov/pubmed/18400738

Howren, M. B., Lamkin, D. M., & Suls, J. (2009). Associations of depression with C-reactive protein, IL-1, and IL-6: A meta-analysis. *Psychosomatic Medicine, 71*(2), 171–186. doi.org/10.1097/PSY.0b013e3181907c1b

Institute of Medicine. (2011). *Dietary reference intakes for calcium and vitamin D health effects of vitamin D and calcium intake*. Washington, DC: National Academies Press.

Jacka, F. N., Maes, M., Pasco, J. A., Williams, L. J., & Berk, M. (2012). Nutrient intakes and the common mental disorders in women. *Journal of Affective Disorders, 141*(1), 79–85. doi.org/10.1016/j.jad.2012.02.018

Jacka, F. N., Mykletun, A., & Berk, M. (2012). Moving towards a population health approach to the primary prevention of common mental disorders. *BMC Medicine, 10*, 149. doi.org/10.1186/1741-7015-10-149

Jacka, F. N., Cherbuin, N., Anstey, K. J., & Butterworth, P. (2015). Does reverse causality explain the relationship between diet and depression? *Journal of Affective Disorders, 175*, 248–250.

Jerneren, F., Elshorbagy, A. K., Oulhaj, A., Smith, S. M., Refsum, H., & Smith, A. D. (2015). Brain atrophy in cognitively impaired elderly: The importance of long-chain-3 fatty acids and B vitamin status in a randomized controlled trial. *The American Journal of Clinical Nutrition, 102*(1), 215–221. doi.org/10.3945/ajcn.114.103283

Jiang, Q. (2012). Natural forms of vitamin E: Metabolism, antioxidant and anti-inflammatory activities and the role in disease prevention and therapy. *Free Radical Biology and Medicine, 72*, 76–90. doi.org/10.1016/j.freeradbiomed.2014.03.035

Kaplan, B. J., Crawford, S. G., Field, C. J., & Simpson, J. S. (2007). Vitamins, minerals, and mood. *Psychological Bulletin, 133*(5), 747–760. doi.org/10.1037/0033-2909.133.5.747

Kennedy, D. O. (2016). B vitamins and the brain: Mechanisms, dose and efficacy—a review. *Nutrients, 8*(2), 68. doi.org/10.3390/nu8020068

Kerns, J. C., Arundel, C., & Chawla, L. S. (2015). Thiamin deficiency in people with obesity. *Advances in Nutrition, 6*(2), 147–153. doi.org/10.3945/an.114.007526

Kim, J., & Wessling-Resnick, M. (2014). Iron and mechanisms of emotional behavior. *The Journal of Nutritional Biochemistry, 25*(11), 1101–1107. doi.org/10.1016/j.jnutbio.2014.07.003

Lang, F., Glocke, M., Schaeffeler, E., Lang, T., Schwab, M., & Lang, U. E. (2013). Impact of vitamin D receptor VDR rs2228570 polymorphism in oldest old. *Kidney and Blood Pressure Research, 3737*. doi.org/10.1159/000350159

Lansdowne, A. T. G., & Provost, S. C. (1998). Vitamin D 3 enhances mood in healthy subjects during winter. *Psychopharmacology, 135*, 319–323.

Leboyer, M., Soreca, I., Scott, J., Frye, M., Henry, C., Tamouza, R., & Kupfer, D. J. (2012). Can bipolar disorder be viewed as a multi-system inflammatory disease? *Journal of Affective Disorders, 141*, 1–10. doi.org/10.1016/j.jad.2011.12.049

Longo, D. L., & Camaschella, C. (2015). Iron-deficiency anemia. *The New England Journal of Medicine, 372*, 1832–1843. doi.org/10.1056/NEJMra1401038

Lozoff, B., De Andraca, I., Castillo, M., Smith, J. B., Walter, T., & Pino, P. (2003). Behavioral and developmental effects of preventing iron-deficiency anemia in healthy full-term infants. *Pediatrics, 112*, 846.

Maes, M., D'Haese, P. C., Scharpé, S., D'Hondt, P., Cosyns, P., & De Broe, M. E. (1994). Hypozincemia in depression. *Journal of Affective Disorders, 31*(2), 135–140. doi.org/10.1016/0165-0327(94)90117-1

Mark, L. P., Prost, R. W., Ulmer, J. L., Smith, M. M., Daniels, D. L., Strottmann, J. M., et al. (2001). Pictorial review of glutamate excitotoxicity: fundamental concepts for neuroimaging. *AJNR: American Journal of Neuroradiology, 22*(10), 1813–1824. Retrieved from http://www.ncbi.nlm.nih.gov/pubmed/11733308

Matteini, A. M., Walston, J. D., Bandeen-Roche, K., Arking, D. E., Allen, R. H., Fried, L. P., Chakravarti, A., Stabler, S. P., & Fallin, M. D. (2010). Transcobalamin-II variants, decreased vitamin B12 availability and increased risk of frailty. *Journal of Nutrition, Health, and Aging, 14*(1), 73–77.

McNamara, R. K., & Strawn, J. R. (2013). Role of long-chain omega-3 fatty acids in psychiatric practice. *PharmaNutrition, 1*(2), 41–49. doi.org/10.1016/j.phanu.2012.10.004

Mech, A. W., & Farah, A. (2016). Correlation of clinical response with homocysteine reduction during therapy with reduced B vitamins in patients with MDD who are positive for MTHFR C677T or A1298C polymorphism. *The Journal of Clinical Psychiatry, 77*(5), 668–671. doi.org/10.4088/JCP.15m10166

Metcalf, S. A., Jones, P. B., Nordstrom, T., Timonen, M., Mäki, P., Miettunen, J., et al. (2016). Serum C-reactive protein in adolescence and risk of schizophrenia in adulthood: A prospective birth cohort study. *Brain, Behavior, and Immunity, 59*, 253–259. doi.org/10.1016/j.bbi.2016.09.008

Michopoulos, V., Powers, A., Gillespie, C. F., Ressler, K. J., & Jovanovic, T. (2016). Inflammation in fear- and anxiety-based disorders: PTSD, GAD, and beyond. *Neuropsychopharmacology, 42*, 254–270. doi.org/10.1038/npp.2016.146

Milaneschi, Y., Bandinelli, S., Penninx, B. W., Vogelzangs, N., Corsi, A. M., Lauretani, F., et al. (2011). Depressive symptoms and inflammation increase in a prospective study of older adults: A protective effect of a healthy (Mediterranean-style) diet. *Molecular Psychiatry, 16*, 589–590. doi.org/10.1038/mp.2010.113

Morris, M. S., Jacques, P. F., Rosenberg, I. H., & Selhub, J. (2007). Folate and vitamin B-12 status in relation to anemia, macrocytosis, and cognitive impairment in older Americans in the age of folic acid fortification. *The American Journal of Clinical Nutrition, 85*(1), 193–200. Retrieved from http://www.ncbi.nlm.nih.gov/pubmed/17209196

Muñoz, F. J., Solé, M., & Coma, M. (2005). The protective role of vitamin E in vascular amyloid beta-mediated damage. *Sub-Cellular Biochemistry, 38*, 147–165. Retrieved from http://www.ncbi.nlm.nih.gov/pubmed/15709477

National Institutes of Health. (2011). Dietary supplements: What you need to know. Retrieved from https://ods.od.nih.gov/HealthInformation/DS_WhatYouNeedToKnow.aspx

Natural Medicines Professional Database. (2016a). Retrieved from https://naturalmedicines.therapeuticresearch.com/databases/food,-herbs-supplements/professional.aspx?productid=993#background

Natural Medicines Professional Database. (2016b). Retrieved from https://natural-medicines-therapeuticresearch-com.proxy1.lib.tju.edu/databases/food,-herbs-supplements/professional.aspx?productid=954#adverseEvents

Natural Medicines Professional Database. (2016c). Retrieved from https://natural-medicines-therapeuticresearch-com.proxy1.lib.tju.edu/databases/food,-herbs-supplements/professional.aspx?productid=912#adverseEvents

Natural Medicines Professional Database. (2016d). Retrieved from https://natural-medicines-therapeuticresearch-com.proxy1.lib.tju.edu/databases/food,-herbs-supplements/professional.aspx?productid=982#dosing

Nemets, H., Nemets, B., Apter, A., Bracha, Z., & Belmaker, R. H. (2006). Omega-3 treatment of childhood depression: A controlled, double-blind pilot study. *The American Journal of Psychiatry, 163*(6), 1098–1100. doi.org/10.1176/ajp.2006.163.6.1098

Niki, E., & Traber, M. G. (2012). A history of vitamin E. *Annals of Nutrition & Metabolism, 61*(3), 207–212. doi.org/10.1159/000343106

Oh, R., & Brown, D. L. (2003). Vitamin B12 deficiency. *American Family Physician, 67*(5), 979–986. doi.org/10.1056/NEJMc1304350#SA2

Parletta, N., Milte, C. M., & Meyer, B. J. (2013). Nutritional modulation of cognitive function and mental health. *Journal of Nutritional Biochemistry, 24*, 725–743. doi.org/10.1016/j.jnutbio.2013.01.002

Patrick, R. P., & Ames, B. N. (2015). Vitamin D and the omega-3 fatty acids control serotonin synthesis and action, part 2: Relevance for ADHD, bipolar disorder, schizophrenia, and impulsive behavior. *The FASEB Journal, 29*(6), 2207–2222. doi.org/10.1096/fj.14-268342

Pottala, J. V., Yaffe, K., Robinson, J. G., Espeland, M. A., Wallace, R., & Harris, W. S. (2014). Higher RBC EPA + DHA corresponds with larger total brain and hippocampal volumes: WHIMS-MRI study. *Neurology, 82*(5), 435–442.

Raederstorff, D., Wyss, A., Calder, P. C., Weber, P., & Eggersdorfer, M. (2015). Vitamin E function and requirements in relation to PUFA. *British Journal of Nutrition, 114*(8), 1113–1122. doi.org/10.1017/S000711451500272X

Rakel, D. (2012). *Integrative medicine*. Philadelphia, PA: Elsevier.

Reynolds, E. (2006). Vitamin B12, folic acid, and the nervous system. *The Lancet: Neurology, 5*(11), 949–960. doi.org/10.1016/S1474-4422(06)70598-1

Rolland, Y., de Souto Barreto, P., van Kan, G. A., Annweiler, C., Beauchet, O., Bischoff-Ferrari, H., et al. (2013). Vitamin D supplementation in older adults: Searching for specific guidelines in nursing homes. *The Journal of Nutrition, Health & Aging, 17*(4), 402–412. doi.org/10.1007/s12603-013-0007-x

Rubio-López, N., Morales-Suárez-Varela, M., Pico, Y., Livianos-Aldana, L., & Llopis-González, A. (2016). Nutrient intake and depression symptoms in Spanish children: The ANIVA study. *International Journal of Environmental Research and Public Health, 13*(3). doi.org/10.3390/ijerph13030352

Samieri, C., Féart, C., Letenneur, L., Dartigues, J.-F., Pérès, K., Auriacombe, S., et al. (2008). Low plasma eicosapentaenoic acid and depressive symptomatology are independent predictors of dementia risk. *The American Journal of Clinical Nutrition, 88*(3), 714–721. Retrieved from http://www.ncbi.nlm.nih.gov/pubmed/18779288

Sanchez-Villegas, A., & Martínez-González, M. A. (2013). Diet, a new target to prevent depression? *BMC Medicine, 11*, 3. doi.org/10.1186/1741-7015-11-3

Sawada, T., & Yokoi, K. (2010). Effect of zinc supplementation on mood states in young women: A pilot study. *European Journal of Clinical Nutrition, 64*(3), 331–333. doi.org/10.1038/ejcn.2009.158

Serefko, A., Szopa, A., Wlaź, P., Nowak, G., Radziwoń-Zaleska, M., Skalski, M., & Poleszak, E. (2013). Magnesium in depression. *Pharmacological Reports, 65*(3), 547–554. doi.org/10.1016/s1734-1140(13)71032-6

Sheikh, M., Hantoushzadeh, S., Shariat, M., Farahani, Z., & Ebrahiminasab, O. (2017). The efficacy of early iron supplementation on postpartum depression: A randomized double-blind placebo-controlled trial. *European Journal of Nutrition, 56*, 901–908. doi.org/10.1007/s00394-015-1140-6

Sikoglu, E. M., Navarro, A. A. L., Starr, D., Dvir, Y., Nwosu, B. U., Czerniak, S. M., et al. (2015). Vitamin D3 supplemental treatment for mania in youth with bipolar spectrum disorders. *Journal of Child and Adolescent Psychopharmacology, 25*(5), 415–424. doi.org/10.1089/cap.2014.0110

Simopoulos, A. P. (2008). The importance of the omega-6/omega-3 fatty acid ratio in cardiovascular disease and other chronic diseases. *Experimental Biology and Medicine, 233*(6), 674–688. doi.org/10.3181/0711-MR-311

Simopoulos, A. P. (2002). Omega-3 fatty acids in inflammation and autoimmune diseases. *Journal of the American College of Nutrition, 21*(6), 495–505.

Siwek, M., Dudek, D., Paul, I. A., Sowa-Kućma, M., Zięba, A., Popik, P., et al. (2009). Zinc supplementation augments efficacy of imipramine in treatment resistant patients: A double blind, placebo-controlled study. *Journal of Affective Disorders, 118*(1), 187–195. doi.org/10.1016/j.jad.2009.02.014

Stoll, A. L., Severus, W. E., Freeman, M. P., Rueter, S., Zboyan, H. A., Diamond, E., et al. (1999). Omega 3 fatty acids in bipolar disorder. *Archives of General Psychiatry, 56*(5), 407–412. doi.org/10.1001/archpsyc.56.5.407

Tartagni, M., Cicinelli, M. V., Tartagni, M. V., Alrasheed, H., Matteo, M., Baldini, D., et al. (2016). Vitamin D supplementation for premenstrual syndrome-related mood disorders in adolescents with severe hypovitaminosis D. *Journal of Pediatric and Adolescent Gynecology, 29*(4), 357–361. doi.org/10.1016/j.jpag.2015.12.006

Turnbull, T., Cullen-Drill, M., & Smaldone, A. (2008). Efficacy of omega-3 fatty acid supplementation on improvement of bipolar symptoms: A systematic review. *Archives of Psychiatric Nursing, 22*(5), 305–311. doi.org/10.1016/j.apnu.2008.02.011

US Department of Agriculture, & US Department of Health and Human Services. (2010). *Dietary guidelines for Americans 2010*. Retrieved from https://health.gov/dietaryguidelines/dga2010/DietaryGuidelines2010.pdf

Valk, E. E., & Hornstra, G. (2000). Relationship between vitamin E requirement and polyunsaturated fatty acid intake in man: A review. *International Journal for Vitamin and Nutrition Research, 70*(2), 31–42. doi.org/10.1024/0300-9831.70.2.31

van Groningen, L., Opdenoordt, S., van Sorge, A., Telting, D., Giesen, A., & de Boer, H. (2010). Cholecalciferol loading dose guideline for vitamin D-deficient adults. *European Journal of Endocrinology, 162*(4), 805–811. doi.org/10.1530/EJE-09-0932

Vieth, R. (1999). Vitamin D supplementation, 25-hydroxyvitamin D concentrations, and safety. *The American Journal of Clinical Nutrition, 69*(5), 842–856. Retrieved from http://ajcn.nutrition.org/cgi/content/long/69/5/842

Witte, A. V., Kerti, L., Hermannstädter, H. M., Fiebach, J. B., Schreiber, S. J., Schuchardt, J. P., et al. (2014). Long-chain omega-3 fatty acids improve brain function and structure in older adults. *Cerebral Cortex, 24*(11), 3059–3068. doi.org/10.1093/cercor/bht163

Zeisel, S. H. (2000). Choline: An essential nutrient for humans. *Nutrition, 16*, 669–671. doi.org/10.1016/S0899-9007(00)00349-X

Zempleni, J. (2007). *Handbook of vitamins*. London: Taylor & Francis.

Zempleni, J., Suttie, J. W., Gregory, J. F. III, & Stover, P. J. (Eds.). (2013). *Handbook of vitamins* (5th ed.). Boca Raton, FL: CRC Press.

3

Effects of Exercise on Mental Health

STEPHEN OLEX AND KRISTA OLEX

> **Key Points**
>
> - There are many different ways to use exercise and body movement to improve mental health.
> - There are numerous possible mechanisms by which exercise improves brain function and mental health including enhanced neuroplasticity, increased cerebral blood flow, and neurotransmitter changes.
> - Aerobic exercise has a beneficial effect on cognition and reduces depression and anxiety symptoms.
> - Less is known about the effects of resistance training, but there is some data supporting its ability to have beneficial effects on cognition and in depression.
> - Yoga has been shown to be beneficial for depression, anxiety, and cognitive function, though more data is needed.
> - Exercise programs might be useful in patients with posttraumatic stress disorder.
> - There is limited data, and hence limited use, of exercise programs in more severe psychiatric disorders such as schizophrenia.

Introduction

The beneficial effects of exercise on the body are well established, but physical activity also has significant benefits on brain function and mental health. There are many ways to move the human body that have the potential to have a positive impact on mental health. Physical activity including aerobic exercise, resistance exercise, yoga, and tai chi can favorably influence mental health through numerous physiological mechanisms. While the evidence is strongest for the effects of aerobic exercise on cognitive dysfunction and depression, there is promising data in the use of aerobic exercise in other populations with mental illness, as well as promising data for the use of the other types of movement for mental health.

Types of Exercise

Aerobic exercise can be thought of as sustained movement that has the potential to improve the efficiency of aerobic energy–producing systems in the body and to increase maximal oxygen uptake and cardiorespiratory endurance (Voss et al., 2013). Well-known examples of aerobic activity include walking, jogging, running, and cycling. Resistance exercise involves exercise that forces a muscle to contract against resistances above that encountered in daily activities and includes the use of elastic bands, resistance machines, and weight lifting (Physical Activity Guidelines Advisory Committee, 2008; Strickland & Smith, 2014).

The physical branch of yoga (Hatha yoga) is an ancient mind-body discipline originating in India in which meditation, breath control, and specific postures are utilized for spiritual growth as well as for mental and physical well-being (Ernst, Pittler, & Wider, 2008). As yoga has been demonstrated to be accessible to those with lower physical tolerance, the practice has the potential to benefit patients with limited functional capacity who may not be able to perform aerobic exercise (Hunink et al., 2016; Olex, Newberg, & Figueredo, 2013). Yoga therapy is the application of yoga for preventive medicine and for therapeutic purposes; the practice of yoga therapy has been increasing in recent years (Khalsa, Telles, & Cohen, 2016).

Tai chi is a mind-body practice and martial art that originated in China with foundations in Taoism that has been described as "a system of movements and postures used to enhance mental and physical health" (Ernst et al., 2008). Tai chi has three components including movement, meditation, and deep breathing; the practice is considered to be low-impact exercise of low to moderate intensity that can be performed by older adults and those with chronic disease (Hartley, Flowers, Lee, Ernst, & Rees, 2014; Lan, Chen, Wong, & Lai, 2013; Olex et al., 2013).

Mechanisms of Psychological Benefit

Exercise is powerful medicine for the mind and body with the potential to exert beneficial effects on multiple levels ranging from the microscopic to the level of behavior and social connection (Box 3.1). The beneficial anatomic, physiologic, and psychosocial changes that result from exercise are incompletely understood and involve significant complexity. An overview of the probable mechanisms whereby physical activity can benefit mental health is presented here. Potential mechanisms are separated here for ease of discussion; however, there is substantial overlap and interaction between the mechanisms described.

In recent decades it has become evident that the brain is not fixed and stable as was previously thought (Cicchetti & Curtis, 2015; Kays, Hurley, & Taber, 2008; Leuner & Gould, 2008). The term *neuroplasticity* refers to the dynamic nature of the brain and includes the capacity of the brain to change structure in response to internal and/or external influences (Kandola, Hendrikse, Yucel, & Lucassen, 2016). The umbrella term *neuroplasticity* includes the process of *neurogenesis*, which involves the formation of new neurons and glial cells in certain parts of the adult brain; neuroplasticity also involves the formation of new neural connections and changes in existing connections (Kays et al., 2008). Neuroplasticity can be adaptive and associated with gains in functioning but can also be maladaptive, contributing to psychiatric and neurological pathology (Kays et al., 2008).

Aging and mental illness are associated with maladaptive changes in brain structure. Aging is associated with gray matter volume loss in regions including

---

Box 3.1 Potential Mechanisms of Benefit of Exercise on Mental Health

Enhanced neuroplasticity
Increased neurotrophic factors (BNDF most crucially)
Epigenetic changes
Increased endorphins
Increased endocannabinoids
Neurotransmitter modulation
Increased cerebral blood flow
Autonomic balance (decreased sympathetic/increased parasympathetic tone)
Beneficial effect on hypothalamus-pituitary-axis
Decreased inflammation and oxidative stress
Improved physical healthEffects on cognition
Increased mindfulness
Decreased anxiety sensitivity/muscular tension
Improved sleep
Increased self-efficacy/active coping
Beneficial effects of social interaction

the prefrontal cortex, caudate nucleus, and medial temporal lobes most significantly; this age-related gray matter volume loss is thought to precede and lead to more severe memory loss and cognitive impairment (Erickson, Leckie, & Weinstein, 2014). A reduction in the volume of the white matter has also been noted with age (Voss et al., 2013).

To some degree, mental illness can be thought of as an abnormality in neuroplasticity (Krystal et al., 2009). The hippocampus, heavily involved in learning, memory, and affective processing (Jarrard, 1993; Phillips, Drevets, Rauch, & Lane, 2003), has a high degree of neuroplasticity (Bavelier & Neville, 2002) and also appears to have a prominent role in mental illness (Kandola et al., 2016). The hippocampus is particularly vulnerable to damage in neuropsychiatric pathology including major depression, anxiety, schizophrenia, and Alzheimer's dementia (Adriano, Caltagirone, & Spalletta, 2012; Bartsch & Wulff, 2015; Kandola et al., 2016; Schmaal et al., 2016). Significant acute or chronic stress is disruptive of hippocampus-dependent memory, and high levels of glucocorticoids induce atrophic changes in hippocampal subregions (McEwen, 2007). In addition, hippocampal damage or atrophy can also result in a prolonged hypothalamus-pituitary axis stress response to psychological stress (Herman & Cullinan, 1997; Wegner et al., 2014). Other areas of the brain have been shown to have pathologic changes in patients with mental illness. For example, depression can lead to atrophy of neurons and cell loss in other limbic structures including the amygdala and the prefrontal cortex (McEwen, 2007). Not merely an imbalance of neurotransmitters, mental illness such as depression alters the structure of the brain propagating psychopathology in both cognitive and affective domains. It follows that targeting adaptive neuroplasticity is an important and even essential component of fully addressing mental illness.

Aerobic exercise has been demonstrated to be a potent inducer of neuroplasticity. The effects of exercise on neuroplasticity are noted throughout the lifespan and is not limited to the young—exercise induced neuroplasticity has been noted in numerous studies in older adults (Erickson et al., 2014; Kandola et al., 2016; Voss et al., 2013). Aerobic exercise has a positive influence on hippocampal volume and hippocampal dependent forms of cognition (Kandola et al., 2016). In addition, regular physical activity is associated with an increase in prefrontal cortex volume (Erickson et al., 2014). Though the majority of the literature has focused on assessing gray matter changes, improvements in white matter integrity have also been noted with aerobic exercise (Kandola et al., 2016). Though other forms of exercise may stimulate neuroplasticity, the vast majority of research on physical activity and neuroplasticity has been done on aerobic exercise. There is limited animal data suggesting resistance exercise stimulates hippocampal neurogenesis (Lee et al., 2013).

Neurotrophic factors are a family of molecules that have an important role in neurogenesis by increasing the rate of cell birth and promoting maturation and survival. Brain-derived neurotrophic factor (BDNF) is a centrally produced neurotrophin that is a crucial mediator of the benefits of exercise on brain health (Huang et al., 2014). BDNF promotes neurogenesis, increases synaptic plasticity, induces long-term potentiation (the cellular mechanism for learning and memory; Ratey & Spark, 2014), enhances learning and memory, and promotes neural repair (Bekinschtein, Cammarota, & Medina, 2013; Cotman, Berchtold, & Christie, 2007; Gomez-Pinilla & Hillman, 2013; Kuipers & Bramham, 2006; Pang & Lu, 2004; Polusny et al., 2008; Yang, Lin, Chuang, Bohr, & Mattson, 2014). In animals BDNF has been shown to be reduced by both acute and chronic psychological stress; studies in humans have noted decreased BDNF levels in mood disorders, significant psychological stress, and schizophrenia (Kandola et al., 2016; Martinowich & Lu, 2008; Murakami, Imbe, Morikawa, Kubo, & Senba, 2005).

In numerous studies, aerobic exercise has been shown to increase BDNF levels acutely after exercise and has been shown to increase baseline levels after regular training (Huang et al., 2014). The increase in BDNF with exercise is not limited to intense exercise in younger populations—a year-long walking program increased BDNF in older adults (Leckie et al., 2014). Vascular endothelial growth factor and insulin-like growth factor are also increased by aerobic exercise (Lorens-Martín, Torres-Alemán, & Trejo, 2010; Schobersberger et al., 2000) and are implicated in central nervous system angiogenesis and neurogenesis (Gomez-Pinilla & Hillman, 2013). Fibroblast growth factor (FGF-2) is also increased by aerobic activity; FGF-2 is also involved in neurogenesis and is important for long-term potentiation (Kandola et al., 2016). Though more research is needed, there is evidence that exercise affects neurotrophin gene expression (Sølvsten, de Paoli, Christensen, & Nielsen, 2016), suggesting that epigenetic changes may mediate some of the effects of exercise on neurotrophins.

Resistance exercise may not have the same effects as aerobic exercise on BDNF (Strickland & Smith, 2014). Although acute increases have been noted after training (Yarrow, White, McCoy, & Borst, 2010), a recent meta-analysis noted that aerobic but not resistance exercise increased resting peripheral blood BDNF concentrations (Dinoff et al., 2016). Resistance exercise has been noted to increase insulin-like growth factor (Cassilhas, Lee, Fernandes, et al., 2012; Cassilhas, Lee, Venâncio, et al., 2012). Though limited, there is data to suggest yoga may increase BDNF (Naveen et al., 2016).

Traditionally, the postaerobic exercise positive mood change has been attributed to endorphins (Boecker et al., 2008), but the endorphin hypothesis has been debated (Heijnen, Hommel, Kibele, & Colzato, 2016). Endocannabinoids (eCB) are molecules produced in the brain and peripherally that are increased with exercise (Raichlen & Polk, 2013). There is animal data to suggest that blocking eCB receptors—but not endorphin receptors—decreases the anxiolytic and analgesic effects of aerobic exercise (Fuss et al., 2015). There is a high density of cannabinoid receptors in areas critical for emotional hemostasis, including the frontal cortex, amygdala, hippocampus, and hypothalamus (Marco et al., 2011).

Exercise has the potential to beneficially affect mental health through modulation of neurotransmitters. Serotonin has numerous functions including involvement in mood, anger, memory, appetite, perception, reward, sexuality, and attention (Berger, Gray, & Roth, 2009; Haider, Khaliq, Ahmed, & Haleem, 2006). Tryptophan, the precursor to serotonin, competes with branched-chain amino acids for transport across the blood–brain barrier. The muscle activity of exercise requires uptake of branched-chain amino acids, therefore reducing the amount of competition tryptophan has for transport to the brain and potentially increasing serotonin through this mechanism (Patrick & Ames, 2015). The changes in serotonin metabolism in the brain from aerobic exercise are complex; increases, decreases, and no change in serotonin metabolism have been noted depending on factors including brain region evaluated, intensity of exercise, and duration of exercise (Dey, Singh, & Dey, 1992; Lin & Kuo, 2013; Raichlen & Polk, 2013). In one study, yoga has been associated with increased plasma serotonin in patients with depression (Devi, Chansauria, & Udupa, 1986).

Dopamine is involved in numerous processes including control of voluntary movement, cognitive processes (attention and memory), and control of motivated behavior including involvement in reward mechanisms (Kurian, Gissen, Smith, Heales, & Clayton, 2011). Norepinephrine is involved in attention, concentration, arousal, and sleep (Klein & Thorne, 2006). In animal studies, aerobic exercise has increased dopamine levels in the striatum, hypothalamus, midbrain, and brainstem (Foley & Fleshner, 2008) and in humans physical stress results in eCB-mediated dopamine boost from the nucleus accumbens (Heyman et al., 2012). Physical activity increases norepinephrine levels in the brain in animals as well (Gordon, Spector, & Sjoerdsma, 1964). There is preliminary data from imaging that yoga can increase endogenous dopamine release in the ventral striatum (Kjaer et al., 2002) and also increase thalamic gamma-aminobutyric acid levels (Streeter et al., 2010), an inhibitory neurotransmitter that is deficient in numerous disorders including anxiety, depression, and posttraumatic stress disorder (PTSD; Khalsa et al., 2016; Streeter, Gerbarg, Saper, Ciraulo, & Brown, 2012).

Aerobic exercise may have beneficial effects on brain health through improving cerebral blood flow acutely and chronically (Kandola et al., 2016). Aerobic exercise has been noted in animal models to stimulate the generation of the new capillaries (angiogenesis) and improve vasculature in the hippocampus (Carro, Trejo, Busiguina, & Torres-Aleman, 2001; van Praag, 2005). Increased cerebral blood flow is of course important in providing oxygen and nutrients that are essential for optimal brain functioning; in addition the increased blood flow may facilitate the release of neurotrophic factors as well as promote increased synaptic plasticity and neurogenesis (Kandola et al., 2016).

As psychiatric illness is associated with autonomic imbalance (increased sympathetic and decreased parasympathetic activity; Alvares, Quintana, Hickie, & Guastella, 2016), aerobic exercise has the potential to improve psychological health through the known beneficial effects of aerobic exercise on sympathovagal balance (Carter, Banister, & Blaber, 2003; Curtis & O'Keefe, 2002). The practice of yoga has beneficial effects on the balance of the autonomic nervous system (Streeter et al., 2010); Tai chi practice appears to have beneficial autonomic effects as well (Motivala, Sollers, Thayer, & Irwin, 2006).

The mental health benefits of improved autonomic balance has the potential to occur through numerous mechanisms including direct central effects of increased vagal tone—many *afferent* vagal fibers project to the nucleus tractus solitarius, a relay station that has connections throughout the brain including to the limbic system and cortex (Khalsa et al., 2016; Streeter et al., 2012). Vagal *afferent* activity, through this network, can influence emotional states and thought processes as well as their expression in the body (Streeter et al., 2012).

Heart rate variability, a measure of the variation of instantaneous heart rate over time, can provide a window into the functioning of the autonomic nervous system and autonomic balance (Olex et al., 2013). Reduced heart rate variability, secondary to reduced vagal *efferent* tone, has been noted in numerous studies in a wide range of psychiatric disorders and also is a risk factor for cardiovascular morbidity and mortality (Alvares et al., 2016; Olex et al., 2013). Pathways have been identified linking cardiac vagal tone to neural networks implicated in emotional and cognitive self-regulation (Park & Thayer, 2014). Higher resting heart rate variability has been associated with more adaptive modulation of emotional stimuli and is thought to provide a greater flexibility in response to stress, while reduced heart rate variability is associated with a hypervigilant, maladaptive cognitive response to emotional stimuli as well as reduced flexibility of response to challenges (Park & Thayer, 2014; Streeter et al., 2012). Exercise training has been has been shown in numerous populations to increase heart rate variability, with aerobic exercise being the most studied type of exercise in regard to heart rate variability (Caruso et al., 2015; Dixon, Kamath, McCartney, & Fallen, 1992; Furlan et al., 1993; Pichot et al., 2005; Tyagi & Cohen, 2016).

Exercise also has a beneficial effect on the hypothalamic-pituitary (HPA) axis. Prolonged hyperactivation of the HPA axis is deleterious to mental and physical health and is common in mental illness (Wegner et al., 2014). A hyperactive HPA axis is common in depression; observations in patients with depression include increased numbers of adrenocorticotropic hormone and cortisol pulses (Rubin, Poland, Lesser, & Winston, 1987), increased corticotropin-releasing factor levels in the cerebrospinal fluid, and increased corticotropin-releasing factor neurons in the limbic area (Raadsheer, Hoogendijk, Stam, Tilders, & Swaab, 1994). Increased HPA axis activity is also seen in patients with anxiety, though to a lesser degree than in depression (Curtis, Cameron, & Nesse, 1982). Patients with panic disorder have elevated cortisol levels accompanying attacks (Bandelow et al., 2000).

As a stressor, physical activity activates the sympathetic nervous system and stress response and results in glucocorticoid secretion (Wegner et al., 2014). However, chronic exercise appears to have the potential to favorably influence the HPA axis and therefore may be able to reduce the negative mind-body consequences of HPA dysfunction and hypercortisolemia. Exercised animals have shown attenuated glucocorticoid responses and less anxious behavior in new situations (Droste, Chandramohan, Hill, Linthorst, & Reul, 2007), and studies in humans suggest that physical fitness is associated with reduced HPA axis reactivity (Rimmele et al., 2007; Traustadóttir, Bosch, & Matt, 2005). The peptide atrial natriuretic peptide (ANP), produced by atrial myocytes, is increased with exercise. ANP inhibits the HPA axis and has been show to result in anxiolytic behavior after central or peripheral administration (Ströhle et al, 1997; Ströhle, Kellner, Holsboer, & Wiedemann, 2001). There is data that resistance exercise modulates the HPA axis as well (Strickland & Smith, 2016). The mind-body practice of yoga is intuitively thought to favorably affect HPA axis dysregulation. Although there is evidence to support this intuition (Danucalov et al., 2013; Devi et al., 1986), reduced cortisol from yoga practice has not been a consistent finding, which may be due to limitations in the current study designs (Li & Goldsmith, 2012).

Acute and chronic psychosocial stress activates the inflammatory response (Haroon, Raison, & Miller, 2012), and increases in inflammatory markers have been reported in patients with depression and bipolar disorder (Mechawar & Savitz, 2016). Inflammation appears to have a role in anxiety disorders as well (Hou & Baldwin, 2012). Chronic inflammation has also been associated with the neurodegenerative process of Alzheimer's disease (Ravari, Mirzaei, Kennedy, & Arababadi, 2017). The neuroinflammatory state has been associated with numerous abnormalities that can contribute to mental illness including neurotransmitter dysfunction, reduced hippocampal neuroplasticity, oxidative stress, and insensitivity to glucocorticoids (Eyre, Papps, & Baune, 2013).

Although exercise can be acutely inflammatory, regular exercise can have anti-inflammatory effects (Petersen & Pedersen, 2005) and therefore can maintain and improve brain health through reducing baseline inflammation (Silverman & Deuster, 2014). The anti-inflammatory effect of exercise appears to be in part secondary to epigenetic changes as well as through improved autonomic balance (Bonaz, Sinniger, & Pellissier, 2011; Horsburgh, Robson-Ansley, Adams, & Smith, 2015; Pongratz & Straub, 2014; Thayer & Sternberg, 2006).

Exercise also results in improvements in physical health, which can concomitantly improve mental health. The diagnosis of a psychiatric disorder is associated with an increased risk of all-cause mortality; approximately 60% of this increase is due to comorbid physical illness with cardiovascular disease being the most common cause of death (Alvares et al., 2016). As physical activity has well-known beneficial effects on physical health (Centers for Disease Control and Prevention, n.d.; Kodama et al., 2009), exercise has the potential to interrupt the vicious cycle of mental illness, resultant comorbid medical disease, and consequential reduced quality of life and worsening of mental illness. Through enhanced feelings of health and well-being, physical activity has the potential to create a positive feedback loop where increased well-being promotes further healthy behavior, which may further uplift mental and physical well-being.

Cognitive dysfunction is a common and significant problem in mental illness (Kandola et al., 2016); cognitive dysfunction and decline can also of course occur independently of mental illness (Barnes, Yaffe, Satariano, & Tager, 2003). In mental illnesses such as depression and schizophrenia, cognitive dysfunction commonly persists despite pharmacologic treatment (Bortolato et al., 2016; Kandola et al., 2016). Similar to its effects on mental health in general, aerobic exercise induces numerous beneficial changes both peripherally and centrally that can result in improved cognition (Hogan & Carstensen, 2013). A proposed conceptual model of the mechanisms for the effect of exercise on cognitive function is seen in Figure 3.1 Stillman, Cohen, Lehman, & Erickson, 2016). Though the majority of the research has been done on aerobic exercise, there is data for improvements in executive function from resistance training, yoga, and tai chi as well (Cassilhas et al., 2007; Gothe, Keswani, & McAuley, 2016; Matthews & Williams, 2008; Ozkaya et al., 2005). Improved executive function, combined with elevated mood and enhanced ability to learn, may create an environment where new, more adaptive patterns of thinking are introduced and utilized (Ratey, 2008). Exercise may create a favorable milieu where approaches such as cognitive behavioral therapy (CBT) can better function.

Through providing additional input on which the mind can focus (including bodily sensations and movement with or without additional sensory input

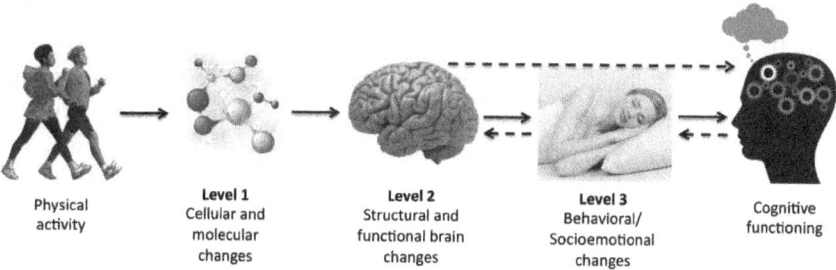

FIGURE 3.1. Conceptual model of mechanisms of physical activity at multiple levels of analysis. As for the effects of exercise on mental health in general, there is significant complexity involved and bidirectional effects between mechanisms.
Figure as originally published in Stillman, C. M., Cohen, J., Lehman, M. E., & Erickson, K. I. (2016). Mediators of physical activity on neurocognitive function: A review at multiple levels of analysis. *Frontiers in Human Neuroscience, 10*, 1–17. doi:10.3389/fnhum.2016.00626

such as music or television) as well as through acute beneficial effects on brain neurotransmission, exercise can also be a diversion from daily stresses and concerns, potentially breaking a cycle of negative affect and depressive rumination and improving short- and long-term mental health in the process (Asmundson et al., 2013).

Mindfulness involves cultivating a present-moment, nonjudgmental awareness of conscious phenomena (Kabat-Zinn, 2003) whether the experience is pleasant, unpleasant, or neutral. Physical activity has the potential to improve an individual's awareness of mind and body, which may in turn contribute to improved mental and physical health (Goyal et al., 2014; Loucks, Britton, Howe, & Eaton, 2015). Though research is needed, the effects of exercise (increased monoamine levels, improved autonomic balance, and reduced muscular tension) may also create an environment in which intentionally cultivated mindfulness can flourish. The beneficial effects of exercise may help allow some individuals to engage in the difficult but healing process of turning toward and experiencing unpleasant and unwanted emotions. This may be one of the mechanisms by which the gentle yoga in the mindfulness-based stress reduction (Kabat-Zinn, 2013) has its beneficial effect. Though limited, there is data to suggest that aerobic exercise may increase dispositional mindfulness (Mothes, Klaperski, Seelig, Schmidt, & Fuchs, 2014). The practice of yoga, in which awareness of mind and body is commonly intentionally cultivated, has been associated with increases in perceived mindfulness (Bowden, Gaudry, An, & Gruzelier, 2012; Brisbon & Lowery, 2011). Tai chi is considered mindful movement and has also been associated with increased mindfulness as well (Caldwell Hooper, Bryan, & Hagger, 2014).

There are additional potential mechanisms of benefit of exercise on mental health. As aerobic exercise can induce physiologic changes that are similar to anxiety, aerobic exercise has the potential to benefit mental health through exposure to anxiety-related sensations and subsequent reduction in anxiety sensitivity (Broman-Fulks, Berman, Rabian, & Webster, 2004; Broman-Fulks & Storey, 2008; Smits et al., 2008). Exercise decreases muscular tension following exercise (DeVries et al., 1982), thereby reducing the subjective feelings of tension and hyperarousal. Exercise may have a beneficial effect on mental health through improvements in sleep (Youngstedt, 2005) and consequential improvements in mental health. In addition, exercise has the potential to increase mental health through increases in a sense of mastery and self-efficacy (Pearlin & Schooler, 1978) as well as providing an active coping strategy. Animal data suggests that an active coping strategy redirects brain signaling, which may reduce a conditioned fear response (Ledoux & Gorman, 2001). Exercise also has the potential to provide social interactions and interrupt the social isolation associated with mental illness and may have a therapeutic effect through this mechanism (Asmundson et al., 2013).

Clinical Effects of Exercise Interventions on Cognitive Function

Poor cognitive function has been associated with the development of numerous adverse outcomes including comorbid disease, dementia, loss of independence, and death (Barnes et al., 2003). Consequently, it is crucial that we identify interventions to preserve and improve cognitive function. A large body of evidence suggests that aerobic exercise has a positive influence on cognition throughout the lifespan (Kandola et al., 2016). Numerous large epidemiologic studies have correlated increased levels of aerobic fitness with cognitive health; increased aerobic fitness has been correlated with higher IQ scores and academic achievement (Howie & Pate, 2012; Sibley & Etnier 2003; Tomporowski et al., 2009; Tomporowski, McCullick, Pendleton, & Pesce, 2014), preservation of cognitive function with aging (Barnes et al., 2003; Middleton, Mitnitski, Fallah, Kirkland, & Rockwood, 2008; Wendell et al., 2014; Yaffe, Barnes, Nevitt, Lui, & Covinsky, 2001), and reduced incidence of dementia (Hamer & Chida, 2009; Kandola et al., 2016).

Beyond mere correlation, the data strongly suggests there is a causal relationship between aerobic exercise and improved cognition. Numerous prospective studies of aerobic exercise have investigated the effects of moderate intensity interventions (e.g., 30 minutes of walking) that generally span 3 to 12 months (Kandola et al., 2016). A recent review noted that meta-analyses of these trials have demonstrated that aerobic exercise interventions improve cognitive function across a variety of domains including attention, executive functioning, processing speed, motor functioning, and memory across the lifespan (Kandola et al., 2016). Meta-analyses found improvements in the aforenoted domains in healthy young and middle-aged adults (Chang, Labban, Gapin, & Etnier, 2012; Etnier, Nowell, Landers, & Sibley, 2006; Roig, Nordbrandt, Geertsen, & Nielsen, 2013; Smith et al., 2011; Verburgh, Konigs, Scherder, & Oosterlaan, 2014) and in older adults (Angevaren, Aufdemkampe, Verhaar, Aleman, & Vanhees, 2008; Chang et al., 2012; Colcombe & Kramer, 2003; Etnier et al., 2006; Smith et al., 2011; Snowden et al, 2011; van Uffelen, Chin, Paw, Hopman-Rock, & van Mechelen, 2008). The benefits have also been noted in those with mild cognitive impairments or dementia (Gates, Fiatarone Singh, Sachdev, & Valenzuela, 2013; Heyn, Abreu, & Ottenbacher, 2004; van Uffelen et al., 2008).

Studies on the effect of other movement and exercise practices on cognition are more limited. However, there is data that resistance exercise is associated with improvements in cognitive performance, particularly in older adults (Cassilhas, Lee, Venâncio, et al., 2012; Chang, Pan, Chen, Tsai, & Huang, 2012; Ozkaya et al., 2005; Strickland & Smith, 2016). There is some data suggesting that yoga can improve cognitive function including short- and long-term memory, though more data is needed (Gothe et al., 2016; Gothe, Pontifex, Hillman, & McAuley, 2013; Khalsa et al., 2016; Rocha et al., 2012) A meta-analysis of nine prospective trials noted that tai chi shows potential to protect cognitive function, but more data is needed (Zheng et al., 2015).

Clinical Effects of Exercise Interventions on Mood

With current estimates of 350 million people of all ages around the world affected (World Health Organization, 2016), major depressive disorder is a significant public health problem that is known to be a major cause of worldwide disability (Whiteford et al., 2010). Best practices treatment generally consists of therapies such as CBT and/or medication management, but 10-% to 30% of patients have been found to demonstrate treatment-resistant symptoms (Al-Harbi, 2012). This has led to interest in adjunctive treatment options, paving the way for exercise to be considered as one such option.

There is substantial evidence documenting the beneficial effects of aerobic exercise in depression. A landmark study by Blumenthal and colleagues in 1999 called SMILE (Standard Medical Intervention and Long-Term Exercise) investigated the effects of 16 weeks of exercise and also the selective serotonin reuptake inhibitor sertraline (Zoloft; Blumenthal et al., 1999). Inclusion criteria were greater than or equal to 50 years of age, clinical diagnosis of depression, and score of at least 13 on the Hamilton Rating Scale for Depression (HAM-D; Hamilton, 1960). The 156 patients were randomly assigned into three groups: sertraline, supervised exercise (walking or jogging), or a combination of sertraline and supervised exercise (walking or jogging). The exercise intervention included a 10-minute warm-up, 30 minutes of exercise at 70% to 85% of heart rate reserve (heart rate reserve measured as the difference between maximum heart rate measured through exercise treadmill testing and resting heart rate), and then a five-minute cool-down. Dropout rates did not vary significantly between the groups. The three groups all showed significant decreases in depression as measured by the HAM-D as well as the Beck Depression Inventory (Beck, Ward, Mendelson, Mock, & Erbaugh, 1961). Greater than 60% of the patients in all three groups no longer met diagnostic criteria for major depressive disorder. Though there were no significant differences between groups at the end of the study, those in the medication arm had more rapid improvement. Six months after the study ended patients in the exercise group who had experienced clinical remission during the trial had significantly lower relapse rates ($p = .01$) than did subjects in the medication group; exercising on one's own after the study was associated with a reduced probability of depression diagnosis at the six-month follow-up (odds ratio = 0.49, $p = 0.0009$; Babyak et al., 2000).

Several recent meta-analyses have investigated the effects of exercise (primarily aerobic) on depression (Catalan-Matamoros, Gomez-Conesa, Stubbs, & Vancampfort, 2016; Kvam, Kleppe, Nordhus, & Hovland, 2016; Schuch et al., 2016). Patients with major depressive disorder as well as minor depression and dysthymia were represented in the meta-analyses; two of the meta-analyses investigated the effects of exercise on adults at varied ages (Kvam et al., 2016; Schuch et al., 2016), and one of the meta-analyses focused on older adults (Catalan-Matamoros et al., 2016). The three meta-analyses noted that exercise is an effective intervention in the treatment of depression (Catalan-Matamoros et al., 2016; Kvam et al., 2016; Schuch et al., 2016). The data suggests that exercise has the potential by itself to be effective treatment for depression and that it may be an effective adjunct treatment in combination with antidepressants (Kvam et al., 2016; Legrand & Neff, 2016).

Though it is difficult to extrapolate firm conclusions from the current data, it is probably best to utilize an intervention that is best supported by data if possible. The majority of studies utilized exercise interventions between 30 and 45 minutes in length three times a week (Nyström; Neely, Hassmén, & Carlbring, 2015). A study with a twice per week exercise intervention was negative (Krogh, Saltin, Gluud, & Nordentoft, 2009) as was a study that utilized a 90-minute three times per week intervention (Krogh, Videbech, Thomsen, Gluud, & Nordentoft, 2012). A recent review concluded that at least 30 minutes of exercise at least three times per week is a reasonable recommendation for patients with depression (Nyström et al., 2015). Moderate and vigorous intensity exercise may be better than light to moderate exercise (Dunn, Trivedi, Kampert, Clark, & Chambliss, 2005; Schuch et al., 2016), a conclusion based on a small number of studies (Schuch et al., 2016). The mode of aerobic activity (i.e., walking, jogging, or cycling) does not seem to have any significant effect (Nyström et al., 2015).

With regard to other programs in depression, there is data to suggest regular resistance training improves depression (Pilu et al., 2007; Singh, Clements, & Fiatarone, 1997; Singh et al., 2005), though the topic is much less studied than the effects of aerobic exercise on depression. There is data to suggest that yoga reduces depression in the context of medical problems (Uebelacker & Broughton, 2016). In addition, there is data on the positive effects of yoga in clinical depression (Cramer, Lauche, Langhorst, & Dobos, 2013; Uebelacker, Lavretsky, & Tremont, 2016). However, authors of a recent review of 16 randomized trials note that firm conclusions cannot be made secondary to limitations in the trials including heterogeneity in the yoga intervention, heterogeneity in the control groups, small sample size, high risk of bias, and an overall lack of safety data (Khalsa et al., 2016). A meta-analysis investigated the effects of tai chi in randomized trials and noted that tai chi had positive psychological benefit on depressive symptoms, although methodological limitations of the study were noted (Wang et al., 2014). Additionally, a limited number of trials investigated the effects of tai chi specifically in individuals diagnosed with major depressive disorder (Wang et al., 2014).

It has been noted that individuals with bipolar disorder are symptomatic for approximately half of their lives, a finding that has been attributed to the longer term persistence of depressive symptoms (Judd et al., 2002). Therefore, at first glance, it might seem that findings from studies investigating exercise interventions in unipolar depression could be extrapolated to bipolar disorder. However, the occurrence of manic episodes in this disorder warrants special attention. Indeed, *the Diagnostic and Statistical Manual of Mental Disorders* (5th ed. [DSM-5]) now recognizes bipolar disorders as separate from depressive disorders (American Psychiatric Association, 2013), a distinction that acknowledges differences between the two in terms of symptomatology and genetics and underscores the need to understand bipolar depression as a distinct condition. Generally treated with pharmacotherapy, often in conjunction with psychological approaches, the illness has the potential to be lifelong and to be associated with a significantly reduced quality of life.

The evidence base is limited on the effects of exercise in bipolar patients. A recent review did note that physical exercise was associated with better functioning, improved quality of life, and reduced depressive symptoms, but no prospective randomized trials of exercise in bipolar disorder were identified (Melo, Daher, Albuquerque, & De Bruin, 2016). While exercise has the potential to be a healthy coping strategy to provide an outlet for increased energy and a distraction during manic episodes, exercise also increases energy, social contact, and self-efficacy and has been postulated to have the potential to also exacerbate manic symptoms. There is some data to suggest frequent exercise is associated with mania in patients with bipolar disorder; it is unknown whether the mania is caused by or is a consequence of the exercise. No studies were identified assessing the effect of resistance exercise in a population of patients with bipolar disorder. Research investigating yoga interventions specifically in individuals with bipolar disorder is currently scant, but one recent study detailed the self-reported benefits and risks of yoga in this patient population (Uebelacker, Weinstock, & Kraines, 2014). Using qualitative data analysis, the most common effects described by the 70 participants, all of whom practiced yoga, were positive in nature (e.g., decreased anxiety, increased cognitive effects such as an enhanced sense of acceptance or increased focus, and positive physical effects such as weight loss). Some negative effects were reported, most commonly physical injury or pain. In addition, five participants provided specific examples of experiencing an increase in agitation and/or manic symptoms, and five reported examples of experiencing an increase in depressive symptoms. Although significant limitations exist, results were interpreted as warranting a pilot study of yoga for this patient population.

Clinical Effects of Exercise Interventions on Anxiety

Anxiety disorders are the most common classification of mental disorders and place a significant burden on patients as well as the healthcare system in terms of utilization of both medical and mental health services. Consequently, a need for practical interventions that both are cost effective and allow the individual to learn tools to self-manage anxiety has become of paramount importance (Vorkapic & Rang, 2014). As the DSM-5 no longer classifies post-traumatic stress disorder and obsessive-compulsive disorder (OCD) under anxiety disorders (American Psychiatric Association, 2013), these illnesses are considered separately.

The literature suggests aerobic exercise has a beneficial effect on anxiety, but the effects of exercise on anxiety have not been as well studied as the effects of exercise on depression. A recent systematic review and analysis included 12 randomized controlled trials and 5 meta-analyses in which participants were preselected as having either a diagnosis of an anxiety disorder or elevated symptoms of anxiety (Stonerock, Hoffman, Smith, & Blumenthal, 2015). The authors concluded that exercise could be a useful, affordable, and accessible treatment for anxiety but there is a lack of data from well-designed randomized trials that preclude definitive conclusions from being made about the effectiveness of exercise in anxiety (Stonerock et al., 2015).

The anxiolytic effects of regular resistance training have been demonstrated in healthy patients and several medical populations. The most robust decreases in anxiety were noted at low to moderate intensities (Strickland & Smith, 2014). However, there is very limited data investigating the effects of resistance exercise in patients with a formal anxiety diagnosis (Herring, Jacob, Suveg, Dishman, & O'Connor, 2012), and more data is needed (Hallgren et al., 2016).

There is encouraging data suggesting the beneficial effects of yoga on anxiety in chronic illnesses such as cancer (Danhauer, Addington, Sohl, Chaoul, & Cohen, 2017) as well as anxiety related to performing a specific task (such as a music performance; Pilkington, Gerbarg, & Brown, 2016). There are a limited number of yoga studies investigating the effects of yoga on specific anxiety disorders, including generalized anxiety disorder (Uebelacker & Broughton, 2016). Two single-arm trials found improvements in anxiety symptoms over time in patients with generalized anxiety disorder (Katzman et al., 2012; Khalsa, Greiner-Ferris, Hofmann, & Khalsa, 2015), one of which utilized a yoga-enhanced CBT intervention (Khalsa et al., 2015). A larger scale randomized trial of yoga versus CBT versus educational control group is underway (ClinicalTrials.gov, 2017).

There is promising data on the effects of tai chi on anxiety. A recent qualitative review included 17 studies that investigated the effects of tai chi on anxiety; the review included those with primary anxiety, those with anxiety comorbid with a specific medical condition, and a general healthy population (Sharma & Haider, 2015). Statistically significant reductions of anxiety were noted in 12 of the studies reviewed. Limitations of the review included less than half of the studies were randomized controlled (8 out of 17), and the review did not include trials published in Chinese. In addition, more data is needed on the effects of tai chi in patients with anxiety diagnoses.

Among anxiety disorders, panic disorder can be particularly debilitating. CBT and pharmacotherapy are considered first-line interventions for panic disorder (Hofmann & Smits, 2008), and a few studies have investigated aerobic exercise either versus or as an add-on to these treatments. In the first randomized controlled trial investigating the effects of exercise in anxiety disorders, individuals with panic disorder who participated in regular aerobic exercise were found to demonstrate greater symptom improvement than those in the placebo group over a 10-week period but were also found to demonstrate less improvement than those treated with clomipramine (Broocks et al., 2003). Building upon this work, a more recent randomized controlled trial investigated aerobic exercise in combination with paroxetine and yielded a similar pattern of results to those of the clomipramine study (Wedekind et al., 2010). In considering results from both studies, the authors concluded that exercise has a greater effect than placebo treatment but less than that of pharmacological treatment. Consequently, exercise was not recommended as a standalone treatment but rather as a potential add-on treatment to standard treatments.

One study compared both the short- and longer term efficacy of physical exercise (including aerobic exercise) directly to CBT (Hovland et al., 2013). Although CBT was found to the superior treatment, exercise alone had at least some effect on panic disorder symptomatology. While the authors noted that it could not be ruled out that the social component of the exercise group was responsible for this effect, they concluded that it nonetheless remains that physical exercise alone resulted in large and significant short- and long-term effects on panic symptoms.

Using a randomized, controlled, double-blind design, a more recent study investigated aerobic exercise as an add-on (versus an alternative) intervention to CBT (Gaudlitz, Plag, Dimeo, & Ströhle, 2015). As predicted, those in combined therapy were found to demonstrate significantly greater improvement in terms of anxiety symptomatology at seven-month follow-up, which led the authors to conclude that aerobic exercise did indeed have an anxiolytic effect. In sum, although limited, the existing body of literature suggests aerobic exercise may be a promising adjunctive treatment for panic disorder.

Compared to aerobic exercise, relatively less research has been conducted that specifically addresses yoga as a treatment option for this disorder. One recent study did investigate the effects of yoga as a standalone treatment and in conjunction with CBT for panic disorder, and participants in the combined yoga and CBT group demonstrated greater symptom reduction over time than did those in the yoga group (Vorkapic & Range, 2014). It was argued that yoga, a contemplative technique, and CBT, a technique that addresses irrational beliefs and cognitive distortions, are in fact complementary techniques that augment one another's efficacy. Although this study had a relatively small sample size, it provides some promise for the application of yoga as a treatment option for this patient population.

Clinical Effects of Exercise Interventions on Posttraumatic Stress Disorder

Although closely related to anxiety disorders and having once been considered an anxiety disorder, PTSD, and other stressor-related disorders are now considered to be a distinct class of disorders in the DSM-5 (American Psychiatric Association, 2013). This separation has underscored the need to consider PTSD as distinct from anxiety disorders, and recent decades have been characterized by an increased awareness of PTSD on a societal level, particularly as it pertains to the return of military personnel from the Middle East. Prolonged exposure therapy (Foa, Dancu, Hembree, Meadows, & Street, 1999) has long been considered a first-line treatment approach for PTSD, and with the efficacy of this modality well established, research efforts have increasingly sought to identify strategies to enhance its effectiveness (Powers et al., 2015). Given research suggesting positive effects of regular aerobic exercise on the mental health of individuals with anxiety disorders (Asmundson et al., 2013), a logical extension is to apply this intervention to PTSD, a disorder that certainly has an anxiety component. Indeed, exercise represents a logical adjunctive intervention given its potential to impact the distressing physiological hyperarousal symptoms characteristic of PTSD.

Recent research has investigated aerobic exercise specifically as an add-on treatment to traditional exposure therapy. Based on studies that indicated nonideal response rates to exposure therapy as a standalone treatment (Foa, Rothbaum, Riggs, & Murdock, 1991), a recent pilot study in which aerobic exercise was combined with exposure therapy yielded promising results (Powers et al., 2015). Among the nine participants diagnosed with PTSD, those randomly assigned to the prolonged exposure therapy and aerobic exercise condition demonstrated a greater improvement in symptom severity than did the exposure therapy-only condition.

Studies have also investigated aerobic exercise as a standalone intervention for PTSD. For example, a recent randomized controlled study investigated the benefits of aerobic exercise in a sample of 33 individuals with PTSD (Fetzner & Asmundson, 2015). Although limitations such as the lack of control over additional activity were noted, aerobic exercise was found to be related to decreased PTSD symptoms, anxiety sensitivity, and depression.

When considering research investigating the effects of aerobic exercise or any other intervention on PTSD symptoms, it is important to recognize that PTSD can result from a wide range of traumatic experiences, from a single event in adulthood to chronic, recurrent events that begin in childhood. Consequently, studies have addressed the effectiveness of exercise interventions in specific subgroups of trauma survivors, such as military veterans. Special focus on this group is certainly warranted given data indicating that veterans of the armed forces demonstrate significantly higher rates of PTSD than the general population (Hines, Sundin, Rona, Wessely, & Fear, 2014) yet have low rates of seeking treatment (Kim, Thomas, Wilk, Castro, & Hoge, 2010). This difference with respect to engagement in treatment has been attributed to factors such as cost, access issues, and the stigma associated with seeking mental health treatment (Ouimette et al., 2011). Therefore, a need for alternatives has become increasingly important for veterans. Exercise is a logical candidate because it does not require a mental health professional, thereby eliminating the impediments caused by stigma, and because military personnel are accustomed to physical activity and the discipline required for consistent participation. A recent, systematic literature review, the first of its kind, found that although the literature in this area is quite sparse, the existing body of research suggests an inverse correlation between PTSD symptoms and exercise in military veterans (Whitworth & Ciccolo, 2016).

Given that PTSD is characterized by re-experiencing symptoms such as intrusive thoughts and flashbacks, the calming effect of yoga combined with a focus on awareness and acceptance of present-moment thoughts, emotions, and physical sensations appears to render it an excellent treatment option for PTSD. Although yoga has not been studied as frequently as aerobic exercise in this patient population, promising data does exist. For example, a recent randomized controlled trial found that yoga significantly reduced the intensity of PTSD symptoms in a sample of 60 women with chronic, treatment-resistant PTSD (Van Der Kolk et al., 2014). Results from a longer term follow-up study suggested that ongoing participation in yoga was predictive of decreases in PTSD and depressive symptoms over time, as well as an increased propensity for no longer qualifying for a PTSD diagnosis (Rhodes, Spinazzola, & Van Der Kolk, 2016). Despite limitations, recent studies such as these have provided a solid foundation for further study.

Although research for the use of tai chi for PTSD is scant, two recent studies have explored the use of this practice in specific subgroups of individuals with PTSD. One involved refugee survivors of torture (Grodin, Piwowarczyk, Fulker, Bazazi, & Saper, 2008), while the second involved veterans (Niles et al., 2016). Both yielded qualitative data that suggested tai chi was not only a feasible intervention but also a beneficial one that requires further study in this patient population. Research for the use of resistance training for PTSD is also scant, but results from one randomized controlled trial involving 30-minute resistance training sessions three times per week for 12 weeks combined with a walking program suggested a positive effect of the intervention on PTSD symptoms, depressive symptoms, waist circumference, sedentary time, and sleep quality (Rosenbaum & Sherrington, 2015).

Clinical Effects of Exercise Interventions on OCD

Many patients with OCD treated with first-line treatments have persistent clinically significant symptoms, leaving room for the identification of adjunctive interventions (Wang et al., 2014). There is limited but promising data on the effects of aerobic exercise on the symptoms of OCD as an adjunct intervention (Brown et al., 2007; Rector, Richter, Lerman, & Regev, 2015). A recent pilot study examined the feasibility and efficacy of adding an exercise program to group CBT in 11 patients with moderate to severe, medication-refractory OCD. Though small, the study noted very large effects and reaffirmed the potential of combining aerobic exercise with CBT (Rector et al., 2015).

Few studies have investigated yoga as a treatment option for OCD. Recently, a yoga therapy module specifically for OCD was developed, validated, and pilot tested in a sample of 10 participants with OCD (Bhat, Varambally, Karmani, Govindaraj, & Gangadhar, 2016). Improvement in OCD symptom severity was demonstrated by the participants after 10 sessions/two weeks of yoga practice. Although preliminary, the results of this study were consistent with older studies (Shannahoff-Khalsa & Beckett, 1996; Shannahoff-Khalsa et al., 1999), each of which provided similar evidence for (a) the feasibility of yoga as an intervention for OCD and (b) the possible positive therapeutic effects of yoga for this population. While the application of yoga as a treatment option for this patient population appears to be in its infancy, efforts thus far have provided promise as well as directions for future research.

Clinical Effects of Exercise Interventions on Schizophrenia

Schizophrenia is one of the most severe mental disorders and is associated with significant functional impairment, disability, morbidity, and stigma. Initial onset is often experienced during important years of life (early to mid-20s for males and late 20s for females; Ochoa, Usall, Cobo, Labad, & Kulkarni, 2012), and the illness course tends to be chronic with waxing and waning of symptoms over time, with most individuals requiring some form of support throughout their lives (American Psychiatric Association, 2013). First-line treatment is generally pharmacotherapy, often in conjunction with nonpharmacological therapies that help individuals cope with their illness and to improve socialization.

Though aerobic exercise has attracted attention as having benefits in patients with schizophrenia, only a handful of studies has systematically investigated the effects of aerobic exercise on cognitive deficits in the disorder. A recent systematic review and meta-analysis has provided evidence of the positive impact of aerobic exercise on cognitive functioning in individuals with schizophrenia (Firth, Cotter, Elliott, French, & Yung, 2017). Of the 10 studies with 385 participants that were eligible for inclusion, pooled effect sizes across all cognitive outcomes demonstrated exercise (mostly aerobic exercise) improved global cognition significantly more than control conditions. Further, exercise participation in which supervision was provided by instructors, as well as higher durations of exercise per week, were found to result in greater cognitive improvements. In terms of specific aspects of cognitive functioning, working memory, social cognition, and attention/vigilance were found to be positively impacted by exercise whereas processing speed verbal memory, visual memory, and reasoning/problem-solving were not found to be positively impacted. In sum, based on this analysis of the existing body of research, there is some promise for aerobic exercise, particularly when applied in higher dosages and in a supervised setting, as a potential intervention for the cognitive aspects of schizophrenia.

Data on resistance exercise in schizophrenia is limited, but results from one recent study suggested that 20 weeks of resistance exercise had a significant beneficial effect on both positive and negative symptoms, muscle strength, and quality of life in a sample of 34 patients with schizophrenia (Silva et al., 2015). Results remained even after the effects of medication were controlled for via statistical analysis. Further study is clearly needed to build on this promising data.

It has been noted that the use of yoga as a therapeutic intervention for this disorder has remained largely unexplored until recently, a fact that was attributed to not only the misperception that most patients are too impaired to engage in meaningful yoga practice but also to reports that forms of meditation practice can worsen or even trigger symptoms of psychosis (Khalsa, Cohen, McCall, & Telles, 2016). Research has increasingly begun to explore the use of yoga in this population, with support for the benefits of yoga on the symptoms of schizophrenia coming from the few randomized control studies that have been conducted. For example, one such study involved random assignment of 61 individuals diagnosed with schizophrenia of moderate severity to either a yoga therapy condition or a physical exercise therapy condition (Duraiswamy, Thirthalli, Nagendra, & Gangadhar, 2007). After four months of therapy, those in the yoga condition were found to exhibit significantly less psychopathology, significantly greater social and occupational functioning, and significantly greater quality of life than those in the physical exercise therapy condition. While a study such as this provides support for possible benefits of yoga for individuals with schizophrenia, it remains unclear if yoga can result in any longer term benefit for this population. Future research could address the feasibility of yoga as a function of schizophrenia symptom severity.

Authors of a 2016 review noted some evidence in favor of yoga over standard-care control in domains including mental state improvement (in terms of Positive and Negative Syndrome Scale scores; Kay, Fiszbein, & Opfer, 1987), social functioning, quality of life, and leaving the study early but encouraged caution as many of the outcomes were based on one study with limited sample size and short follow-up (Broderick, Knowles, Chadwick, & Vancampfort, 2016). The authors concluded that the evidence is of low to moderate quality and is too weak to assert that yoga is superior to standard care control for schizophrenia.

The emphasis of tai chi on motor coordination and relaxation seems well suited to the needs of individuals with schizophrenia. Although data is limited, recent studies have provided promising results. For example, data has suggested a benefit from this practice in terms of movement functioning and interpersonal functioning in residential patients (Ho et al., 2012). More recent data from a randomized, one-year study has supported the use of tai chi in the community setting to improve clinical symptoms, quality of life, and even medication compliance (Kang et al., 2016).

Clinical Effects of Exercise Interventions on ADHD

Emerging in childhood or adolescence (American Psychiatric Association, 2013), attention deficit hyperactivity disorder (ADHD) has been associated with several neurobiological abnormalities but not with a clear etiology. Treatment has generally consisted of pharmacotherapy alone or in conjunction with psychosocial or behavioral interventions. With the negative side effects, unfavorable response rates, and discontinuation rates associated with pharmacological treatment of ADHD in children (Connor, 2006), as well as the controversy associated with the use of stimulants in children, attention has turned to novel, nonpharmacological interventions. In a disorder characterized by excessive motor activity and/or impaired concentration, the use of interventions that require physical energy and promote relaxation of the mind and body certainly appears reasonable.

In a review and meta-analysis of only randomized control trials, the first known effort of its kind, seven studies up to November 2014 were identified that evaluated the effects of aerobic exercise in children with ADHD (Cerrillo-Urbina et al., 2015). Although the overall quality of these studies was characterized as low by the authors, statistical analysis revealed that aerobic exercise reduced inattention, impulsivity, and hyperactivity in children with ADHD. Pooled effects also demonstrated that exercise improved anxiety, executive functioning, and impulsivity. Given the small number of studies included as well as the heterogeneity of outcome measures used by the included studies, results were interpreted with caution but did suggest that further investigation is warranted.

Another recent review explored the evidence for the effectiveness of aerobic exercise in not only children but also in adults (Klil-Drori & Hechtman, 2009). Results of the studies reviewed were found generally to provide evidence of the social and neurocognitive benefits of aerobic exercise in children and adults with ADHD. Further, clinical trials of aerobic exercise in children with ADHD have generally found it to be an adjunctive treatment to medication. Limitations of the existing body of research were noted, such as the existence of few randomized controlled studies on the effectiveness of aerobic exercise in children and the use of small and heterogeneous samples in the existing studies. The authors also raised the important point that no randomized controlled studies of exercise interventions with adults with ADHD have been conducted. In conclusion, further attention to the clinical effectiveness of aerobic exercise in both adults and children appears warranted.

Research assessing the efficacy of yoga on the symptoms of ADHD is fairly limited and has generally occurred in the context of children stabilized on medication. The first known such study found that yoga had a greater effect on several ADHD symptoms than did a cooperative activity control condition (Jensen & Kenny, 2004). Results are not interpreted as strong support for the use of this intervention for ADHD due to the small sample size and other study limitations, but further investigation in larger groups was deemed warranted, paving the way for larger, more controlled studies of yoga as an intervention for ADHD.

Clinical Implications

With data increasingly supporting the use of various forms of exercise as an adjuvant treatment approach for an array of mental illnesses (see Table 3.1 for summary), the question becomes how these interventions can be implemented in clinical practice. This question is particularly important given that

Table 3.1. Summary of the Evidence for the Use of Exercise in Mental Health

	Aerobic	Resistance	Yoga	Tai Chi
Cognition	Large body of evidence for beneficial effect	Evidence for beneficial effect; much less evidence than for aerobic	Promising; more high-quality data needed	Promising; more high-quality data needed
Depression	Large body of evidence for beneficial effect	Evidence for beneficial effect; much less evidence than for aerobic	Promising; more high-quality data needed	Promising effects on depressive symptoms; more data needed in major depression
Bipolar disorder	Promising but limited and less than for unipolar depression; larger controlled studies needed	No data identified	No randomized trials; benefit suggested by qualitative data, more data needed including assessment of safety	No data identified
Anxiety	Evidence suggests positive effect; less evidence than for depression	Reduced anxiety noted in several populations; more data needed in patients with primary anxiety disorders	Reduced anxiety noted in several populations; more data needed in patients with primary anxiety disorders	Reduced anxiety noted in several populations; more data needed in patients with primary anxiety disorders
Panic disorder	Promising; more data needed	No data identified	Very limited but promising data	No data identified

(continued)

Table 3.1. Continued

	Aerobic	Resistance	Yoga	Tai Chi
PTSD	Very limited but promising; more data needed particularly with regard to subgroups of PTSD	Very limited data; one trial had promising result when combined with aerobic; more data needed	Promising; less data than for aerobic exercise; more data needed	Limited data in specific subgroups of PTSD patients; larger controlled studies needed
OCD	Limited but promising data; more data needed	No data identified	Very limited but promising data; larger controlled studies needed	No data identified
Schizophrenia	Limited but promising especially for cognitive symptoms; more data needed	One study with encouraging findings; more data needed	Very limited but promising data; more data needed	Limited but promising data; more data needed
ADHD	Promising; more data needed	No data identified	Limited data with promising results; larger controlled studies needed	No data identified

Note: PTSD = posttraumatic stress disorder; OCD = obsessive-compulsive disorder; ADHD = attention deficit hyperactivity disorder.

there are several potential barriers to employing exercise interventions in individuals with mental illnesses. For example, symptoms such as low energy, fatigue, and anhedonia are often experienced by individuals with a range of illnesses, and a sedentary lifestyle is common in modern society (Wasfy & Baggish, 2016). A recent systematic review and meta-analysis of motivating factors and barriers toward exercise in severe mental illness found that across 12 independent studies of 6,431 patients with severe mental illness, low mood and stress were cited as the most commonly expressed barriers toward exercise (61% of patients) followed by a lack of social support (50% of patients; Firth et al., 2016). In addition, practical issues regarding access to appropriate classes, equipment, or even a safe outdoor place in which to exercise may exist, further impeding implementation of these interventions. Funding issues have also been raised; it has been noted that lack of funding represents the greatest challenge to the wide implementation of evidence-based services for people with serious mental illnesses (Pratt et al., 2016).

Given these potential obstacles, it is critical to consider exactly how these interventions can be implemented in practice. One recent study employed interdisciplinary group medical visits with an integrated physical activity component to promote physical activity among a sample of 15 patients with either unipolar or bipolar depression (Adams, Remick, Davis, Vazirian, & Khan, 2015). Fourteen weekly, two-hour group medical visits, which combined specific medical advice, medication management, group discussion of individual concerns, education, and 50 minutes of physical activity (alternating weeks of a brisk walk and exercise in a gym), were conducted by a psychiatrist and exercise therapist. Additionally, study participants attended 11 weekly hatha yoga classes that were conducted by a certified yoga therapist, thereby creating an interdisciplinary treatment model. At three-month poststudy follow-up of the 14 participants who completed the study, median scores on an objective measure of depression decreased by 38%, median scores on an objective measure of anxiety decreased by 50%, and median daily steps increased by 71%. It was noted that at the time of three-month follow-up, study participants had moved from a sedentary lifestyle to a daily step count average more in line with those for adults in general population in the United States. Despite this study's limitations of a small sample size and the absence of a control group, it offers promising results in terms of the ability of an organized program to increase both the psychological and physical well-being of adults with depression.

While this study investigated the implementation of exercise interventions on a larger scale, it is also important to consider the issue in terms of a typical clinical practice. That is, what can the individual clinician do to increase physical activity in a patient with depression, for example? In the absence of the ability to implement a formal program such as that of the aforementioned study, clinicians can certainly apply the key components of that study in daily practice. For example, the use of psychoeducation to increase a patient's understanding of the importance of physical activity to recovery, the use of techniques such as motivational interviewing to enhance a patient's impetus to be physically active, the use of a prescription for exercise, or detailing a specific target frequency and duration of activity are each reasonable approaches that can be readily employed in clinical practice.

Current guidelines for physical activity for adults 18 to 64 years old (Office of Disease Prevention and Health Promotion, 2017) recommend a weekly target of at least 150 minutes of moderate aerobic physical activity or 75 minutes of vigorous aerobic activity or a combination of moderate and vigorous aerobic activity. In addition, muscle-strengthening activities should be included. For additional benefits, the guidelines recommend increasing the weekly amount of aerobic exercise to at least 300 minutes of moderate or 150 minutes of vigorous aerobic activity or a combination of moderate and vigorous activity. Though the guidelines are important, they should not foster all-or-nothing thinking as physical and mental health benefits have been noted with levels of physical activity less than what is recommended (Nyström; et al., 2015; Sparling, Howard, Dunstan, & Owen, 2015). Even everyday activities such as walking or going up steps can provide a simple method for increasing body activity, which has the potential to improve overall physical and mental health.

With any form of physical activity to be used or prescribed in patient care, caution is warranted to minimize the risk of the intervention having the opposite of its intended effect: *primum non nocere* (first do no harm). For certain patients, a medical evaluation including assessment of cardiovascular risk (and potentially exercise stress testing) is warranted before undertaking an exercise regimen. Psychological ramifications of an exercise prescription should also be considered. For example, recommending one hour of aerobic exercise per day to an individual with depression, who may already be experiencing low self-esteem and low self-efficacy, could potentially cause damage if the person is unable to meet the goal. More specifically, failing to meet a behavioral exercise goal could negatively impact self-esteem and self-efficacy, thereby creating a decreased likelihood of the patient attempting exercise in the future and even increased depression. Additionally, there is the possibility of too much exercise. An exercise regimen with intensity and frequency that exceeds an individual's capacity for rest, repair, and homeostasis has the potential to result in autonomic nervous system dysfunction, inflammation, and HPA axis dysfunction (Meeusen et al., 2013; Müssigbrodt et al., 2016), all of which would of course have the potential to exert deleterious effects on mental health.

In order to maximize the likelihood of the effectiveness of any exercise-based intervention, a thorough assessment and understanding of the patient is recommended, including the patient's capabilities, readiness for change, motivation, and physical health status. For some patients, gradual implementation of an exercise intervention may be prudent, allowing self-efficacy and self-esteem to grow as incremental, easily attainable goals are achieved by the patient. Other patients may not need a gradual approach and may derive faster and more significant psychological benefit from a program that begins immediately with frequent and more intense exercise.

The type of movement and frequency is almost certainly not a one-size-fits-all approach; what is best for an individual person at a certain time is likely affected by numerous factors including age, autonomic nervous system balance, HPA axis activity, hormonal factors, degree of inflammation, brain structure and function, genetic factors, psychological factors, and social connections, as well as the state of a person's life when not exercising. One individual with an illness such as depression may find joy and remission in a daily running routine and strength training; another may find personal transformation through frequent moderate intensity yoga practice and following a healthy and active lifestyle based on the principles and philosophy of yoga. Yet another may find relief of suffering through frequent walks with a close friend or partner, combining a healing connection with exercise. Another may find that gentle yoga helps foster mindfulness and acceptance of unpleasant thoughts and feelings, thereby helping to break the cycle of low mood and rumination (Williams, Teasdale, Segal, & Kabat-Zinn, 2007).

It is of paramount importance that the patient's capabilities are understood and that any exercise-related treatment goals are not only realistic but also collaboratively set and agreed upon by both clinician and patient. Further, it is important that a sound therapeutic alliance be established to increase the patient's trust in the clinician and the likelihood of complying with treatment recommendations, including recommendations for physical activity. Ideally, an individual will be attuned to how he or she feels mentally and physically and consequently will be able to evaluate how an exercise program is supporting mind and body health. A clinician can help guide the process based on the data, through evaluation of the patient over time, and through encouraging mindfulness to help allow a patient to know what works for him or her as of now. If possible, it is helpful for a clinician to have a basic, preferentially experiential familiarity with the different types of movement and exercise described in this chapter.

Conclusion and Future Directions

Research on exercise and mental health, as reviewed in this chapter, is essential to document the objective benefits of movement, which is crucial for legitimizing exercise as a valuable therapy in mental illness. Future studies are needed to help clarify and identify psychological, physiological, anatomic, and genetic factors that could guide clinicians and patients in selecting an exercise regimen that will have the greatest mental health benefits. In addition, future studies could look at the effects of combining known powerful interventions such as aerobic exercise and formal mindfulness practice in both healthy populations as well as patients with mental illness. It is hoped that as the body of research in this area continues to grow and as these areas are explored, clinicians will increasingly consider exercise interventions and will have a database that helps support an individualized, nuanced approach to recommending exercise for mental health.

For some time it has been impossible to deny the significant beneficial effects of exercise on the body; we are now at a point where it is impossible to deny the significant beneficial effects of exercise on mental health. The data has demonstrated numerous diverse mechanisms through which physical activity can potentially positively influence mental processes. In addition, a large body of clinical data now exists that confirms that exercise is an effective medicine to improve mental health. Clinicians should be aware of physical activity as a powerful tool in their clinical toolbox with the potential for tremendous benefit on mind and body.

REFERENCES

Adams, D. J., Remick, R. A., Davis, J. C., Vazirian, S., & Khan, K. M. (2015). Exercise as medicine—the use of group medical visits to promote physical activity and treat chronic moderate depression: A preliminary 14-week pre-post study. *BMJ Open Sport & Exercise Medicine, 1*(1). doi:10.1136/bmjsem-2015-000036

Adriano, F., Caltagirone, C., & Spalletta, G. (2012). Hippocampal volume reduction in first-episode and chronic schizophrenia: A review and meta-analysis. *Neuroscientist, 18*(2), 180–200. doi:10.1177/1073858410395147

Al-Harbi, K. S. (2012). Treatment-resistant depression: Therapeutic trends, challenges, and future directions. *Patient Preference and Adherence, 6*, 369–388. doi:10.2147/PPA.S29716

Alvares, G. A., Quintana, D. S., Hickie, I. B., & Guastella, A. J. (2016). Autonomic nervous system dysfunction in psychiatric disorders and the impact of psychotropic medications: A systematic review and meta-analysis. *Journal of Psychiatry & Neuroscience, 41*(2), 89–104. doi:10.1503/jpn.140217

American Psychiatric Association. (2013). *Diagnostic and statistical manual of mental disorders* (5th ed.). Washington, DC: American Psychiatric Publishing.

Angevaren, M., Aufdemkampe, G., Verhaar, H. J., Aleman, A., & Vanhees, L. (2008). Physical activity and enhanced fitness to improve cognitive function in older people without known cognitive impairment. *Cochrane Database of Systematic Reviews, 3*, CD005381. doi:10.1002/14651858.CD005381.pub3

Asmundson, G. J. G., Fetzner, M. G., Deboer, L. B., Powers, M. B., Otto, M. W., & Smits, J. A. J. (2013). Let's get physical: A contemporary review of the anxiolytic effects of exercise for anxiety and its disorders. *Depression and Anxiety, 30*(4), 362–373. doi:10.1002/da.22043

Babyak, M., Blumenthal, J. A., Herman, S., Khatri, P., Doraiswamy, M., Moore, K., et al. (2000). Exercise treatment for major depression: Maintenance of therapeutic benefit at 10 months. *Psychosomatic Medicine, 62*(5), 633–638.

Bandelow, B., Wedekind, D., Pauls, J., Broocks, A., Hajak, G., & Ruther, E. (2000). Salivary cortisol in panic attacks. *American Journal of Psychiatry, 157*(3), 454–456. doi:10.1176/appi.ajp.157.3.454

Barnes, D. E., Yaffe, K., Satariano, W., & Tager, I. B. (2003). A longitudinal study of cardiorespiratory fitness and cognitive function in healthy older adults. *Journal of the American Geratrics Society, 51*(4), 459–465. doi:10.1046/j.1532-5415.2003.51153

Bartsch, T., & Wulff, P. (2015). The hippocampus in aging and disease: From plasticity to vulnerability. *Neuroscience, 309*, 1–16. doi:10.1016/j.neuroscience.2015.07.084

Bavelier, D., & Neville, H. J. (2002). Cross-modal plasticity: Where and how? *Nature Reviews Neuroscience, 3*(6), 443–452. doi:10.1038/nrn848

Beck, A. T., Ward, C. H., Mendelson, M., Mock, J., & Erbaugh, J. (1961). An inventory for measuring depression. *Archives of General Psychiatry, 4*, 561–571.

Bekinschtein, P., Cammarota, M., & Medina, J. H. (2014). BDNF and memory processing. *Neuropharmacology, 76*(Pt C), 677–683. doi:10.1016/j.neuropharm.2013.04.024

Berger, M., Gray, J. A., & Roth, B. L. (2009). The expanded biology of serotonin. *Annual Review of Medicine, 60*, 355–366. doi:10.1146/annurev.med.60.042307.110802

Bhat, S., Varambally, S., Karmani, S., Govindaraj, R., & Gangadhar, B. N. (2016). Designing and validation of a yoga-based intervention for obsessive compulsive disorder. *International Review of Psychiatry, 261*, 1–7. doi:10.3109/09540261.2016.1170001

Blumenthal, J. A., Babyak, M. A., Moore, K. A., Craighead, W. E., Herman, S., Khatri, P., et al. (1999). Effects of exercise training on older patients with major depression. *Archives of Internal Medicine, 159*(19), 2349–2356.

Boecker, H., Sprenger, T., Spilker, M. E., Henriksen, G., Koppenhoefer, M., Wagner, K. J., et al. (2008). The runner's high: Opioidergic mechanisms in the human brain. *Cerebral Cortex, 18*(11), 2523–2531. doi:10.1093/cercor/bhn013

Bonaz, B., Sinniger, V., & Pellissier, S. (2011). Anti-inflammatory properties of the vagus nerve: Potential therapeuitc implications of vagus nerve stimulation. *Journal of Physiology, 82*(6), 1496–1514. doi:10.1113/JP271539

Bortolato, B., Miskowiak, K. W., Köhler, C. A., Maes, M., Fernandes, B., Berk, M., & Carvalho, A. (2016). Cognitive remission: A novel objective for the treatment of major depression? *BMC Medicine, 14*(1), 9. doi:10.1186/s12916-016-0560-3

Bowden, D., Gaudry, C., An, S. C., & Gruzelier, J. (2012). A comparative randomised controlled trial of the effects of brain wave vibration training, Iyengar yoga, and mindfulness on mood, well-being, and salivary cortisol. *Evidence-Based Complementary and Alternative Medicine, 2012*, 234713. doi:10.1155/2012/234713

Brisbon, N. M., & Lowery, G. A. (2011). Mindfulness and levels of stress: A comparison of beginner and advanced hatha yoga practitioners. *Journal of Religion and Health, 50*(4), 931–941. doi:10.1007/s10943-009-9305-3

Broderick, J., Knowles, A., Chadwick, J., & Vancampfort, D. (2016). Yoga vs standard care for schizophrenia. *Schizophrenia Bulletin, 42*(1), 15–17. doi:10.1093/schbul/sbv165

Broman-Fulks, J. J., Berman, M. E., Rabian, B. A., & Webster, M. J. (2004). Effects of aerobic exercise on anxiety sensitivity. *Behaviour Research and Therapy, 42*(2), 125–136. doi:10.1016/S0005-7967(03)00103-7

Broman-Fulks, J. J., & Storey, K. M. (2008). Evaluation of a brief aerobic exercise intervention for high anxiety sensitivity. *Anxiety, Stress, & Coping, 21*(2), 117–128. doi:10.1080/10615800701762675

Broocks, A., Meyer, T., Opitz, M., Bartmann, U., Hillmer-Vogel, U., George, A., et al. (2003). 5-HT(1A) responsivity in patients with panic disorder before and after treatment with aerobic exercise, clomipramine or placebo. *European Neuropsychopharmacology, 13*(3), 153–164.

Brown, R., Abrantes, A. M., Strong, D. R., Mancebo, M., Menard, J., Rasmussen, S., & Greenberg, B. (2007). A pilot study of moderate-intensity aerobic exercise for obsessive compulsive disorder. *Journal of Nervous and Mental Disorders, 195*(6), 514–520. doi:10.1097/01.nmd.0000253730.31610.6c

Caldwell Hooper, A. E., Bryan, A. D., & Hagger, M. S. (2014). What keeps a body moving? The brain-derived neurotrophic factor val66met polymorphism and intrinsic motivation to exercise in humans. *Journal of Behavioral Medicine, 37*(6), 1180–1192. doi:10.1007/s10865-014-9567-4

Carro, E., Trejo, J. L., Busiguina, S., & Torres-Aleman, I. (2001). Circulating insulin-like growth factor I mediates the protective effects of physical exercise against brain insults of different etiology and anatomy. *Journal of Neuroscience, 21*(15), 5678–5684. doi:21/15/5678

Carter, J. B., Banister, E. W., & Blaber, A. P. (2003). Effect of endurance exercise on autonomic control of heart rate. *Sports Medicine, 33*(1), 33–46. doi:10.2165/00007256-200333010-00003

Caruso, F. R., Arena, R., Phillips, S. A., Bonjorno, J. C. Jr., Mendes, R. G., Arakelian, V. M., et al. (2015). Resistance exercise training improves heart rate variability and muscle performance: A randomized controlled trial in coronary artery disease patients. *European Journal of Physical and Rehabilitation Medicine, 51*(3), 281–289. Retrieved from http://www.ncbi.nlm.nih.gov/pubmed/25384514.

Cassilhas, R. C., Lee, K. S., Fernandes, J., Oliveira, M. G. M., Tufik, S., Meeusen, R., & de Mello, M. T. (2012). Spatial memory is improved by aerobic and resistance exercise through divergent molecular mechanisms. *Neuroscience, 202*, 309–317. doi:10.1016/j.neuroscience.2011.11.029

Cassilhas, R. C., Lee, K. S., Venâncio, D. P., Oliveira, M. G. M., Tufk, S., & de Mello, M. T. (2012). Resistance exercise improves hippocampus-dependent memory. *Brazilian Journal of Medical and Biological Research, 45*(12), 1215–1220. doi:10.1590/S0100-879X2012007500138

Cassilhas, R. C., Viana, V. A. R., Grassmann, V., Santos, R. T., Santos, R. F., Tufik, S., & Mello, M. T. (2007). The impact of resistance exercise on the cognitive function of the elderly. *Medicine & Science in Sports & Exercise, 39*(8), 1401–1407. doi:10.1249/mss.0b013e318060111f

Catalan-Matamoros, D., Gomez-Conesa, A., Stubbs, B., & Vancampfort, D. (2016) Exercise improves depressive symptoms in older adults: An umbrella review of systematic reviews and meta-analyses. *Psychiatry Research, 244*, 202–209. doi:10.1016/j.psychres.2016.07.028

Chang, Y. K., Pan, C. Y., Chen, F. T., Tsai, C. L., & Huang, C. C. (2012). Effect of resistance-exercise training on cognitive function in healthy older adults: A review. *Journal of Aging and Physical Activity, 20*(4), 497–517.

Centers for Disease Control and Prevention. (n.d.). Benefits of physical activity. Retrieved from https://www.cdc.gov/physicalactivity/basics/pa-health/

Cerrillo-Urbina, A. J., García-Hermoso, A., Sánchez-López, M., Pardo-Guijarro, M. J., Santos Gómez, J. L., & Martínez-Vizcaíno, V. (2015). The effects of physical exercise in children with attention deficit hyperactivity disorder: A systematic review and meta-analysis of randomized control trials. *Child: Care, Health and Development, 41*(6), 779–788. doi:10.1111/cch.12255

Chang, Y. K., Labban, J. D., Gapin, J. I., & Etnier, J. L. (2012). The effects of acute exercise on cognitive performance: A meta-analysis. *Brain Research, 1453*, 87–101. doi:10.1016/j.brainres.2012.02.068

Cicchetti, D., & Curtis, W. J. (2015). The developing brain and neural plasticity: Implications for normality, psychopathology, and resilience. In *Developmental psychopathology* (pp. 1–64). Hoboken, NJ: John Wiley. doi:10.1002/9780470939390.ch1

ClinicalTrials.gov. (n.d.). GATE: generalized anxiety—a treatment evaluation. Retrieved from https://clinicaltrials.gov/ct2/show/NCT01912287?term=yoga+AND+anxiety&rank=2.

Colcombe, S. J., & Kramer, A. F. (2003). Fitness effects on the cognitive function of older adults. *Psychological Science, 14*, 125. doi:10.1111/1467-9280.t01-1-01430

Connor, D. (2006). Stimulants. In R. Barkley (Ed.), *Attention-deficit hyperactivity disorder: A handbook for diagnosis and treatment* (3rd ed., pp. 608–648). New York: Guilford Press.

Cotman, C. W., Berchtold, N. C., & Christie, L. A. (2007). Exercise builds brain health: Key roles of growth factor cascades and inflammation. *Trends in Neuroscience, 30*(9), 464–472. doi:10.1016/j.tins.2007.06.011

Cramer, H., Lauche, R., Langhorst, J., & Dobos, G. (2013). Yoga for depression: A systematic review and meta-analysis. *Depression and Anxiety, 30*(11), 1068–1083. doi:10.1002/da.22166

Curtis, B. M., & O'Keefe, J. H. J. (2002). Autonomic tone as a cardiovascular risk factor: The dangers of chronic fight or flight. *Mayo Clinic Proceedings, 77*(1), 45–54. doi:10.4065/77.1.45

Curtis, G. C., Cameron, O. G., & Nesse, R. M. (1982). The dexamethasone suppression test in panic disorder and agoraphobia. *American Journal of Psychiatry, 139*(8), 1043–1046. doi:10.1176/ajp.139.8.1043

Danhauer, S. C., Addington, E. L., Sohl, S. J., Chaoul, A., & Cohen, L. (2017). Review of yoga therapy during cancer treatment. *Supportive Care in Cancer, 25*(4), 1357–1372. doi:10.1007/s00520-016-3556-9

Danucalov, M. A. D., Kozasa, E. H., Ribas, K. T., Galduróz, J. C. F., Garcia, M. C., Verreschi, I. T. N., et al. (2013). A yoga and compassion meditation program reduces stress in familial caregivers of Alzheimer's disease patients. *Evidence-Based Complementary and Alternative Medicine, 2013*, 513149. doi:10.1155/2013/513149

Devi, S. K., Chansauria, J. P., & Udupa, K. N. (1986). Mental depression and kundalini yoga. *Ancient Science of Life, 6*(2), 112–118. doi:10.1161/01.CIR.101.3.329.

DeVries, H. A., Simard, C. P., Wiswell, R. A., Heckathorne, E., & Carabetta, V. (1982). Fusimotor System Involvement in the Tranquilizer Effect of Exercise. *American Journal of Physical Medicine & Rehabilitation, 61*(3). Retrieved from http://journals.lww.com/ajpmr/Fulltext/1982/06000/FUSIMOTOR_SYSTEM_INVOLVEMENT_IN_THE_TRANQUILIZER.1.aspx

Dey, S., Singh, R. H., & Dey, P. K. (1992). Exercise training: Significance of regional alterations in serotonin metabolism of rat brain in relation to antidepressant effect of exercise. *Physiology & Behavior, 52*(6), 1095–1099. doi:10.1016/0031-9384(92)90465-E

Dinoff, A., Herrmann, N., Swardfager, W., Liu, C. S., Sherman, C., Chan, S., & Lanctôt, K. L. (2016). The effect of exercise training on resting concentrations of peripheral brain-derived neurotrophic factor (BDNF): A meta-analysis. *PLoS One, 11*(9), 1–21. doi:10.1371/journal.pone.0163037

Dixon, E. M., Kamath, M. V., McCartney, N., & Fallen, E. L. (1992). Neural regulation of heart rate variability in endurance athletes and sedentary controls. *Cardiovascular Research, 26*(7), 713–719.

Droste, S. K., Chandramohan, Y., Hill, L. E., Linthorst, A. C. E., & Reul, J. M. H. M. (2007). Voluntary exercise impacts on the rat hypothalamic-pituitary-adrenocortical axis mainly at the adrenal level. *Neuroendocrinology, 86*(1), 26–37. doi:10.1159/000104770

Dunn, A. L., Trivedi, M. H., Kampert, J. B., Clark, C. G., & Chambliss, H. O. (2005). Exercise treatment for depression: Efficacy and dose response. *American Journal of Preventative Medicine, 28*(1), 1–8. doi:10.1016/j.amepre.2004.09.003

Duraiswamy, G., Thirthalli, J., Nagendra, H. R., & Gangadhar, B. N. (2007). Yoga therapy as an add-on treatment in the management of patients with schizophrenia—a randomized controlled trial. *Acta Psychiatrica Scandinavica, 116*(3), 226–232. doi:10.1111/j.1600-0447.2007.01032.x

Erickson, K. I., Leckie, R. L., & Weinstein, A. M. (2014). Physical activity, fitness, and gray matter volume. *Neurobiology of Aging, 35*(Suppl 2), S20–S28. doi:10.1016/j.neurobiolaging.2014.03.034

Ernst, E., Pittler, M. H., & Wider. B. K (Eds.). (2008). *Oxford handbook of complimentary medicine.* New York: Oxford University Press.

Etnier, J. L., Nowell, P. M., Landers, D. M., & Sibley, B. A. (2006). A meta-regression to examine the relationship between aerobic fitness and cognitive performance. *Brain Research Reviews, 52*(1), 119–130. doi:10.1016/j.brainresrev.2006.01.002

Eyre, H. A., Papps, E., & Baune, B. T. (2013). Treating depression and depression-like behavior with physical activity: An immune perspective. *Frontiers in Psychiatry, 4.* doi:10.3389/fpsyt.2013.00003

Fetzner, M. G., & Asmundson, G. J. G. (2015). Aerobic exercise reduces symptoms of posttraumatic stress disorder: A randomized controlled trial. *Cognitive Behaviour Therapy, 44*(4), 301–313. doi:10.1080/16506073.2014.916745

Firth, J., Cotter, J., Elliott, R., French, P., & Yung, A. R. (2017). A systematic review and meta-analysis of exercise interventions in schizophrenia patients. *Psychological Medicine, 45*(7), 1343–1361. doi:10.1017/S0033291714003110

Firth, J., Rosenbaum, S., Stubbs, B., Gorczynski, P., Yung, A. R., & Vancampfort, D. (2016). Motivating factors and barriers towards exercise in severe mental illness: A systematic review and meta- analysis. *Psychological Medicine, 46*(14), 2869–2881. doi:10.1017/S0033291716001732

Foa, E. B., Rothbaum, B. O., Riggs, D. S., & Murdock T. B. (1991). Treatment of posttraumatic stress disorder in rape victims: A comparison between cognitive-behavioral procedures and counseling. *Journal of Consulting and Clinical Psychology, 59*(5), 715–723.

Foa, E. B., Dancu, C. V., Hembree, E. A., Meadows, E. A., & Street, G. (1999). A comparison of exposure therapy, stress inoculation training, and their combination for reducing posttraumatic stress disorder in female assault victims. *Journal of Consulting and Clinical Psychology, 67*(2), 194–200.

Foley, T. E., & Fleshner, M. (2008). Neuroplasticity of dopamine circuits after exercise: Implications for central fatigue. *NeuroMolecular Medicine, 10*(2), 67–80. doi:10.1007/s12017-008-8032-3

Furlan, R., Piazza, S., Orto, S. D., Gentile, E., Cerutti, S., Pagani, M., & Malliani, A. (1993). Early and late effects of exercise and athletic training on neural mechanisms controlling heart rate. *Cardiovascular Research, 27*(3), 482–488. doi:10.1093/cvr/27.3.482

Fuss, J., Steinle, J., Gass, P., Fuss, J., Bindila, L., Lutz, B., et al. (2015). A runner's high depends on cannabinoid receptors in mice. *Proceedings of the National Academy of Sciences of the United States of America, 112*(42), 13105–13108. doi:10.1073/pnas.1514996112

Gates, N., Fiatarone Singh, M. A., Sachdev, P. S., & Valenzuela, M. (2013). The effect of exercise training on cognitive function in older adults with mild cognitive impairment: A meta-analysis of randomized controlled trials. *American Journal of Geriatric Psychiatry, 21*(11), 1086–1097. Retrieved from http://dx.doi.org/10.1016/j.jagp.2013.02.018

Gaudlitz, K., Plag, J., Dimeo, F., & Ströhle, A. (2015). Aerobic exercise training facilitates the effectiveness of cognitive behavioral therapy in panic disorder. *Depression and Anxiety, 32*(3), 221–228. doi:10.1002/da.22537

Gomez-Pinilla, F., & Hillman, C. (2013). The influence of exercise on cognitive abilities. *Comprehensive Physiology, 3*(1), 403–428. doi:10.1002/cphy.c110063

Gordon, R., Spector, S., & Sjoerdsma, A. (1964). Increased synthesis of norepinephrine and in the intact rat during exercise and exposure tocold. *The Journal of Pharmacology and Experimental Therapeutics, 153*(3), 440–447.

Gothe, N. P., Keswani, R. K., & McAuley, E. (2016). Yoga practice improves executive function by attenuating stress levels. *Biological Psychology, 121*, 109–116. doi:10.1016/j.biopsycho.2016.10.010

Gothe, N., Pontifex, M. B., Hillman, C., & McAuley, E. (2013). The acute effects of yoga on executive function. *Journal of Physical Activity & Health, 10*(4), 488–495.

Goyal, M., Singh, S., Sibinga, E. M. S., Gould, N. F., Rowland-Seymour, A., Sharma, R., et al. (2014). Meditation programs for psychological stress and well-being. *JAMA Internal Medicine, 174*(3), 357. doi:10.1001/jamainternmed.2013.13018

Grodin, M. A., Piwowarczyk, L., Fulker, D., Bazazi, A. R., & Saper, R. B. (2008). Treating survivors of torture and refugee trauma: A preliminary case series using qigong and t'ai chi. *Journal of Alternative and Complementary Medicine, 14*(7), 801–806. doi:10.1089/acm.2007.0736

Haider, S., Khaliq, S., Ahmed, S. P., & Haleem, D. J. (2006). Long-term tryptophan administration enhances cognitive performance and increases 5HT metabolism in the hippocampus of female rats. *Amino Acids, 31*(4), 421–425. doi:10.1007/s00726-005-0310-x

Hallgren, M., Herring, M. P., Owen, N., Dunstan, D., Ekblom, O., Helgadottir, B., et al. (2016). Exercise, physical activity, and sedentary behavior in the treatment of depression: Broadening the scientific perspectives and clinical opportunities. *Frontiers in Psychiatry, 7*, 1–5. doi:10.3389/fpsyt.2016.00036.

Hamer, M., & Chida, Y. (2009). Physical activity and risk of neurodegenerative disease: A systematic review of prospective evidence. *Psychological Medicine, 39*(1), 3–11. doi:10.1017/S0033291708003681

Hamilton, M. (1960). A rating scale for depression. *Journal of Neurology, Neurosurgery, and Psychiatry, 23*, 56–62.

Haroon, E., Raison, C. L., & Miller, A. H. (2012). Psychoneuroimmunology meets neuropsychopharmacology: Translational implications of the impact of inflammation on behavior. *Neuropsychopharmacology, 37*(1), 137–162. doi:10.1038/npp.2011.205

Hartley, L., Flowers, N., Lee, M. S., Ernst, E., & Rees, K. (2014). Tai chi for primary prevention of cardiovascular disease. *Cochrane Database of Systematic Reviews, 4*, CD010366. doi:10.1002/14651858.CD010366.pub2

Heijnen, S., Hommel, B., Kibele, A., & Colzato, L. S. (2016). Neuromodulation of aerobic exercise: A review. *Frontiers in Psychology, 6*, 1–6. doi:10.3389/fpsyg.2015.01890

Herman, J. P., & Cullinan, W. E. (1997). Neurocircuitry of stress: Central control of the hypothalamo-pituitary-adrenocortical axis. *Trends in Neuroscience, 20*(2), 78–84.

Herring, M. P., Jacob, M. L., Suveg, C., Dishman, R. K., & O'Connor, P. J. (2012). Feasibility of exercise training for the short-term treatment of generalized anxiety disorder: a randomized controlled trial. *Psychotherapy and Psychosomatics, 81*(1), 21–28. doi:10.1159/000327898

Heyman, E., Gamelin, F. X., Goekint, M., Piscitelli, F., Roelands, B., Leclair, E., et al. (2012). Intense exercise increases circulating endocannabinoid and BDNF levels in humans: Possible implications for reward and depression. *Psychoneuroendocrinology, 37*(6), 844–851. doi:10.1016/j.psyneuen.2011.09.017

Heyn, P., Abreu, B. C., & Ottenbacher, K. J. (2004). The effects of exercise training on elderly persons with cognitive impairment and dementia: A meta-analysis.

Archives of Physical Medicine and Rehabilitation, 85(10), 1694–1704. doi:10.1016/j.apmr.2004.03.019

Hines, L. A., Sundin, J., Rona, R. J., Wessely, S., & Fear, N. T. (2014). Posttraumatic stress disorder post Iraq and Afghanistan: Prevalence among military subgroups. *Canadian Journal of Psychiatry, 59*(9), 468–479.

Ho, R. T. H., Au Yeung, F. S. W., Lo, P. H. Y., Law, K. Y., Wong, K. O. K., Cheung, I. K. M., & Nget, S. M. (2012). Tai-chi for residential patients with schizophrenia on movement coordination, negative symptoms, and functioning: A pilot randomized controlled trial. *Evidence-Based Complementary and Alternative Medicine, 2012*(2), 1–10. doi:10.1155/2012/923925

Hofmann, S. G., & Smits, J. (2008).Cognitive-behavioral therapy for adult anxiety disorders: A meta-analysis of randomized placebo-controlled trials. *Journal of Clinical Psychiatry, 69*(4), 621–632.

Hogan, C. L., Mata, J., & Carstensen, L. L. (2013). Exercise holds immediate benefits for affect and cognition in younger and older adults. *Psychology and Aging, 28*(2), 587–594. doi:10.1037/a0032634.Exercise

Horsburgh, S., Robson-Ansley, P., Adams, R., & Smith, C. (2015). Exercise and inflammation-related epigenetic modifications: Focus on DNA methylation. *Exercise Immunology Review, 21*(C), 26–41.

Hou, R., & Baldwin, D. S. (2012). A neuroimmunological perspective on anxiety disorders. *Human Psychopharmacology, 27*(1), 6–14. doi:10.1002/hup.1259

Hovland, A., Nordhus, I. H., Sjøbø, T., Gjestad, B. A., Birknes, B., Martinsen, E. W., et al. (2013). Comparing physical exercise in groups to group cognitive behaviour therapy for the treatment of panic disorder in a randomized controlled trial. *Behavioural and Cognitive Psychotherapy, 41*, 408–432. doi:10.1017/S1352465812000446

Howie, E. K., & Pate, R. R. (2012). Physical activity and academic achievement in children: A historical perspective. *Journal of Sport and Health Science, 1*(3), 160–169. doi:10.1016/j.jshs.2012.09.003

Huang, T., Larsen, K. T., Ried-Larsen, M., Møller, N. C., Andersen, L. B., & Huang, T. (2014). The effects of physical activity and exercise on brain-derived neurotrophic factor in healthy humans: A review. *Scandinavian Journal of Medicine & Science in Sports, 24*(1), 1–10. doi:10.1111/sms.12069

Hunink, M. G. M., Yeh, G. Y., Goldie, S. J., Gotink, R. A., & Chu, P. (2016). The effectiveness of yoga in modifying risk factors for cardiovascular disease and metabolic syndrome: A systematic review and meta-analysis of randomized controlled trials. *European Journal of Preventive Cardiology, 23*(3), 291–307. doi:10.1177/2047487314562741

Jarrard, L. E. (1993). On the role of the hippocampus in learning and memory in the rat. *Behavioral and Neural Biology, 60*(1), 9–26.

Jensen, P. S., & Kenny, D. T. (2004). The effects of yoga on the attention and behavior of boys with attention-deficit/hyperactivity disorder (ADHD). *Journal of Attention Disorders, 7*(4), 205–216. doi:10.1177/108705470400700403

Judd, L. L., Akiskal, H. S., Schettler, P. J., Endicott, J., Maser, J., Solomon, D. A., et al. (2002). The long-term natural history of the weekly symptomatic status of bipolar I disorder. *Archives of General Psychiatry, 59*(6), 530–537. doi:10.1001/archpsyc.59.6.530

Kabat-Zinn, J. (2013). *Full catastrophe living—Using the wisdom of your body and mind to face stress, pain, and illness.* New York: Bantam Books.

Kabat-Zinn, J. (2003). Mindfulness-based interventions in context: Past, present, and future. *Clinical Psychology: Science and Practice, 10*(2), 144–156. doi:10.1093/clipsy/bpg016

Kandola, A., Hendrikse, J., Lucassen, P. J., & Yücel, M. (2016). Aerobic exercise as a tool to improve hippocampal plasticity and function in humans: Practical implications for mental health treatment. *Frontiers in Human Neuroscience, 10*, 373. doi:10.3389/fnhum.2016.00373

Kang, R., Wu, Y., Li, Z., Jiang, J., Gao, Q., Yu, Y., et al. (2016). Effect of community-based social skills training and tai-chi exercise on outcomes in patients with chronic schizophrenia: A randomized, one-year study. *Psychopathology, 49*(5), 345–355. doi:10.1159/000448195

Katzman, M. A., Vermani, M., Gerbarg, P. L., Tsirgielis, D., Iorio, C., Gerbarg, P. L., et al. (2012). A multicomponent yoga-based, breath intervention program as an adjunctive treatment in patients suffering from generalized anxiety disorder with or without comorbidities. *International Journal of Yoga, 5*(1), 57–65. doi:10.4103/0973-6131.91716

Kay, S. R., Fiszbein, A., & Opfer, L. A. (1987). The Positive and Negative Syndrome Scale (PANSS) for schizophrenia. *Schizophrenia Bulletin, 13*(2), 261–276. doi:10.1093/schbul/13.2.261

Kays, J. L., Hurley, R. A., & Taber, K. H. (2012). The dynamic brain: Neuroplasticity and mental health. *Journal of Neuropsychiatry and Clinical Neurosciences, 24*(2), 118–124.

Khalsa, M. K., Greiner-Ferris, J. M., Hofmann, S. G., & Khalsa, S. B. S. (2015). Yoga-enhanced cognitive behavioural therapy (Y-CBT) for anxiety management: A pilot study. *Clinical Psychology & Psychotherapy, 22*(4), 364–371. doi:10.1002/cpp.1902

Khalsa, S. B. S., Cohen, L., McCall, T., & Telles, S. (Eds.). (2016). *The principles and practice of yoga in health care.* Edinburgh, UK: Handspring.

Khalsa, S., Telles, S., & Cohen, L. (2016). Introduction to yoga in health care. In S. B. S. Khalsa, L. Cohen, T. McCall, & S. Telles (Eds.), *The principles and practice of yoga in health care* (pp. 5–14). Edinburgh, UK: Handspring.

Kim, P. Y., Thomas, J. L., Wilk, J. E., Castro, C., & Hoge, C. W. (2010). Stigma, barriers to care, and use of mental health services among active duty and National Guard soldiers after combat. *Psychiatric Services, 61*(6), 582–588. doi:10.1176/appi.ps.61.6.582

Kjaer, T. W., Bertelsen, C., Piccini, P., Brooks, D., Alving, J., & Lou, H. C. (2002). Increased dopamine tone during meditation-induced change of consciousness. *Cognitive Brain Research, 13*(2), 255–259. doi:10.1016/S0926-6410(01)00106-9

Klein, S., & Thorne, M. (2006). *Biological psychology* (1st ed.). New York: Worth.

Klil-Drori, S., & Hechtman, L. (2009). Potential social and neurocognitive benefits of aerobic exercise as adjunct treatment for patients with ADHD. *Journal of Attention Disorders,* 1–15.

Kodama, S., Saito, K., Tanaka, S., Maki, M., Yachi, Y., Asumi, M., et al. (2009). Clinician's corner: Cardiorespiratory fitness as a quantitative predictor of all-cause mortality and cardiovascular events. *Journal of the American Medical Association, 301*(19), 2024–2035.

Krogh, J., Saltin B., Gluud, C., & Nordentoft, M. (2009). The DEMO trial: A randomized, parallel-group, observer-blinded clinical trial of strength versus aerobic versus relaxation training for patients with mild to moderate depression. *Journal of Clinial Psychiatry, 70*(6), 790–800.

Krogh, J., Videbech, P., Thomsen, C., Gluud, C., Nordentoft, M., & DEMO-II Trial. (2012). Aerobic exercise versus stretching exercise in patients with major depression—a randomised clinical trial. *PLoS One, 7*(10). doi:10.1371/journal.pone.0048316

Krystal, J. H., Tolin, D. F., Sanacora, G., Castner, S. A., Williams, G. V., Aikins, D. E., et al. (2009). Neuroplasticity as a target for the pharmacotherapy of anxiety disorders, mood disorders, and schizophrenia. *Drug Discovery Today, 14*(13–14), 690–697. doi:10.1016/j.drudis.2009.05.002

Kuipers. S. D., & Bramham, C. R. (2006). Brain-derived neurotrophic factor mechanisms and function in adult synaptic plasticity: New insights and implications for therapy. *Current Opinion in Drug Discovery & Development, 9*(5), 580–586.

Kurian, M. A., Gissen, P., Smith, M., Heales, S. J. R., & Clayton, P. T. (2011). The monoamine neurotransmitter disorders: An expanding range of neurological syndromes. *Lancet Neurolology, 10*(8), 721–733. doi:10.1016/S1474-4422(11)70141-7

Kvam, S., Kleppe, C. L., Nordhus, I. H., & Hovland, A. (2016). Exercise as a treatment for depression: A meta-analysis. *Journal of Affective Disorders, 202*, 67–86. doi:10.1016/j.jad.2016.03.063

Lan, C., Chen, S.-Y., Wong, M.-K., & Lai, J. S. (2013). Tai chi chuan exercise for patients with cardiovascular disease. *Evidence-Based Complementary and Alternative Medicine, 2013*, 983208. doi:10.1155/2013/983208

Leckie, R. L., Oberlin, L. E., Voss, M. W., Prakash, R. S., Szabo-Reed, A., Chaddock-Heyman, L.et al. (2014). BDNF mediates improvements in executive function following a 1-year exercise intervention. *Frontiers in Human Neuroscience, 8*, 985. doi:10.3389/fnhum.2014.00985

Ledoux, J. E., & Gorman, J. M. (2001). A call to action: Overcoming anxiety through active coping. *American Journal of Psychiatry, 158*(12), 1953–1955. doi:10.1176/appi.ajp.158.12.1953

Lee, M. C., Inoue, K., Okamoto, M., Liu, Y. F., Matsui, T., Yook, J. S., & Soya, H. (2013). Voluntary resistance running induces increased hippocampal neurogenesis in rats comparable to load-free running. *Neuroscience Letters, 537*, 6–10. doi:10.1016/j.neulet.2013.01.005

Legrand, F. D., & Neff, E. M. (2016). Efficacy of exercise as an adjunct treatment for clinically depressed inpatients during the initial stages of antidepressant pharmacotherapy: An open randomized controlled trial. *Journal of Affective Disorders, 191*, 139–144. doi:10.1016/j.jad.2015.11.047

Leuner, B., & Gould, E. (2008). Structural plasticity and hippocampal function. *Annual Review of Pscyhology, 61,* 111–140. doi:10.1146/annurev.psych.093008.100359. Structural

Li. A. W., & Goldsmith, C. A. (2012). The effects of yoga on anxiety and stress. *Alternative Medicine Review, 17*(1), 21–35. Retrieved from http://www.ncbi.nlm.nih.gov/pubmed/22502620.

Lin, T.-W., & Kuo, Y.-M. (2013). Exercise benefits brain function: The monoamine connection. *Brain Science, 3*(1), 39–53. doi:10.3390/brainsci3010039

Lorens-Martín, M., Torres-Alemán, I., & Trejo, J. L. (2010). Exercise modulates insulin-like growth factor 1-dependent and -independent effects on adult hippocampal neurogenesis and behaviour. *Molecular and Cellular Neurosciences, 44*(2), 109–117. doi:10.1016/j.mcn.2010.02.006

Loucks, E. B., Britton, W. B., Howe, C. J., & Eaton, C. B. (2015). Cardiovascular health: The New England Family Study. *International Journal of Behavioral Medicine, 22*(4), 540–550. doi:10.1007/s12529-014-9448-9.Positive

Marco, E. M., Garcia-Gutierrez, M. S., Bermudez-Silva, F. J., Silva, B., Javier, F., Moreira, F. A., et al. (2011). Endocannabinoid system and psychiatry: In search of a neurobiological basis for detrimental and potential therapeutic effects. *Frontiers in Behavioral Neuroscience, 5,* 63. doi:10.3389/fnbeh.2011.00063

Martinowich, K., & Lu, B. (2008). Interaction between BDNF and serotonin: Role in mood disorders. *Neuropsychopharmacology, 33*(1), 73–83. doi:10.1038/sj.npp.1301571

Matthews. M. M., & Williams, H. G. (2008). Can Tai chi enhance cognitive vitality? A preliminary study of cognitive executive control in older adults after a tai chi intervention. *Journal of the South Carolina Medical Association, 104*(8), 255–257.

McEwen, B. S. (2007). Physiology and neurobiology of stress and adaptation: Central role of the brain. *Physiology Review, 87*(3), 873–904. doi:10.1152/physrev.00041.2006

Mechawar, N., & Savitz, J. (2016). Neuropathology of mood disorders: Do we see the stigmata of inflammation? *Translational Psychiatry, 6*(11), e946. doi:10.1038/tp.2016.212

Meeusen, R., Duclos, M., Foster, C., Fry, A., Nieman, D., Raglin, J., et al. (2013). Prevention, diagnosis, and treatment of the overtraining syndrome: Joint consensus statement of the European College of Sport Science and the American College of Sports Medicine. *Medicine and Science in Sports and Exercise, 45*(1), 186–205. doi:10.1249/MSS.0b013e318279a10a

Melo, M. C. A., Daher, E. D. F., Albuquerque, S. G. C., & De Bruin, V. M. S. (2016). Exercise in bipolar patients: A systematic review. *Journal of Affective Disorders, 198,* 32–38. doi:10.1016/j.jad.2016.03.004

Middleton, L. E., Mitnitski, A., Fallah, N., Kirkland, S. A., & Rockwood, K. (2008). Changes in cognition and mortality in relation to exercise in late life: A population based study. *PLoS One, 3*(9), 1–7. doi:10.1371/journal.pone.0003124

Mothes, H., Klaperski, S., Seelig, H., Schmidt, S., & Fuchs, R. (2014). Regular aerobic exercise increases dispositional mindfulness in men: A randomized controlled trial. *Mental Health and Physical Activity, 7*(2), 111–119. doi:http://dx.doi.org/10.1016/j.mhpa.2014.02.003

Motivala, S. J., Sollers, J., Thayer, J., & Irwin, M. R. (2006). Tai chi chih acutely decreases sympathetic nervous system activity in older adults. *Journals of Gerontology. Series A, Biological Sciences and Medical Sciences*, 61(11), 1177–1180.

Murakami, S., Imbe, H., Morikawa, Y., Kubo, C., & Senba, E. (2005). Chronic stress, as well as acute stress, reduces BDNF mRNA expression in the rat hippocampus but less robustly. *Neuroscience Research*, 53(2), 129–139. doi:http://dx.doi.org/10.1016/j.neures.2005.06.008

Müssigbrodt, A., Weber, A., Mandrola, J., van Belle, Y.; Richter, S., Döring, M., et al. (2017). Excess of exercise increases the risk of atrial fibrillation. *Scandinavian Journal of Medicine & Science in Sports*, 27(9), 910–917. doi:10.1111/sms.12830

Naveen, G. H., Varambally, S., Thirthalli, J., Rao, M., Christopher, R., & Gangadhar, B. N. (2016). Serum cortisol and BDNF in patients with major depression—effect of yoga. *International Review of Psychiatry*, 261, 1–6. doi:10.1080/09540261.2016.1175419

Niles, B. L., Mori, D. L., Polizzi, C. P., Pless Kaiser, A., Ledoux, A. M., & Wang. C. (2016). Feasibility, qualitative findings and satisfaction of a brief tai chi mind–body programme for veterans with post-traumatic stress symptoms. *BMJ Open*, 6(11). Retrieved from http://bmjopen.bmj.com/content/6/11/e012464.abstract

Nyström, M. B. T., Neely, G., Hassmén, P., & Carlbring, P. (2015). Treating major depression with physical activity: A systematic overview with recommendations. *Cognitive Behaviour Therapy*, 44(4), 341–352.

Ochoa, S., Usall, J., Cobo, J., Labad, X., & Kulkarni, J. (2012). Gender differences in schizophrenia and first-episode psychosis: A comprehensive literature review. *Schizophrrenia Research and Treatment*, 2012, 1–9. doi:10.1155/2012/916198

Office of Disease Prevention and Health Promotion. (2017). Appendix 1. Physical activity guidelines for Americans. Retrieved from https://health.gov/dietaryguidelines/2015/guidelines/appendix-1/

Olex, S., Newberg, A., & Figueredo, V. M. (2013). Meditation: Should a cardiologist care? *International Journal of Cardiology*, 168(3), 1805–1810.

Ouimette, P., Vogt, D., Wade, M., Tirone, V., Greenbaum, M. A., Kimerling, R., et al. (2011). Perceived barriers to care among veterans health administration patients with posttraumatic stress disorder. *Psychological Services*, 8(3), 212–223. doi:10.1037/a0024360

Ozkaya, G. Y., Aydin, H., Toraman, F. N., Kizilay, F., Ozdemir, O., & Cetinkaya, V. (2005). Effect of strength and endurance training on cognition in older people. *Journal of Sports Science & Medicine*, 4(3), 300–313. Retrieved from http://www.pubmedcentral.nih.gov/articlerender.fcgi?artid=3887334&tool=pmcentrez&rendertype=abstract

Pang, P. T., & Lu, B. (2004). Regulation of late-phase LTP and long-term memory in normal and aging hippocampus: Role of secreted proteins tPA and BDNF. *Ageing Research Review*, 3(4), 407–430. doi:http://dx.doi.org/10.1016/j.arr.2004.07.002

Park, G., & Thayer, J. F. (2014). From the heart to the mind: Cardiac vagal tone modulates top-down and bottom-up visual perception and attention to emotional stimuli. *Frontiers in Psychology*, 5, 1–8. doi:10.3389/fpsyg.2014.00278

Patrick, R. P., & Ames, B. N. (2015). Vitamin D and the omega-3 fatty acids control serotonin synthesis and action, part 2: Relevance for ADHD, bipolar disorder, schizophrenia, and impulsive behavior. *FASEB Journal, 29*(6), 2207–2222. doi:10.1096/fj.14-268342

Pearlin. L. I., & Schooler, C. (1978). The structure of coping. *Journal of Health and Social Behavior, 19*(1), 2–21.

Petersen, M. W., & Pedersen, B. K. (2005). The anti-inflammatory effect of exercise. *Journal of Applied Physiology, 98,* 1154–1162. doi:10.1152/japplphysiol.00164.2004

Phillips, M. L., Drevets, W. C., Rauch, S. L., & Lane, R. (2003). Neurobiology of emotion perception I: The neural basis of normal emotion perception. *Biological Psychiatry, 54*(5), 504–514. doi:10.1016/S0006-3223(03)00168-9

Physical Activity Guidelines Advisory Committee. (2008). Physical Activity Guidelines Advisory Committee report. *Nutrition Review, 67*(2), 114–120. doi:10.1111/j.1753-4887.2008.00136.x

Pichot, V., Roche, F., Denis, C., Garet, M., Duverney, D., Costes, F., & Barthélémy, J.-C. (2005). Interval training in elderly men increases both heart rate variability and baroreflex activity. *Clinical Autonomic Research, 15*(2), 107–115. doi:10.1007/s10286-005-0251-1

Pilkington, K., Gerbarg, P. L., & Brown, R. (2016). Yoga therapy for anxiety. In S. B. S. Khalsa, L. Cohen, T. McCall, & S. Telles (Eds.), *The principles and practice of yoga in health care* (pp. 95–113). Edinburgh, UK: Handspring.

Pilu, A., Sorba, M., Hardoy, M. C., Floris, A. L., Mannu, F., Seruis, M. L., et al. (2007). Efficacy of physical activity in the adjunctive treatment of major depressive disorders: Preliminary results. *Clinical Practice and Epidemiology in Mental Health, 3,* 8. doi:10.1186/1745-0179-3-8

Polusny, M. A., Ries, B. J., Schultz, J. R., Calhoun, P., Clemensen, L., & Johnsen, I. R. (2008). PTSD symptom clusters associated with physical health and health care utilization in rural primary care patients exposed to natural disaster. *Journal of Traumatic Stress, 21*(1), 75–82. doi:10.1002/jts

Pongratz, G., & Straub, R. H. (2014). The sympathetic nervous response in inflammation. *Arthritis Research & Therapy, 16,* 504–516. doi:10.1186/s13075-014-0504-2

Powers, M. B., Medina, J. L., Burns, S., Kauffman, B. Y., Monfils, M., Asmundson, G.J. G., et al. (2015). Exercise augmentation of exposure therapy for PTSD: Rationale and pilot efficacy data. *Cognitive Behaviour Therapy, 44*(4), 314–327. doi:10.1080/16506073.2015.1012740

Pratt, S. I., Jerome, G. J., Schneider, K. L., Craft, L. L., Buman, M. P., Stoutenberg, M., et al. (2016). Increasing US health plan coverage for exercise programming in community mental health settings for people with serious mental illness: A position statement from the Society of Behavior Medicine and the American College of Sports Medicine. *Translational Behavioral Medicine, 6*(3), 478–481. doi:10.1007/s13142-016-0407-7

Raadsheer, F. C., Hoogendijk, W. J., Stam, F. C., Tilders, F. J., & Swaab, D. F. (1994). Increased numbers of corticotropin-releasing hormone expressing neurons in the hypothalamic paraventricular nucleus of depressed patients. *Neuroendocrinology, 60*(4), 436–444.

Raichlen, D. A., & Polk, J. D. (2013). Linking brains and brawn: Exercise and the evolution of human neurobiology. *Proceedings of the Royal Society of London B, 280*(1750), 2250. Retrieved from http://rspb.royalsocietypublishing.org/content/280/1750/20122250.full.html#ref-list-1

Ratey, J. (2008). *Spark the revolutionary new science of exercise and the brain.* New York: Litte, Brown.

Ravari, A., Mirzaei, T., Kennedy, D., & Arababadi, M. K. (2017). Chronoinflammaging in Alzheimer: A systematic review on the roles of toll like receptor 2. *Life Sciences, 171*, 16–20. doi:10.1016/j.lfs.2017.01.003

Rector, N. A., Richter, M. A., Lerman, B., & Regev, R. (2015). A pilot test of the additive benefits of physical exercise to CBT for OCD. *Cognitive Behavioral Therapy, 44*(4), 328–340.

Rhodes, A., Spinazzola, J., & Van Der Kolk, B. (2016). Yoga for adult women with chronic PTSD: A long-term follow-up study. *Journal of Alternative and Complementary Medicine, 22*(3), 189–196. doi:10.1089/acm.2014.0407

Rimmele, U., Zellweger, B. C., Marti, B., Seiler, R., Mohiyeddini, C., Ehlert, U., & Heinrich, M. (2007). Trained men show lower cortisol, heart rate and psychological responses to psychosocial stress compared with untrained men. *Psychoneuroendocrinology, 32*(6), 627–635. doi:10.1016/j.psyneuen.2007.04.005

Rocha, K. K. F., Ribeiro, A. M., Rocha, K. C. F., Sousa, M. B. C., Albuquerque, F. S., Ribeiro, S., & Silva, R. H. (2012). Improvement in physiological and psychological parameters after 6months of yoga practice. *Conscious Cognition, 21*(2), 843–850. doi:10.1016/j.concog.2012.01.014

Roig, M., Nordbrandt, S., Geertsen, S. S., & Nielsen, J. B. (2013). The effects of cardiovascular exercise on human memory: A review with meta-analysis. *Neuroscience and Biobehavorial Reviews, 37*(8), 1645–1666. doi:http://dx.doi.org/10.1016/j.neubiorev.2013.06.012

Rosenbaum, S., & Sherrington, C. T. A. (2015). Exercise augmentation compared with usual care for post-traumatic stress disorder: A randomized controlled trial. *Acta Psychiatrica Scandinavica, 131*(5), 350–359.

Rubin, R. T., Poland, R. E., Lesser, I. M., Winston, R. A., & Blodgett, A. L.N. (1987). Neuroendocrine aspects of primary endogenous depression. *Archives of General Psychiatry, 44*, 328–336. doi:10.1001/archpsyc.1992.01820070052008

Schmaal, L., Veltman, D., Van Erp, T., Saemann, P. G., Frodl, T., Jahanshad, N., et al. (2016). Subcortical brain alterations in major depressive disorder: Findings from the ENIGMA Major Depressive Disorder Working Group. *Molecular Psychiatry, 21*(6), 806–812. doi:10.1038/mp.2015.69

Schobersberger, W., Hobisch-Hagen, P., Fries, D., Wiedermann, F., Rieder-Scharinger, J., Villiger, B., et al. (2000). Increase in immune activation, vascular endothelial growth factor and erythropoietin after an ultramarathon run at moderate altitude. *Immunobiology, 201*(5), 611–620. doi:10.1016/S0171-2985(00)80078-9

Schuch, F. B., Vancampfort, D., Richards, J., Rosenbaum, S., Ward, P. B., & Stubbs, B. (2016). Exercise as a treatment for depression: A meta-analysis adjusting for publication bias. *Journal of Psychiatric Research, 77,* 42–51. doi:10.1016/j.jpsychires.2016.02.023

Shannahoff-Khalsa, D. S., & Beckett, L. (1996). Clinical case report: Efficacy of yogic techniques in the treatment of obsessive compulsive disorders. *International Journal of Neuroscience, 85*(1–2), 1–17.

Shannahoff-Khalsa, D. S., Ray, L. E., Levine, S., Gallen, C. C., & Schwartz, B. J., & Sidorowich, J. J. (1999). Randomized controlled trial of yogic meditation techniques for patients with obsessive-compulsive disorder. *CNS Spectrums, 4*(12), 34–47. doi:10.1017/S1092852900006805

Sharma, M., & Haider, T. (2015). Tai chi as an alternative and complimentary therapy for anxiety: A systematic review. *Journal of Evidence-Based Complementary & Alternative Medicine, 20*(2), 143–153. doi:10.1177/2156587214561327

Sibley, B. A., & Etnier, J. L. (2003). The relationship between physical activity and cognition in children: A meta-analysis. *Pediatric Exercise Science, 15*(3), 243–256. doi:10.1123/pes.15.3.243

Silva, B. A., Cassilhas, R. C., Attux, C., Gadelha, A. L., Telles, B. A., Bressan, R. A., et al. (2015). A 20-week program of resistance or concurrent exercise improves symptoms of schizophrenia: Results of a blind, randomized controlled trial. *Revista Brasileira de Psiquiatria, 37*(4), 271–279. doi:10.1590/1516-4446-2014-1595

Silverman, M. N., & Deuster, P. A. (2014). Biological mechanisms underlying the role of physical fitness in health and resilience. *Interface Focus, 4*(5), 20140040. doi:10.1098/rsfs.2014.0040

Singh, N. A., Clements, K. M., & Fiatarone, M. A. (1997). A randomized controlled trial of progressive resistance training in depressed elders. *Journals of Gerontology. Series A, Biological Sciences and Medical Sciences, 52*(1), M27–M35. Retrieved from http://ovidsp.ovid.com/ovidweb.cgi?T=JS&CSC=Y&NEWS=N&PAGE=fulltext&D=med4&AN=9008666%5Cnhttp://openurl.man.ac.uk/sfxlcl3?sid=OVID:medline&id=pmid:9008666&id=doi:&issn=1079-5006&isbn=&volume=52&issue=1&spage=M27&pages=M27-35&date=1997&title=Journals+of+Ger

Singh, N. A., Stavrinos, T. A., Scarbek, Y., Galambos, G., Liber, C., & Singh, M. A. F. (2005). A randomized controlled trial of high versus low intensity weight training versus general practitioner care for clinical depression in older adults. *Journals of Gerontology. Series A, Biological Sciences and Medical Sciences, 60*(6), 768–776. doi:10.1093/gerona/60.6.768

Smith, P. J., Blumenthal, J. A., Hoffman, B. M., Cooper, H., Strauman, T. A., Welsh-Bohmer, K., et al. (2011). Aerobic exercise and neurocognitive performance: A meta-analytic review of randomized controlled trials. *Psychosomatic Medicine, 72*(3), 239–252. doi:10.1097/PSY.0b013e3181d14633.Aerobic

Smits, J. A. J., Berry, A. C., Rosenfield, D., Powers, M. B., Behar, E., & Otto, M. W. (2008). Reducing anxiety sensitivity with exercise. *Depression and Anxiety, 25*(8), 689–699. doi:10.1002/da.20411

Snowden, M., Steinman, L., Mochan, K., Grodstein, F., Prohaska, T. R., Thurman, D. J., et al. (2011). Effect of exercise on cognitive performance in community-dwelling older adults: Review of intervention trials and recommendations for public health practice and research. *Journal of the American Geriatrics Society, 59*(4), 704–716. doi:10.1111/j.1532-5415.2011.03323.x

Sølvsten, C. A. E., de Paoli, F., Christensen, J. H., & Nielsen, A. L. (2016). Voluntary physical exercise induces expression and epigenetic remodeling of VegfA in the rat hippocampus. *Molecular Neurobiology.* doi:10.1007/s12035-016-0344-y

Sparling, P. B., Howard, B. J., Dunstan, D. W., & Owen, N. (2015). Recommendations for physical activity in older adults. *British Medical Journal, 350,* h100. doi:10.1136/bmj.h100

Stillman, C. M., Cohen. J., Lehman, M. E., & Erickson, K. I. (2016). Mediators of physical activity on neurocognitive function: A review at multiple levels of analysis. *Frontiers in Human Neuroscience, 10,* 1–17. doi:10.3389/fnhum.2016.00626

Stonerock, G. L., Hoffman, B. M., Smith, P. J., & Blumenthal, J. A. (2015). Exercise as treatment for anxiety: Systematic review and analysis. *Annals of Behavioral Medicine.* doi:10.1007/s12160-014-9685-9

Streeter, C. C., Gerbarg, P. L., Saper, R. B., Ciraulo, D. A., & Brown, R. P. (2012). Effects of yoga on the autonomic nervous system, gamma-aminobutyric-acid, and allostasis in epilepsy, depression, and post-traumatic stress disorder. *Medical Hypotheses, 78*(5), 571–579. doi:10.1016/j.mehy.2012.01.021

Streeter, C. C., Whitfield, T. H., Owen, L., Whitfield, T. H., Owen, L., Karri, S. K., et al. (2010). Effects of yoga versus walking on mood, anxiety, and brain GABA levels: A randomized controlled MRS study. *Journal of Alterative and Complementary Medicine, 16*(11), 1145–1152. doi:10.1089/acm.2010.0007

Strickland, J. C., & Smith, M. A. (2014). The anxiolytic effects of resistance exercise. *Frontiers in Psychology, 5,* 753. doi:10.3389/fpsyg.2014.00753

Strickland, J. C., & Smith, M. A. (2016). Animal models of resistance exercise and their application to neuroscience research. *Journal of Neuroscience Methods, 273,* 191–200. doi:10.1016/j.jneumeth.2016.08.003

Ströhle, A., Jahn, H., Montkowski, A., Liebsch, G., Boll, E., Landgraf, R., et al. (1997). Central and peripheral administration of atriopeptin is anxiolytic in rats. *Neuroendocrinology, 65*(3), 210–215. Retrieved from http://www.karger.com/DOI/10.1159/000127274

Ströhle, A., Kellner, M., Holsboer, F., & Wiedemann, K. (2001). Anxiolytic activity of atrial natriuretic peptide in patients with panic disorder. *American Journal of Psychiatry, 158*(9), 1514–1516. Retrieved from http://www.ncbi.nlm.nih.gov/pubmed/11532742

Thayer, J. F., & Sternberg, E. (2006). Beyond heart rate variability: Vagal regulation of allostatic systems. *Annals of the New York Academy of Sciences, 1088,* 361–372. doi:10.1196/annals.1366.014

Tomporowski, P. D., Davis, C. L., Miller, P. H., Naglieri, J. A., Miller, P. D. T. P. H., & Road, R. (2009). Exercise and children's intelligence, cognition, and academic achievement. *Educational Psychology Review, 20*(2), 111–131. doi:10.1007/s10648-007-9057-0.Exercise

Tomporowski, P. D., McCullick, B., Pendleton, D. M., & Pesce, C. (2014). Exercise and children's cognition: The role of exercise characteristics and a place for metacognition. *Journal of Sport and Health Science, 4*(1), 47–55. doi:10.1016/j.jshs.2014.09.003

Traustadóttir, T., Bosch, P. R., & Matt, K. S. (2004). The HPA axis response to stress in women: Effects of aging and fitness. *Psychoneuroendocrinology, 30*(4), 392–402. doi:10.1016/j.psyneuen.2004.11.002

Tyagi, A., & Cohen, M. (2016). Yoga and heart rate variability: A comprehensive review of the literature. *International Journal of Yoga, 9*(2), 97–113. doi:10.4103/0973-6131.183712

Uebelacker, L. A., & Broughton, M. K. (2016). Yoga for depression and anxiety: A review of published research and implications for healthcare providers. *Rhode Island Medical Journal, 99*(3), 20. Retrieved from https://www.rimed.org/rimedicaljournal/2016/03/2016-03-20-intmed-uebelacker.pdf%5Cnhttp://www.ncbi.nlm.nih.gov/pubmed/26929966

Uebelacker, L. A., Weinstock, L. M., & Kraines, M. A. (2014). Self-reported benefits and risks of yoga in individuals with bipolar disorder. *Journal of Psychiatric Practice, 20*(5), 345–352. doi:10.1097/01.pra.0000454779.59859.f8

Uebelacker, L., Lavretsky, H., & Tremont, G. (2016). Yoga therapy for depression. In S. B. S. Khalsa, L. Cohen, T. McCall. & S. Telles (Eds.), *The principles and practice of yoga in health care* (pp. 73–93). Edinburgh, UK: Handspring.

Van Der Kolk, B. A., Stone, L., West, J., Rhodes, A., Emerson, D., Spinazzola, J., et al. (2014). Yoga as an adjunctive treatment for posttraumatic stress disorder: A randomized controlled trial. *Journal of Clinical Psychiatry, 75*(6), e559–e565. doi:10.4088/JCP.13m08561

van Praag, H. (2005). Exercise enhances learning and hippocampal neurogenesis in aged mice. *Journal of Neuroscience, 25*(38), 8680–8685. doi:10.1523/JNEUROSCI.1731-05.2005

van Uffelen, J., Chin, A., Paw, M., Hopman-Rock, M., & van Mechelen, W. (2008). The effects of exercise on cognition in older adults with and without cognitive decline: A systematic review. *Clinical Journal of Sport Medicine, 18*(6), 486–500.

Verburgh, L., Konigs, M., Scherder, E. J. A., & Oosterlaan, J. (2012). Physical exercise and executive functions in preadolescent children, adolescents and young adults: A meta-analysis. *Britich Journal of Sports Medicine, 48*(12), 973–979. doi:10.1136/bjsports-2012-091441

Vorkapic, C. F., & Range, B. (2014). Reducing the symptomatology of panic disorder: The effects of a yoga program alone and in combination with cognitive-behavioral therapy. *Frontiers in Psychiatry, 5*. doi:10.3389/fpsyt.2014.00177

Voss, M. W., Erickson, K. I., Prakash, R. S., Chaddock, L., Kim, J. S., Alves, H., et al. (2013). Neurobiological markers of exercise-related brain plasticity in older adults. *Brain, Behavior and Immunity, 28*, 90–99. doi:10.1016/j.bbi.2012.10.021

Voss, M. W., Heo, S., Prakash, R. S., Erickson, K. I., Alves, H., Chaddock, L., et al. (2013). The influence of aerobic fitness on cerebral white matter integrity and cognitive function in older adults: Results of a one-year exercise intervention. *Human Brain Mapping*, *34*(11), 2972–2985. doi:10.1002/hbm.22119

Wang, F., Othelia Lee, E.-K., Wu, T., Benson, H., Fricchione, G., Wang, W., & Yeung, A. S. (2014). The effects of tai chi on depression, anxiety, and psychological well-being: A systematic review and meta-analysis. *International Journal of Behavioral Medicine*, *21*(4), 605–617. doi:10.1007/s12529-013-9351-9

Wasfy. M. M., & Baggish, A. L. (2016). Exercise dose in clinical practice. *Circulation*, *133*(23), 2297–2313. doi:10.1161/CIRCULATIONAHA.116.018093

Wedekind, D., Broocks, A., Weiss, N., Engel, K., Neubert, K., & Bandelow, B. (2010). A randomized, controlled trial of aerobic exercise in combination with paroxetine in the treatment of panic disorder. *The World Journal of Biological Psychiatry*, *11*(7). doi:10.3109/15622975.2010.489620

Wegner, M., Helmich, I., Machado, S., Nardi, A. E., Arias-Carrión, O., & Budde, H. (2014). Effects of exercise on anxiety and depression disorders: Review of meta-analyses and neurobiological mechanisms. *CNS and Neurological Disorders—Drug Targets*, *13*(6), 1002–1014.

Wendell, C. R., Gunstad, J., Waldstein, S. R., Wright, J. G., Ferrucci, L., & Zonderman, A. B. (2014). Cardiorespiratory fitness and accelerated cognitive decline with aging. *Journals of Gerontology. Series A, Biological Sciences and Medical Sciences*, *69*(4), 455–462. doi:10.1093/gerona/glt144

Whiteford, H. A., Degenhardt, L., Rehm, J., Baxter, A. J., Ferrari, A. J., Erskine, H. E., et al. (2013). Global burden of disease attributable to mental and substance use disorders: Findings from the Global Burden of Disease Study 2010. *Lancet*. *382*(9904), 1575–1586.

Whitworth. J. W., & Ciccolo, J. T. (2016). Exercise and post-traumatic stress disorder in military veterans: A systematic review. *Military Medicine*, *181*(9), 953–960. doi:10.7205/MILMED-D-15-00488

Williams, M., Teasdale, J., Segal, Z., & Kabat-Zinn, J. (2007). *The mindful way through depression: Freeing yourself from chronic unhappiness*. New York: Guilford Press.

World Health Organization. (2016). Depression fact sheet. Retrieved from http://www.who.int/mediacentre/news/releases/2016/depression-anxiety-treatment/en/.

Yaffe, K., Barnes, D., Nevitt, M., Lui, L.-Y., & Covinsky, K. (2001). A prospective study of physical activity and cognitive decline in elderly women: Women who walk. *Archives of Internal Medicine*, *161*, 1703–1708.

Yang, J. L., Lin, Y. T., Chuang, P. C., Bohr, V. A., & Mattson, M. P. (2014). BDNF and exercise enhance neuronal DNA repair by stimulating CREB-mediated production of apurinic/apyrimidinic endonuclease 1. *NeuroMolecular Medicine*, *16*(1), 161–174. doi:10.1007/s12017-013-8270-x

Yarrow, J. F., White, L. J., McCoy, S. C., & Borst, S. E. (2005). Training augments resistance exercise induced elevation of circulating brain derived neurotrophic factor (BDNF). *Neuroscience Letters*, *479*(2), 161–165. doi:10.1016/j.neulet.2010.05.058

Youngstedt, S. D. (2005). Effects of exercise on sleep. *Clinics in Sports Medicine, 24*(2), 355–365. doi:10.1016/j.csm.2004.12.003

Zheng, G., Liu, F., Li, S., Huang, M., Tao, J., & Chen, L. (2013). Tai chi and the protection of cognitive ability: A systematic review of prospective studies in healthy adults. *American Journal of Preventive Medicine, 49*(1), 89–97. doi:10.1016/j.amepre.2015.01.002

4

The Neurobiology of Meditation and Stress Reduction

ANDREW B. NEWBERG AND DAVID B. YADEN

Key Points

- Meditation is a complex mental process that involves changes in cognition, sensory perception, emotions, hormones, and autonomic activity.
- Many different neurotransmitter systems, including dopamine, serotonin, glutamate, and opiates, are likely affected by meditation practices.
- Meditation has also become widely used, either alone or combined with other therapies, for stress reduction, as well as for a variety of physical and mental disorders.
- There has been an increasing understanding of the overall biological mechanism of meditation practices in terms of their effects on both the brain and the body.
- Recent studies using clinical tools and functional neuroimaging have substantially augmented the knowledge of the biology of meditative practices.

Introduction

The study of meditation, a complex mental task, remains an expanding area of research. Meditation practices offer a window into aspects of human consciousness, psychology, and subjective experience, as well as the relationship between mental states and body physiology, emotional and cognitive processing, and the biological correlates of religious experience. The past 30 years have marked important scientific progress on the neurobiological effects and mechanisms of meditation. Initial studies measured changes in autonomic activity, such as heart rate and blood pressure, and electroencephalographic (EEG) changes. More recent studies have utilized functional neuroimaging as well as explored changes in hormonal and immunological function associated with meditation practices. A number of studies have also explored the clinical effects of meditation in both physical and psychological disorders.

Functional neuroimaging, in particular, has opened a new window into the investigation of meditative states by exploring the neurological correlates of these experiences. Over 100 neuroimaging studies of meditative practices are currently available in the medical literature. The neuroimaging techniques used in these studies include positron emission tomography (PET; Herzog et al., 1990–1991; Lou et al., 1999), single photon emission computed tomography (SPECT; Newberg et al., 2001; Newberg, Pourdehnad, Alavi, & d'Aquili, 2003), and functional magnetic resonance imaging (fMRI; Beauregard & Paquette, 2006; Brefczynski-Lewis, Lutz, Schaefer, Levinson, & Davidson, 2007; Lazar et al., 2000). Each of these techniques provides different advantages and disadvantages in the study of meditation. Functional MRI has improved resolution over SPECT and the ability of immediate anatomic correlation. However, fMRI can be difficult to utilize for the study of meditation because of noise from the machine and the problem of requiring the subject to lie down, an atypical posture for many forms of meditation. The advantage of SPECT cerebral blood flow imaging is that the subject can be in a variety of positions and postures while keeping an intravenous catheter in the arm for injection of the radioactive tracer. When the tracer is injected, it is taken up in the brain over a relatively short time period (i.e. three to five minutes), thus capturing cerebral function of the person's state at the time of injection. If a person is injected while meditating, he or she can complete the meditation session and then be brought into the scanner for image acquisition. The images obtained reveal the cerebral blood flow pattern around the time of the injection, thus capturing the meditation state in this case. The downside of this approach is that only a single brain state can be observed during a SPECT scan acquisition. Functional MRI allows for the ability to measure multiple time points, and hence multiple brain states, during meditation practices. A major potential strength of PET and SPECT is that they offer the opportunity to evaluate neurotransmitter systems such as dopamine or serotonin (ST). Thus functional brain imaging offers important techniques for studying meditation, although the best approach may depend on a number of factors related to the meditation practice as well as the specific aims of the study.

This chapter reviews the existing data on neurophysiology and physiology with regard to meditation practices and attempts to integrate this data into a comprehensive neurobiological model of such practices. There are many possible neurochemical changes that may occur during meditation, even though they may not occur in every type of practice or in each individual. We aim to provide a framework of the neurological and physiological correlates of meditative practices with respect to mental health and stress reduction that will help guide future research. Within this model, specific structures, including the prefrontal cortex (PFC), parietal lobe, limbic system, and autonomic nervous system (ANS), appear to interact in an integrated manner.

Types of Meditation

There are many specific approaches to meditation, and several taxonomies to organize various meditation practices have been attempted. Early approaches to categorizing meditation practices divided them into two primary types. The first category consists of practices that involve clearing all thought from the sphere of attention (d'Aquili & Newberg, 1993). This form of meditation is an attempt to reach a subjective state characterized by a loss of one's usual sense of space, time, and thought. Further, this state is cognitively experienced as fully integrated and unified, such that there is no sense of a boundary between one's self and "other." The second category consists of focused attention on a particular object, image, phrase, or word—such as mantra meditations. This form of meditation is designed to lead to a subjective experience of absorption with the object of focus. Mindfulness meditation (Kabat-Zinn, 2005) is another popular meditation practice in which attention is focused on whatever thoughts or feelings enter into the mind, and this has sometimes been referred to as "open monitoring" to denote a different type of meditation. The goal is to be more aware of one's inner mental processes.

A more recent reworking of the meditation taxonomy has focused along two dimensions. One has to do with goal of the practice, that is, the enhanced mental state that is achieved. These mental states can refer to an enhanced cognitive state, an enhanced emotional or affective state, or a null state that is noncognitive and nonaffective. Many concentration-based practices would fall into the enhanced cognitive state category since they ask the person to focus on a particular object such as a mantra or prayer. Practices such as lovingkindness meditation lead to an enhanced emotional state in which the person feels overwhelming love or compassion. Practices such as Tibetan or Zen Buddhism that lead to a "void consciousness" reflect the null state.

The second aspect of meditation practices has to do with explicit directions that are part of the method and overall approach that is employed (Nash & Newberg, 2013). These "taxonomic keys" include employing specific cognitive strategies, using conceptual or physical objects of focus, having the eyes opened or closed, being stationary or moving (i.e., tai chi), making verbalizations or being in silence, maintaining certain postures or positions, controlling breathing, and meditating based on intrinsic or extrinsic processes (i.e., meditating on one's own volition or following a teacher or tape). Each of these elements can affect the meditative experience as well as the brain in different ways.

Overall, it appears that the end result of many practices of meditation is similar or at least converges on a limited set of outcomes such as reduction in stress and anxiety. Therefore, it seems reasonable that while the initial neurophysiological activation occurring during any given practice may differ, there may eventually be a convergence of experiences and neurophysiological correlates. This chapter focuses on a description of volitional meditation in which subjects focus on an object that, hopefully, will provide an overall framework from which other types of meditation can be considered (see Figure 4.1). The

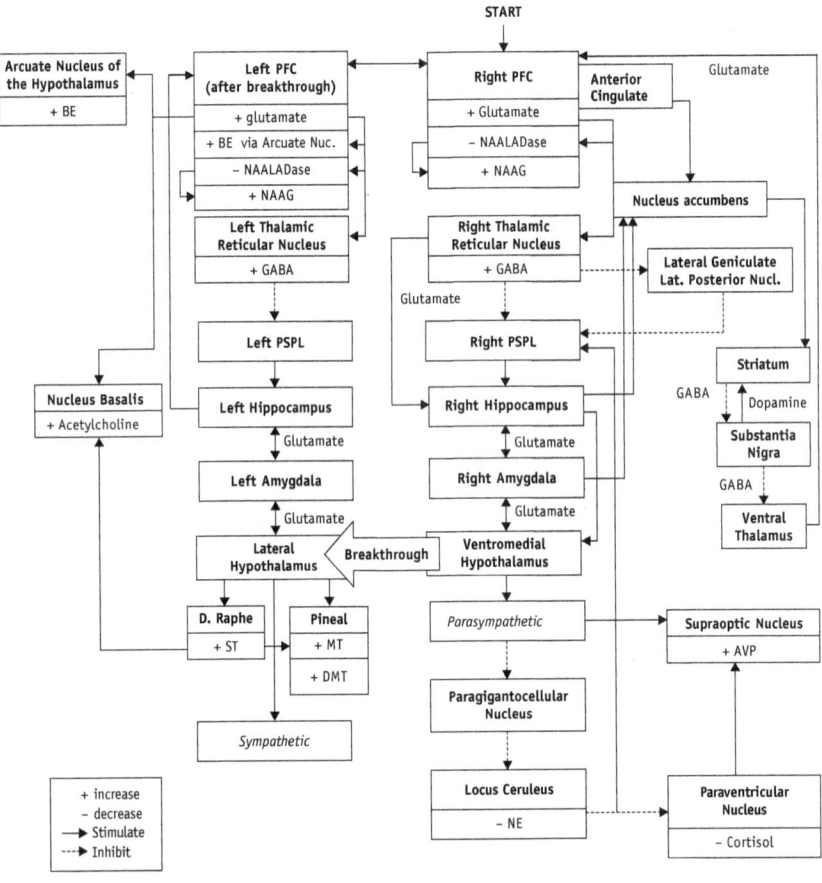

FIGURE 4.1. Schematic overview of the neurophysiological network possibly associated with meditative states. The circuits generally apply to both hemispheres; however, much of the initial activity is likely on the right.

Activation of the Prefrontal and Cingulate Cortex

Brain imaging studies suggest that willful acts and tasks that require sustained attention are initiated via activity in the PFC, particularly in the right hemisphere (Frith, Friston, Liddle, & Frackowiak, 1991; Ingvar, 1994; Pardo, Fox, & Raichle, 1991; Posner & Petersen, 1990). The cingulate gyrus has also been shown to be involved in focusing attention, probably in conjunction with the PFC (Vogt, Finch, & Olson, 1992). Since most meditation practices require intense focus of attention, it seems appropriate that a model for meditation begin with activation of the PFC (particularly in the right hemisphere) as well as the cingulate gyrus. This notion is supported by the increased activity observed in these regions on several of the brain imaging studies of volitional types of meditation (Herzog et al., 1990–1991; Lazar et al., 2000; Newberg et al., 2001; Zeidan et al., 2011, 2014). In a study of Tibetan Buddhist meditators (see Figures 4.2 and 4.3), there was increased activity in the PFC bilaterally (greater on the right) and in the cingulate gyrus during meditation. Therefore, meditation appears to start by activating the prefrontal and cingulate cortex, associated with the will or intent to clear the mind of thoughts or to focus on

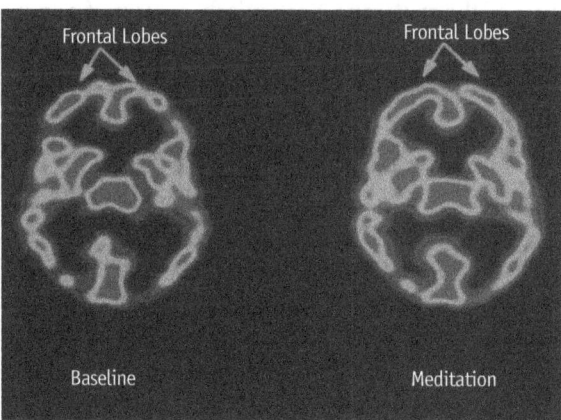

FIGURE 4.2. The SPECT images were obtained during a study of the neurophysiological correlates of Tibetan Buddhist meditation. These axial images show the results from a baseline scan on the left (i.e., at rest) and during a "peak" of meditation shown on the right. The images demonstrate that the frontal lobes, usually involved in focusing attention, are more active during meditation (increased red activity).

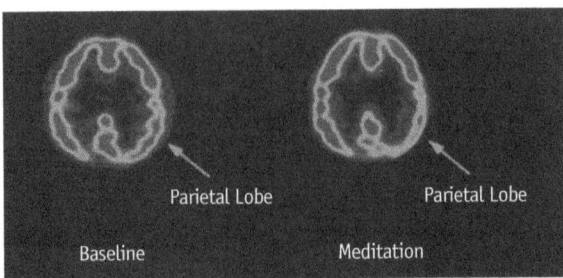

FIGURE 4.3. Axial SPECT images, slightly higher up in the brain, demonstrate decreased activity in the superior parietal lobe (lower right shows up as yellow rather than the red on the left image) during meditation compared to the resting state.

an object. One PET study of a guided type of meditation did not demonstrate increased prefrontal activity; however, a recent study showed decreased frontal activity during externally guided word generation compared to internal or volitional word generation (Crosson et al., 2001). Thus prefrontal and cingulate activation may be associated with the volitional aspects of meditation.

Thalamic Activation

A number of studies have shown that the PFC, when activated, innervates the reticular nucleus of the thalamus, particularly as part of a more global attentional network (Portas et al., 1998; Zikopoulos & Barbas, 2006). Such activation may be accomplished by the PFC's production and distribution of the excitatory neurotransmitter glutamate, which the PFC neurons use to communicate among themselves and to innervate other brain structures (Cheramy, Romo, & Glowinski, 1987). The thalamus itself governs the flow of sensory information to cortical processing areas via its interactions with the lateral geniculate and lateral posterior nuclei and also probably uses the glutamate system in order to activate neurons in other structures (Armony & LeDoux, 2000). The lateral geniculate nucleus receives raw visual data from the optic tract and routes it to the striate cortex for processing (Andrews, Halpern, & Purves, 1997). The lateral posterior nucleus of the thalamus provides the parietal lobe with the sensory information it needs to determine the body's spatial orientation (Bucci, Conley, & Gallagher, 1999).

When excited, the reticular nucleus secretes the inhibitory neurotransmitter gamma aminobutyric acid (GABA) onto the lateral posterior and geniculate nuclei, cutting off input to the superior parietal lobe and visual centers in proportion to the reticular activation (Destexhe, Contreras, & Steriade, 1998). During meditation, because of the increased activity in the PFC, particularly on the right, there should be a concomitant increase in the activity in the reticular nucleus of the thalamus. While brain imaging studies of meditation have not had the resolution to distinguish the reticular nuclei, several studies have demonstrated increases in thalamic and PFC activity (Newberg & Iversen, 2003; Farb, Anderson, & Segal, 2012). This is consistent with, but does not confirm, the specific interaction between the PFC and reticular nuclei during meditation practices. However, if the activation of the right PFC causes increased activity in the reticular nucleus during meditation, the result may be decreased sensory input entering into the parietal lobe. Several studies have demonstrated an increase in GABA during meditation including a recent magnetic resonance spectroscopy study (see Table 4.1 for an overview of neurochemical changes observed during meditation; Elias, Guich, & Wilson, 2000; Guglietti, Daskalakis, Radhu, Fitzgerald, & Ritvo, 2013; Streeter et al., 2007). This functional deafferentation related to increased GABA would mean that fewer distracting outside stimuli would arrive at the visual cortex and parietal lobe. This might enhance the sense of focus of the meditator and contribute to the overall experience.

It should also be noted that the dopaminergic system, via the basal ganglia, is believed to participate in regulating the glutamatergic system and the interactions between the PFC and subcortical structures. A PET study utilizing 11C-Raclopride to measure the dopaminergic tone during yoga nidra

Table 4.1. Summary of Neurochemically Related Changes in Serum Concentration Observed During Meditation Techniques and the Central Nervous System Structures Typically Involved in Their Production

Neurochemical	Observed change	CNS structure
Arginine vasopressin	Increased	Supraoptic nucleus
GABA	Increased	Thalamus, other inhibitory structures
Melatonin	Increased	Pineal gland
Serotonin	Increased	Dorsal raphe
Cortisol	Decreased	Paraventricular nucleus
Norepinephrine	Decreased	Locus ceruleus
β-Endorphin	Rhythm changed; levels unaltered	Arcuate nucleus

Note: GABA = gamma aminobutyric acid.

meditation demonstrated a significant increase in dopamine levels during the meditation practice (Kjaer et al., 2002). The authors hypothesized that this increase may be associated with the gating of cortical-subcortical interactions that leads to an overall decrease in readiness for action that is associated with this particular type of meditation. Future studies will be necessary to elaborate on the role of dopamine during meditative practices, as well as the interactions between dopamine and other neurotransmitter systems.

Parietal Lobe Deafferentation

The parietal lobe is heavily involved in the analysis and integration of higher order visual, auditory, and somaesthetic information (Adair, Gilmore, Fennell, Gold, & Heilman, 1995). It is also involved in a complex attentional network that includes the PFC and thalamus (Fernandez-Duque & Posner, 2001). Through the reception of auditory and visual input from the thalamus, the parietal lobe is able to help generate a three-dimensional image of the body in space, provide a sense of spatial coordinates in which the body is oriented, help distinguish between objects, and exert influences in regard to objects that may be directly grasped and manipulated (Lynch, 1980; Mountcastle, Motter, & Anderson, 1980). These functions of the parietal lobe might be critical for distinguishing between the self and the external world. It should be noted that a recent study has suggested that the superior temporal lobe may play a more important role in body spatial representation, although this has not been confirmed by other reports (Karnath, Ferber, & Himmelbach, 2001). However, it remains to be seen what the actual relationship is between the parietal and temporal lobes in terms of spatial representation.

Regardless, deafferentation of these orienting areas of the brain has been suggested as an important mediator in the physiology of meditation (Newberg & Iversen, 2003). If, for example, deafferentation of the parietal lobe occurs by the reticular nucleus's GABAergic effects, the person may begin to lose his or her usual ability to define the self spatially and to help orient the self. Such a notion is supported by clinical findings in patients with parietal lobe damage who have difficulty orienting themselves. A more recent study of brain tumor patients undergoing surgery found that those patients with parietal lobe lesions/surgery were more likely to report feelings of self-transcendence compared to lesions in other parts of the brain. Again, abnormal function in the parietal lobes appears to be associated with alterations in the person's sense of self that might be related to similar effects during meditation. Deafferentation of the parietal lobe has also been supported by several imaging studies demonstrating decreased activity in this region during intense meditation (Herzog et al., 1990–1991; Newberg et al., 2001; Newberg et al., 2003). The lateralization of these decreases has not been fully elucidated, although it is reasonable that, depending on the practice and experience, greater decreases might be observed in either the right or left hemisphere. Noninvasive brain stimulation technologies, such as transcranial magnetic stimulation, may be helpful in establishing which cortical regions are capable of enhancing or inhibiting some of meditation's effects (Yaden, Anderson, Mattar, & Newberg, 2015; Yaden & Newberg, 2014). However, more studies will be needed to determine the precise relationship between changes in each of the hemispheres and other cortical regions.

Hippocampal and Amygdalar Activation

In addition to the complex cortical-thalamic activity, meditation might also be expected to alter activity in the limbic system, especially since the limbic system is associated with emotional responses. Thus the limbic structures are associated with experiences similar to those described during meditation (Fish, Gloor, Quesney, & Oliver, 1993; Newberg & Iverson, 2003; Saver & Rabin, 1997). The hippocampus acts to modulate and moderate cortical arousal and responsiveness, via rich and extensive interconnections with the PFC, other neocortical areas, the amygdala, and the hypothalamus (Joseph, 1996). Hippocampal stimulation has been shown to affect cortical responsiveness and arousal (Cromwell, Mears, Wan, & Boutros, 2008; Redding, 1967).

The ability of the hippocampus to stimulate or inhibit neuronal activity in other structures probably relies upon the glutamate and GABA systems, respectively (Armony & LeDoux, 2000). The partial deafferentation of the right parietal lobe during meditation may result in stimulation of the right hippocampus because of the inverse modulation of the hippocampus in relation to cortical activity. If, in addition, there is simultaneous direct stimulation of the right hippocampus via the thalamus (as part of the known attentional network) and mediated by glutamate, then a powerful recruitment of stimulation of the right hippocampus could theoretically occur. Right hippocampal activity may ultimately enhance the stimulatory function of the PFC on the thalamus via the nucleus accumbens, which gates the neural input from the PFC to the thalamus via the neuromodulatory effects of dopamine (Chow & Cummings, 1999; Newman & Grace, 1999).

The hippocampus greatly influences the amygdala, such that they interact reciprocally in the generation of attention, emotion, and certain types of imagery (Canbeyli, 2010; Richter-Levin & Akirav, 2000). It seems that much of the prefrontal modulation of emotion is via the hippocampus and its connections with the amygdala (McEwen, 2006; Poletti & Sujatanond, 1980; Richter-Levin & Akirav, 2000). Because of this reciprocal interaction between the amygdala and hippocampus, the activation of the right hippocampus probably stimulates the right lateral amygdala as well. The results of the fMRI study by Lazar et al. (2000) support the notion of increased activity in the regions of the amygdala and hippocampus during meditation. Other neuroimaging studies of meditation practices have shown increased activity in limbic structures especially in relation to strong emotional responses (Lutz et al., 2008; Sperduti, Martinelli, & Piolino, 2012).

Hypothalamic and ANS Changes

The hypothalamus is interconnected extensively with the limbic system. Increased activity in the right amygdala has been shown to result in activation of the ventromedial portion of the hypothalamus, with a subsequent activation of the peripheral parasympathetic system (Davis, 1992). Increased parasympathetic activity should be associated with the subjective sensation first of relaxation and, eventually, of a more profound quiescence. Activation of the parasympathetic system would also cause a reduction in heart rate and respiratory rate. All of these physiological responses have been observed during meditation (Jevning, Wallace, & Beidebach, 1992).

Typically, when breathing and heart rate slow down, the paragigantocellular nucleus of the medulla ceases to innervate the locus ceruleus (LC) of the pons. The LC produces and distributes norepinephrine (NE; Foote, 1987), a neuromodulator that increases the susceptibility of brain regions to sensory input by amplifying strong stimuli, while simultaneously gating out weaker activations and cellular "noise" that fall below the activation threshold (Waterhouse, Moises, & Woodward, 1998). Decreased stimulation of the LC results in a decrease in the level of NE (Van Bockstaele & Aston-Jones, 1995). Some studies show that the breakdown products of catecholamines, such as NE and epinephrine, are reduced in the urine and plasma during meditation (Infante et al., 2001; Walton, Pugh, Gelderloos, & Macrae, 1995), which may simply reflect the systemic change in autonomic balance. Similarly, meditation decreases heart rate and blood pressure. During a meditative practice, the reduced firing of the paragigantocellular nucleus probably cuts back its innervation of the locus ceruleus, which densely and specifically supplies the parietal lobe and the lateral posterior nucleus with NE (Foote, 1987). Thus a reduction in NE would decrease the impact of sensory input on the parietal lobe, potentially contributing to its deafferentation.

The LC would also deliver less NE to the hypothalamic paraventricular nucleus. The paraventricular nucleus of the hypothalamus typically secretes corticotropin-releasing hormone (CRH) in response to innervation by NE from the LC (Ziegler, Cass, & Herman, 1999). This CRH stimulates the anterior pituitary to release adrenocorticotropic hormone (ACTH; Livesey, Evans, Mulligan, & Donald, 2000). ACTH, in turn, stimulates the adrenal cortex to produce cortisol, one of the body's stress hormones (Davies, Kenyon, & Fraser, 1985). Decreasing NE from the LC during meditation would probably decrease the production of CRH by the paraventricular nucleus and ultimately decrease cortisol levels. Most studies have found that cortisol levels are decreased during meditation (Jevning, Wilson, & Davidson, 1978; Ray et al., 2014; Sudsuang, Chentanez, & Veluvan, 1991; Walton et al., 1995).

The drop in blood pressure associated with parasympathetic activity during meditation practices would be expected to relax the arterial baroreceptors, leading the caudal ventral medulla to decrease its GABAergic inhibition of the supraoptic nucleus of the hypothalamus. This lack of inhibition can provoke the supraoptic nucleus to release the vasoconstrictor arginine vasopressin (AVP), thereby tightening the arteries and returning blood pressure to normal (Renaud, 1996). AVP has also been shown to contribute to the general maintenance of positive affect (Pietrowsky et al., 1991), decrease fatigue, and significantly improve the consolidation of new memories (Weingartner et al., 1981). In fact, plasma AVP has been shown to increase dramatically during meditation (O'Halloran et al., 1985). The sharp increase in AVP should result in a decreased subjective feeling of fatigue and increased sense of arousal. It could also help to enhance the meditator's memory of his or her experience, perhaps explaining the subjective phenomenon that meditative experiences are remembered and described in very vivid terms.

PFC Effects on Other Neurochemical Systems

As a meditation practice continues, continued activity in the PFC could be due to the persistent will to focus attention that is often required. PFC activity might be particularly associated with meditations in which individuals focus on nothing, though this has not been fully studied. In general, as PFC activity increases, it produces ever-increasing levels of free synaptic glutamate in the brain. Increased glutamate can stimulate the hypothalamic arcuate nucleus to release beta-endorphin (BE; Kiss, Kocsis, Csaki, Gorcs, & Halasz, 1997).

BE is an opioid produced primarily by the arcuate nucleus of the medial hypothalamus and distributed to the brain's subcortical areas (Yadid, Zangen, Herzberg, Nakash, & Sagen, 2000). BE is known to depress respiration, reduce fear, reduce pain, and produce sensations of joy and euphoria (Janal, Colt, Clark, & Glusman, 1984). That such effects have been described during meditation may implicate some degree of BE release related to the increased PFC activity. Meditation has been found to disrupt diurnal rhythms of BE and ACTH, while not affecting diurnal cortisol rhythms (Infante et al., 1998). However, it is probable that BE is not solely responsible for meditative experiences, because simply taking morphine-related substances does not produce equivalent experiences to those in meditation. Furthermore, one very limited study demonstrated that blocking the opiate receptors with naloxone did not affect the experience or EEG associated with meditation (Sim & Tsoi, 1992).

Glutamate activates N-methyl d-aspartate receptors (NMDAr), but excess glutamate can kill these neurons through excitotoxic processes (Albin & Greenamyre, 1992). We have previously proposed that if glutamate levels approach excitotoxic concentrations during intense states of meditation, the brain might limit its production of N-acetylated-alpha-linked-acidic dipeptidase, which converts the endogenous NMDAr antagonist N-acetylaspartylglutamate (NAAG) into glutamate (Thomas, Vornov, Olkowski, Merion, & Slusher, 2000). The resultant increase in NAAG would protect cells from excitotoxic damage. Since the NMDAr inhibitor NAAG is functionally analogous to the disassociative hallucinogens ketamine, phencyclidine, and nitrous oxide (Jevtovic-Todorovic Wozniak, Benshoff, & Olney, 2001), it might help in eliciting a variety of altered states of consciousness such as out-of-body and near-death experiences (Vollenweider et al., 1997).

Autonomic-Cortical Activity

In the early 1970s, Gellhorn and Kiely (1972) developed a model of the physiological processes involved in meditation based almost exclusively on ANS activity. This model is somewhat limited because of the heavy reliance on the ANS, but their work indicated the importance of the ANS during meditative experiences. These authors suggested that intense stimulation of either the sympathetic or parasympathetic system, if continued, could ultimately result in simultaneous discharge of both systems (what might be considered a "breakthrough" of the other system). Several studies have demonstrated predominant parasympathetic activity during meditation associated with decreased heart rate and blood pressure, decreased respiratory rate, and decreased oxygen metabolism (Jevning et al., 1992; Sudsuang et al., 1991; Travis, 2001). However, two studies of different meditative techniques suggested a mutual activation of parasympathetic and sympathetic systems by demonstrating an increase in the variability of heart rate during meditation (Peng et al., 1999; Peng et al., 2004).

The increased variation in heart rate was hypothesized to reflect activation of both arms of the ANS. This notion also fits the characteristic description of meditative states in which there is a sense of overwhelming calmness as well as significant alertness. Also, the notion of mutual activation of both arms of the ANS is consistent with recent developments in the study of autonomic interactions (Hugdahl, 1996).

Serotonergic Activity

Activation of the ANS can result in intense stimulation of structures in the lateral hypothalamus and median forebrain bundle, which are known to produce both ecstatic and blissful feelings when directly stimulated (Olds & Forbes, 1981). Stimulation of the lateral hypothalamus can also result in changes in serotonergic activity. In fact, several studies have shown that, after meditation, the breakdown products of ST in urine are significantly increased, suggesting an overall elevation in ST during meditation (Walton et al., 1995). A more recent study showed that meditation is associated with activation of the ST system (Yu et al., 2011). ST is a neuromodulator that densely supplies the visual centers of the temporal lobe, where it strongly influences the flow of visual associations generated by this area (Foote, 1987). The cells of the dorsal raphe produce and distribute ST when innervated by the lateral hypothalamus (Aghajanian, Sprouse, & Rasmussen, 1987) and also when activated by the PFC (Juckel, Mendlin, & Jacobs, 1999). Moderately increased levels of ST appear to correlate with positive affect, while low ST often signifies depression (Van Praag & De Haan, 1980). This relationship has clearly been demonstrated with regard to the effects of the selective serotonin reuptake inhibitor medications that are widely used for the treatment of depression. When cortical ST_2 receptors (especially in the temporal lobes) are activated, however, the stimulation can result in a hallucinogenic effect.

Tryptamine psychedelics such as psylocybin and LSD seem to take advantage of this mechanism to produce their extraordinary visual associations and mystical or religious experiences (Aghajanian & Marek, 1999; Griffiths, Richards, McCann, & Jesse, 2006). The mechanism by which this appears to occur is that ST inhibits the lateral geniculate nucleus, greatly reducing the amount of visual information that can pass through (Funke & Eysel, 1995; Yoshida, Sasa, & Takaori, 1984). If combined with reticular nucleus inhibition of the lateral geniculate, ST may increase the fluidity of temporal visual associations in the absence of sensory input, possibly resulting in the internally generated imagery that has been described during certain meditative states.

Increased ST levels can affect several other neurochemical systems. An increase in ST has a modulatory effect on dopamine, suggesting a link between the serotonergic and dopaminergic system, which may enhance feelings of euphoria (Vollenweider, Vontobel, Hell, & Leenders, 1999) frequently described during meditative states. ST, in conjunction with the increased glutamate, has been shown to stimulate the nucleus basalis to release acetylcholine, which has important modulatory influences throughout the cortex (Manfridi, Brambilla, & Mancia, 1999; Zhelyazkova-Savova, Giovannini, & Pepeu, 1997). Increased acetylcholine in the frontal lobes has been shown to augment the attentional system and in the parietal lobes to enhance orienting without altering sensory input (Fernandez-Duque & Posner, 2001). While no studies have evaluated the specific role of acetylcholine in meditation, it appears that this neurotransmitter may enhance the attentional component as well as the orienting response in the face of progressive deafferentation of sensory input into the parietal lobes during meditation.

Increased ST combined with lateral hypothalamic innervation of the pineal gland may lead the latter to increase production of the neurohormone melatonin (MT) from the conversion of ST (Moller, 1992). MT has been shown to depress the central nervous system and reduce pain sensitivity (Shaji & Kulkarni, 1998). During meditation, blood plasma MT has been found to increase sharply (Tooley, Armstrong, Norman, & Sali, 2000), which may contribute to the feelings of calmness and decreased awareness of pain (Dollins, Lynch, Wurtman, Deng, & Lieberman, 1993). Under circumstances of heightened activation, pineal enzymes can also endogenously synthesize the powerful hallucinogen 5-methoxy-dimethyltryptamine (DMT; Monti & Christian, 1981). Several studies have linked DMT to a variety of mystical states, including out-of-body experiences, distortion of time and space, and interaction with supernatural entities (Gallimore & Strassman, 2016; Strassman & Clifford, 1994; Strassman, Clifford, Qualls, & Berg, 1996). Hyperstimulation of the pineal at this step, then, could also lead to DMT production, which can be associated with the wide variety of mystical-type experiences associated with that hallucinogen.

Conclusion

Much work still needs to be done to better elucidate the intricate neurobiological mechanisms underlying meditative practices. Most studies of the biological correlates of meditation currently available suffer from a low number of subjects, lack of control conditions, and difficulty in factoring out confounding variables. Furthermore, knowledge of neurotransmitter systems is highly complex and continually being refined. Thus it may be very difficult to assess if all of the systems would function in the integrated manner described here. However, the neurophysiological effects that have been observed during meditative states seem to outline a consistent pattern of changes involving certain key cerebral structures in conjunction with autonomic and hormonal changes. These changes are also reflected in neurochemical changes involving the endogenous opioid, GABA, NE, and serotonergic receptor systems. The current research studies have begun to elucidate the mechanism underlying the physical and psychological effects of meditative practices and provide an impetus for future studies of these and other complex mental tasks.

References

Adair, K. C., Gilmore, R. L., Fennell, E. B., Gold, M., & Heilman, K. M. (1995). Anosognosia during intracarotid barbiturate anaesthesia: Unawareness or amnesia for weakness. *Neurology, 45,* 241–243.

Aghajanian, G., Sprouse, J., & Rasmussen, K. (1987). Physiology of the midbrain serotonin system. In H. Meltzer (Ed.), *Psychopharmacology, the third generation of progress* (pp. 141–149). New York: Raven Press.

Aghajanian, G. K., & Marek, G. J. (1999). Serotonin and hallucinogens. *Neuropsychopharmacology, 21,* 16S–23S.

Albin, R., & Greenamyre, J. (1992). Alternative excitotoxic hypotheses. *Neurology, 42,* 733–738.

Andrews, T. J., Halpern, S. D., & Purves, D. (1997). Correlated size variations in human visual cortex, lateral geniculate nucleus, and optic tract. *Journal of Neuroscience, 17,* 2859–2868.

Armony, J. L., & LeDoux, J. E. (2000). How danger is encoded: Toward a systems, cellular, and computational understanding of cognitive-emotional interactions in fear. In M. S. Gazzaniga (Ed.), *The new cognitive neurosciences* (pp. 1067–1079). Cambridge, MA: MIT Press.

Beauregard, M., & Paquette, V. (2006). Neural correlates of a mystical experience in Carmelite nuns. *Neuroscience Letters, 405*(3), 186–190.

Brefczynski-Lewis, J. A., Lutz, A., Schaefer, H. S., Levinson, D. B., & Davidson, R. J. (2007). Neural correlates of attentional expertise in long-term meditation practitioners. *Proceedings of National Academy of Sciences USA, 104*(27), 11483–11488.

Bucci, D. J., Conley, M., & Gallagher, M. (1999). Thalamic and basal forebrain cholinergic connections of the rat posterior parietal cortex. *Neuroreport, 10,* 941–945.

Canbeyli, R. (2010). Sensorimotor modulation of mood and depression: An integrative review. *Behavior and Brain Research, 207*(2), 249–264.

Cheramy, A., Romo, R., & Glowinski, J. (1987). Role of corticostriatal glutamatergic neurons in the presynaptic control of dopamine release. In M. Sandler, C. Feuerstein, & B. Scatton (Eds.), *Neurotransmitter interactions in the basal ganglia.* New York: Raven Press.

Chow, T. W., & Cummings, J. L. (1999). Frontal-subcortical circuits. In B. L. Miller & J. L. Cummings (Eds.), *The human frontal lobes* (pp. 3–26). New York: Guilford Press.

Cromwell, H. C., Mears, R. P., Wan, L., & Boutros, N. N. (2008). Sensory gating: A translational effort from basic to clinical science. *Clinical EEG and Neuroscience, 39*(2), 69–72.

Crosson, B., Sadek, J. R., & Maron, L., Gökçay, D., Mohr, C., Auerbach, E., et al. (2001). Relative shift in activity from medial to lateral frontal cortex during internally versus externally guided word generation. *Journal of Cognitive Neuroscience, 13*, 272–283.

d'Aquili, E. G., & Newberg, A. B. (1993). Religious and mystical states: A neuropsychological model. *Zygon, 28*, 177–200.

Davies, E., Kenyon, C. J., & Fraser, R. (1985). The role of calcium ions in the mechanism of ACTH stimulation of cortisol synthesis. *Steroids, 45*(6), 551–560.

Davis, M. (1992). The role of the amygdala in fear and anxiety. *Annual Review of Neuroscience, 15*, 353–375.

Destexhe, A., Contreras, D., & Steriade, M. (1998). Mechanisms underlying the synchronizing action of corticothalamic feedback through inhibition of thalamic relay cells. *Journal of Neurophysiology, 79*, 999–1016.

Dollins, A. B., Lynch, H. J., Wurtman, R. J., Deng, M. H., & Lieberman, H. R. (1993). Effect of pharmacological daytime doses of melatonin on human mood and performance. *Psychopharmacology, 112*, 490–496.

Elias, A. N., Guich, S., & Wilson, A. F. (2000). Ketosis with enhanced GABAergic tone promotes physiological changes in transcendental meditation. *Medical Hypotheses, 54*, 660–662.

Farb, N. A., Anderson, A. K., & Segal, Z. V. (2012). The mindful brain and emotion regulation in mood disorders. *Canadian Journal of Psychiatry, 57*(2), 70–77.

Fernandez-Duque, D., & Posner, M. I. (2001). Brain imaging of attentional networks in normal and pathological states. *Journal of Clinical and Experimental Neuropsychology, 23*, 74–93.

Fish, D. R., Gloor, P., Quesney, F. L., & Oliver, A. (1993). Clinical responses to electrical brain stimulation of the temporal and frontal lobes in patients with epilepsy. *Brain, 116*, 397–414.

Foote, S. (1987). Extrathalamic modulation of cortical function. *Annual Review of Neuroscience, 10*, 67–95.

Frith, C. D., Friston, K., Liddle, P. F., & Frackowiak, R. S. J. (1991). Willed action and the prefrontal cortex in man: A study with PET. *Proceedings of the Royal Society of London, 244*, 241–246.

Funke, K., & Eysel, U. T. (1995). Possible enhancement of GABAergic inputs to cat dorsal lateral geniculate relay cells by serotonin. *Neuroreport, 6*, 474–476.

Gallimore, A. R., & Strassman, R. J. (2016). A model for the application of target-controlled intravenous infusion for a prolonged immersive dmt psychedelic experience. *Frontiers in Pharmacology, 7*, 211. doi:10.3389/fphar.2016.00211

Gellhorn, E., & Kiely, W. F. (1972). Mystical states of consciousness: Neurophysiological and clinical aspects. *Journal of Nervous and Mental Disease, 154*, 399–405.

Griffiths, R. R., Richards, W. A., McCann, U., & Jesse, R. (2006). Psilocybin can occasion mystical-type experiences having substantial and sustained personal meaning and spiritual significance. *Psychopharmacology, 187*(3), 268–283.

Guglietti, C. L., Daskalakis, Z. J., Radhu, N., Fitzgerald, P. B., & Ritvo, P. (2013). Meditation-related increases in GABAB modulated cortical inhibition. *Brain Stimulation, 6*(3), 397–402.

Herzog, H., Lele, V. R., Kuwert, T., Langen, K., Kops, E. R., & Feinendegenen, L. E. (1990–1991). Changed pattern of regional glucose metabolism during yoga meditative relaxation. *Neuropsychobiology, 23,* 182–187.

Hugdahl, K. (1996). Cognitive influences on human autonomic nervous system function. *Current Opinion in Neurobiology, 6,* 252–258.

Infante, J. R., Peran, F., Martinez, M., Roldan, A., Poyatos, R., Ruiz, C., et al. (1998). ACTH and beta-endorphin in transcendental meditation. *Physiology & Behavior, 64,* 311–315.

Infante, J. R., Torres-Avisbal, M., Pinel, P., Vallejo, J. A., Peran, E., Gonzalez, E., et al. (2001). Catecholamine levels in practitioners of the transcendental meditation technique. *Physiology & Behavior, 72,* 141–146.

Ingvar, D. H. (1994). The will of the brain: Cerebral correlates of willful acts. *Journal of Theoretical Biology, 171,* 7–12.

Janal, M., Colt, E., Clark, W., & Glusman, M. (1984). Pain sensitivity, mood and plasma endocrine levels in man following long-distance running: Effects of naxalone. *Pain, 19,* 13–25.

Jevning, R., Wallace, R. K., & Beidebach, M. (1992). The physiology of meditation: A review. A wakeful hypometabolic integrated response. *Neuroscience Biobehavioral Review, 16,* 415–424.

Jevning, R., Wilson, A. F., & Davidson, J. M. (1978). Adrenocortical activity during meditation. *Hormones and Behavior, 10,* 54–60.

Jevtovic-Todorovic, V., Wozniak, D. F., Benshoff, N. D., & Olney J. W. (2001). A comparative evaluation of the neurotoxic properties of ketamine and nitrous oxide. *Brain Research, 895,* 264–267.

Joseph, R. (1996). *Neuropsychology, neuropsychiatry, and behavioral neurology.* New York: Williams & Wilkins.

Juckel, G. J., Mendlin, A., & Jacobs, B. L. (1999). Electrical stimulation of rat medial prefrontal cortex enhances forebrain serotonin output: implications for electroconvulsive therapy and transcranial magnetic stimulation in depression. *Neuropsychopharmacology, 21,* 391–398.

Kabat-Zinn, J. (2005). *Wherever you go, there you are: Mindfulness meditation in everyday life.* New York: Hyperion.

Karnath, H. O., Ferber, S., & Himmelbach, M. (2001). Spatial awareness is a function of the temporal not the posterior parietal lobe. *Nature, 411,* 950–953.

Kiss, J., Kocsis, K., Csaki, A., Gorcs, T. J., & Halasz, B. (1997). Metabotropic glutamate receptor in GHRH and beta-endorphin neurons of the hypothalamic arcuate nucleus. *Neuroreport, 8,* 3703–3707.

Kjaer, T. W., Bertelsen, C., Piccini, P., Brooks, D., Alving, J., & Lou, H. C. (2002). Increased dopamine tone during meditation-induced change of consciousness. *Cognitive Brain Research, 13*(2), 255–259.

Lazar, S. W., Bush, G., Gollub, R. L., Fricchione, G. L., Khalsa, G., & Benson, H. (2000). Functional brain mapping of the relaxation response and meditation. *Neuroreport, 11,* 1581–1585.

Livesey, J. H., Evans, M. J., Mulligan, R., & Donald, R. A. (2000). Interactions of CRH, AVP and cortisol in the secretion of ACTH from perifused equine anterior pituitary cells: "Permissive" roles for cortisol and CRH. *Endocrine Research, 26,* 445–463.

Lou, H. C., Kjaer, T. W., Friberg, L., Wildschiodtz, G., Holm, S., & Nowak, M. (1999). A 15O-H2O PET study of meditation and the resting state of normal consciousness. *Human Brain Mapping, 7,* 98–105.

Lutz, A., Brefczynski-Lewis, J., Johnstone, T., & Davidson, R. J. (2008). Regulation of the neural circuitry of emotion by compassion meditation: effects of meditative expertise. *PLoS One, 3*(3), e1897. doi:10.1371/journal.pone.0001897

Lynch, J.C. (1980). The functional organization of posterior parietal association cortex. *Behavioral and Brain Sciences, 3,* 485–499.

Manfridi, A., Brambilla, D., & Mancia, M. (1999). Stimulation of NMDA and AMPA receptors in the rat nucleus basalis of Meynert affects sleep. *American Journal of Physiology, 277,* R1488–R1492.

McEwen, B. S. (2006). Protective and damaging effects of stress mediators: Central role of the brain. *Dialogues in Clinical Neuroscience, 8*(4), 367–381.

Moller, M. (1992). Fine structure of pinealopetal innervation of the mammalian pineal gland. *Microscopy Research and Technique, 21,* 188–204.

Monti, J. A., & Christian, S. T. (1981). N-N-Dimethyltryptamine: an endogenous hallucinogen. *International Review of Neurobiology, 22,* 83–110.

Mountcastle, V. B., Motter, B. C., & Anderson, R. A. (1980). Some further observations on the functional properties of neurons in the parietal lobe of the waking monkey. *Behavioral and Brain Sciences, 3,* 520–523.

Nash, J. D., & Newberg, A. (2013). Toward a unifying taxonomy and definition for meditation. *Frontiers in Psychology, 4,* 806. doi:10.3389/fpsyg.2013.00806

Newberg, A., Pourdehnad, M., Alavi, A., & d'Aquili, E. G. (2003). Cerebral blood flow during meditative prayer: Preliminary findings and methodological issues. *Perceptual and Motor Skills, 97*(2), 625–630.

Newberg, A. B., Alavi. A., Baime, M., Pourdehnad, M., Santanna, J., & d'Aquili, E. (2001). The measurement of regional cerebral blood flow during the complex cognitive task of meditation: A preliminary SPECT study. *Psychiatric Research: Neuroimaging, 106,* 113–122.

Newberg, A. B., & Iversen, J. (2003). The neural basis of the complex mental task of meditation: Neurotransmitter and neurochemical considerations. *Medical Hypotheses, 61*(2), 282–291.

Newman, J., & Grace, A. A. (1999). Binding across time: The selective gating of frontal and hippocampal systems modulating working memory and attentional states. *Consciousness and Cognition, 8,* 196–212.

O'Halloran, J. P., Jevning, R., Wilson, A. F., Skowsky, R., Walsh, R. N., & Alexander, C. (1985). Hormonal control in a state of decreased activation: Potentiation of arginine vasopressin secretion. *Physiology & Behavior, 35,* 591–595.

Olds, M. E., & Forbes, J. L. (1981). The central basis of motivation, intracranial self-stimulation studies. *Annual Review of Psychology, 32,* 523–574.

Pardo, J. V., Fox, P. T., & Raichle, M. E. (1991). Localization of a human system for sustained attention by positron emission tomography. *Nature, 349,* 61–64.

Peng, C. K., Henry, I. C., Mietus, J. E., Hausdorff, J. M., Khalsa, G., Benson, H., & Goldberger, A. L. (2004). Heart rate dynamics during three forms of meditation. *International Journal of Cardiology, 95*(1), 19–27.

Peng, C. K., Mietus, J. E., Liu, Y., Khalsa, G., Douglas, P. S., Benson, H., & Goldberger, A. L. (1999). Exaggerates heart rate oscillations during two meditation techniques. *International Journal of Cardiology, 70,* 101–107.

Pietrowsky, R., Braun, D., Fehm, H. L., Pauschinger, P., & Born, J. (1991). Vasopressin and oxytocin do not influence early sensory processing but affect mood and activation in man. *Peptides, 12,* 1385–1391.

Poletti, C. E., & Sujatanond, M. (1980). Evidence for a second hippocampal efferent pathway to hypothalamus and basal forebrain comparable to fornix system: A unit study in the monkey. *Journal of Neurophysiology, 44,* 514–531.

Portas, C. M., Rees, G., Howseman, A. M., Josephs, O., Turner, R., & Frith, C. D. (1998). A specific role for the thalamus in mediating the interaction attention and arousal in humans. *Journal of Neuroscience, 18,* 8979–8989.

Posner, M. I., & Petersen, S. E. (1990). The attention system of the human brain. *Annual Review of Neuroscience, 13,* 25–42.

Ray, I. B., Menezes, A. R., Malur, P., Hiltbold, A. E., Reilly, J. P., & Lavie, C. J. (2014). Meditation and coronary heart disease: A review of the current clinical evidence. *Ochsner Journal, 14*(4), 696–703.

Redding, F. K. (1967). Modification of sensory cortical evoked potentials by hippocampal stimulation. *Electroencephalography and Clinical Neurophysiology, 22,* 74–83.

Renaud, L. P. (1996). CNS pathways mediating cardiovascular regulation of vasopressin. *Clinical and Experimental Pharmacology & Physiology, 23,* 157–160.

Richter-Levin, G., & Akirav, I. (2000). Amygdala-hippocampus dynamic interaction in relation to memory. *Molecular Neurobiology, 22*(1–3), 11–20.

Saver, J. L., & Rabin J. (1997). The neural substrates of religious experience. *Journal of Neuropsychiatry and Clinical Neurosciences, 9,* 498–510.

Shaji, A. V., & Kulkarni, S. K. (1998). Central nervous system depressant activities of melatonin in rats and mice. *Indian Journal of Experimental Biology, 36,* 257–263.

Sim, M. K., & Tsoi, W. F. (1992). The effects of centrally acting drugs on the EEG correlates of meditation. *Biofeedback Self Regulation, 17,* 215–220.

Sperduti, M., Martinelli, P., & Piolino, P. (2012). A neurocognitive model of meditation based on activation likelihood estimation (ALE) meta-analysis. *Consciousness and Cognition, 21*(1), 269–276.

Strassman, R. J., & Clifford, R. (1994). Dose–response study of N, N-Dimethyltrypamine in humans. I: Neuroendocrine, autonomic, and cardiovascular effects. *Archives of General Psychiatry, 51*, 85–97.

Strassman, R. J., Clifford, R., Qualls, R., & Berg, L. (1996). Differential tolerance to biological and subjective effects of four closely spaced doses of N, N-Dimethyltrypamine in humans. *Biological Psychiatry, 39*, 784–795.

Streeter, C. C., Jensen, J. E., Perlmutter, R. M., Cabral, H. J., Tian, H., Terhune, D. B, et al. (2007). Yoga Asana sessions increase brain GABA levels: A pilot study. *Journal of Alternative and Complementary Medicine, 13*(4), 419–426.

Sudsuang, R., Chentanez, V., & Veluvan, K. (1991). Effects of Buddhist meditation on serum cortisol and total protein levels, blood pressure, pulse rate, lung volume and reaction time. *Physiology & Behavior, 50*, 543–548.

Thomas, A. G., Vornov, J. J., Olkowski, J. L., Merion, A. T., & Slusher, B. S. (2000). N-Acetylated alpha-linked acidic dipeptidase converts N-acetylaspartylglutamate from a neuroprotectant to a neurotoxin. *Journal of Pharmacology and Experimental Therapeutics, 295*, 16–22.

Tooley, G. A., Armstrong, S. M., Norman, T. R., & Sali, A. (2000). Acute increases in night-time plasma melatonin levels following a period of meditation. *Biological Psychology, 53*, 69–78.

Travis, F. (2001). Autonomic and EEG patterns distinguish transcending from other experiences during transcendental meditation practice. *International Journal of Psychophysiology, 42*, 1–9.

Van Bockstaele, E. J., & Aston-Jones, G. (1995). Integration in the ventral medulla and coordination of sympathetic, pain and arousal functions. *Clinical and Experimental Hypertension, 17*, 153–165.

Van Praag, H., & De Haan, S. (1980). Depression vulnerability and 5-hydroxytryptophan prophylaxis. *Psychiatric Research, 3*, 75–83.

Vogt, B. A., Finch, D. M., & Olson, C. R. (1992). Functional heterogeneity in cingulate cortex: The anterior executive and posterior evaluative regions. *Cerebral Cortex, 2*, 435–443.

Vollenweider, F. X., Leenders, K. L., Scharfetter, C., Antonini, A., Maguire, P., Missimer, J., & Angst, J. (1997). Metabolic hyperfrontality and psychopathology in the ketamine model of psychosis using positron emission tomography (PET) and [18F]fluorodeoxyglucose (FDG). *European Neuropsychopharmacology, 7*, 9–24.

Vollenweider, F. X., Vontobel, P., Hell, D., & Leenders, K. L. (1999). 5-HT modulation of dopamine release in basal ganglia in psilocybin-induced psychosis in man—a PET study with [11C]raclopride. *Neuropsychopharmacology, 20*, 424–433.

Walton, K. G., Pugh, N. D., Gelderloos, P., & Macrae, P. (1995). Stress reduction and preventing hypertension: Preliminary support for a psychoneuroendocrine mechanism. *Journal of Alternative and Complementary Medicine, 1*, 263–283.

Waterhouse, B. D., Moises, H. C., & Woodward, D. J. (1998). Phasic activation of the locus coeruleus enhances responses of primary sensory cortical neurons to peripheral receptive field stimulation. *Brain Research, 790*, 33–44.

Weingartner, H., Gold, P., Ballenger, J. C., Smallberg, S., Post, R. M. & Goodwin, F. D. (1981). Effects of vasopressin on human memory functions. *Science, 211*, 601–603.

Yaden, D. B., Anderson, D. A., Mattar, M., & Newberg, A. B. (2015). Psychoactive stimulation and psychoactive substances: Ethical and conceptual considerations. In J. H. Ellens & T. J. Roberts (Eds.), *Psychedelic policy quagmire: Health, law, freedom, and society* (pp. 219–236). Santa Barbara, CA: Praeger.

Yaden, D. B., & Newberg, A. B. (2014). A new means for perennial ends: Self-transcendent experiences & direct neural stimulation. In J. H. Ellens (Ed.), *Seeking the sacred with psychoactive substances* (pp. 303–324). Santa Barbara, CA: Praeger.

Yadid, G., Zangen, A., Herzberg, U., Nakash, R., & Sagen, J. (2000). Alterations in endogenous brain beta-endorphin release by adrenal medullary transplants in the spinal cord. *Neuropsychopharmacology, 23*, 709–716.

Yoshida, M., Sasa, M., & Takaori, S. (1984). Serotonin-mediated inhibition from dorsal raphe neurons nucleus of neurons in dorsal lateral geniculate and thalamic reticular nuclei. *Brain Research, 290*, 95–105.

Yu, X., Fumoto, M., Nakatani, Y., Sekiyama, T., Kikuchi, H., Seki, Y., et al. (2011). Activation of the anterior prefrontal cortex and serotonergic system is associated with improvements in mood and EEG changes induced by Zen meditation practice in novices. *International Journal of Psychophysiology, 80*(2), 103–111.

Zeidan, F., Martucci, K. T., Kraft, R. A., Gordon, N. S., McHaffie, J. G., & Coghill, R. C. (2011). Brain mechanisms supporting the modulation of pain by mindfulness meditation. *Journal of Neuroscience, 31*(14), 5540–5548.

Zeidan, F., Martucci, K. T., Kraft, R. A., McHaffie, J. G., & Coghill, R. C. (2014). Neural correlates of mindfulness meditation-related anxiety relief. *Social, Cognitive, and Affective Neuroscience, 9*(6), 751–759.

Zhelyazkova-Savova, M., Giovannini, M. G., & Pepeu, G. (1997). Increase of cortical acetylcholine release after systemic administration of chlorophenylpiperazine in the rat: An in vivo microdialysis study. *Neuroscience Letters, 236*, 151–154.

Ziegler, D. R., Cass, W. A., & Herman, J. P. (1999). Excitatory influence of the locus coeruleus in hypothalamic-pituitary-adrenocortical axis responses to stress. *Journal of Neuroendocrinology, 11*, 361–369.

Zikopoulos, B., & Barbas, H. (2006). Prefrontal projections to the thalamic reticular nucleus form a unique circuit for attentional mechanisms. *Journal of Neuroscience, 26*(28), 7348–7361.

5

The Interaction of Religion and Health

DAVID B. YADEN AND ANDREW B. NEWBERG

Key Points

- Religion and spirituality are an important part of many patients' lives and influence healthcare and healthcare-related decisions.
- Measuring religious and spiritual beliefs is difficult and relies mostly on self-report.
- Religion and spirituality overlap but also are distinct concepts that can play varying roles in a person's life.
- Religiousness and spirituality include multiple domains such as beliefs, practices, and behaviors.
- Religious beliefs can influence dietary practices such as Kosher laws, being a vegetarian for religious beliefs, or fasting rituals.
- Religions often have specific rules or guidelines regarding sexual behavior, diet, drugs, and alcohol.
- Religiousness has generally correlated with improved overall physical and mental health outcomes.
- Religion and spirituality are sources of support and coping for many people.
- Religiousness can sometimes have negative influences such as in the case of cults or terrorism.
- Specific spiritual practices such as prayer, meditation, and yoga can have a direct effect on the brain and body.

Introduction

Religion and healthcare have a history of oscillating between cooperation and antagonism. In ancient times, many of the world's most advanced civilizations (such as the Assyrians, Chinese, Egyptians,

Mesopotamians, and Persians) equated physical illnesses with evil spirits and demonic possessions and devised treatments to exorcize these spirits. Since then, religious groups have labeled physicians and other healthcare providers as everything from evil sorcerers to charlatans to conduits of God's healing powers. Similarly, views on religion of physicians, scientists, and healthcare providers have ranged from interest to disinterest to disdain.

In recent years, the medical and scientific communities have grown increasingly interested in the effects of religion on health (Levin, 1996). Coverage of the interplay of religion and health has become much more frequent in popular magazines, such as *Time* and *Newsweek*, and on television shows (Begley, 2001a, 2001b; Greenwald, 2001; Woodward, 2001). There has been a surge in the popularity of spiritual activities, such as yoga, that aim to improve or maintain health (Corliss, 2001; van Montfrans, Karemaker, Wieling, & Dunning, 1990b). Moreover, many patients consider religion to be very important and have indicated that they would like their physicians to discuss religious issues with them.

In this chapter, we review what is currently known about the clinical effects of religious and spiritual practices. We also discuss some of the challenges that researchers and healthcare practitioners may face in designing appropriate studies and translating results to clinical practice. Finally, we outline some future directions for research regarding the roles that religion and spirituality play in healthcare.

The Importance of Religion and Spirituality to Patients and Physicians

Religion and spirituality play significant roles in many people's lives. Over 90% of Americans believe in God or a higher power, 90% pray, 67% to 75% pray on a daily basis, 69% are members of a church or synagogue, 40% attend a church or synagogue regularly, 60% consider religion to be very important in their lives, and 82% acknowledge a personal need for spiritual growth (Bezilla, 1992–1993; Miller, & Thoresen, 2003; Poloma & Pendleton, 1991; Shuler, Gelberg, & Brown, 1994; The Gallup Report, 1994). Additionally, many patients seem interested in integrating religion with their healthcare. Over 75% of surveyed patients want physicians to include spiritual issues in their medical care, approximately 40% want physicians to discuss their religious faith with them, and nearly 50% would like physicians to pray with them (Daaleman & Nease, 1994; King & Bushwick, 1994; King, Hueston, & Rudy, 1994; Matthews et al., 1998). Although many physicians seem to agree that spiritual well-being is an important component of health that should be addressed with patients, only a minority (less than 20%) do so with any regularity (MacLean et al., 2003; Monroe et al., 2003). According to surveyed physicians, lack of time, inadequate training, discomfort in addressing the topics, and difficulty in identifying patients who want to discuss spiritual issues are responsible for this discrepancy (Armbruster, Chibnall, & Legett, 2003; Chibnall & Brooks, 2001; Ellis, Vinson, & Ewigman, 1999).

Educators have responded by offering courses, conferences, and curricula in medical schools, postgraduate training, and continuing medical education on the topic of understanding the religious and spiritual needs of many patients (Pettus, 2002). However, some still question the relevance and appropriateness of discussing religion and spirituality in healthcare settings, fearing that healthcare workers may impose personal religious beliefs on others and replace necessary medical interventions with religious interventions. Sloan and colleagues (Sloan & Bagiella, 2002; Sloan, Bagiella, & Powell, 1999) cautioned that patients may be forced to believe that their illnesses are due solely to poor faith. Moreover, there is considerable debate over how religion should be integrated with healthcare and who should be responsible, especially when healthcare providers are agnostic or atheist (Levin, Larson, & Puchalski, 1997).

The Role of Religion in Healthcare

Despite this controversy, the role of religion in healthcare seems to be growing. For instance, the *Diagnostic and Statistical Manual of Mental Disorders* (fifth ed.) recognizes religion and spirituality as relevant sources of either emotional distress or support (Kutz, 2002; Lukoff, Lu, & Turner, 1992; Turner, Lukoff, Barnhouse, & Lu, 1995). Also, the guidelines of the Joint Commission on Accreditation of Health care Organizations require hospitals to meet the spiritual needs of patients (La Pierre, 2003). The medical literature reflects this trend as well. The frequency of studies on religion and spirituality and health has increased over the past decade (Levin et al., 1997). Stefanek, McDonald, and Hess (2004) tallied a 600% increase in spirituality and health publications and a 27% increase in religion and health publications from 1993 to 2002.

Some have recommended that physicians and other healthcare providers routinely take religious and spiritual histories of their patients to better understand the patient's religious background, determine how he or she may be using religion to cope with illness, open the door for future discussions about any spiritual or religious issues, and help detect potentially deleterious side effects from religious and spiritual activities (Kuhn, 1988; Lo et al., 2002; Lo, Quill, & Tulsky, 1999; Matthews & Clark, 1998). It may also be a way of detecting spiritual distress (Abrahm, 2001). There has also been greater emphasis in integrating various religious resources and professionals into patient care, especially when the patient is near the end-of-life (Lo et al., 2002). Some efforts have been made to train healthcare providers to listen appropriately to patients' religious concerns, perform clergy-like duties when religious professionals are not available, and better understand spiritual practices (Morse, & Proctor, 1998; Proctor, Morse, & Khonsari, 1996).

Methodological Issues with Clinical Studies

Like most nascent research areas, the study of religion and health has had to contend with lack of adequate funding, institutional support, and training for investigators. These challenges have helped limit the number of well-designed studies in the medical literature. Rather than true scientific studies, many "studies" actually have been anecdotes and editorials, which can galvanize discussions, germinate ideas, and fuel future studies but cannot establish causality or scientifically justify the use of specific interventions. In fact, many of these studies have only been correlational, and while they have demonstrated interesting associations, they have not always controlled for potentially confounding variables, such as socioeconomic status, ethnicity, or different lifestyles or diets. As a result, many such studies have not clearly established causality. In some cases, religious variables were included in a larger study that did not focus on the effects of religion. Since these studies were not necessarily designed and powered primarily to study the religious variables, results must be considered cautiously. There have been a limited number of randomized controlled trials (RCTs). For example, in a systematic review of studies from 1966 to 1999, Townsend, Kladder, Ayele, and Mulligan (2002) counted nine RCTs. But as the study of religion and health progresses, the number and sophistication of scientific studies should continue to grow.

In addition to external challenges, the clinical study of religion has some inherent challenges as well. Understanding these inherent challenges is crucial when either designing or interpreting studies. Otherwise, one may conduct significantly flawed studies, draw inappropriate conclusions, administer unnecessary or even dangerous interventions, pursue the wrong research questions, or neglect to pursue further necessary research. Some common questions include the following.

1. **How do you do you define religion and spirituality?**

"Religion" and "spirituality" are two distinct yet difficult to define terms that many often mistakenly use synonymously (Powell, Shahabi, & Thoresen, 2003; Tanyi, 2002). Even if universal definitions were established, which specific practices would be classified as either or neither? For example, where does one draw the line between religions and cults? In fact, the Merriam Webster Dictionary defines cult as "a religion regarded as unorthodox or spurious." What then is the criterion for being "unorthodox and spurious"? In fact, as history has often demonstrated, what formerly was considered a cult and spurious can eventually become a major religion and vice versa.

2. **Can you recruit and retain enough study subjects?**

Finding appropriate and compliant subjects is not easy. The beliefs and practices relevant to your study may be rare in your vicinity. The further a subject has to travel, the less likely that subject is to participate in your study. Some beliefs and practices may be incompatible with your study design or environment (e.g., some religions do not allow subjects to travel or use electronic devices on certain days). Subjects may be unwilling or unable to alter their religious beliefs and practices for your study.

3. **How do you monitor and maintain subject compliance?**

Many religious and spiritual activities such as prayer and meditation are private, silent, subtle, integrated with, or indistinguishable from social interactions. How do you verify if and how often a subject prays or meditates? How do you ensure that a subject performs a religious or spiritual activity in a "proper" or certain manner? A subject may inadvertently be noncompliant. The environment and other people may influence whether and how a subject behaves. For example, a subject may be more likely to pray when he or she is in a church or surrounded by others who frequently pray.

4. **Which measures of religiousness or spirituality should you use?**

Many possible measures of religiousness and spirituality exist. Someone who scores high in one dimension of religiousness may not necessarily score high in others. For example, individuals who describe themselves as "very religious" (high *subjective religiosity*) may not necessarily score high on more objective measures (low *religious commitment/motivation*). An individual may not participate significantly in formal church, synagogue, or temple activities (low *organizational religiosity*) but may regularly perform private religious activities, such as praying, reading religious scriptures, and watching religious television (high *nonorganizational religiosity*). A number of other potential measures exist, including how closely an individual's beliefs conform to the established doctrines of a religious body (*religious belief*), how knowledgeable or informed an individual is about the doctrines of his or her religion (*religious knowledge*) and how well his or her actions, such as working for the church and acts of altruism, support his or her religion (*religious consequences*). Finally, spirituality and religiousness are not always commensurate, with some individuals considering themselves spiritual and not religious or religious and not spiritual. Thus studies should always clearly state the exact measures used and avoid making claims about measures not used.

5. Is your measure of religiousness accurate and valid?

Directly observing a subject's behavior frequently is the most accurate and valid way of measuring religiousness. For example, you may determine organizational religiosity by measuring how often a person attends church, reads religious scriptures, and prays over a period of time. However, direct observation may not be practical or easy. Shadowing each of your subjects throughout the duration of the study would be incredibly time consuming and expensive. Even if you were able to follow and observe a subject's every move, counting and interpreting such activities can be challenging. You may miss subtle religious displays (e.g., a momentary pause or gesture can represent prayer, meditation, or a religious thought). Moreover, what are the correct units of measure? Is the duration or intensity of an activity more important than the frequency? Is reading scriptures everyday for an hour equivalent to reading scriptures five days a week for four hours? What if someone reads the scriptures as a rote ritual instead of truly feeling connected with what is being read? To establish a true cause and effect relationship, it would be helpful to elicit a dose-response curve, that is, determine if increased religiosity corresponds to better health. Many studies simply divide patients into dichotomous groups (e.g., do they belong to a church?), which do not account for significant variation within each of the two groups. Should certain religious activities be considered more important than others? Someone who does not belong to a church but regularly prays and follows religious doctrine may in fact have greater religious commitment than a person who belongs to a church but does not believe in, or care to comprehend, religious doctrine.

Since direct observation is difficult or impossible across many of these constructs, many investigators have relied on questionnaires or interviews of subjects. As you can imagine, depending on subjects' self-report is problematic. People may consciously or unconsciously misrepresent their actual behavior. Subjects may be forgetful or distracted. Dutifully keeping track of one's activities and thoughts requires significant organization, focus, and compulsiveness. Some patients may be unwilling to admit lapses in religiousness. Moreover, the quality of data depends on the quality of the instrument collecting the data. Poorly worded questions and vague instructions can mislead or confuse subjects. Some questions may not elicit the information they are supposed to produce. Unfortunately, many studies do not indicate whether and how their questionnaires or interviews were tested and validated.

6. How do you treat the positive externalities of religion?

Participating in religious activities can alter a person's life in many ways. Church groups often provide a social support network. Many church activities also function as social and recreational activities. They may offer opportunities for people to exercise and to stay away from unhealthy environments. Through church activities people may meet future spouses, physicians, other healthcare workers, exercise partners, nutritionists, potential employers, or any other individuals that may help their professional and personal lives. Participating in religious activities may offer a reprieve from daily stress. Religion can provide structure and discipline to a person's life. These favorable secondary effects of religious activities (i.e., "positive externalities" of religion) may be responsible for some health benefits. So when a study shows a positive effect of religion, differentiating what is truly responsible for the effect can be difficult.

7. Is a patient's religious activity causing the observed effects on his or her health, or is the patient's health status affecting his or her religious activity?

Establishing the direction of causality can be challenging. A person's health status may influence whether he or she participates in a religious activity. Physical disabilities or problems may prevent a person from traveling to or engaging in certain activities. A person with a contagious disease may not want to expose others. Someone depressed or anxious may feel unmotivated or embarrassed to see others. Conversely, serious health problems may motivate patients to attend religious activities to seek solace or healing.

8. How do you handle the variability among and within different religious affiliations and denominations?

People practice religion in many different ways. For example, prayers may be silent or vocal, restrained or demonstrative, short or long in duration, and performed alone or in groups. Some groups may require specific words to be said or garments to be worn. What constitutes devoted religious behavior in one sect or denomination may be inadequate or irreverent in other sects or denominations. For example, proper dress in one denomination may be sacrilegious in more orthodox denominations.

9. How do you handle hierarchical social aspects of some religions?

Some religions are more hierarchical than others. A person's status within a religious group may affect his or her psychological and physical well-being. Those near the top of the organization may feel more powerful and have many benefits, while those near the bottom may feel more stress or be forced to do unpleasant work. Religious groups vary in how their leaders treat and take care of their members. Different members do not receive equal treatment. A person's degree of acceptance by a given religious group may depend on his or her socioeconomic status, gender, ethnicity, or appearance.

10. What is the role of the cultural context?

Different religions hold different social statuses in different countries during different times. Practically all religions have faced persecution, discrimination, and isolation at some time and place during history. Belonging to the dominant religion in a society can confer greater social acceptance, a stronger and more extensive social network, and more access to resources, all of which can have subtle psychological and physical consequences. Minority religious sects may endure psychological or physical stress or, in some severe cases, physical punishment. Moreover, minority or fringe religious sects that are unable to convince mainstream individuals to join their cause may have to recruit among societal outcasts, many of whom could have psychological or physical illness. Therefore, any study of a specific religious sect should account for the location of the study group, and the sect's relationship with the ambient society.

11. What is a proper time frame for the study?

How long should you follow and observe individuals or populations before seeing any effects? Some spiritual activities, such as prayer, yoga, and meditation, may have immediate effects on physical parameters, such as heart rate and blood pressure. But the potential effects of other religious and spiritual activities may take longer to manifest. Therefore, observing subjects over only a short period of time may miss findings. However, the longer the follow-up, the more difficult the study is to perform and the greater chance that more confounders will enter the picture.

12. Should the research or clinical team be multidisciplinary?

The study of religion and health involves individuals from different disciplines and professions. Ultimately, interdisciplinary research can be more productive than research confined to a single discipline. People from different fields and professions bring different interests, experiences, perspectives, and abilities to the table. However, multidisciplinary research must confront and overcome communicative, administrative, and cultural hurdles. Every discipline and profession has its own language, culture, structure, and motivations. Health researchers and religion researchers often are not familiar with important publications in each other's specialty journals. Separate meetings, separate departments, different methodologies, and different lexicons have hindered collaboration. However, the emergence of interdisciplinary journals and conferences has alleviated this problem.

The Positive Effects of Religion on Health

DISEASE INCIDENCE AND PREVALENCE

Various systematic reviews and meta-analyses have demonstrated that religious involvement correlates with decreased morbidity and mortality (Ball, Armistead, & Austin, 2003; Braam, Beekman, Deeg, Smit, & Van Tilburg, 1999; Brown, 2000; Kark et al., 1996; Kune, Kune, & Watson, 1993; McCullough, Hoyt, Larson, Koenig, & Thoresen, 2000; McCullough & Larson, 1999; Oman, Kurata, Strawbridge, & Cohen, 2002), and high levels of religious involvement may be associated with slightly longer life expectancy (Helm, Hays, Flint, Koenig, & Blazer, 2000; Hummer, Rogers, Nam, & Ellison, 1999; Koenig, 2015; Koenig et al., 1999; Lucchetti, Lucchetti, & Koenig, 2011; Oman & Reed, 1998; Strawbridge, Cohen, Shema, & Kaplan, 1997). A study by Kark and colleagues (1996) over a 16-year period revealed that belonging to a religious collective in Israel was associated with lower mortality. In Comstock and Partridge's (1972) analysis of 91,000 people in a Maryland county, those who regularly attended church had a lower prevalence of cirrhosis, emphysema, suicide, and death from ischemic heart disease. Several studies have implied that religious participation and higher religiosity may have a beneficial effect on blood pressure (Armstrong, van Merwyk, & Coates, 1977; Hixson, Gruchow, & Morgan, 1998; Koenig et al., 1998; Walsh, 1998).

Some studies have suggested that religious individuals may have different mortality and morbidity, even when adjusting for major biological, behavioral, and socioeconomic differences (Rasanen, Kauhanen, Lakka, Kaplan, & Salonen, 1996; Van Poppel, Schellekens, & Liefbroer, 2002). However, as mentioned previously, the experience of individuals within a given religion can depend significantly on the local environment, the person's status within the religious group, and the religious group's status within the surroundings. Therefore, one should interpret the results of such comparisons with caution. For instance, a study of contemplative monks in the Netherlands showed that mortality compared with the general population varied with time during the 1900s (de Gouw, Westendorp, Kunst, Mackenbach, & Vandenbroucke, 1995). Greater morbidity and mortality have been reported among Irish Catholics in Britain, which may reflect their disadvantaged socioeconomic status in that country (Abbotts, Williams, & Ford, 2001; Abbotts, Williams, Ford, Hunt, & West, 1997). A study in Holland suggested that smaller religious groups may be less susceptible to infectious disease because of social isolation (Van Poppel et al., 2002). In general, there have not been enough studies looking at how mortality and morbidity for different religions vary over time and place. Moreover, many religions and religious sects have received little attention from investigators. Consequently, the body of literature comparing morbidity and mortality rates among religions is not large enough to draw any definitive conclusions.

As a whole, broad epidemiological studies that use crude outcome measures such as morbidity and mortality cannot establish causality but suggest that something about religion may protect health. Many study populations may have been too large to account for all possible confounders. Religious participation may be associated with a number of socioeconomic, lifestyle, ethnic, and geographic factors that may affect health. Further, epidemiological studies looking at different subgroups may help refine and define associations.

DISEASE AND SURGICAL OUTCOMES

Many studies have shown that people with higher religiousness may have better outcomes after major illnesses and medical procedures (Koenig, 2015). In Oxman, Freeman, and Manheimer's (1995) analysis of 232 patients following elective open heart surgery, lack of participation in social or community groups, and absence of strength and comfort from religion, were consistent predictors of mortality. In Pressman, Lyons, Larson, and Strain's (1990) look at 30 elderly women after hip repair, religious belief was associated with lower levels of depressive symptoms and better ambulation status. Contrada and colleagues (2004) found that in patients who underwent heart surgery, stronger religious beliefs were associated with shorter hospital stays and fewer complications, but attendance at religious services predicted longer hospitalizations.

On the other hand, Hodges, Humphreys, and Eck (2002) did not find spiritual beliefs to significantly affect recovery from spinal surgery.

Studies have examined whether religiosity improves the survival of patients with different illnesses as well. In a study of African American women with breast cancer, patients who did not belong to a religion tended not to survive as long (Van Ness, Kasl, & Jones, 2003). In a study by Zollinger, Phillips, and Kuzma (1984), Seventh-day Adventists had better breast cancer survival than non-Seventh-day Adventists, but this was probably due to earlier diagnosis and treatment. Several other studies of various cancers, including colorectal, lung, and breast cancer, showed no statistically significant effect of religious involvement on cancer survival (Kune, Kune, & Watson, 1992; Loprinzi et al., 1994; Ringdal, Gotestam, Kaasa, Kvinnsland, & Ringdal, 1996; Yates, Chalmer, St. James, Follansbee, & McKegney, 1981). A study by Blumenthal and colleagues (2007) showed no correlation between post-myocardial infarction outcomes and self-reported spirituality, frequency of church attendance, or frequency of prayer.

GENERAL BEHAVIOR AND LIFESTYLES

Studies have looked at whether people with high religiosity live generally healthier and less risky lifestyles than those with lower religiosity, which may account for some of the observed health benefits of religion. One hypothesis is that religion may provide structure, teaching, role models, and support to individuals, so that they do not have the desire or time to engage in risky behavior. Some studies have supported this hypothesis. The study of Texas adults by Hill, Burdette, Ellison, and Musick (2006) showed that regular religious activity attendance correlated with use of preventive care, vitamins, and seatbelts, decreased bar attendance, and decreased smoking and drinking, walking, strenuous exercise, and sound sleep quality. Oleckno and Blacconiere's (1991) study of college students revealed an inverse correlation between religiosity and behaviors that adversely affect health. Religious involvement is associated with greater use of seat belts (Oleckno & Blacconiere, 1991) and preventative services (Comstock & Partridge, 1972). Compared to the general population, Mormons and Seventh-day Adventists have been found to have lower incidence of and mortality rates from cancers that have been linked to tobacco and alcohol (Fraser, 1999; Grundmann, 1992). A study of diabetic patients in Iran indicated that those individuals who more actively engaged religious practices had improved self care activities (Heidari et al., 2017). Furthermore, the social support derived from religious involvement can help people maintain appropriate diet and nutrition as well as other health related behaviors that can be beneficial (Watkins et al., 2013). However, other studies have shown no relationship, or even an inverse relationship, between religiosity and certain risky behaviors (Hasnain, Sinacore, Mensah, & Levy, 2005; Poulson, Eppler, Satterwhite, Wuensch, & Bass, 1998).

DIET AND NUTRITION

Could dietary differences explain some of the observed health benefits of religion? A 2005 study found that African American women with high religiosity consumed more fruits and vegetables than those with low religiosity (Holt, Haire-Joshu, Lukwago, Lewellyn, & Kreuter, 2005). Studies in Israel showed that compared to religious residents, secular residents had diets higher in total fat and saturated fatty acids (Friedlander, Kark, Kaufmann, & Stein, 1985), and higher plasma levels of cholesterol, triglyceride, and low-density lipoprotein (Friedlander, Kark, & Stein, 1987). Some religions enforce certain specific diets, such as periodic fasting or vegetarianism (Roky, Houti, Moussamih, Qotbi, & Aadil, 2004; Sarri, Linardakis, Codrington, & Kafatos, 2007). For example, a large, prospective epidemiologic study of Seventh-day Adventists revealed that a diet rich in nuts, as advocated by Adventists, was associated with a lower risk of cardiovascular disease (Sabate, 1999). However, the benefits and harms of specific religious diets have not been clearly established.

ALCOHOL, TOBACCO, AND DRUG ABUSE

Religion can affect alcohol and substance use at several stages. It may affect whether a person initiates use, how significant the use becomes, how the use affects the person's life, and whether the person is able to quit and recover (Miller, 1998). The attitudes of religions toward alcohol and substance use vary considerably. Some religious sects strictly prohibit alcohol and substance use (Enstrom & Breslow, 2007). Others are less stringent but discourage excessive use. Some allow the use of alcohol and have incorporated drinking wine into their rituals, and others use psychoactive substances, such as peyote, khat, and hashish to achieve spiritual goals (Lyttle, 1988).

Indeed, some evidence suggests that individuals involved in religion are less likely to use alcohol and other substances (Heath et al., 1999; Luczak, Shea, Carr, Li, & Wall, 2002; Stewart, 2001). Even among alcohol and drug users, religiously involved individuals are more likely to use them moderately and not heavily (Gorsuch & Butler, 1976; Miller, 1998). Leigh, Bowen, and Marlatt's (2005) study of college students revealed that students with higher spirituality scores smoked and binge-drank less frequently. In a nationally representative sample of adolescents, Miller, Davies, and Greenwald (2000) determined that personal devotion—which they defined as a personal relationship with the Divine—and affiliation with more fundamentalist denominations were inversely associated with alcohol and illicit drug use. This effect was seen outside the United States as well, in Latin America (Chen, Dormitzer, Bejarano, & Anthony, 2004). There are a number of possible reasons for these findings. Fear of violating religious principles and doctrines can have a powerful effect. Religions can play a role in educating people about the dangers of alcohol and drugs (Stylianou, 2004). Religious involvement and the accompanying positive externalities may keep people occupied and prevent idleness and boredom that can lead to substance abuse. There may be peer pressure from other members of the church to remain abstinent and an absence of peer pressure to try alcohol and other substances. Moreover, religious involvement could be the effect rather than the cause. Substance abuse may prevent religious involvement. Larson and Wilson (1980) noted that alcoholics compared to nonalcoholic subjects had less involvement in religious practices, less exposure to religious teachings, and fewer religious experiences.

Many, including patients, believe that incorporating religion and spirituality into alcohol, tobacco, and drug cessation programs may enhance their efficacy (Arnold, Avants, Margolin, & Marcotte, 2002; Dermatis, Guschwan, Galanter, & Bunt, 2004). Indeed, spirituality already permeates many established programs, such as Alcoholics Anonymous (AA; Brush & McGee, 2000; Forcehimes, 2004; Li, Feifer, & Strohm, 2000; Moriarity, 2001). Studies have suggested that religious and spiritual practices may aid recovery (Aron & Aron, 1980; Avants, Warburton, & Margolin, 2001; Carter, 1998). A significant number of recovering intravenous drug abusers seem to use religious healing, relaxation techniques, and meditation (Manheimer, Anderson, & Stein, 2003). Data suggests that patients often experience spiritual awakenings or religious conversion during recovery (Green, Fullilove, & Fullilove, 1998). However, not all studies showed that religiously involved patients have better outcomes. The first RCTs failed to demonstrate sufficient clinical benefit from meditation (Murphy, Pagano, & Marlatt, 1986) or intercessory prayer (Walker, Tonigan, Miller, Corner, & Kahlich, 1997). In a study by Tonigan, Miller, and Schermer (2002), while subjects self-labeled as religious were more likely than agnostics and atheists to initiate and continue attending AA meetings, their outcomes were not better.

SEXUAL BEHAVIOR

Some religions may play a role in preventing risky sexual behavior. In a study of African American adolescent females, religiosity correlated with more frank discussions about the risks of sex and avoidance of unsafe sexual situations (McCree, Wingood, DiClemente, Davies, & Harrington, 2003). Miller and Gur's (2002) study of over 3,000 adolescent girls found positive associations between personal devotion and fewer sexual partners outside a romantic relationship, religious event attendance and proper birth control use, and religious event attendance and a better understanding of human immunodeficiency virus or pregnancy risks from unprotected intercourse.

But these findings are not universal. Some have found no relationship between religiosity and sexual practices (Dunne, Lucke, & Raphael, 1994; McCormick, Izzo, & Folcik, 1985). Based on data from the 1995 National Survey of Family Growth, Jones, Darroch, and Singh (2005) concluded that young women with more frequent religious service attendance tended to have delayed first intercourse but did not exhibit significantly different sexual behavior from others once they began having sex. In fact, religious traditions or environments may actually suppress open discussion of sex and contraception. Lefkowitz, Boone, Au, and Sigman (2003) found that adolescents who discussed safe sex with their mothers tended to be less religious.

EXERCISE

Some religious or spiritual practices promote or involve exercise. Religious activities can motivate people to leave their homes, walk to different locations, and participate in physical activities. Some church-related activities, such as softball leagues or dances, involve even more strenuous exercise. Among Utah residents, Merill and Thygerson (2001) found that people who attended church weekly were more likely to exercise regularly. However, differences in smoking and general health status seemed to account for this effect. A study by McLane Lox, Butki, and Stern (2003) suggested incorporating faith-based practices in exercise programs may be attractive to certain people and improve participation in physical activity. To date, church-based initiatives to promote exercise have yielded mixed results (Wilcox et al., 2007; Young & Stewart, 2006).

ACCESS TO HEALTHCARE RESOURCES

Along with encouraging healthy lifestyles, religious groups may promote or provide access to better healthcare and sponsor health improvement programs (e.g., blood pressure screening, blood drives, soup kitchens, and food drives; Heath et al., 1999; Koenig et al., 1998; Stewart, 2001; Zaleski & Schiaffino, 2000). Groups, such as the Catholic Church, have substantial resources and positions that allow them to influence people positively in ways that many secular organizations cannot. Additionally, many hospitals and healthcare clinics are supported by, affiliated with, or even owned by religious groups.

GENERAL MENTAL HEALTH

The impact of religion on mental health has been studied more extensively than the impact of religion on physical health. Studies have demonstrated religiosity to be positively associated with feelings of well-being in White American, Mexican American (Markides, Levin, & Ray, 1987), and African American populations (Coke, 1992), as well as in different age groups (Yoon & Lee, 2007). Krause (2003) observed that older African American individuals were more likely than similarly aged White Americans to derive life satisfaction from religion. Religious service attendance was predictive of higher life satisfaction among elderly Chinese Hong Kong residents (Ho et al., 1995) and elderly Mexican American women (Levin & Markides, 1988). Members of religious kibutzes in Israel reported a higher sense of coherence and less hostility and were more likely to engage in volunteer work than nonmembers (Kark, Carmel, Sinnreich, Goldberger, & Friedlander, 1996). Similar findings occurred in a population of nursing home residents (House, Robbins, & Metzner, 1982). Hope and optimism seemed to run higher among religious individuals than nonreligious individuals in some study populations (Idler & Kasl, 1997a, 1997b; Raleigh, 1992). Using religious attendance as one of the markers of social engagement, Bassuk, Glass, and Berkman (1999) determined that social disengagement was linked with cognitive decline in the noninstitutionalized elderly.

A few studies compared different religions. For example, one study showed that among elderly women in Hong Kong, Catholics and Buddhists enjoyed better mental health status than Protestants (Boey, 2003). However, not enough data exist to generate meaningful conclusions.

Experiences often considered religious, spiritual, or mystical (RSMEs) have also been shown to relate to mental health in complex ways. While RSMEs can sometimes have pathological features, they seem to result in positive outcomes more often (Yaden, McCall, Ellens, 2015; Yaden et al., 2015; Yaden, Iwry, et al., 2016; Yaden, Le Nguyen, et al., 2016). Neurobiological aspects of RSMEs have also been investigated (Newberg et al., 2001; Newberg et al., 2015), with a consistent finding that parietal regions related to spatial awareness are affected, among many others (for reviews see Newberg & Iversen, 2003; Yaden, Iwry, & Newberg, 2016).

DEPRESSION

A number of investigators have looked at the effects of religion on depression. Prospective cohort studies have shown religious activity to be associated with remission of depression in Protestant and Catholic Netherlanders (Braam, Beekman, Deeg, Smit, van Tilburg, 1997) and in ill older adults (Koenig, George, & Peterson, 1998). Prospective studies have also found religious activity to be strongly protective against depression in Protestant and Catholic offspring who share the same religion as their mother (Miller, Warner, Wickramaratne, & Weissman, 1997) and weakly protective in female twins (Kennedy, Kelman, Thomas, & Chen, 1996). Cross-sectional studies have yielded significant (Koenig et al., 1997) and nonsignificant (Bienenfeld, Koenig, Larson, & Sherrill, 1997; Koenig, 1998; Musick, Koenig, Hays, & Cohen, 1998) associations between different indicators of religiosity and a lower prevalence of depression in various populations. Chen, Cheal, McDonel Herr, Zubritsky, and Levkoff (2007) found that in patients already diagnosed with depression, religious participation may lead to better outcomes.

Studies also have suggested an inverse correlation between religiosity and suicide. This was found to be the case in Nisbet, Duberstein, Conwell, and Seidlitz's (2000) analysis of 1993 National Mortality Followback Survey data and Neeleman and Lewis's (1999) analysis of cross-sectional data of Judaeo-Christian older adults from 26 countries. Suicide may be less acceptable to people with high religious devotion and orthodox religious beliefs (Neeleman, Halpern, Leon, & Lewis, 1997; Neeleman, Wessely, & Lewis, 1998). But again, it is unclear whether suicidal individuals are less likely to hold strong religious beliefs or individuals with strong religious beliefs are less likely to be suicidal.

Several RCTs have been performed. One RCT demonstrated that directed and nondirected intercessory prayer correlated favorably with multiple measures of self-esteem, anxiety, and depression but did not clearly state the randomization technique and did not account for multiple confounders (O'Laoire, 1997). Another RCT suggested that using religion-based cognitive therapy had a favorable impact on Christian patients with clinical depression but may have contained too many comparison groups for strong cause-and-effect relationships to be established (Propst, Ostrom, Watkins, Dean, & Mashburn, 1992). Three RCTs suggested that religious (Islamic-based) psychotherapy appeared to speed recovery from anxiety and depression in Muslim Malays but did not control for the use of antidepressants and benzodiazepines (Azhar & Varma, 1995; Azhar, Varma, & Dharap, 1994; Razali, Hasanah, Aminah, & Subramaniam, 1998).

COPING WITH MEDICAL PROBLEMS

Religious belief may provide meaning to and, in turn, help patients better cope with their diseases (Autiero, 1987; Foley, 1988; Patel, Shah, Peterson, & Kimmel, 2002). Although many major religions have deemed illness and suffering the result of sin, many believe that pain and suffering can be strengthening, enlightening, and purifying. According to various religious teachings, pain and suffering are inevitable and can be cleansing, test virtue, educate, readjust priorities, stimulate personal growth, and define human life (Amundsen, 1982).

Different religions may differ in how they confront suffering. While generalizations are difficult to draw since considerable variability exists within each religion, many Buddhists believe in enduring pain matter-of-factly (Tu, 1980), many Hindus stress understanding and detachment from pain (Shaffer, 1978), many Muslims and Jews favor resisting or fighting pain (Bowker, 1978), and many Christians stress seeking atonement and redemption (Amundsen, 1982). Though it is worth reiterating that substantial differences exist within each group, limiting the value of broad generalizations.

Evidence suggests that religion provides more than just a distraction from suffering. The "diverting attention" and "praying" factors on the Coping Strategies Questionnaire have correlated with pain levels (Geisser et al., 1994; Swartzman, Gwadry, Shapiro, & Teasell, 1994; Swimmer, Robinson, & Geisser, 1992). The social network and support provided by religions may be associated with lower pain levels, and religious belief may improve self-esteem and sense of purpose (Hays et al., 1998; Musick et al., 1998; Swimmer et al., 1992). After following 720 adults, Williams, Larson, Buckler, Heckmann, and Pyle (1991) concluded that religious attendance buffered the effects of stress on mental health. In Coward's (1991) study of 107 women with advanced breast cancer, spirituality appeared to improve emotional well-being.

The Negative Effects of Religion on Health

Although most studies have shown positive effects, religion and spirituality also may negatively impact health. For example, religious groups may directly oppose certain healthcare interventions, such as transfusions or contraception, and convince patients that their ailments are due to noncompliance with religious doctrines rather than to organic disease (Donahue, 1985). Asser and Swan (1998) demonstrated that a large number of child fatalities could have been prevented had medical care not been withheld for religious reasons. After interviewing 682 North Carolina women, Mitchell, Lannin, Mathews, and Swanson (2002) concluded that belief in religious intervention may delay African American women from seeing their physicians for breast lumps. In addition, religions can stigmatize those with certain diseases to the point that they do not seek proper medical care (Lichtenstein, 2003; Madru, 2003).

Moreover, as history has shown, religion can be the source of military conflicts, prejudice, violent behaviors, and other social problems. Religions may ignore, sterotype, ostracize, or abuse those who do not belong to their church. Those not belonging to a dominant religion may face obstacles to obtaining resources hardships, and stress that deleteriously affect their health (Bywaters, Ali, Fazil, Wallace, & Singh, 2003; Walls & Williams, 2004). Religious leaders may abuse their own members physically, emotionally, or sexually (Rossetti, 1995; Tieman, 2002). Religious laws or dictums may be invoked to justify harmful, oppressive, and injurious behavior (Kernberg, 2003).

Additionally, perceived religious transgressions can cause emotional and psychological anguish, manifesting as physical discomfort. This "religious" and "spiritual pain" can be difficult to distinguish from pure physical pain (Satterly, 2001). In extreme cases, spiritual abuse—convincing people that they are going to suffer eternal purgatory—and spiritual terrorism—an extreme form of spiritual abuse—can occur either overtly or insidiously; that is, it can be implied, though not actually stated, that a patient will be doomed (Purcell, 1998a, 1998b). When a mix of religious, spiritual, and organic sources is causing physical illness, treatment can become complicated. Healthcare workers must properly balance treating each source.

The Effects of Specific Religious and Spiritual Activities

Religious and spiritual activities have become highly prevalent and may be practiced in either a religious or a secular manner. Although many of these activities have been correctly or incorrectly linked to specific religions, practicing them does not necessarily connote certain beliefs. In fact, hundreds of variations of each spiritual activity exist, since many have been altered and combined with other activities, such as aerobics, to develop hybrid techniques.

As a result, some forms barely resemble the original versions. Thus investigators must be very specific in describing the technique or activity that they are examining. Results from one form of meditation or yoga may not apply to other forms. A review of literature shows that many studies do not clearly describe the form of spiritual activity under investigation.

PRAYER

In Eisenberg and colleagues' (1998) survey of alternative medicine usage among Americans, one-fourth of respondents used prayer to cope with physical illness. There is evidence that prayer may be associated with less muscle tension, improved cardiovascular and neuroimmunologic parameters, psychologic and spiritual peace, a greater sense of purpose, enhanced coping skills, less disability, and better physical function in patients with knee pain (Rapp, Rejeski, & Miller, 2000) and a lower incidence of coronary heart disease (Gupta, 1996; Gupta, Prakash, Gupta, & Gupta, 1997).

Poloma and Pendleton (1991) found that *petitionary* and *ritualistic prayers* were associated with lower levels of well-being and life satisfaction, while *colloquial prayers* were associated with higher levels. Leibovici (2001) reported on a double-blinded RCT that showed that remote, retroactive intercessory prayer was associated with shorter length of fever and hospital stay in patients with bloodstream infection. A very small, limited double-blind study showed that intercessory prayer used as adjunct therapy appeared to decrease mortality among children with leukemia (Collipp, 1969). In Byrd's (1988) double-blind study of patients admitted to a coronary care unit, *intercessory prayer* was linked to significantly more "good" outcomes (163 versus 147) than "bad" outcomes (27 versus 44). Harris and colleagues (1999) found similar outcomes with remote *intercessory prayer*. However, similar subsequent studies were not able to replicate these findings (Aviles et al., 2001; Matthews, Conti, & Sireci, 2001; Matthews, Marlowe, & MacNutt, 2000; Townsend, Kladder, Ayele, Mulligan, 2002). Interestingly, the Study of the Therapeutic Effects of Intercessory Prayer, a multicenter randomized clinical trial, showed that patients who knew that they were receiving intercessory prayer had worse postcoronary artery bypass graft surgery outcomes than patients who did not receive intercessory prayer. The same study showed no difference between patients who unknowingly received intercessory prayer and patients who did not receive intercessory prayer (Benson et al., 2006). In fact, a Cochrane systematic review of all major studies on intercessory prayer yielded equivocal results, precluding any definitive conclusions (Roberts, Ahmed, & Hall, 2007).

MEDITATION

Meditation and meditation-related practices are widely used as alternative therapy for physical ailments (Eisenberg et al., 1998). Many physicians routinely recommend meditation techniques to their patients and include them as part of integrated health programs, such as Dean Ornish's popular heart disease programs and a Stanford arthritis self-care course. Meditative and relaxation techniques are often part of childbirth preparation classes.

While evidence is not yet definitive, preliminary studies suggest that meditation may have a number of health benefits, helping people achieve a state of restful alertness with improved reaction time, creativity, and comprehension (Domino, 1977; Solberg, Berglund, Engen, Ekeberg, & Loeb, 1996); decreasing anxiety, depression, irritability, and moodiness; and improving learning ability, memory, self-actualization, feelings of vitality and rejuvenation, and emotional stability (Astin, 1977; Astin et al., 2003; Bitner, Hillman, Victor, & Walsh, 2003; Jain et al., 2007; Solberg et al., 1996; Walton, Pugh, Gelderloos, & Macrae, 1995). Preliminary studies suggest that meditative practices may benefit and provide acute and chronic support for patients with hypertension, psoriasis, irritable bowel disease, anxiety, epilepsy, premenstrual symptoms, menopausal symptoms, and depression (Arias, Steinberg, Banga, & Trestman, 2006; Barrows & Jacobs, 2002; Castillo-Richmond et al., 2000; Jacobs, Carlson, Ursuliak, Goodey, Angen, & Speca, 2001; Kabat-Zinn et al., 1992, 1998; Kaplan, Goldenberg, & Galvin-Nadeau, 1993; Keefer & Blanchard, 2002; King, Carr, & D'Cruz, 2002; Manocha, Marks, Kenchington, Peters, & Salome, 2002; Reibel, Greeson, Brainard, & Rosenzweig, 2001; Williams, Kolar, Reger, & Pearson, 2001). There is also evidence that meditation can improve chronic pain (Kabat-Zinn, 1982; Kabat-Zinn, Lipworth, & Burney, 1985). In a study by Kaplan and colleagues, all 77 men and women with fibromyalgia who completed a 10-week stress-reduction program using meditation had symptom improvement. Moreover, in several studies, meditators had better respiratory function (vital capacity, tidal volume, expiratory pressure, and breath holding), cardiovascular parameters (diastolic blood pressure and heart rate), and lipid profiles than nonmeditators (Cooper & Aygen, 1979; Wallace, Silver, Mills, Dillbeck, & Wagoner, 1983; Wenneberg et al., 1997).

Unfortunately, many studies did not specify or describe the type of meditation used. A wide variety of methods may be used, including some in which the body is immobile (e.g., Zazen, Vipassana), others in which the body is let free (e.g., siddha yoga, the Latihan, the chaotic meditation of Rajneesh), and still others in which the person participates in daily activities while meditating (e.g., Mahamudra, Shikan Taza, Gurdjieff's "self-remembering"). So it is not clear which forms may be beneficial and what aspects of meditation are providing the benefits.

Although physically noninvasive, meditation can be harmful in patients with psychiatric illness, potentially aggravating and precipitating psychotic episodes in delusional or strongly paranoid patients and heightening anxiety in patients with overwhelming anxiety. Moreover, it can trigger the release of repressed memories. Therefore, all patients using meditative techniques should be monitored, especially when a patient first starts using meditation.

YOGA

Yoga has become a popular practice and is often used for physical exercise as well as spiritual or religious practice. The American Yoga Association emphasizes that it can be compatible with all major religions since yoga practice does not specify particular higher powers or religious doctrines. In fact, many religions, including many Christian denominations, have adopted yoga techniques.

Yoga practitioners use a series of stretching, breathing, and relaxation techniques to prepare for meditation and use stretching movements or postures (*asanas*) that aim to increase blood supply and *prana* (vital force) as well as increase the flexibility of the spine, which is thought to improve the nerve supply. They also use breathing techniques (*pranayamas*) to try to improve brain function, eliminate toxins, and store reserve energy in the solar plexus region.

Some clinical studies on yoga have been encouraging, showing reduced serum total cholesterol, LDL cholesterol, and triglyceride levels; decreased basal metabolic rates; and improved pulmonary function tests in yoga practitioners (Arambula, Peper, Kawakami, & Gibney, 2001; Birkel, & Edgren, 2000; Chaya, Kurpad, Nagendra, & Nagarathna, 2006; Sarang & Telles, 2006; Schell, Allolio, & Schonecke, 1994; Selvamurthy et al., 1998; Stancak, Kuna, Srinivasan, Dostalek, & Vishnudevananda, 1991; Stanescu, Nemery, Veriter, & Marechal, 1981; Udupa, Singh, & Yadav, 1973). They also suggest that yoga may be associated with acute- and long-term decreases in blood pressure (Murugesan, Govindarajulu, & Bera, 2000; Sundar et al., 1984) and acute increases in brain gamma-aminobutyric levels (Streeter et al., 2007). Preliminary evidence indicates that yoga may benefit patients with asthma, hypertension, heart failure, mood disorders, insomnia, migraine headaches, irritable bowel syndrome, end-stage renal disease, and diabetes (Jain, Uppal, Bhatnagar, & Talukdar, 1993; John, Sharma, Sharma, & Kankane, 2007; Khalsa, 2004; Kuttner et al., 2006;

Malhotra, Singh, Singh, et al., 2002; Malhotra, Singh, Tandon, et al., 2002; Manocha et al., 2002; van Montfrans, Karemaker, Wieling, & Dunning, 1990a; Yurtkuran, Alp, & Dilek, 2007) and improve pregnancy outcomes (Narendran, Nagarathna, Narendran, Gunasheela, & Nagendra, 2005). Two small controlled but nondouble-blinded studies showed hatha yoga to significantly alleviate pain in osteoarthritis of the fingers and in carpal tunnel syndrome (Garfinkel et al., 1998; Garfinkel, Schumacher, Husain, Levy, & Reshetar, 1994). However, yoga is not completely benign, as certain asanas may be strenuous and cause injury. In fact, yoga practitioners believe some asanas cause disease.

More studies are needed to determine the benefits (and potential dangers) of yoga. Like meditation, many forms of yoga have emerged. Some involve significant aerobic exercise. Others involve significant strength and conditioning work. Many yoga practices include changes in diet and lifestyles. It may be difficult to draw the line between yoga and other practices that have established health benefits, such as exercise. Therefore, future studies should focus on specific yoga forms and movements and avoid making general conclusions about all yoga practices.

FAITH HEALING

Faith healers use prayer or other religious practices to combat disease. Surveys have found that a fair number of patients in rural (21%) and inner city (10%) populations have used faith healers, and many physicians (23%) believe that faith healers can heal patients (McKee & Chappel, 1992). Despite numerous anecdotes of healing miracles, there has been no convincing scientific proof that faith healers are effective (King & Bushwick, 1994). Additionally, it has not been determined whether faith healers affect patients psychologically or physiologically through mechanisms such as the placebo effect.

Conclusion and Future Directions

Existing evidence suggests that religious and spiritual practices may have beneficial effects on health. But the reasons behind these findings are not clearly understood. It appears that religious and spiritual practices can bring social and emotional support, motivation, healthy lifestyles, and healthcare resources to their practitioners. However, are there other mechanisms involved? The medical world is just starting to answer this question.

In general, performing clinical studies that can establish cause-and-effect relationships is difficult. This is especially true in the study of religion and health. Confounding factors abound. Religious and spiritual doctrines and practices vary significantly among and within different sects and denominations. Other challenges include measuring religious and spiritual activity and monitoring and ensuring compliance among study subjects. Moreover, available resources, properly-trained investigators, and institutional support for clinical studies have been scarce. As a result, the current body of medical literature lacks many well-designed clinical studies.

Future studies should address a number of different issues. What are the roles of different potential confounding factors? What physiologic mechanisms may be involved? What are the clinical implications of existing physiologic studies? How much does a person's health affect his or her ability to engage in religious and spiritual activities? Do findings hold across different practices, sects, and denominations? Existing studies have only looked at a limited population of religious groups and sects. What are the effects of varying demographic parameters, such as age, gender, and location? Do different practices affect disease progression? Many practices and diseases have not been studied. How should religious and spiritual issues be incorporated into the healthcare system?

The findings to date already have clinical implications. Religion and spirituality are clearly important to many patients. Healthcare providers may need to better address patients' religious concerns and be aware of how religious involvement can affect patients' symptoms, quality of life, and willingness to receive treatment. Moreover, religious and spiritual activities may serve as adjunct therapy in various disease and addiction treatment programs. The future may see the development of more specific spiritual interventions for particular medical problems.

In the coming years, the study of religion and health, as well as the integration of religion into healthcare, should continue to grow. New research methods, designs, techniques, and instruments may emerge. As long as the worlds of religion, science, and healthcare cooperate, many exciting new findings may appear in coming decades, hopefully for the betterment of all.

REFERENCES

Abbotts, J., Williams, R., & Ford, G. (2001). Morbidity and Irish Catholic descent in Britain: Relating health disadvantage to socio-economic position. *Social Science & Medicine, 52,* 999–1005.

Abbotts, J., Williams, R., Ford, G., Hunt, K., & West, P. (1997). Morbidity and Irish Catholic descent in Britain, an ethnic and religious minority 150 years on. *Social Science & Medicine, 45,* 3–14.

Abrahm, J. (2001). Pain management for dying patients: How to assess needs and provide pharmacologic relief. *Postgraduate Medicine, 110*, 99–100, 108–109, 113–114.

Amundsen, D. W. (1982). Medicine and faith in early Christianity. *Bulletin of the History of Medicine, 56*, 326–350.

Arambula, P., Peper, E., Kawakami, M., & Gibney, K. H. (2001). The physiological correlates of Kundalini Yoga meditation: A study of a yoga master. *Applied Psychophysiology and Biofeedback. 26*, 147–153.

Arias, A. J., Steinberg, K., Banga, A., & Trestman, R. L. (2006). Systematic review of the efficacy of meditation techniques as treatments for medical illness. *Journal of Alternative and Complementary Medicine, 12*, 817–832.

Armbruster, C. A., Chibnall, J. T., & Legett, S. (2003). Pediatrician beliefs about spirituality and religion in medicine: Associations with clinical practice. *Pediatrics, 111*, e227–e235.

Armstrong, B., van Merwyk, A. J., & Coates, H. (1977). Blood pressure in Seventh-day Adventist vegetarians. *American Journal of Epidemiology, 105*, 444–449.

Arnold, R., Avants, S. K., Margolin, A., & Marcotte, D. (2002). Patient attitudes concerning the inclusion of spirituality into addiction treatment. *Journal of Substance Abuse Treatment, 23*, 319–326.

Aron, A., & Aron, E. N. (1980). The transcendental meditation program's effect on addictive behavior. *Addictive Behaviors, 5*, 3–12.

Asser, S. M., & Swan, R. (1998). Child fatalities from religion-motivated medical neglect. *Pediatrics, 101*, 625–629.

Astin, J. A. (1997). Stress reduction through mindfulness meditation: Effects on psychological symptomatology, sense of control, and spiritual experiences. *Psychotherapy and Psychosomatics, 66*, 97–106.

Astin, J. A., Berman, B. M., Bausell, B., Lee, W. L., Hochberg, M., & Forys, K. L. (2003). The efficacy of mindfulness meditation plus Qigong movement therapy in the treatment of fibromyalgia: A randomized controlled trial. *Journal of Rheumatology, 30*, 2257–2262.

Autiero, A. (1987). The interpretation of pain: The point of view of Catholic theology. *Acta Neurochirurgica Supplement, 38*, 123–126.

Avants, S. K., Warburton, L. A., & Margolin, A. (2001). Spiritual and religious support in recovery from addiction among HIV-positive injection drug users. *Journal of Psychoactive Drugs, 33*, 39–45.

Aviles, J. M., Whelan, S. E., Hernke, D. A., Williams, B. A., Kenny, K. E., O'Fallon, W. M., & Kopecky, S. L. (2001). Intercessory prayer and cardiovascular disease progression in a coronary care unit population: A randomized controlled trial. *Mayo Clinic Proceedings, 76*, 1192–1198.

Azhar, M. Z., & Varma, S. L. (1995). Religious psychotherapy in depressive patients. *Psychotherapy and Psychosomatics, 63*, 165–168.

Azhar, M. Z., Varma, S. L., & Dharap, A. S. (1994). Religious psychotherapy in anxiety disorder patients. *Acta Psychiatrica Scandinavica, 90*, 1–3.

Ball, J., Armistead, L., & Austin, B. J. (2003). The relationship between religiosity and adjustment among African-American, female, urban adolescents. *Journal of Adolescence, 26*, 431–446.

Barrows, K. A., & Jacobs, B. P. (2002). Mind-body medicine: An introduction and review of the literature. *Medical Clinics of North America, 86,* 11–31.

Bassuk, S. S., Glass, T. A., & Berkman, L. F. (1999). Social disengagement and incident cognitive decline in community-dwelling elderly persons. *Annals of Internal Medicine, 131,* 165–173.

Begley, S. (2001a). Religion and the brain. *Newsweek, 137,* 50–57.

Begley, S. (2001b). Searching for the God within. *Newsweek, 137,* 59.

Benson, H., Dusek, J. A., Sherwood, J. B., Lam, P., Bethea, C. F., Carpenter, W., et al. (2006). Study of the Therapeutic Effects of Intercessory Prayer (STEP) in cardiac bypass patients: A multicenter randomized trial of uncertainty and certainty of receiving intercessory prayer. *American Heart Journal, 151,* 934–942.

Bezilla, R. (Ed.). (1992–1993). *Religion in America.* Princeton, NJ: Princeton Religious Center.

Bienenfeld, D., Koenig, H. G., Larson, D. B., & Sherrill, K. A. (1997). Psychosocial predictors of mental health in a population of elderly women: Test of an explanatory model. *American Journal of Geriatric Psychiatry, 5,* 43–53.

Birkel, D. A., & Edgren, L. (2000). Hatha yoga: Improved vital capacity of college students. *Alternative Therapies in Health and Medicine, 6,* 55–63.

Bitner, R., Hillman, L., Victor, B., & Walsh, R. (2003). Subjective effects of antidepressants: A pilot study of the varieties of antidepressant-induced experiences in meditators. *Journal of Nervous and Mental Disease, 191,* 660–667.

Blumenthal, J. A., Babyak, M. A., Ironson, G., Thoresen, C., Powell, L., Czajkowski, S., et al. (2007). Spirituality, religion, and clinical outcomes in patients recovering from an acute myocardial infarction. *Psychosomatic Medicine, 69,* 501–508.

Boey, K. W. (2003). Religiosity and psychological well-being of older women in Hong Kong. *International Journal of Psychiatric Nursing Research, 8,* 921–935.

Bowker, D. (1978). Pain and suffering: Religious perspective. In W. T. Reich (Ed.), *Encyclopedia of bioethics* (pp. 1185–1189). New York: Free Press.

Braam, A. W., Beekman, A. T., Deeg, D. J., Smit, J. H., & van Tilburg, W. (1997). Religiosity as a protective or prognostic factor of depression in later life: Results from a community survey in The Netherlands. *Acta Psychiatrica Scandinavica, 96,* 199–205.

Braam, A., Beekman, A. T., Deeg, D. J., Smit, J. H., & van Tilburg, W. (1999). Religiosity as a protective factor in depressive disorder. *American Journal of Psychiatry, 156,* 809; author reply 10.

Brown, C. M. (2000). Exploring the role of religiosity in hypertension management among African Americans. *Journal of Health Care for the Poor and Underserved, 11,* 19–32.

Brush, B. L., & McGee, E. M. (2000). Evaluating the spiritual perspectives of homeless men in recovery. *Applied Nursing Research, 13,* 181–186.

Byrd, R. C. (1988). Positive therapeutic effects of intercessory prayer in a coronary care unit population. *Southern Medical Journal, 81,* 826–829.

Bywaters, P., Ali, Z., Fazil, Q., Wallace, L. M., & Singh, G. (2003). Attitudes towards disability amongst Pakistani and Bangladeshi parents of disabled children in the

UK: Considerations for service providers and the disability movement. *Journal of Health Care for the Poor and Underserved, 11*, 502–509.

Carlson, L. E., Ursuliak, Z., Goodey, E., Angen, M., & Speca, M. (2001). The effects of a mindfulness meditation-based stress reduction program on mood and symptoms of stress in cancer outpatients: 6-month follow-up. *Support Care Cancer, 9*, 112–123.

Carter, T. M. (1998). The effects of spiritual practices on recovery from substance abuse. *Journal of Psychiatric and Mental Health Nursing, 5*, 409–413.

Castillo-Richmond, A., Schneider, R. H., Alexander, C. N., Cook, R., Myers, H., Nidich, S., et al. (2000). Effects of stress reduction on carotid atherosclerosis in hypertensive African Americans. *Stroke, 31*, 568–573.

Chaya, M. S., Kurpad, A. V., Nagendra, H. R., & Nagarathna, R. (2006). The effect of long term combined yoga practice on the basal metabolic rate of healthy adults. *BMC Complementary and Alternative Medicine, 6*, 28.

Chen, C. Y., Dormitzer, C. M., Bejarano, J., & Anthony, J. C. (2004). Religiosity and the earliest stages of adolescent drug involvement in seven countries of Latin America. *American Journal of Epidemiology, 159*, 1180–1188.

Chen, H., Cheal, K., McDonel Herr, E. C., Zubritsky, C., & Levkoff, S. E. (2007). Religious participation as a predictor of mental health status and treatment outcomes in older persons. *International Journal of Geriatric Psychiatry, 22*, 144–153.

Chibnall, J. T., & Brooks, C. A. (2001). Religion in the clinic: The role of physician beliefs. *Southern Medical Journal, 94*, 374–379.

Coke, M. M. (1992). Correlates of life satisfaction among elderly African Americans. *Journal of Gerontology, 47*, P316–P320.

Collipp, P. J. (1969). The efficacy of prayer: A triple-blind study. *Medical Times, 97*, 201–204.

Comstock, G. W., & Partridge, K. B. (1972). Church attendance and health. *Journal of Chronic Diseases, 25*, 665–672.

Contrada, R. J., Goyal, T. M., Cather, C., Rafalson, L., Idler, E. L., & Krause, T. J. (2004). Psychosocial factors in outcomes of heart surgery: The impact of religious involvement and depressive symptoms. *Health Psychology, 23*, 227–238.

Cooper, M. J., & Aygen, M. M. (1979). A relaxation technique in the management of hypercholesterolemia. *Journal of Human Stress, 5*, 24–27.

Corliss, R. (2001). The power of yoga. *Time, 157*, 54–63.

Coward, D. D. (1991). Self-transcendence and emotional well-being in women with advanced breast cancer. *Oncology Nursing Forum, 18*, 857–863.

Daaleman, T. P., & Nease, D. E. Jr. (1994). Patient attitudes regarding physician inquiry into spiritual and religious issues. *Journal of Family Practice, 39*, 564–568.

de Gouw, H. W., Westendorp, R. G., Kunst, A. E., Mackenbach, J. P., & Vandenbroucke, J. P. (1995). Decreased mortality among contemplative monks in The Netherlands. *American Journal of Epidemiology, 141*, 771–775.

Dermatis, H., Guschwan, M. T., Galanter, M., & Bunt, G. (2004). Orientation toward spirituality and self-help approaches in the therapeutic community. *Journal of Addictive Diseases, 23*, 39–54.

Domino, G. (1977). Transcendental meditation and creativity: An empirical investigation. *Journal of Applied Psychology, 62,* 358–362.

Donahue, M. J. (1985). Intrinsic and extrinsic religiousness: Review and meta-analysis. *Journal of Personality and Social Psychology, 48,* 400–419.

Dunne, M. P., Edwards, R., Lucke, J., Donald, M., & Raphael, B. (1994). Religiosity, sexual intercourse and condom use among university students. *Australian Journal of Public Health, 18,* 339–341.

Eisenberg, D. M., Davis, R. B., Ettner, S. L., Appel, S., Wilkey, S., Van Rompay, M., & Kessler, R. C. (1998). Trends in alternative medicine use in the United States, 1990-1997: Results of a follow-up national survey. *Journal of American Medical Association, 280,* 1569–1575.

Ellis, M. R., Vinson, D. C., & Ewigman, B. (1999). Addressing spiritual concerns of patients: Family physicians' attitudes and practices. *Journal of Family Practice, 48,* 105–109.

Enstrom, J. E., & Breslow, L. (2007). Lifestyle and reduced mortality among active California Mormons, 1980-2004. *Preventive Medicine, 46*(2), 133–136.

Foley, D. P. (1988). Eleven interpretations of personal suffering. *Journal of Religion and Health, 27,* 321–328.

Forcehimes, A. A. (2004). De profundis: Spiritual transformations in Alcoholics Anonymous. *Journal of Clinical Psychology, 60,* 503–517.

Fraser, G. E. (1999). Associations between diet and cancer, ischemic heart disease, and all-cause mortality in non-Hispanic white California Seventh-day Adventists. *American Journal of Clinical Nutrition, 70,* 532S–538S.

Friedlander, Y., Kark, J. D., Kaufmann, N. A., & Stein, Y. (1985). Coronary heart disease risk factors among religious groupings in a Jewish population sample in Jerusalem. *American Journal of Clinical Nutrition, 42,* 511–521.

Friedlander, Y., Kark, J. D., & Stein, Y. (1987). Religious observance and plasma lipids and lipoproteins among 17-year-old Jewish residents of Jerusalem. *Preventive Medicine, 16,* 70–79.

Garfinkel, M. S., Schumacher, H. R., Jr., Husain, A., Levy, M., & Reshetar, R. A. (1994). Evaluation of a yoga based regimen for treatment of osteoarthritis of the hands. *Journal of Rheumatology, 21,* 2341–2343.

Garfinkel, M. S., Singhal, A., Katz, W. A., Allan, D. A., Reshetar, R., & Schumacher, H. R. Jr. (1998). Yoga-based intervention for carpal tunnel syndrome: A randomized trial. *Journal of American Medical Association, 280,* 1601–1603.

Geisser, M. E., Robinson, M. E., & Henson, C. D. (1994). The Coping Strategies Questionnaire and chronic pain adjustment: A conceptual and empirical reanalysis. *Clinical Journal of Pain, 10,* 98–106.

Gorsuch, R. L., & Butler, M. C. (1976). Initial drug abuse: A review of predisposing social psychological factors. *Psychological Bulletin, 83,* 120–137.

Green, L. L., Fullilove, M. T., & Fullilove, R. E. (1998). Stories of spiritual awakening: The nature of spirituality in recovery. *Journal of Substance Abuse Treatment, 15,* 325–331.

Greenwald, J. (2001). Alternative medicine: A new breed of healers. *Time, 157,* 62–65, 68–69.

Grundmann, E. (1992). Cancer morbidity and mortality in USA Mormons and Seventh-day Adventists. *Archives d'Anatomie Et De Cytologie Pathologiques, 40*, 73–78.

Gupta, R. (1996). Lifestyle risk factors and coronary heart disease prevalence in Indian men. *Journal of the Association of Physicians of India, 44*, 689–693.

Gupta, R., Prakash, H., Gupta, V. P., & Gupta, K. D. (1997). Prevalence and determinants of coronary heart disease in a rural population of India. *Journal of Clinical Epidemiology, 50*, 203–209.

Harris, W. S., Gowda, M., Kolb, J. W., Strychacz, C. P., Vacek, J. L., Jones, P. G., et al. (1999). A randomized, controlled trial of the effects of remote, intercessory prayer on outcomes in patients admitted to the coronary care unit. *Archives of Internal Medicine, 159*, 2273–2278.

Hasnain, M., Sinacore, J. M., Mensah, E. K., & Levy, J. A. (2005). Influence of religiosity on HIV risk behaviors in active injection drug users. *AIDS Care, 17*, 892–901.

Hays, J. C., Landerman, L. R., George, L. K., Flint, E. P., Koenig, H. G., et al. (1998). Social Correlates of the Dimensions of Depression in the Elderly. *The Journal of Gerontology: Series B, Psychological Sciences and Social Sciences, 53*, P31–39.

Heath, A. C., Madden, P. A., Grant, J. D., McLaughlin, T. L, Todorov, A. A., & Bucholz, K. K. (1999). Resiliency factors protecting against teenage alcohol use and smoking: Influences of religion, religious involvement and values, and ethnicity in the Missouri Adolescent Female Twin Study. *Twin Research, 2*, 145–155.

Heidari, S., Rezaei, M., Sajadi, M., Ajorpaz, N. M., & Koenig, H. G. (2017). Religious practices and self-care in Iranian patients with type 2 diabetes. *Journal of Religion and Health, 56*(2), 683–696.

Helm, H. M., Hays, J. C., Flint, E. P., Koenig, H. G., & Blazer, D. G. (2000). Does private religious activity prolong survival? A six-year follow-up study of 3,851 older adults. *Journals of Gerontology. Series A Biological Sciences and Medical Sciences, 55*, M400–M405.

Hill, T. D., Burdette, A. M., Ellison, C. G., & Musick, M. A. (2006). Religious attendance and the health behaviors of Texas adults. *Preventive Medicine, 42*, 309–312.

Hixson, K. A., Gruchow, H. W., & Morgan, D. W. (1998). The relation between religiosity, selected health behaviors, and blood pressure among adult females. *Preventive Medicine, 27*, 545–552.

Ho, S. C., Woo, J., Lau, J., Chan, S. G., Yuen, Y. K., & Chan, Y. K., & Chi, I. (1995). Life satisfaction and associated factors in older Hong Kong Chinese. *Journal of the American Geriatrics Society, 43*, 252–255.

Hodges, S. D., Humphreys, S. C., & Eck, J. C. (2002). Effect of spirituality on successful recovery from spinal surgery. *Southern Medical Journal, 95*, 1381–1384.

Holt, C. L., Haire-Joshu, D. L., Lukwago, S. N., Lewellyn, L. A., & Kreuter, M. W. (2005). The role of religiosity in dietary beliefs and behaviors among urban African American women. *Cancer Control, 12*(Suppl 2), 84–90.

House, J. S., Robbins, C., & Metzner, H. L. (1982). The association of social relationships and activities with mortality: Prospective evidence from the Tecumseh Community Health Study. *American Journal of Epidemiology, 116*, 123–140.

Hummer, R. A., Rogers, R. G., Nam, C. B., & Ellison, C. G. (1999). Religious involvement and U.S. adult mortality. *Demography, 36*, 273–285.

Idler, E. L., & Kasl, S. V. (1997a). Religion among disabled and nondisabled persons I: Cross-sectional patterns in health practices, social activities, and well-being. *Journals of Gerontology. Series B Psychological Sciences and Social Sciences, 52*, S294–S305.

Idler, E. L., & Kasl, S. V. (1997b). Religion among disabled and nondisabled persons II: Attendance at religious services as a predictor of the course of disability. *Journals of Gerontology. Series B Psychological Sciences and Social Sciences, 52*, S306–S316.

Jain, S., Shapiro, S. L., & Swanick, S., Roesch, S. C., Mills, P. J., Bell, I., & Schwartz, G. E. (2007). A randomized controlled trial of mindfulness meditation versus relaxation training: Effects on distress, positive states of mind, rumination, and distraction. *Annals of Behavioral Medicine, 33*, 11–21.

Jain, S. C., Uppal, A., Bhatnagar, S. O., & Talukdar, B. (1993). A study of response pattern of non-insulin dependent diabetics to yoga therapy. *Diabetes Research and Clinical Practice, 19*, 69–74.

John, P. J., Sharma, N., Sharma, C. M., & Kankane, A. (2007). Effectiveness of yoga therapy in the treatment of migraine without aura: A randomized controlled trial. *Headache, 47*, 654–661.

Jones, R. K., Darroch, J. E., & Singh, S. (2005). Religious differentials in the sexual and reproductive behaviors of young women in the United States. *Journal of Adolescent Health, 36*, 279–288.

Kabat-Zinn, J. (1982). An outpatient program in behavioral medicine for chronic pain patients based on the practice of mindfulness meditation: Theoretical considerations and preliminary results. *General Hospital Psychiatry, 4*, 33–47.

Kabat-Zinn, J., Lipworth, L., & Burney, R. (1985). The clinical use of mindfulness meditation for the self-regulation of chronic pain. *Journal of Behavioral Medicine, 8*, 163–190.

Kabat-Zinn, J., Massion, A. O., Kristeller, J., Peterson, L. G., Fletcher, K., Pbert, L., et al. (1992). Effectiveness of a meditation-based stress reduction program in the treatment of anxiety disorders. *American Journal of Psychiatry, 149*, 936–943.

Kabat-Zinn, J., Wheeler, E., Light, T., Skillings, A., Scharf, M.S., Cropley, T. G., et al. (1998). Influence of a mindfulness meditation-based stress reduction intervention on rates of skin clearing in patients with moderate to severe psoriasis undergoing phototherapy (UVB) and photochemotherapy (PUVA). *Psychosomatic Medicine, 60*, 625–632.

Kaplan, K. H., Goldenberg, D. L., & Galvin-Nadeau, M. (1993). The impact of a meditation-based stress reduction program on fibromyalgia. *General Hospital Psychiatry, 15*, 284–289.

Kark, J. D., Carmel, S., Sinnreich, R., Goldberger, N., & Friedlander, Y. (1996). Psychosocial factors among members of religious and secular kibbutzim. *Israel Journal of Medical Sciences, 32*, 185–194.

Kark, J. D., Shemi, G., Friedlander, Y., Martin, O., Manor, O., & Blondheim, S. H. (1996). Does religious observance promote health? Mortality in secular vs religious kibbutzim in Israel. *American Journal of Public Health, 86*, 341–346.

Keefer, L., & Blanchard, E. B. (2002). A one year follow-up of relaxation response meditation as a treatment for irritable bowel syndrome. *Behaviour Research and Therapy, 40,* 541–546.

Kennedy, G. J., Kelman, H. R., Thomas, C., & Chen, J. (1996). The relation of religious preference and practice to depressive symptoms among 1,855 older adults. *Journals of Gerontology. Series B Psychological Sciences and Social Sciences, 51,* P301–P308.

Kernberg, O. F. (2003). Sanctioned social violence: A psychoanalytic view. Part II. *International Journal of Psycho-analysis, 84,* 953–968.

Khalsa, S. B. (2004). Treatment of chronic insomnia with yoga: A preliminary study with sleep-wake diaries. *Applied Psychophysiology and Biofeedback, 29,* 269–278.

King, D. E., & Bushwick, B. (1994). Beliefs and attitudes of hospital inpatients about faith healing and prayer. *Journal of Family Practice, 39,* 349–352.

King, D. E., Hueston, W., & Rudy, M. (1994). Religious affiliation and obstetric outcome. *Southern Medical Journal, 87,* 1125–1128.

King, M. S., Carr, T., & D'Cruz, C. (2002). Transcendental meditation, hypertension and heart disease. *Australian Family Physician, 31,* 164–168.

Koenig, H. G. (1998). Religious attitudes and practices of hospitalized medically ill older adults. *International Journal of Geriatric Psychiatry, 13,* 213–224.

Koenig, H. G. (2015). Religion, spirituality, and health: A review and update. *Advances in Mind Body Medicine, 29(3),* 19–26.

Koenig, H. G., George, L. K., Cohen, H. J., Hays, J. C., Larson, D. B., & Blazer, D. G. (1998). The relationship between religious activities and cigarette smoking in older adults. *Journals of Gerontology. Series A Biological Sciences and Medical Sciences, 53,* M426–M434.

Koenig, H. G., George, L. K., Hays, J. C., Larson, D. B., Cohen, H. J., & Blazer, D. G. (1998). The relationship between religious activities and blood pressure in older adults. *International Journal of Psychiatry in Medicineicine, 28,* 189–213.

Koenig, H. G., George, L. K., & Peterson, B. L. (1998). Religiosity and remission of depression in medically ill older patients. *American Journal of Psychiatry, 155,* 536–542.

Koenig, H. G., Hays, J. C., George, L. K., Blazer, D. G., Larson, D. B., & Landerman, L. R. (1997). Modeling the cross-sectional relationships between religion, physical health, social support, and depressive symptoms. *American Journal of Geriatric Psychiatry, 5,* 131–144.

Koenig, H. G., Hays, J. C., Larson, D. B., George, L. K., Cohen, H. J., McCullough, M. E., et al. (1999). Does religious attendance prolong survival? A six-year follow-up study of 3,968 older adults. *Journals of Gerontology. Series A Biological Sciences and Medical Sciences, 54,* M370–M376.

Krause, N. (2003). Religious meaning and subjective well-being in late life. *Journals of Gerontology. Series B Psychological Sciences and Social Sciences, 58,* S160–S170.

Kuhn, C. C. (1988). A spiritual inventory of the medically ill patient. *Psychiatric Medicine, 6,* 87–100.

Kune, G. A., Kune, S., & Watson, L. F. (1992). The effect of family history of cancer, religion, parity and migrant status on survival in colorectal cancer. The Melbourne Colorectal Cancer Study. *European Journal of Cancer, 28A,* 1484–1487.

Kune, G. A., Kune, S., & Watson, L. F. (1993). Perceived religiousness is protective for colorectal cancer: Data from the Melbourne Colorectal Cancer Study. *Journal of the Royal Society of Medicine, 86*, 645–647.

Kuttner, L., Chambers, C. T., Hardial, J., Israel, D. M., Jacobson, K., & Evans, K. (2006). A randomized trial of yoga for adolescents with irritable bowel syndrome. *Pain Research and Management, 11*, 217–223.

Kutz, I. (2002). Samson, the Bible, and the DSM. *Archives of General Psychiatry, 59*, 565; author reply, 6.

La Pierre, L. L. (2003). JCAHO safeguards spiritual care. *Holistic Nursing Practice, 17*, 219.

Larson, D. B., & Wilson, W. P. (1980). Religious life of alcoholics. *Southern Medical Journal, 73*, 723–727.

Lefkowitz, E. S., Boone, T. L., Au, T. K., & Sigman, M. (2003). No sex or safe sex? Mothers' and adolescents' discussions about sexuality and AIDS/HIV. *Health Education and Research, 18*, 341–351.

Leibovici, L. (2001). Effects of remote, retroactive intercessory prayer on outcomes in patients with bloodstream infection: Randomised controlled trial. *British Medical Journal, 323*, 1450–1451.

Leigh, J., Bowen, S., & Marlatt, G. A. (2005). Spirituality, mindfulness and substance abuse. *Addictive Behaviors, 30*, 1335–1341

Levin, J., & Markides, K. (1988). Religious attendance and psychological well-being in middle-aged and older Mexican Americans. *Sociological Analysis, 49*, 66–72.

Levin, J. S. (1996). How religion influences morbidity and health: Reflections on natural history, salutogenesis and host resistance. *Social Science & Medicine, 43*, 849–864.

Levin, J. S., Larson, D. B., & Puchalski, C. M. (1997). Religion and spirituality in medicine: Research and education. *Journal of American Medical Association, 278*, 792–793.

Li, E. C., Feifer, C., & Strohm, M. (2000). A pilot study: Locus of control and spiritual beliefs in alcoholics anonymous and smart recovery members. *Addictive Behaviors, 25*, 633–640.

Lichtenstein, B. (2003). Stigma as a barrier to treatment of sexually transmitted infection in the American deep south: Issues of race, gender and poverty. *Social Science & Medicine, 57*, 2435–2445.

Lo, B., Quill, T., & Tulsky, J. (1999). Discussing palliative care with patients. ACP-ASIM End-of-Life Care Consensus Panel. American College of Physicians-American Society of Internal Medicine. *Annals of Internal Medicine, 130*, 744–749.

Lo, B., Ruston, D., & Kates, L. W., Arnold, R. M., Cohen, C. B., Faber-Langendoen, K., et al. (2002). Discussing religious and spiritual issues at the end of life: A practical guide for physicians. *Journal of American Medical Association, 287*, 749–754.

Loprinzi, C. L., Laurie, J. A., Wieand, H. S., Krook, J. E., Novotny, P. J., Kugler, J. W., et al. (1994). Prospective evaluation of prognostic variables from patient-completed questionnaires. North Central Cancer Treatment Group. *Journal of Clinical Oncology, 12*, 601–607.

Lucchetti, G., Lucchetti, A. L., & Koenig, H. G. (2011). Impact of spirituality/religiosity on mortality: Comparison with other health interventions. *Explore, 7*(4), 234–238.

Luczak, S. E., Shea, S. H., Carr, L. G., Li, T. K., & Wall, T. L. (2002). Binge drinking in Jewish and non-Jewish White college students. *Alcoholism, Clinical and Experimental Research, 26*, 1773–1778.

Lukoff, D., Lu, F., & Turner, R. (1992). Toward a more culturally sensitive DSM-IV. Psychoreligious and psychospiritual problems. *Journal of Nervous and Mental Disease, 180*, 673–682.

Lyttle, T. (1988). Drug based religions and contemporary drug taking. *Journal of Drug Issues, 18*, 271–284.

MacLean, C. D., Susi, B., Phifer, N., Schultz, L., Bynum, D., Franco, M., et al. (2003). Patient preference for physician discussion and practice of spirituality. *Journal of General Internal Medicine, 18*, 38–43.

Madru, N. (2003). Stigma and HIV: Does the social response affect the natural course of the epidemic? *Journal of the Association of Nurses in AIDS Care, 14*, 39–48.

Malhotra, V., Singh, S., Singh, K. P., Gupta, P., Sharma, S. B., Madhu, S. V., & Tandon, O. P. (2002). Study of yoga asanas in assessment of pulmonary function in NIDDM patients. *Indian Journal of Physiology and Pharmacology, 46*, 313–320.

Malhotra, V., Singh, S., Tandon, O. P., Madhu, S. V., Prasad, A., & Sharma, S. B. (2002). Effect of yoga asanas on nerve conduction in type 2 diabetes. *Indian Journal of Physiology and Pharmacology, 46*, 298–306.

Manheimer, E., Anderson, B. J., & Stein, M. D. (2003). Use and assessment of complementary and alternative therapies by intravenous drug users. *American Journal of Drug Alcohol Abuse, 29*, 401–413.

Manocha, R., Marks, G. B., Kenchington, P., Peters, D., & Salome, C. M. (2002). Sahaja yoga in the management of moderate to severe asthma: A randomised controlled trial. *Thorax, 57*, 110–115.

Markides, K. S., Levin, J. S., & Ray, L. A. (1987). Religion, aging, and life satisfaction: An eight-year, three-wave longitudinal study. *Gerontologist, 27*, 660–665.

Matthews, D. A., & Clark, C. (1998). *The faith factor: Proof of the healing power of prayer.* New York: Viking.

Matthews, D. A., Marlowe, S. M., & MacNutt, F. S. (2000). Effects of intercessory prayer on patients with rheumatoid arthritis. *Southern Medical Journal, 93*, 1177–1186.

Matthews, D. A., McCullough, M. E., Larson, D. B., Koenig, H. G., Swyers, J. P., & Milano, M. G. (1998). Religious commitment and health status: A review of the research and implications for family medicine. *Archives of Family Medicine, 7*, 118–124.

Matthews, W. J., Conti, J. M., & Sireci, S. G. (2001). The effects of intercessory prayer, positive visualization, and expectancy on the well-being of kidney dialysis patients. *Alternative Therapies in Health and Medicine, 7*, 42–52.

McCormick, N., Izzo, A., & Folcik, J. (1985). Adolescents' values, sexuality, and contraception in a rural New York county. *Adolescence, 20*, 385–395.

McCree, D. H., Wingood, G. M., DiClemente, R., Davies, S., & Harrington, K. F. (2003). Religiosity and risky sexual behavior in African-American adolescent females. *Journal of Adolescent Health, 33*, 2–8.

McCullough, M. E., & Larson, D. B. (1999). Religion and depression: A review of the literature. *Twin Research, 2*, 126–136.

McCullough, M. E., Hoyt, W. T., Larson, D. B., Koenig, H. G., & Thoresen, C. (2000). Religious involvement and mortality: A meta-analytic review. *Health Psychology, 19*, 211–222.

McKee, D. D., & Chappel, J. N. (1992). Spirituality and medical practice. *Journal of Family Practice, 35*, 201, 205–208.

McLane, S., Lox, C. L., Butki, B., & Stern, L. (2003). An investigation of the relation between religion and exercise motivation. *Perceptual and Motor Skills, 97*, 1043–1048.

Merrill, R. M., & Thygerson, A. L. (2001). Religious preference, church activity, and physical exercise. *Preventive Medicine, 33*, 38–45.

Miller, L., Davies, M., & Greenwald, S. (2000). Religiosity and substance use and abuse among adolescents in the National Comorbidity Survey. *Journal of the American Academy of Child and Adolescent Psychiatry, 39*, 1190–1197.

Miller, L., & Gur, M. (2002). Religiousness and sexual responsibility in adolescent girls. *Journal of Adolescent Health, 31*, 401–406.

Miller, L., Warner, V., Wickramaratne, P., & Weissman, M. (1997). Religiosity and depression: Ten-year follow-up of depressed mothers and offspring. *Journal of the American Academy of Child and Adolescent Psychiatry, 36*, 1416–1425.

Miller, W. R. (1998). Researching the spiritual dimensions of alcohol and other drug problems. *Addiction, 93*, 979–990.

Miller, W. R., & Thoresen, C.E. (2003). Spirituality, religion, and health: An emerging research field. *American Psychologist, 58*, 24–35.

Mitchell, J., Lannin, D. R., Mathews, H. F., & Swanson, M. S. (2002). Religious beliefs and breast cancer screening. *Journal of Womens Health, 11*, 907–915.

Monroe, M. H., Bynum, D., Susi, B., Phifer, N., Schultz, L., Franco, M., et al. (2003). Primary care physician preferences regarding spiritual behavior in medical practice. *Archives of Internal Medicine, 163*, 2751–2756.

Moriarity, J. (2001). The spiritual roots of AA. *Minnesota Medicine, 84*, 10.

Morse, J. M., & Proctor, A. (1998). Maintaining patient endurance: The comfort work of trauma nurses. *Clinical Nursing Research, 7*, 250–274.

Murphy, T. J., Pagano, R. R., & Marlatt, G. A. (1986). Lifestyle modification with heavy alcohol drinkers: Effects of aerobic exercise and meditation. *Addictive Behaviors, 11*, 175–186.

Murugesan, R., Govindarajulu, N., & Bera, T. K. (2000). Effect of selected yogic practices on the management of hypertension. *Indian Journal of Physiology and Pharmacology, 44*, 207–210.

Musick, M. A., Koenig, H. G., Hays, J. C., & Cohen, H. J. (1998). Religious activity and depression among community-dwelling elderly persons with cancer: The moderating effect of race. *Journals of Gerontology. Series B Psychological Sciences and Social Sciences, 53*, S218–S227.

Narendran, S., Nagarathna, R., Narendran, V., Gunasheela, S., & Nagendra, H. R. (2005). Efficacy of yoga on pregnancy outcome. *Journal of Alternative and Complementary Medicine, 11*, 237–244.

Neeleman, J., Halpern, D., Leon, D., & Lewis, G. (1997). Tolerance of suicide, religion and suicide rates: An ecological and individual study in 19 Western countries. *Psychological Medicine, 27,* 1165–1171.

Neeleman, J., & Lewis, G. (1999). Suicide, religion, and socioeconomic conditions: An ecological study in 26 countries, 1990. *Journal of Epidemiology and Community Health, 53,* 204–210.

Neeleman, J., Wessely, S., & Lewis, G. (1998). Suicide acceptability in African- and White Americans: The role of religion. *Journal of Nervous and Mental Disease, 186,* 12–16.

Newberg, A., Alavi, A., Baime, M., Pourdehnad, M., Santanna, J., & d'Aquili, E. (2001). The measurement of regional cerebral blood flow during the complex cognitive task of meditation: A preliminary SPECT study. *Psychiatry Research: Neuroimaging, 106*(2), 113–122.

Newberg, A. B., & Iversen, J. (2003). The neural basis of the complex mental task of meditation: Neurotransmitter and neurochemical considerations. *Medical hypotheses, 61*(2), 282–291.

Newberg, A. B., Wintering, N. A., Waldman, M. R., Yaden, D. B., & Alavi, A. (2015). A case series study of the neurophysiological effects of intense Islamic prayer. *Journal of Physiology, 109*(4–6), 214–220.

Nisbet, P. A., Duberstein, P. R., Conwell, Y., & Seidlitz, L. (2000). The effect of participation in religious activities on suicide versus natural death in adults 50 and older. *Journal of Nervous and Mental Disease, 188,* 543–546.

O'Laoire, S. (1997). An experimental study of the effects of distant, intercessory prayer on self-esteem, anxiety, and depression. *Alternative Therapies in Health and Medicine, 3,* 38–53.

Oleckno, W. A., & Blacconiere, M. J. (1991). Relationship of religiosity to wellness and other health-related behaviors and outcomes. *Psychological Reports, 68,* 819–826.

Oman, D., Kurata, J. H., Strawbridge, W. J., & Cohen, R. D. (2002). Religious attendance and cause of death over 31 years. *International Journal of Psychiatry in Medicine, 32,* 69–89.

Oman, D., & Reed, D. (1998). Religion and mortality among the community-dwelling elderly. *American Journal of Public Health, 88,* 1469–1475.

Oxman, T. E., Freeman, D. H. Jr., & Manheimer, E. D. (1995). Lack of social participation or religious strength and comfort as risk factors for death after cardiac surgery in the elderly. *Psychosomatic Medicine, 57,* 5–15.

Patel, S. S., Shah, V. S., Peterson, R. A., & Kimmel, P. L. (2002). Psychosocial variables, quality of life, and religious beliefs in ESRD patients treated with hemodialysis. *American Journal of Kidney Disease, 40,* 1013–1022.

Pettus, M. C. (2002). Implementing a medicine-spirituality curriculum in a community-based internal medicine residency program. *Academic Medicine, 77,* 745.

Poloma, M., & Pendleton, B. (1991). The effects of prayer and prayer experience on measures of general well being. *Journal of Psychology and Theology, 10,* 71–83.

Poulson, R. L., Eppler, M. A., Satterwhite, T. N., Wuensch, K. L., & Bass, L. A. (1998). Alcohol consumption, strength of religious beliefs, and risky sexual behavior in college students. *Journal of American College Health, 46,* 227–232.

Powell, L. H., Shahabi, L., & Thoresen, C. E. (2003). Religion and spirituality: Linkages to physical health. *American Psychologist, 58*, 36–52.

Pressman, P., Lyons, J. S., Larson, D. B., & Strain, J. J. (1990). Religious belief, depression, and ambulation status in elderly women with broken hips. *American Journal of Psychiatry, 147*, 758–760.

Proctor, A., Morse, J. M., & Khonsari, E. S. (1996). Sounds of comfort in the trauma center: How nurses talk to patients in pain. *Social Science & Medicine, 42*, 1669–1680.

Propst, L. R., Ostrom, R., Watkins, P., Dean, T., & Mashburn, D. (1992). Comparative efficacy of religious and nonreligious cognitive-behavioral therapy for the treatment of clinical depression in religious individuals. *Journal of Consulting and Clinical Psychology, 60*, 94–103.

Purcell, B. C. (1998a). Spiritual abuse. *American Journal of Hospice & Palliative Care, 15*, 227–231.

Purcell, B. C. (1998b). Spiritual terrorism. *American Journal of Hospice & Palliative Care, 15*, 167–173.

Raleigh, E. D. (1992). Sources of hope in chronic illness. *Oncology Nursing Forum, 19*, 443–448.

Rapp, S. R., Rejeski, W. J., & Miller, M. E. (2000). Physical function among older adults with knee pain: The role of pain coping skills. *Arthritis Care and Research, 13*, 270–279.

Rasanen, J., Kauhanen, J., Lakka, T. A., Kaplan, G. A., & Salonen, J. T. (1996). Religious affiliation and all-cause mortality: A prospective population study in middle-aged men in eastern Finland. *International Journal of Epidemiology, 25*, 1244–1249.

Razali, S. M., Hasanah, C. I., Aminah, K., & Subramaniam, M. (1998). Religious-sociocultural psychotherapy in patients with anxiety and depression. *Australian and New Zealand Journal of Psychiatry, 32*, 867–872.

Reibel, D. K., Greeson, J. M., Brainard, G. C., & Rosenzweig, S. (2001). Mindfulness-based stress reduction and health-related quality of life in a heterogeneous patient population. *General Hospital Psychiatry, 23*, 183–192.

Ringdal, G. I., Gotestam, K. G., Kaasa, S., Kvinnsland, S., & Ringdal, K. (1996). Prognostic factors and survival in a heterogeneous sample of cancer patients. *British Journal of Cancer, 73*, 1594–1599.

Roberts, L., Ahmed, I., & Hall, S. (2007). Intercessory prayer for the alleviation of ill health. *Cochrane Database of Systematic Reviews, 2007*, CD000368.

Roky, R., Houti, I., Moussamih, S., Qotbi, S., & Aadil, N. (2004). Physiological and chronobiological changes during Ramadan intermittent fasting. *Annals of Nutrition & Metabolism, 48*, 296–303.

Rossetti, S. J. (1995). The impact of child sexual abuse on attitudes toward God and the Catholic Church. *Child Abuse & Neglect, 19*, 1469–1481.

Sabaté, J. (1999). Nut consumption, vegetarian diets, ischemic heart disease risk, and all-cause mortality: evidence from epidemiologic studies. *American Journal of Clinical Nutrition, 70*(3 Suppl), 500S–503S.

Sarang, P. S., & Telles, S. (2006). Oxygen consumption and respiration during and after two yoga relaxation techniques. *Applied Psychophysiology and Biofeedback, 31,* 143–153.

Sarri, K., Linardakis, M., Codrington, C., & Kafatos, A. (2007). Does the periodic vegetarianism of Greek Orthodox Christians benefit blood pressure? *Preventive Medicine, 44,* 341–348.

Satterly, L. (2001). Guilt, shame, and religious and spiritual pain. *Holistic Nursing Practice, 15,* 30–39.

Schell, F. J., Allolio, B., & Schonecke, O. W. (1994). Physiological and psychological effects of Hatha-Yoga exercise in healthy women. *International Journal of Psychosomatics, 41,* 46–52.

Selvamurthy, W., Sridharan, K., Ray, U. S., Tiwary, R. S., Hegde, K. S., Radhakrishan, U., & Sinha, K. C. (1998). A new physiological approach to control essential hypertension. *Indian Journal of Physiology and Pharmacology, 42,* 205–213.

Shaffer, J. A. (1978). Pain and suffering: Philosophical perspectives. In W. T. Reich (Ed.), *Encyclopedia of bioethics* (pp. 1181–1185). New York: Free Press.

Shuler, P. A., Gelberg, L., & Brown, M. (1994). The effects of spiritual/religious practices on psychological well-being among inner city homeless women. *Nurse Practitioner Forum, 5,* 106–113.

Sloan, R. P., & Bagiella, E. (2002). Claims about religious involvement and health outcomes. *Annals of Behavioral Medicine, 24,* 14–21.

Sloan, R. P., Bagiella, E., & Powell, T. (1999). Religion, spirituality, and medicine. *Lancet, 353,* 664–667.

Solberg, E. E., Berglund, K. A., Engen, O., Ekeberg, O., & Loeb, M. (1996). The effect of meditation on shooting performance. *British Journal of Sports Medicine, 30,* 342–346.

Stancak, A., Jr., Kuna, M., Srinivasan, Dostalek, C., & Vishnudevananda, S. (1991). Kapalabhati—yogic cleansing exercise. II. EEG topography analysis. *Homeostasis in Health and Disease, 33,* 182–189.

Stanescu, D. C., Nemery, B., Veriter, C., & Marechal, C. (1981). Pattern of breathing and ventilatory response to CO_2 in subjects practicing hatha-yoga. *Journal of Applied Physiology, 51,* 1625–1629.

Stefanek, M., McDonald, P. G., & Hess, S. A. (2004). Religion, spirituality and cancer: Current status and methodological challenges. *Psychooncology, 14,* 450–463.

Stewart, C. (2001). The influence of spirituality on substance use of college students. *Journal of Drug Education, 31,* 343–351.

Strawbridge, W. J., Cohen, R. D., Shema, S. J., & Kaplan, G. A. (1997). Frequent attendance at religious services and mortality over 28 years. *American Journal of Public Health, 87,* 957–961.

Streeter, C. C., Jensen, J. E., Perlmutter, R. M., Cabral, H. J., Tian, H., Terhune, D. B., et al. (2007). Yoga Asana sessions increase brain GABA levels: A pilot study. *Journal of Alternative and Complementary Medicine, 13,* 419–426.

Stylianou, S. (2004). The role of religiosity in the opposition to drug use. *International Journal of Offender Therapy and Comparative Criminology, 48,* 429–448.

Sundar, S., Agrawal, S. K., Singh, V. P., Bhattacharya, S. K., Udupa, K. N., & Vaish, S. K. (1984). Role of yoga in management of essential hypertension. *Acta Cardiologica, 39,* 203–208.

Swartzman, L. C., Gwadry, F. G., Shapiro, A. P., & Teasell, R. W. (1994). The factor structure of the Coping Strategies Questionnaire. *Pain, 57,* 311–316.

Swimmer, G. I., Robinson, M. E., & Geisser, M. E. (1992). Relationship of MMPI cluster type, pain coping strategy, and treatment outcome. *Clinical Journal of Pain, 8,* 131–137.

Tanyi, R. A. (2002). Towards clarification of the meaning of spirituality. *Journal of Advanced Nursing, 39,* 500–509.

The Gallup Report: Religion in America: 1993–1994. (1994). Princeton, NJ: Gallup Poll.

Tieman, J. (2002). Priest scandal hits hospitals. As pedophilia reports grow, church officials suspend at least six hospital chaplains in an effort to address alleged sexual abuse. *Modern Healthcare, 32,* 6–7, 14, 1.

Tonigan, J. S., Miller, W. R., & Schermer, C. (2002). Atheists, agnostics and Alcoholics Anonymous. *Journal of Studies on Alcohol, 63,* 534–541.

Townsend, M., Kladder, V., Ayele, H., & Mulligan, T. (2002). Systematic review of clinical trials examining the effects of religion on health. *Southern Medical Journal, 95,* 1429–1434.

Tu, W. (1980). A religiophilosophical perspective on pain. In H. W. Koster, D. Kosterlitz, & L. Y. Terenius (Eds.), *Pain and society* (pp. 63–78). Deerfield Beach, FL and Weinhem: Verlag Chemie.

Turner, R. P., Lukoff, D., Barnhouse, R. T., & Lu, F. G. (1995). Religious or spiritual problem: A culturally sensitive diagnostic category in the DSM-IV. *Journal of Nervous and Mental Disease, 183,* 435–444.

Udupa, K. N., Singh, R. H., & Yadav, R. A. (1973). Certain studies on psychological and biochemical responses to the practice in Hatha Yoga in young normal volunteers. *Indian Journal of Medical Research, 61,* 237–244.

van Montfrans, G. A., Karemaker, J. M., Wieling, W., & Dunning, A. J. (1990a). Relaxation therapy and continuous ambulatory blood pressure in mild hypertension: A controlled study. *British Medical Journal, 300,* 1368–1372.

van Montfrans, G. A., Karemaker, J. M., Wieling, W., & Dunning, A. J. (1990b). Yoga and massage: If it's physical, it's therapy. *Newsweek, 140,* 74–75.

Van Ness, P. H., Kasl, S. V., & Jones, B. A. (2003). Religion, race, and breast cancer survival. *International Journal of Psychiatry in Medicineicine, 33,* 357–375.

Van Poppel, F., Schellekens, J., & Liefbroer, A. C. (2002). Religious differentials in infant and child mortality in Holland, 1855–1912. *Population Studies, 56,* 277–289.

Walker, S. R., Tonigan, J. S., Miller, W. R., Corner, S., & Kahlich, L. (1997). Intercessory prayer in the treatment of alcohol abuse and dependence: A pilot investigation. *Alternative Therapies in Health and Medicine, 3,* 79–86.

Wallace, R. K., Silver, J., Mills, P. J., Dillbeck, M. C., & Wagoner, D. E. (1983). Systolic blood pressure and long-term practice of the transcendental meditation and TM-Sidhi program: Effects of TM on systolic blood pressure. *Psychosomatic Medicine, 45,* 41–46.

Walls, P., & Williams, R. (2004). Accounting for Irish Catholic ill health in Scotland: A qualitative exploration of some links between "religion," class and health. *Sociology of Health & Illness, 26*, 527–556.

Walsh, A. (1998). Religion and hypertension: Testing alternative explanations among immigrants. *Behavioral Medicine, 24*, 122–130.

Walton, K. G., Pugh, N. D., Gelderloos, P., & Macrae, P. (1995). Stress reduction and preventing hypertension: Preliminary support for a psychoneuroendocrine mechanism. *Journal of Alternative and Complementary Medicine, 1*, 263–283.

Watkins, Y. J., Quinn, L. T., Ruggiero, L., Quinn, M. T., & Choi, Y. K. (2013). Spiritual and religious beliefs and practices and social support's relationship to diabetes self-care activities in African Americans. *Diabetes Education, 39*(2), 231–239.

Weaver, A. J., Koenig, H. K., Flannelly, K. J., et al. (2003). Spiritual assessment required in all settings. *Hospital Peer Review, 28*, 55–56.

Wenneberg, S. R., Schneider, R. H., MacLean, C., Levitsky, D. K., Walton, K. G., Mandarino, J. V., et al. (1997). A controlled study of the effects of the transcendental meditation program on cardiovascular reactivity and ambulatory blood pressure. *International Journal of Neuroscience, 89*, 15–28.

Wilcox, S., Laken, M., & Bopp, M., Gethers, O., Huang, P., McClorin, L., et al. (2007). Increasing physical activity among church members: Community-based participatory research. *American Journal of Preventive Medicine, 32*, 131–138.

Williams, D. R., Larson, D. B., Buckler, R. E., Heckmann, R. C., & Pyle, C. M. (1991). Religion and psychological distress in a community sample. *Social Science & Medicine, 32*, 1257–1262.

Williams, K. A., Kolar, M. M., Reger, B. E., & Pearson, J. C. (2001). Evaluation of a wellness-based mindfulness stress reduction intervention: A controlled trial. *American Journal of Health Promotion, 15*, 422–432.

Woodward, K. L. (2001). Faith is more than a feeling. *Newsweek, 137*, 58.

Yaden, D. B., Eichstaedt, J. C., Schwartz, H. A., Kern, M, L., Le Nguyen, K., Wintering, N. A., et al. (2015). The language of ineffability: Linguistic analysis of mystical experiences. *Journal of Religion and Spirituality, 8*(3), 244–252.

Yaden, D. B., Iwry, J., & Newberg, A. B., (2016). Neurochemistry and religion: Surveying the field. In J. Kripal, A. DeConick, & T. Pinn (Eds.), *MacMillan interdisciplinary handbooks on religion: The brain, cognition, and culture.* New York: Macmillan.

Yaden, D. B., Iwry, J., Slack, K. J., Eiechstaedt, J. C., Zhao, Y., Vaillant, G. E., & Newberg, A. B. (2016). The overview effect: Awe and self-transcendent experience in space flight. *Psychology of Consciousness: Theory, Research, and Practice, 3*(1), 1–11.

Yaden, D. B., Le Nguyen, K. D., Kern, M. L., Belser, A. B., Eichstaedt, J. C., Iwry, J., et al. (2016). Of roots and fruits: A comparison of psychedelic and non-psychedelic mystical experiences. *The Journal of Humanistic Psychology, 57*(4), 338–353.

Yaden, D. B., McCall, T., & Ellens, J. H. (Eds.). (2015). *Being called: Secular, scientific, and sacred perspectives.* Santa Barbara, CA: Praeger.

Yates, J. W., Chalmer, B. J., St. James, P., Follansbee, M., & McKegney, F. P. (1981). Religion in patients with advanced cancer. *Medical and Pediatric Oncology, 9*, 121–128.

Yoon, D. P., & Lee, E. K. (2007). The impact of religiousness, spirituality, and social support on psychological well-being among older adults in rural areas. *Journal of Gerontology and Social Work, 48,* 281–298.

Young, D. R., & Stewart, K. J. (2006). A church-based physical activity intervention for African American women. *Family Community Health, 29,* 103–117.

Yurtkuran, M., Alp, A., & Dilek, K. (2007). A modified yoga-based exercise program in hemodialysis patients: A randomized controlled study. *Complementary Therapies in Medicine, 15,* 164–171.

Zaleski, E. H., & Schiaffino, K. M. (2000). Religiosity and sexual risk-taking behavior during the transition to college. *Journal of Adolescence, 23,* 223–227.

Zollinger, T. W., Phillips, R. L., & Kuzma, J. W. (1984). Breast cancer survival rates among Seventh-day Adventists and non-Seventh-day Adventists. *American Journal of Epidemiology, 119,* 503–509.

6

Behavioral Strategies for Happiness and Satisfaction

CATHY GREENBERG AND RELLY NADLER

Key Points

- The neural circuitry associated with experiencing emotional pleasure such as from spiritual fulfillment, happiness, or love is likely the same or closely replicative of the neural circuitry associated with experiencing physical pleasure such as from sex, music, or warmth.
- The neural circuitry associated with experiencing physical pain such as from a headache, injury, or disease is likely the same or closely replicative of the neural circuitry associated with experiencing emotional pain such as social rejection, depression, or self-criticism.
- Attention management is essential for developing happiness and satisfaction, while the opposite, attention mismanagement, is a catalyst for unhappiness and dissatisfaction.
- Happiness is believed to have a set point in each person—a base level in a similar way that each person has a foundational level of intelligence—and by all indications this set point can be enhanced through deliberate and supportive constructs.
- "Being on your side" yields more sustainable degrees of happiness and satisfaction than does "being on your case."

Introduction

Happiness is difficult to quantify though the field of study is gaining tools to better assess the emotion. The Positive and Negative Affect Scale (PANAS), the Oxford Happiness Inventory, the Subjective

Happiness Scale, and the Satisfaction with Life Scale are among the most recognizable batteries. Along with those are subdivision measurements including the Fordyce Emotions Questionnaire, which measures current happiness, and the Subjective Happiness Scale, which measures happiness relative to changing variables.

Just as important to understanding happiness itself is the study of unhappiness. Research reveals the role that regret plays in unhappiness—most notably the greater the feeling of regret, the more miserable a person feels for a longer period of time (Kahneman, 2011; Tversky & Kahneman, 1992).

Thus the natural tendency toward an avoidance of pain offers comfort and a subjective feeling of happiness. A patient who suffers from chronic arthritis will feel a sense of relief if she has a good day with minimized pain. That relief may be experienced as happiness. An employee passed over for a promotion may feel vindicated if the winning candidate eventually goes on to fail in his new position. This vindication, however, may be experienced as happiness too.

In each of these two examples, a diminishment of pain can be misconstrued to be an increase in happiness. Most healthcare providers define authentic happiness as being based more on character traits such as those advanced by the positive psychology movement's three dimensions of happiness: positive emotion, engagement, and meaning (Seligman & Csikszentmihalyi, 2014).

Positive psychology was founded on the principles of engaging happiness and fulfillment in a person's life. Martin Seligman, considered to be one of the pioneers of the movement, though Abraham Maslow coined the term, invigorated mental health research with a view that rather than focusing on a patient's illness as a means to healing, practitioners should instead shift more attention to the patient's strengths. Seligman (2003) defined these strengths in terms of character traits, not skill sets. For example, patience, tolerance, and compassion were strengths he sought to uncover and then build upon in patient treatment programs.

In some sense, his approach echoed the adage "success breeds success" so that by building on what is working in a patient's life, that individual becomes more adept at improving upon troublesome areas. What has evolved from Seligman's early theory is now an evidence-based model that combines ancient philosophy from Aristotle, Confucius, and others with modern-day treatments for increasing happiness, motivation, and a sense of community to arrive at a "meaningful life" in which one's strengths and virtues are applied for the greater good of humanity (Seligman, 2012). Beyond the positive psychology model, these same tenets for authentic happiness are taught by spiritual leaders, career counselors, families, and more. Some critics claim though the approach glosses over the reality of life's interconnected physical and emotional pains.

Indeed, brain imaging studies show that the neural circuitry associated with experiencing physical pain such as from a headache, injury, or disease is likely the same or closely replicative of the neural circuitry associated with experiencing emotional pain such as social rejection, depression, or self-criticism (Eisenberger, 2012). Studies suggest that the regions of the brain where this overlapping pain is processed is in the anterior insula and dorsal anterior cingulate cortex (Eisenberger, 2015).

A potential corollary to this is research that additionally shows the neural circuity of the brain is likely replicative or the same too with regard to emotional pleasure, such as from spiritual fulfillment, happiness, and love, and physical pleasure such as from sex, music, and warmth as indicated by neuroimaging showing shared activation in the brain regions of the bilateral nucleus accumbens, frontal attentional, and ventromedial prefrontal cortical loci (Ferguson et al., 2016).

In work with leadership training for private sector CEOs, federal and state government administrators, and military and paramilitary officers, the application of happiness theory is directly related to priming peak performance through fostering a conscious shift from ordinary thought processing to an inspired one. The bridge between the two is often characterized as "flow" (Csikszentmihalyi, 1990) in which a person feels as if he or she is channeling large amounts of energy and thought through the body with very little, if any, effort.

Models for personal fulfillment and happiness often are based upon concepts of self-leadership (Neck & Houghton, 2006) in which each individual's self-awareness, or emotional and social intelligence (Goleman, 1995), is developed. With this approach, individuals can more deeply understand their decision-making and attention-focusing processes. This includes making conscious decisions, versus being on autopilot, and thus reduces unconscious biases, self-delusions, and errors in judgement. Focusing on self-awareness offers individuals more choices resulting in having greater potential to develop into better listeners, among other aspirations, particularly in the workplace, and thus be more effective at communicating with colleagues, with those they serve, as well as with adversaries. The goal is to enable their brain to be better attuned to empathy, creativity, and intuition in addition to cognitive and higher thought functioning (Goleman & Boyatzis, 2008).

Striking this balance between feeling and thinking suggests one of the greatest opportunities to advance not only individuals and organizations but society as a whole. It is through this advancement that compassion and empathy, reason and analysis, can bring happiness to greater numbers of people. The validity of this claim is supported by functional magnetic resonance imaging studies illustrating the effects this integration has on the brain as does pioneering work in the new field named interpersonal neurobiology (Siegel & Daniel, 2012). This approach encompasses earlier work indicating that cognition and emotion may not be distinctly separate entities as has been a long-held theory. Instead, new evidence indicates that there is a constant interaction between the two that is often influenced by environmental and personal factors (Pessoa, 2008). Furthermore, several neural networks are involved in this process. For example, the "salience" network is activated in empathizing as well as in executive brain functioning (Fan, Duncan, de Greck, & Northoff, 2011).

This chapter explores methods on how to create that balance. The process's end goal is to create happiness and satisfaction, both measured in terms of genuine well-being. While accruing greater wealth or influence may result, these are by-products of the conscientious lifestyle. More central than these externalities are the internal personal transformations such as self-compassion and self-forgiveness—both of which can lead to greater fulfillment that begets greater performance in the workplace and at home (Ornish, 1998).

Conscious Attentional Deployment

A major review of 128 studies on emotional regulation strategies revealed strong empirical support for attentional deployment being at the center of many positive interventions (Quoidbach, Mikolajczak, & Gross, 2015). Quoidbach et al. assert "the way we direct [or deploy] our attention within a situation can powerfully influence our emotional experience" (p. 658).

In support of this attentional deployment hypothesis is the work of Robert Cialdini, who outlines in his book *Pre-Suasion: A Revolutionary Way to Influence and Persuade* the importance of preframing or priming other people in a conscious manner. Cialdini (2016) states that, "Channeled attention leads to pre-suasion: the human tendency to assign undue levels of importance to an idea as soon as one's attention is turned to it."

Additionally, we have adapted some constructive "pre-suasion" strategies in our own work that were originally developed by Sonya Lyubomirsky (2013) and Stephen Covey (1989) such as

> Start the day by counting your blessings.
>
> Contemplate how you can grow from situations, even unfortunate ones.
>
> Mitigate negative self-talk by deliberately limiting the time allowed for it.

As Covey advises in *The 7 Habits of Highly Effective People*:

Start conversations with the end in mind.

Hold meetings with a set agenda and purpose.

Focus on individual strengths before beginning a new initiative or project.

Reframe stress into a more positive outlook as a challenge or opportunity.

Attention management thus facilitates a path toward happiness and satisfaction (Figure 6.1). Attention mismanagement can lead to unhappiness and dissatisfaction, which can lead to physical symptoms euphemistically referred to as "pain in the brain" (Figure 6.2). Furthermore, Naomi Eisenberger (2012) suggests that there may be an overlap in the neural circuitry that is involved in the experience of physical pain and that involved with 'social pain'. Social pain refers to the painful feelings following social rejection or social loss. However, individuals usually mediate physical pain, for example by resting the injured body part. But people often exacerbate social or emotional pain, by engaging in self-criticism, self-punishment, and a general lack of self-compassion, among other unhealthy coping mechanisms. This mismanagement of attention, then, is, in effect, reinjuring the person. Thus by increasing self-awareness of overall painful experiences, individuals can advance their ability to apply conscious attention to grieving, healing, and resurrecting.

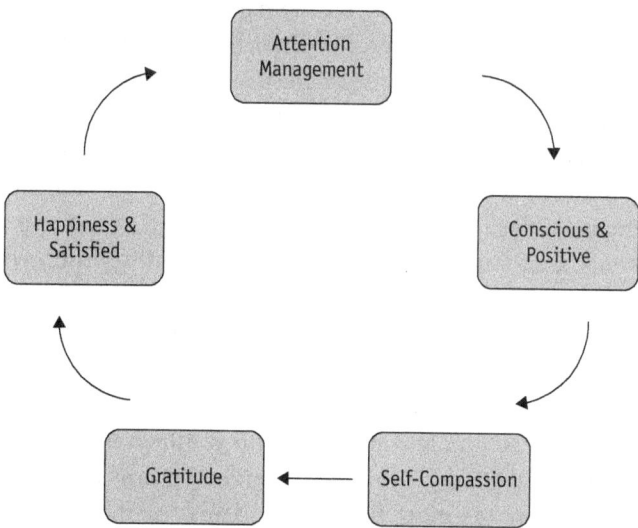

FIGURE 6.1. Constructive characteristics of attention management.

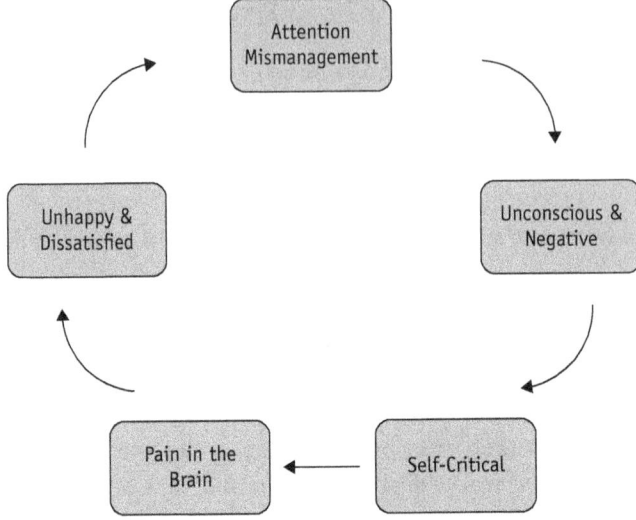

FIGURE 6.2. Harmful characteristics of attention mismanagement.

Studies also reveal that, through reframing, individuals can shift from experiencing a situation as negative to viewing it as positive—or at least change from a negative viewpoint to a point of acceptance where pain is lessened (Butler, Chapman, Froman, & Beck, 2006). The natural tendency to avoid this emotional pain is considered in theories about an individual's awareness of rational and irrational choices (Tversky & Kahneman, 1986) as well as theories on reframing negative experiences to a more positive view (Zettle et al., 2005). Advances in the treatment of chronic physical pain such as from backache, degenerative diseases, and arthritis include similar techniques as those applied to emotional pain. Guided imagery, positive self-talk, and self-compassion can all play vital roles in helping patients cope (Turk, Swanson, & Tunks, 2008). According to the American Academy of Pain Medicine, an estimated 100 million Americans suffer from chronic pain. Thus there is great opportunity to apply this model of conscious attention management to bring relief, and in turn, greater degrees of happiness and satisfaction.

The diagrams in this chapter illustrate feedback loops associated with constructive attention management and harmful attention mismanagement. When individuals are conscious of the direction of their attention, they are apt to treat themselves with more compassion and gratitude and in turn feel more happiness and satisfaction. In contrast, when individuals are unconscious of the direction of their attention they are apt to mistreat themselves with more self-criticism and "brain pain" and in turn feel more unhappiness and dissatisfaction. The loop aspect indicates that as the attention management or mismanagement cycles through its sequences, each step strengthens successive steps. In the case of attention management, the positive effects are self-regenerating. Unfortunately, without some intervention, harmful attention mismanagement perpetuates itself too.

The Happiness Focus

The concept of attention management has found support from a longitudinal research study with more than 200 executives from across the globe that showed how understanding oneself was essential for effective leadership (Greenberg-Walt & Robertson, 2001). The findings from the study revealed that along with the distinctly positive attributes of understanding oneself were the distinctly deleterious outcomes from a lack of self-understanding. These resulted in leaders moving off task and the organization's focus on its mission thus being derailed. Other key leadership behaviors identified included technological savvy, embracing diversity of style, and a networked approach to leadership (Goldsmith, Greenberg, Robertson, & Hu-Chan, 2003). Technological savvy is defined as the capacity to understand and strategically apply computer and web-based solutions for management, communications, media relations, marketing, and client support among other areas of organizational focus. Embracing diversity of style reflects the ability to be aware of and to seek out and understand different perspectives that may impact innovation. For example, the idea of thinking globally but acting locally demonstrates how diversity of experiences can be collected, integrated, and evaluated to best fit within an organization's activities while maintaining relevance to both the entity's culture and its client base. A networked approach to leadership addresses the challenges of leading in a complex, constantly evolving 24/7 environment that requires more than traditional top-down management strategies. "Networked leadership" teams or an interchangeable leadership team of advisory council members who can step in or out of their roles when appropriate is a means to adjust to these needs.

An outgrowth of this study was an extensive synthesis of original and existing research from behavioral sciences, anthropology, neuroscience, leadership development, and positive psychology including the subsets of emotional and social intelligence. Three themes emerged: "personal mastery," "happiness traps," and "happiness tips" (Baker, Greenberg, & Hemingway, 2006).

Personal mastery is the capacity to know oneself well through ongoing objective self-assessments, self-awareness, and conscious action-taking. Understanding and managing oneself before understanding and managing others was deemed by the researchers to be essential to the level of interpersonal skills required, including stress tolerance and overall levels of life satisfaction, to make accurate and timely decisions.

Happiness traps refer to that which individuals believe will bring them greater happiness, joy, and life satisfaction. An example is an individual believing that having a status symbol such as a luxury automobile or expensive jewelry will result in happiness. The consequence is often a sense of confusion about the source and nature of happiness.

Happiness tips are aids to support individual needs for balance as well as achievement of goals. These tips are centered around the belief that happiness comes from within and often can be described as the "simple things in life"—a child's smile, the touch of a reaffirming hand, or the affection of a pet. These tips also serve in overcoming challenges, staying on course, and inspiring one to do one's best.

In total, this year-long research project conducted across four continents with two generations of leaders and future leaders from a range of industries established a baseline for the application of personal mastery and to date is still the most comprehensive research on the subject. These findings were later included in research conducted across the top Fortune 100 companies that resulted in the HAPIE model—**H**eartfelt (the organization's leaders are heartfelt); **A**daptive (the organization flexes when needed); **P**rofit with People (the organization works on behalf of people rather than at their expense); **I**nvigorated stakeholders (the organization cultivates its own first-line marketers); **E**ngaged Community Partners (the organization commits to being socially responsible)—as well as proved instrumental in forming foundations for iterations directed at the educated layperson such as popular literature on emotional and social intelligence. The research is also utilized broadly across studies on attention management and mindfulness.

Based on the original formula for happiness as defined by psychologist Daniel Gilbert (2007)—frequent positive feelings accompanied by an overall sense that one's life has meaning—50% of happiness is postulated to be related to genetics with the remaining 50% broken into two key elements: 40% focused on individual habits of mind and body and 10% remaining outside of one's immediate control such as external stressors related to financial, relationship, and health issues (Gilbert, 2007).

Happiness is therefore deemed to have a *set point* in a similar way that each person has a foundational level of intelligence, and by all indications this set point can be enhanced through deliberate and supportive constructs including reciting positive affirmations, talking about feelings, expressing gratitude, giving of oneself through compassion and kindness, and adopting behaviors that reduce anxiety (Brickman, Coates, & Janoff-Bulman, 1978). Expressions of gratitude are particularly fertile areas of study today in relation to happiness theory development (Krakauer, Ruscio, Froh, & Bono, 2017). These practices and others that are focused on growing happiness have been shown to have a direct correlation to an overall sense of well-being (Easterlin, 2005). The inverse appears to be true as well—a sense of well-being generates greater levels of happiness. In a study on self-reported health status, in all age groups, mean levels of happiness were greater with increased degrees of healthiness. For example, those age 27 to 55 self-reporting as being in excellent health scored at a computed mean level of happiness of 2.37, whereas those in good health scored at a mean level of happiness of 2.17, in fair health scored at 1.92, and in poor health scored at 1.74 (Davis, Smith, & Marsden, 2002). Further research suggests an individual's sense of wellness is tied to his or her sense of an authentic autonomous self, which "emphasizes the individual's self-governing abilities, the independence of one's deliberation from manipulation and the capacity to decide for oneself" (Varga & Guignon, 2016) as opposed to a sense of an inauthentic unfree self experienced when feeling manipulated and controlled (Habron, 2008).

When awareness about happiness is understood to be influenced largely by individual choices, those variables can be incorporated into daily practices for sustaining happiness and well-being. Yet, when those choices are ignored or withheld, happiness and its influence on well-being can become diminished, thereby setting up a domino effect through which overall life satisfaction can decrease as well (Kushlev et al., 2017).

Therefore focus and deliberate action become important components of happiness. This conclusion is at the core of the present-day interest in mindfulness as an outgrowth of pioneering work by Jon Kabat-Zinn and in particular his founding of the mindfulness-based stress reduction program. Mindfulness, as a separate and distinct method, adds yet another critical component for developing happiness and overall life satisfaction (Carmody & Baer, 2008).

Individuals can more effectively maintain a state of mindfulness even when facing adversity by drawing on their self-confidence as well as sense of courage. This is in large part due to a mindfulness-based disarming of a "fight or flight" response and instead activating higher level brain functioning that calms, assesses, and takes appropriate actions (Greenberg & North, 2014). Furthermore, studies show that those with a higher level of overall happiness and satisfaction are also more resilient due to their propensity for a homeostatic psychological and physiological system that supports well-being. This includes an increase in circulating "feel good" neurotransmitters such as endorphins and dopamine (Cohn, Fredrickson, Brown, Mikels, & Conway, 2008).

Taken in total, self-awareness is crucial to resolving subconscious barriers to happiness and satisfaction, as well as to supporting rapid behavioral changes to adapt to the demands of society and the realities of human limitations and vulnerabilities (Connor & Davidson, 2003). Indeed, happiness, mindfulness, and resilience have become *de rigueur* of popular psychology as evidenced by the currently available thousands of books, studies, workshops, and more for both professionals and lay people seeking a means to greater fulfillment (Seligman, 2012).

Yet there is also a growing skepticism about some of the motivations behind the happiness movement—one critique characterizes it as being fueled by behavioral economists and their big-business underwriters seeking new ways to stimulate individuals to buy more of their products (Davies, 2015). Among these stimulants is the encouragement of a "keeping up with the Joneses" rat race that awards happiness only if one measures up favorably to others. This is a significant concern because it can adulterate the reception to well-intentioned findings such as those that show there are indeed economic factors at play. Namely, people experiencing personal transformations leading to more happiness and satisfaction are linked to higher performance levels in the workplace, thus generating more opportunities for prosperity (Baker, Greenberg, & Yalof, 2007). This prosperity can also be linked to how an individual spends his or her money—particularly through generosity that enhances the lives of others—to thus fuel greater degrees of happiness and satisfaction (Dunn, Gilbert, & Wilson, 2011).

Return on Investment

The economic benefits of happiness are bolstering a societal movement toward income equality, which can then help stabilize national economies (Schneider, 2016). Research indicates that companies engaging in more employee happiness expenditures trend toward having a return on investment as much as three times higher than companies that do not substantially engage in employee happiness expenditures (Seligman, 2007). Other research suggests that happiness is tied to job satisfaction by as much as 93% (Pryce-Jones, 2010). Additionally, a theory long-held to be central in philosophical teachings dating back to thousands of years ago (e.g., Plato, 380 BCE) is making its way into modern-day boardrooms: happiness creates success. This is in opposition to the traditional idea that success creates happiness. Furthermore, happy employees engage more in organizational enterprises, are more productive, and are viewed by supervisors as being more trustworthy than those who display unhappiness (Achor, 2010). Though happiness is typically thought of as an intangible, these findings reveal its measurable correlation with generating prosperity.

Being on Your Side Versus Being on Your Case

Self-evaluations of happiness reveal that more than half of reporting individuals demonstrate unreliable self-evaluations (Seligman, 2003). Specifically, they most often rate themselves as having performed unsatisfactorily even when they have been quantifiably measured to have been successful. This may be linked to what is termed the *impostor syndrome* (Clance & Imes, 1978) in that these individuals fear they will be discovered as incompetent and thus may push themselves mercilessly to establish their own sense of competency; it may also be linked to these individuals identifying themselves as feeling low in confidence as a result of unrealistic expectations and hyper-self-criticism (Seligman, 2006).

Yet many people view this distortion as a positive in that they claim their self-criticalness motivates them to drive for greater successes. Oftentimes, however, these same individuals acknowledge an equally harmful result in that their self-criticalness leads them to feel as if they are torturing themselves, and eventually this "motivator" becomes burdensome, even disruptive, as they continually try harder but always fall short in their own eyes (Nadler, 2011). They scold themselves for failing to live up to their abilities. For them, a better effort, a larger result, a faster delivery is a panacea such that nothing will be good enough to earn their self-praise.

These individuals readily admit they are hard on themselves, yet for many "the stick" rather than "the carrot" has given them their best performances, and thus they are reluctant, in their view, to "fix what isn't broken." Yet, to the observant eye, their system is indeed in need of repair.

Specifically, we have ascertained three major unintended consequences of this behavior (Nadler, 2011):

- Damaged self-esteem
- Pervasive tension, unhappiness, and sense of disappointment.
- Unconscious harsh treatment of others similar to how they treat themselves

We have found that breaking through to these individuals requires both direct, strong communications, as well as engaging them in the habitual type of critical thinking, risk versus reward assessment, and data analysis that they apply in pushing themselves to greater heights. Nadler (2011) terms this latter approach "Being on Your Side versus Being on Your Case."

The neurological component to this approach is illustrated in the research findings from *Having a Word With Yourself: Neural Correlates of Self-Criticism and Self-Reassurance* by Olivia Longe et al. (2010):

> Self-criticism was associated with activity in lateral prefrontal cortex (PFC) regions and dorsal anterior cingulate (dAC), therefore linking self-critical thinking to error processing and resolution, and also behavioral inhibition. Self-reassurance was associated with left temporal pole and insula activation, suggesting that efforts to be self-reassuring engage similar regions to expressing compassion and empathy towards others. Additionally, we found a dorsal/ventral PFC divide between an individual's tendency to be self-critical or self-reassuring. (abstract 1849)

Tools to Encourage Being on Your Side

In light of these findings on the dominating roles of self-criticism and its opposite, self-compassion, a variety of evaluative batteries can be administered to bring more clarity to an individual's behavioral patterns in regard to happiness. Among the most recognizable of these tools are the PANAS, the Oxford Happiness Inventory, the Subjective Happiness Scale, and the Satisfaction with Life Scale. Along with those are subdivision measurements including the Fordyce Emotions Questionnaire, which measures current happiness, and the Subjective Happiness Scale, which measures happiness relative to changing variables.

We have also developed tools to help individuals become more aware of their unconscious patterns of hyper-self-critiques, as well as hypervigilance in looking for errors. Through "redirecting," a synonym for reframing, individuals can evolve to being more compassionate toward themselves and others. An important part of the plan is to track on a weekly basis the amount of time they spend being "on their case" as well as the time they spend curtailing that behavior and redirecting their self-talk to being on their side (Nadler, 2011).

We have determined from our own work that the most effective way to change from being on your case to being on your side is first to take notice of and then nonjudgmentally observe the self-disparagement, which we refer to as whipping, and next turn that awareness into constructive action. This observant-self theory is supported by extensive academic research most often based on the benefits of mindfulness (Rolnick, Oren, & Bassett, 2016) as well as through more accessible outreach directed toward the educated layperson such as in *Super Brain: Unleashing the Explosive Power of Your Mind to Maximize Health, Happiness, and Spiritual Well-Being* by Deepak Chopra and

Rudolph Tanzi (2012). The following are some examples of whipping statements and redirecting statements.

On Your Case Whipping

- How could I be so dumb?
- Don't I know better than this?
- I'm an idiot for doing that!
- Why didn't I start this sooner?
- I could have done a much better job!
- What's wrong with me?
- I should have known better!

On Your Side Redirecting

- Which parts of this performance went well?
- What didn't turn out the way I wanted?
- Is there anything I could have done differently?
- What will I have to do to accept this performance and not beat myself up?
- What can I learn from this performance?
- Is there any learning, training, or help I need to improve my performance?
- What is my next step?

The redirecting statements are designed to elicit a tempered, thoughtful review that is compatible with the redirecting process of first acknowledging and then validating what went well as a way to build a healthier overall self-evaluation process and thus disrupt the "more, better, faster" whipping pattern.

Table 6.1 provides key words in defining the differences between being on your case and being on your side.

Table 6.1. Differences Between Being On Your Case and On Your Side

	On Your Case	On Your Side
Quality	• Demanding • Damaging • Irrational • Overgeneralized	• Respectful • Constructive • Rational • Realistic
Results	• Dissatisfied • Less confident • Overwhelmed	• Encouraged • Action plan for future • Energized

Additional approaches for probing clients and patients for insight include asking the following:

- How accurate do you believe your self-evaluation is?
- What percentage of the time are you on your case on a scale of 1 to 100?
- How do you feel after you've been on your case?
- What are the consequences for you and others for being on your case?
- Do you treat others as harshly as yourself?
- Is being on your case an effective pattern for you to continue with?
- If you don't change this, what do you lose out on?
- Are you keeping track of the times you've stopped being on your case and instead redirected to being on your side?
- What is most difficult about being on your side?
- What helps you to be on your side?
- What percentage of the time you are on your side each day on a scale of 1 to 100?

Further Strategies for Developing Happiness and Satisfaction

Using the tools associated with the being on your case versus being on your side behavioral model is one approach for helping individuals develop greater levels of happiness and life satisfaction. Other research shows that the efficacy of self-evaluations can be clouded by culturally influenced biases, levels of self-esteem, and other emotional and psychological factors including shame, guilt, degrees of social support, and fear of social ostracism (Zell & Krizan, 2014).

Thus the self-evaluative questions themselves are as important as the answers they are intended to generate. Neutral, cogent questions devoid as much as possible of the self-contamination and unconscious predispositions as discussed yield a more accurate self-evaluation as does a deeply analytical approach to stating the goals that are hoped to be realized through these self-evaluations (Judge & Kammeyer-Mueller, 2011). Examples of these types of questions include

- What goals would you be interested in working toward?
- What are your personal strengths?
- How could you build and broaden these strengths?
- How do you remain motivated?
- How do you reward yourself for doing well?

Conclusion

The emergence of a distinct field of research into happiness is anticipated to progress as new studies reveal the neurobiological functioning behind the emotion. One of the most groundbreaking related discoveries is that the brain responds similarly to emotional pain as it does to physical pain. With physical pain, there are usually clear treatment protocols in place—take an aspirin, apply an icepack, or undergo surgery. With emotional pain though, the protocols have been less defined. A potential corollary to these findings involves research suggesting similarities in neural activity for both emotional pleasure and physical pleasure. Thus a greater acceptance of, and subsequent application of, evidence that supports self-awareness, self-expression, empathy, and other components of emotional intelligence offers hope for advances in understanding happiness and overall brain health.

Central to this scientific movement that builds on Goleman's emotional intelligence model (1995) is the value of being on your side versus being on your case. The former can be arrived at first through self-awareness and then through cognitive reappraisals redirecting perspectives on misfortune and disappointment toward an outlook of optimism and well-being. The alternative with the latter is a cyclical pattern that can self-injure and even self-traumatize.

In terms of enhanced quality of life, being kind, compassionate, and loving toward one's own self, or being on your side, results in increased happiness as expressed through greater degrees of creativity, a stronger sense of closeness in relationships, better overall social skills, more readied resilience, sharper decision-making skills, and deeper stress tolerance levels.

REFERENCES

Achor, S. (2010). *The happiness advantage: The seven principles of positive psychology that fuel success and performance at work*. New York: Crown.

Baker, D., Greenberg, C. L., & Hemingway, C. (2006). *What happy companies know: How the new science of happiness can change your company for the better*. Upper Saddle River, NJ: Pearson Education.

Baker, D., Greenberg, C. L., & Yalof, I. (2007). *What happy women know: How new findings in positive psychology can change women's lives for the better*. New York: Rodale Books.

Brickman, P., Coates, D., & Janoff-Bulman, R. (1978). Lottery winners and accident victims: Is happiness relative? *Journal of Personality and Social Psychology, 36*(8), 917–927.

Butler, A. C., Chapman, J. E., Froman, E. M., & Beck, A. T. (2006). The empirical status of cognitive-behavioral therapy: A review of meta-analyses. *Clinical Psychology Review, 26*(1), 17–31.

Carmody, J., & Baer, R. A. (2008). Relationships between mindfulness practice and levels of mindfulness: Medical and psychological symptoms and well-being in a mindfulness-based stress reduction program. *Journal of Behavioral Medicine, 31*(1), 23–33.

Chopra, D., & Tanzi, R. E. (2012). *Super brain: Unleashing the explosive power of your mind to maximize health, happiness, and spiritual well-being.* New York: Harmony Books.

Cialdini, R. (2016). *Pre-suasion: A revolutionary way to influence and persuade.* New York: Simon & Schuster.

Clance, P. R., & Imes, S. A. (1978). The imposter phenomenon in high achieving women: Dynamics and therapeutic intervention. *Psychotherapy: Theory, Research and Practice, 15*(3), 241–247.

Cohn, M. A., Fredrickson, B. L., Brown, S. L., Mikels, J. A., & Conway, A. M. (2009). Happiness unpacked: Positive emotions increase life satisfaction by building resilience. *Emotion, 9*(3), 361–368.

Connor, K. M., & Davidson, J. R. T. (2003). Development of a new resilience scale: The Connor-Davidson Resilience Scale (CD-RISC). *Depression and Anxiety, 18*(2), 76–82.

Covey, S. (1989). *The 7 habits of highly effective people.* New York: Free Press.

Csikszentmihalyi, M. (1990). *Flow: The psychology of optimal experience.* New York: HarperCollins.

Davies, W. (2015). *The happiness industry: How the government and big business sold us wellbeing.* New York: Verso.

Davis, J. A., Smith, T. W., & Marsden, P. V. (2002). *General social survey, 1972–2000 (United States).* Chicago: National Opinion Research Center, University of Chicago.

Dunn, E. W., Gilbert, D. T., & Wilson, T. D. (2011). If money doesn't make you happy, then you probably aren't spending it right. *Journal of Consumer Psychology, 21*(2), 115–125.

Easterlin, R. A. (2005). Building a better theory of well-being. In L. Bruni & P. Porta (Eds.), *Economics and happiness: Framing the analysis* (pp. 29–64). Oxford: Oxford University Press.

Eisenberger, N. I. (2012). The neural bases of social pain: Evidence for shared representations with physical pain. *Psychosomatic Medicine, 74*(2), 126–135.

Eisenberger, N. I. (2015). Social pain and the brain: Controversies, questions, and where to go from here. *Annual Review of Psychology, 66*, 601–629.

Fan, Y., Duncan, N. W., de Greck, M., & Northoff, G. (2011). Is there a core neural network in empathy? An fMRI based quantitative meta-analysis. *Neuroscience & Biobehavioral Reviews, 35*, 903–911.

Ferguson, M. A., Nielsen, J. A., King, J. B., Dai, L., Giangrasso, D. M., Holman, R., et al. (2016). Reward, salience, and attentional networks are activated by religious experience in devout Mormons. *Social Neuroscience.* Retrieved from http://www.tandfonline.com/doi/full/10.1080/17470919.2016.1257437

Gilbert, D. (2007). *Stumbling on happiness.* New York: Knopf.

Goldsmith, M., Greenberg, C., Robertson, A., & Hu-Chan, M. (2003). *Global leadership: The next generation.* New York: Pearson.

Goleman, D. (1995). *Emotional intelligence.* New York: Bantam Books.

Goleman, D., & Boyatzis, R. (2008). Social intelligence and the biology of leadership. *Harvard Business Review, 86*(9), 74–81.

Greenberg, C. L., & North, T. C. (2014). *Fearless leaders: Sharpen your focus: How the new science of mindfulness can help you reclaim your confidence.* San Diego, CA: Waterfront.

Habron, D. M. (2008). Philosophy and the science of subjective well-being. In M. Eid & R. J. Larson (Eds.), *The science of subjective well-being* (pp. 17–43). New York: Guilford Press.

Judge, T. A., & Kammeyer-Meuller, J. D. (2011). Implications of core self-evaluations for a changing organizational context. *Human Resource Management Review, 21*, 331–341.

Kahneman, D. (2011). *Thinking, fast and slow.* New York: Farrar, Straus and Giroux.

Krakauer, M., Ruscio, D., Froh, J., & Bono, G. (2017). *Handbook of Australian school psychology: Integrating positive psychology and gratitude to work in schools* (pp. 691–706). Springer International Publishing, Gewerbestrasse, Switzerland.

Kushlev, K., Heintzelmana, S. J., Lutesb, L. D., Wirtzb, D., Oishia, S., & Dienera, E. (2017). ENHANCE: Design and rationale of a randomized controlled trial for promoting enduring happiness & well-being. *Contemporary Clinical Trials, 52*, 62–74.

Longe, O., Maratos, F., Gilbert, P., Evans, G., Voler, F., Rockliff, H., & Rippon, G. (2010). Having a word with yourself: Neural correlates of self-criticism and self-reassurance. *NeuroImage, 49*(2), 1849–1856.

Lyubomirsky, S. (2013). *The myths of happiness: What should make you happy, but doesn't, what shouldn't make you happy, but does.* New York: Penguin Press.

Nadler, R. S. (2011). *Leading with emotional intelligence: Hands-on strategies for building confident and collaborative star performers.* New York: McGraw-Hill.

Neck, C. P., & Houghton, J. D. (2006). Two decades of self-leadership theory and research: Past developments, present trends, and future possibilities. *Journal of Managerial Psychology, 21*(4), 270–295.

Ornish, D. (1998). *Love & survival: The scientific basis for the healing power of intimacy.* New York: HarperCollins.

Pessoa, L. (2008). On the relationship between emotion and cognition. *Nature Reviews Neuroscience, 9*, 148–158.

Pryce-Jones, J. (2010). *Happiness at work: Maximizing your psychological capital for successs.* Hoboken, NJ: John Wiley.

Quoidbach, J., Mikolajczak, M., & Gross, J. (2015). Positive interventions: An emotion regulation perspective. *Psychological Bulletin, 141*(3), 655–693. doi:10.1037/a0038648

Greenberg-Walt, C. L., & Robertson, A. G. (2001). The evolving role of executive leadership. In W. Bennis, G. M. Spreitzer, & T. G. Cummings (Eds.), *The future of leadership* (pp. 139–157). San Francisco: Jossey-Bass.

Rolnick, A., Oren, N. T., & Bassett, D. (2016). Developing acceptance with the help of sensors—Embracing the me that I can see. *Biofeedback, 44*(3), 148–151.

Schneider, S. M. (2016). Income inequality and subjective wellbeing: Trends, challenges, and research directions. *Journal of Happiness Studies, 17*(4), 1719–1739.

Seligman, M. (2003). *Authentic happiness: Using the new positive psychology to realize your potential for fulfillment.* New York: Simon & Schuster.

Seligman, M. (2006). *Learned optimism: How to change your mind and your life.* New York: Pocket Books.

Seligman, M. (2007). *What you can change and what you can't: The complete guide to successful self-improvement.* New York: Vintage.

Seligman, M. (2012). *Flourish: A visionary new understanding of happiness and well-being.* New York: Free Press.

Seligman, M. E. P., & Csikszentmihalyi, M. (2014). Positive psychology: An introduction. In Csikszentmihalyi M (ed.). *Flow and the foundations of positive psychology* (pp. 279-298). Springer, Dordrecht.

Siegel, M. D., & Daniel, J. (2012). *Pocket guide to interpersonal neurobiology: An integrative handbook of the mind* (Norton Series on Interpersonal Neurobiology). New York: W. W. Norton.

Turk, D. C., Swanson, K. S., & Tunks, E. R. (2008). Psychological approaches in the treatment of chronic pain patients—when pills, scalpels, and needles are not enough. *The Canadian Journal of Psychiatry, 53*(4), 213-223.

Tversky, A., & Kahneman, D. (1986). Rational choice and the framing of decisions. *The Journal of Business, 59*(4, Part 2), S251-S278.

Tversky, A., & Kahneman, D. (1992). Advances in prospect theory: Cumulative representation of uncertainty. *Journal of Risk and Uncertainty, 5,* 297-323.

Varga, S., & Guignon, C. (2016). Authenticity. In E. N. Zalta (Ed.), *The Stanford encyclopedia of philosophy* (Summer 2016 ed.). Retrieved from https://plato.stanford.edu/archives/sum2016/entries/authenticity

Zell, E., & Krizan, Z. (2014). Do people have insight into their abilities? A meta-synthesis. *Perspectives on Psychological Science, 9,* 111-125.

Zettle, R. D., Hocker, T. R., Mick, K. A., Scofield, B. E., Petersen, C. L., Song, H., & Sudarijanto, R. P. (2005). Differential strategies in coping with pain as a function of level of experiential avoidance. *The Psychological Record, 55*(4), 511-524.

SECTION 2

Healing Systems: Theory and Evidence

7

Botanicals of Interest to Psychiatrists

DANIEL A. MONTI AND ANDREW B. NEWBERG

> **Key Points**
>
> - Nature provides a rich menu of herbal medicines for the treatment of psychiatric disorders. Because each medicine derives from a different source, contains different active principles, and has a different application, each must be studied thoroughly and used carefully.
> - The use of herbal medicines differs from that of chemical pharmaceuticals, which are usually tested, packaged, and administered as single agents in defined dosages.
> - Clinical evidence of effectiveness and toxicity of natural agents varies greatly as do methods for assessing their efficacy. Systems of evaluation have developed in a rather unsystematic fashion in the United States. The regulation, legality, standards, and control of their use also vary greatly throughout the world.
> - An account of the most frequently used phytopsychopharmaceuticals with their biologic effects, indications, side effects, and interactions can be useful to the clinician.

Introduction

Psychoactive plant substances are so ubiquitous in nature that it is impossible to walk through an ordinary backyard garden without encountering plants with central nervous system effects. Our knowledge of these plants have come from serendipitous discovery by traditional healers, as well as from practitioners with sophisticated theories of disease: the imbalance of vital forces in Chinese and Ayurvedic medicine or humeral imbalance theories originating in Greco-Roman medicine that formed the basis of medical practice until recent times.

In psychiatry, as in all areas of medicine, botanicals were the chief sources of treatment until the first third of the 20th century when they began to be supplanted by synthetic chemicals. Even now, a quarter of all prescription medications are derived from herbal sources. By the second third of the past century, disappointment with the failures and toxicity of synthetic drugs, together with a wish for more authentic natural treatments, led to an upsurge in the use of herbal medicines in the West. In developing countries, herbal remedies administered by traditional practitioners never lost favor.

Regulations and Control

There are significant differences between the regulation and use of herbal preparations in the United States and in other parts of the world. In the United States regulation of herbal preparations is unsatisfactory as no governmental agency has undertaken to evaluate their effectiveness. A succession of federal laws endeavored to correct the problems of the previous legislation. The Federal Food and Drugs Act of 1906 and the Federal Food, Drug, and Cosmetic Act of 1938 were enacted to remedy egregious abuse of drugs. The federal Food and Drug Administration (FDA), authorized to oversee pharmaceuticals, hewed to increasingly rigid evaluation procedures, refusing to modify the strict criteria used for new synthetic chemical drugs in evaluating natural products (Davis, 1999). This approach meant that herbal medicines were marketed as foodstuffs without need for evaluation of effectiveness. The Dietary Supplement and Health Education Act of 1994 was enacted to remedy these failures of regulation. The FDA was empowered not only to protect against dangerous, toxic, and unsanitary products but also to monitor safety, evaluate the truthfulness of advertising claims, and set standards in processing of botanicals. Product labels were required to contain lists of ingredients, potential side effects and contraindications, and special warnings. Manufacturers were not permitted to claim effectiveness of their products for specific diseases or symptoms. The methods designed to evaluate new chemical drugs from the pharmaceutical industry often do not transfer well to natural products (Weill, 1999). It seems unfortunate that, while older chemical drugs are used without proof of efficacy because of their long history of use, natural products have not been granted this latitude. Most botanicals continue to be sold in the United States as medical food rather than medicine. Supplements are found in retail stores in such abundance that it might be almost impossible to inspect all of them.

In Europe and Asia, the regulation and evaluation of herbal medicines took a less rigid, more practical course (DeSmet, 2005). France and Germany acted to accept bibliographic and anecdotal evidence in preparations with a long history of use and with demonstrated plausible pharmacologic effects. Agencies have simplified the registration process and specified dose and potency. In 1978, Commission E of the German Institute for Drugs and Medical Products began to evaluate botanicals, publishing monographs covering description of the plants involved, methods of preparation, chemical content and action of the principle components, standards of purity and content of active principles, and allowable adulterants (Blumenthal & Busse, 1998). The resulting formulary is accepted by herbal practitioners in many places including the United States. An English translation and a more recent revision have been published (Blumenthal, Goldberg, & Brinkmann, 2000). Although there were considerable differences among European countries, the European community has begun to harmonize the disparate standards. The European Scientific Cooperative on Phytotherapy has published monographs on 50 botanicals. The World Health Organization (WHO) has also issued drug monographs (1999) covering botanicals from many areas of the world. The character of the herb, methods of preparation, purity, and uses are specified comprehensively by the WHO. Six of the WHO monographs cover herbals useful in psychiatry.

Problems in Evaluation of Botanicals

Evaluation of the efficacy of natural products has not been easy. National differences in diagnosis and evaluation procedures often lead to different outcomes. For example, the first procedures used for evaluation of Hypericum in Germany were emphatically rejected by American researchers. Even now, there are many criticisms of the scientific validity of clinical trials (Gagnier, DeMelo, Boon, Rochon, & Bombardier, 2006). Herbal medicines contain many constituents. Growing conditions, harvesting procedures, and methods of preparation may account for considerable variation in the products. Confronting these difficulties, the Commission E created three categories based on proven effectiveness and safety: safe and effective, neutral, unsafe. The neutral category described drugs whose therapeutic effectiveness had not been evaluated by scientific methods but posed no significant risk to the user.

Botanicals in Current Practice

Botanical medicines have been used in many psychiatric and neurological disorders including insomnia, anxiety, depression, psychosis, dementia, and fatigue/exhaustion syndromes. In addition to single botanical agents, the practitioner will encounter many combinations of herbal medicines designed to achieve a desired result. Because of the lack of coherent regulation, the phrase *caveat emptor* applies in the United States. The purchaser must be aware of the source of the product, its stated composition and strength, and the various side effects and warnings on the label. Combinations of various botanicals, and the interaction of botanicals with other phytochemicals and synthetic prescription medicines, may be important. This is particularly so in the many remedies that combine different herbs to achieve the desired response. Even after careful reading, the consumer may be at risk from a wide discrepancy in strength of preparations from those that are listed on the label (Beaubrin & Gray, 2000; Straus, 2002). Toxic adulterants have also been a problem for the herbal medicine industry (Marcus & Grollman, 2002). As a further caveat, some researchers and clinicians have pointed out potential dangers of consumer self-diagnosis and treatment (Ernst, 2007).

With increased clinical trials and basic scientific exploration, the field of herbal medicine is changing rapidly. There are improved sources of data and information about the many available botanicals (Baek, Nierenberg, & Kinrys, 2014). These include the PDR for Herbal Medicine (2007) and the Natural Medicines Comprehensive Database (2003). Even more timely information can be obtained on Internet sites, including www.naturaldatabase.com, which is said to be updated on a daily basis, and the National Institute of Health Center for Comprehensive and Alternative Medicine's website (www.nccam.nih.gov).

Although some of these remedies are both powerful and specific, many have milder, more general actions. Unlike pharmaceutical drugs, natural remedies tend not to have specific, strong effects on patients such as inducing desired states of alertness, sleep, or calmness. Further, many botanicals are considered more effective when combined with other alternative methods such as improved diet and nutrition, meditation, or acupuncture. The following accounts are intended to be descriptive rather than prescriptive. The practitioner and user should evaluate the package label for strength, dose, side effects, and possible interactions. Because of the diversity of phytopharmaceuticals, it may be helpful to classify the herbal medicines described here into three groups: those with at least some evidence of clinical effectiveness, those that have been found ineffective or have not been tested, and a final group that the psychiatrist may encounter as a result of their addictive or neurotoxic properties or legal status (Baek et al., 2014). This classification is somewhat arbitrary; members may belong in more than one category. In addition, assignment to either effective or ineffective/safe or unsafe categories will change with further investigation. It should be noted that even many of those listed as unproven contain substances with central nervous system activity. Three of the botanicals listed are refined by pharmaceutical manufacturers and sold as prescription medications.

BOTANICALS WITH SOME EVIDENCE OF CLINICAL EFFECTIVENESS

Coffea arabica, Coffea robusta

Botany

These botanicals are derived from a small tree in the tropics with handsome glossy leaves. The red berries are fermented or dried, then roasted. Production of coffee forms the basis of the economy in many tropical areas. The principle active component, caffeine, a methylxanthene, acts as a central stimulant, increasing monoamines through antagonism of adenosine. At the usual doses (90–140 mg in a cup of coffee), the effect is of heightened alertness, increased reaction speed, and a mild euphoria. Caffeine stimulates gastric acid and is diuretic. Other methylxanthene compounds including theophylline and theobromine have similar effects. Caffeine is found in a number of botanicals, including *Cola acumenata* (cola soft drinks), *Ilex paraguariensis* (mate), *Camellia sinensis* (tea), and *Theobroma cacao* (chocolate). Each of these stimulants have different proportions of various methylxanthenes.

Use

Coffee and other caffeine containing substances are a common antidote to fatigue. They have been used universally as social beverages in Europe and the Americas since the 15th century. Tea has been accepted in Asia for many centuries. There is suggestion that coffee has a beneficial effect in Parkinson's disease. Commission E has approved coffee charcoal for use in intestinal disorders, but not the roasted berry, for reasons that seem obscure.

Cautions

These substances may cause anxiety, insomnia, cardiac arrhythmias, and gastric irritation (Cappelletti et al., 2015). Increased amounts of caffeine result in increasing anxiety. Tolerance develops, and there may be withdrawal symptoms (fatigue, headache). When combined with other stimulants, an additive effect may cause complications. Caffeine crosses the placenta and is secreted in breast milk where it may cause restlessness and poor sleep in nursing infants.

Ginkgo biloba

Pharmacology
Ginkgo biloba is derived from a deciduous tree of China, planted as a shade tree throughout the world. It is dioecious, and the fruits have a strong odor that offends some people, but the nuts are highly prized as both foodstuff and medicine in Asia. The active principles are found in the leaves, which contain a complex mixture of phytochemicals, including flavonoids, bioflavonoids, sesquiterpenes, and diterpenes (Mohanta, Tamboli, & Zubaidha, 2014). Ginkgolides are believed to account for much of the biologic activities. Ginkgolide B inhibits platelet activating factor, which is responsible for many inflammatory processes. Flavonoids are antioxidants and protect against ischemic damage. Ginkgo acts to relax vascular smooth muscle.

Use
Standardized extracts of dried Ginkgo leaves are available for administration with a usual dose of 120 to 240 mg of dry extract or 1.5 ml of fluid extract daily. The WHO and Commission E approve Ginkgo for the symptomatic relief of organic brain dysfunction, intermittent claudication, vertigo, and tinnitus of vascular origin. Ginkgo extract may slow the cognitive and social deterioration in mild cognitive impairment, Alzheimer's, and multi-infarct dementia. However, its ability to slow progression to dementia has been questioned in recent studies (DeKosly et al., 2008). It increases exercise tolerance in vascular conditions of the lower extremity. It is possibly effective when used in premenstrual syndrome, altitude sickness, and age-related macular degeneration.

Cautions
The inhibition of platelet aggregation suggests caution in patients with bleeding disorders. Interaction with anticoagulant and platelet-inhibiting drugs may occur. Interactions with anticonvulsants and antidepressants have been reported. Its safety in pregnancy and nursing has not been documented.

Humulus lupulus *(Hops)*

Biology
Humulus lupulus is a tall, dieocious perennial vine cultivated for commercial use of the inflorescence and fruit cones, which contain the aromatic, bitter-tasting elements used in brewing. Hops contains a complex mixture of acylphoroglucinols, humulones, lupulones humulene, myrcene, flavonoids, and others. The volatile oil has been noted to induce excitement followed by sleep in experimental animals. The active agents induce sleep and reduce anxiety. The extract of hops has antimicrobial activity and binds to estrogen receptors.

Uses
Hops is approved by Commission E for nervousness and insomnia. The use of hops in flavoring beer has a long tradition. It is difficult to separate the effect of hops from that of ethanol in producing the disinhibiting and sedating effects of beer. Nevertheless, hops is an effective sedative and calming agent (Koetter et al., 2007). A tea is prepared by infusion of 1 g of cone with 0.3 L of boiling water for 15 minutes. Capsules, standardized liquid, and alcoholic extracts are available.

Cautions
Excessive dose of hops, in combination with ethanol or other sedative agents, may reduce alertness to dangerous levels. Its safety in pregnancy has not been established.

Hypericum perforatum *(St. John's wort)*

Biology
Hypericum perforatum is a perennial plant with attractive yellow flower, blooming in late June at about the time of St. John's day. Indigenous to Europe, it has been planted throughout the world. It is a prolific plant. Ranchers in America have attempted to eradicate it because it is felt to sensitize cattle to sunburn. The flowers and leaves are collected for drying. Hypericum is produced by many sources and sold in large quantities and has been extensively studied. Hypericum contains the naphthodianthones hypericin and pseudohypericin, the flavonoids hyperocide, quercitrin, isoquecitrin, the acylphoroglucinol hyperforin, and numerous other compounds (Oliveira et al., 2016). The antidepressant effect was at first attributed to hypericin, but now hyperforin is felt to be the active agent. Actually a combination of several compounds

may better explain its activity. The herb has been shown to inhibit monoamine reuptake and downregulate monoamine receptors in the brain. St John's wort has some antiviral and antibacterial properties.

Uses
St. John's wort is approved by Commission E for anxiety and depressive moods. Studies have demonstrated antidepressant activity in mild to moderated depression (Ng, Venkatanarayanan, & Ho, 2017). However, other studies demonstrated its lack of effectiveness in major depression (Hypericum Depression Trial Study Group, 2002). Effectiveness in other conditions is controversial. It has been shown to reduce anxiety. The herb has a long history of use for skin conditions and wounds and is still recommended for that purpose. It is available in many forms including capsules, pellets, tablets, tincture, fluidextract, injection, transdermal patches, and dried herb in doses ranging from 125 to 1000 mg. The most common dose is a 300 mg capsule or tablet three times per day. The growing conditions, preparation, and storage can have marked effect on potency of the product. St. John's wort capsules have been standardized to contain 0.3% hyperforin.

Cautions
Photosensitization is observed in large doses. Hypericum induces cytochrome P450 enzymes. Thus one can expect reduction in blood levels of drugs metabolized by this enzyme system. These include cyclosporine, indinavir, barbiturates, estrogens, and theophylline. There may be a tendency for toxic interactions with a number of antidepressants, and its safety in pregnancy has not been documented.

Panax ginseng, Panax cinquifolium

Biology
Panax are perennial plants native to northern Asia. *Panax cinquifolium* is a North American native with similar properties. The roots of both varieties are harvested in the wild and cultivated and dried as part of a brisk commercial trade. *Panax* should not be confused with Siberian Ginseng, which is an entirely different plant, although with some similar qualities. The principal active components are the ginsenosides, a group of several dozen triterpene saponins with different biologic activities. In addition, the root contains many other compounds with biologic activity. Different components both bind to and block nicotinic acetylcholine receptors. There are antineoplastic, antioxidant, anticoagulant, and antiviral effects. Ginseng induces the alcohol

oxidizing system, activates lipoprotein lipase-lowering blood lipids, and stimulates insulin to hypoglycemic effect. Many of the components of Ginseng have a steroidal nucleus and mimic endogenous steroid hormones.

Use
Controlled studies of the effect of Ginseng on cognitive function have yielded mixed results (Smith et al., 2014). Studies confirm hypoglycemic and antiviral properties (Kachur & Suntres, 2016). The WHO monograph lists Ginseng as restorative agent for enhancement of mental and physical capacities in cases of weakness, exhaustion, tiredness, loss of concentration, and during convalescence. Commission E approves Ginseng for lack of stamina. Accounts of Ginseng's enhancement of sexual virility may account for its enormous popularity in Asia and the West. It may be beneficial for exhaustion and debility. The dried root may be made into tea. More common are the many types of fluidextract and capsules containing dried root supplied in numerous sizes.

Cautions
Side effects include mastalgia, vaginal bleeding, and arterial hypertension. Side effects are dose related. Combination with caffeine containing drugs may raise blood pressure. Interactions with antidiabetic drugs, warfarin, nonsteroidal anti-inflammatory drugs, monoamine oxidase inhibitors (MAOIs), and loop diuretics have been reported. Ginseng is not recommended in pregnancy.

Piper methysticum *(Kava)*

Botany
Piper methysticum is a deciduous bush of the South Pacific. It has been long used in Polynesian rituals aimed at dissipating hostility. The rhizome contains lactones and chalcones. The pyrones—including kavain, dihydrokavain, methysticin, yangonine, and desmethylyangonine—have central muscle relaxant, anticonvulsant, sedative, and analgesic properties through inhibition at neuronal ion channels. They potentiate gamma-aminobutyric acid (GABA)-alpha, inhibit norepinephrine uptake, and increase serotonin and dopamine.

Use
The rhizomes are prepared by maceration, in native culture by mastication. The drug is prepared by several manufacturers as a powder or extract. Controlled studies have demonstrated a reduction of anxiety symptoms

equal to that obtained with the standard benzodiazepines (Sarris, LaPorte, & Schweitzer, 2011).

Cautions
Kava may increase the risk of suicide in depressed patients, but this has not been fully confirmed (PDR for Herbal Medicine). Dose-related side effects include weight loss, liver conditions, depressed alertness, impaired reflexes, skin rash, and discoloration. Kava potentiates the effects of alcohol, benzodiazepines, and barbiturates. It should be discontinued after three months use. The National Institutes of Health discontinued research on kava because of a number of cases of liver damage resulting from use of the herb. Kava is contraindicated in pregnancy.

Rauwolfia serpentina

Botany
Rauwolfia serpentine is a small shrub native to South Asia. The root is collected and dried commercially. Its use in medicine has so depleted the supply that the pharmaceutical industry has been forced to turn to a related species, *Rauwolfia vomitoria*, or else synthesis to obtain the active alkaloid. The active alkaloids include reserpine, reserpinine, serpentine, serpetenine, ajmaline, and others. The effect of reserpine is to deplete both the peripheral and the central nervous system of all catecholamines by limiting their reabsorption. Rauwolfia is dispensed as the alkaloid, reserpine, or preparations containing the powdered whole root.

Use
Rauwolfia is currently used to treat essential hypertension but was one of the first agents shown to be effective in the treatment of acute schizophrenia. It has a sedative effect and gradually ameliorates agitation, delusions, hallucinations, and other psychotic symptoms. Rauwolfia was gradually replaced in psychiatry by synthetic drugs because of its side effects (Nur & Adams, 2016). It is obtainable through prescription. Dose of the refined alkaloid varies from 0.1 mg to 1 mg.

Cautions
Snakeroot (another name for Rauwolfia) causes severe nasal congestion, somnolence, erectile dysfunction, and depression. In depressed patients it increases the severity of symptoms. It increases the depressant effects of alcohol, barbiturates, and benzodiazepines and antagonizes the effects of levodopa

and other anti-Parkinson medicines. Administration with digitalis glycosides results in marked bradycardia. Long-term use may lead to breast tumors, some of which become malignant.

Valeriana officinalis

Biology
Valeriana officinalis is a European native shrub of moderate height that is cultivated for its medicinal uses. The roots are dried in preparation of the medicine. The active components include iridoids, sesqueterpines, pyridine alkaloids, and caffeic acid derivatives. The combination of compounds is central depressant, sedative, and anxiolytic. The herb appears to cause an increase of central GABA. Controlled trials indicate decreased sleep latency and improved quality of sleep (Oxman et al., 2007).

Use
The botanical is supported as a mild sedative by the WHO monograph. Commission E approves this herb for use in patients with nervousness and insomnia. Recent publications have reported Valerian to be ineffective when compared to placebo in double-blind studies on anxiety (Miyasaka, Atallah, & Soares, 2006).

Cautions
Valerian may potentiate other central nervous system depressants. Long-term use may cause headaches, restlessness, insomnia, and cardiac dysfunction.

Cannabis sativa *(Marijuana)*

Biology
The hemp plant is a large shrub reaching considerable height in warm climates. Pictures of the characteristic leaf pattern have been so widely circulated that by now it must be one of our more familiar plants. The plant is dioecious, and the inflorescence of the female plant is the richest source of resin-containing active ingredients. The plant is now bred for maximum cannabinol production. Cannabinoids characterize the plant, and 9-tetrahydrocannabinol is the most thoroughly studied of these; however, there are many other cannabinoids as well as flavinoids and other elements in this plant. Cannabinoid receptors have been demonstrated in several areas of the brain (Bhattacharyya et al., 2012). Naturally occurring neuromodulators of these receptors, such as

anandamide, stimulate release of dopamine in the mesolimbic reward system, as does cannabinol. The usual dose produces a reduction of drive, concentration, thinking, memory, and perception of time. Sensory impressions are heightened or altered. The usual mood is euphoric but can be anxious. In larger amounts, cannabis may be hallucinogenic. The drug stimulates appetite and reduces nausea. It reduces intraocular pressure.

Use
The recreational use of cannabis is the basis of an enormous underground agriculture. The plant has been bred for enhanced content of alkaloids. Marijuana may be taken by mouth as tea or extract but the most common route is inhalation of smoke. More recently, cannabis has been widely studied for medical purposes, and its medical use has been approved in a number of states (Baron, 2015). Cannabis has been studied and utilized in a variety of chronic pain syndromes such as headache and cancer-related pain. Cannabis has been used for symptoms of AIDS and certain malignancies due to its antiemetic and appetite-stimulating properties. A preparation of one of its components, delta-9-tetrahydrocannabinol (Marinol), is manufactured for that purpose. The use of cannabis has been the ground for ongoing political debate.

Cautions
Side effects include dry mouth and a pathognomonic conjunctival injection. Long-term use of smoked cannabis may cause bronchial and pulmonary inflammation and neoplasm (Schrot & Hubbard, 2016). Reports have suggested the occurrence of an amotivational syndrome consequent to heavy long-term use. There may also be an association between cannabis and psychosis (Gage, Hickman, & Zammit, 2016). A number of studies report permanent changes in the structure of the brain. The reports of permanent changes with occasional use are less convincing than those with chronic or excessive use. Cannabinols cross the placental barrier and are secreted in breast milk. They may impair fetal development and, hence, are contraindicated in pregnancy and breastfeeding.

Lavender *angustifolia* (English Lavender)

Biology
Lavender oils derive from several different plants including *Lavender angustifolia,* an aromatic branched perennial evergreen shrub indigenous to the Mediterranean but cultivated in all temperate regions. The fresh and dried

flowers are processed to extract the aromatic oil. Lavender is used in cosmetics and food as well as medicine. The herb contains 160 different compounds including the volatile oils linalool, linalyl acetate, acimene, cineole, and other elements. Central nervous system depressant effects have been demonstrated in animals. An effect on the limbic system of the brain can be demonstrated in humans upon inhalation. The active ingredients shorten sleep latency and increase duration of sleep.

Uses
Lavender is approved by Commission E for loss of appetite, nervousness and insomnia, circulatory disorders, and dyspeptic complaints. A number of studies have shown that Lavender can be beneficial for anxiety including patients with generalized anxiety disorder (Kasper et al., 2010; Kasper et al., 2014). Lavender may be taken as tea prepared by infusing 3 g of dried flowers in 300 mL of boiling water for 15 minutes. In addition, inhalation of the essential oil may give a therapeutic effect. Lavender has also been used in baths as an oil.

Cautions
No ill effects have noted at ordinary quantities.

Passiflora incarnata *(Passionflower)*

Biology
Passionflower is a tall, perennial vine native to the Americas. It is grown as an ornamental. The fruits are edible. Medicine is made of the dried leaves and shoots. Biologically active ingredients include many flavonoids and the glycoside gynocardine. Studies have been unable to prove sedative efficacy.

Use
Although more data is clearly needed, there are a number of studies that have shown that passionflower is beneficial in reducing anxiety. It has been evaluated for reducing anxiety in patients undergoing surgical procedures and in patients with generalized anxiety disorder showing comparable efficacy to benzodiazepines (Akhondzadeh et al., 2001; Movafegh et al., 2008). Commission E approves this botanical for nervousness and insomnia. Passionflower has been given for insomnia, hysterical agitation, and anxiousness. It is prepared as capsules and fluid extract. A tea may be prepared by infusion of the dried leaves. Clinical studies to confirm its effectiveness are lacking.

Cautions
No side effects are reported at the ordinary doses.

Matricaria chamomilla, Matricaria recutita *(Chamomile)*

Botany
Chamomile derives from several related plants such as Matricaria chamomilla *Matricaria recutita* (German Chamomile). The plants typically grow about 1 foot tall, bearing daisy-like flowers with white petals and yellow centers. Diverse components account for the variety of effects of these herbs. Chamazulene and apigenen have anti-inflamatory effects. Chamazulene is an antioxidant. Flavonoids such as apigenen exert anxiolytic effects. On the body surface, the herb inhibits bacteria, tumor formation, and inflammation.

Use
Although the Commission E approval is limited to oral, dermatologic, and infectious problems, the WHO monograph (1999) mentions its usefulness in the restlessness and insomnia associated with nervous disorders. Chamomile has a long history of use as an anxiolytic and sedative and is one of the most commonly used herbal remedies. Recently, there have been several large randomized controlled trials supporting the use of chamomile in patients with generalized anxiety disorder at doses of 1500 mg/day for up to eight weeks (Keefe et al., 2016).

Cautions
Matricaria may potentiate the effects of sedative and anticoagulant herbs. It may precipitate violent allergic reactions in persons sensitive to other members of the composite family.

Rhodiola rosea *(Goldenroot)*

Botany
Rhodiola rosea (R. rosea) is a perennial flowering plant in the family Crassulaceae. It grows naturally in wild Arctic regions of Europe, Asia, and North America and can be propagated as a groundcover. Phenylpropanoids are derived from the *R. rosea* root and contribute to physical and mental endurance. But over 140 molecules have been found in extracts of *R. rosea* including nonpolar monoterpene hydrocarbons, monoterpene and aliphatic alcohols, geraniol, cyanogenic glycosides, phenylpropanoids, flavonoids, flavolignans, gallic acid derivatives,

and rosiridin which is an inhibitor of monoamine oxidase A and B (Panossian. Wikman, & Sarris, 2010).

Use
R. rosea contains adaptogens that can help protect people from mental and physical stress, various toxins, and infections (Amsterdam & Panossian, 2016). *R. rosea* is a plant with a "stimulant" action and can help increase mental work capacity during stress; it is also a general adaptogen. Several randomized controlled trials have demonstrated a benefit from *R. rosea* in patients with depression (Mao et al., 2015).

Cautions
R. rosea may cause several side effects such as agitation, irritability, insomnia, anxiety, brain fog, and dry mouth.

BOTANICALS THAT HAVE NOT DEMONSTRATED CLINICAL EFFECTIVENESS OR HAVE NOT BEEN ADEQUATELY TESTED

Artemesia absinthium *(Wormwood)*

Biology
Artemesia absinthium is a small shrub with deeply incised silvery grey leaves, an aromatic odor, and a bitter taste; it is found throughout the world. Its leaves and stems are the source of medicinal elements, and the volatile oils include thujone, cis-, anabsinthine, and matricine. The leaf is said to have a cholegogic effect epoxy ocimeme and chrysanthenyl acetate. The flavoring elements include absinthine which also inhibits the growth of some bacteria and protozoa. A related species has found to be active against malaria.

Use
The leaf and extracts are approved by Commission E for use in loss of appetite, dyspepsia, and liver and gall bladder complaints. The folk use of wormwood as a vermifuge, appetite stimulant, and digestive has never been demonstrated. The liqueur beverage, absinthe, was banned for most of the 20th century because it was thought to cause seizures, brain damage, and addiction (Lachenmeier et al., 2006). While it is true that thujone precipitates seizures, it is difficult to determine what proportion of the notorious effects were the result of ethanol. Wormwood continues to be used as a flavoring agent in various bitter wines such as Vermouth. The dried leaf may be used in tea at 1 g per cup.

Cautions
A distilled oil preparation is dangerous because of the high levels of active substances. Wormwood may cause gastrointestinal symptoms. Chronic, excessive use leads to central nervous system disorders. Its use in pregnancy is contraindicated.

Artemisia vulgaris *(Mugwort)*

Biology
Mugwort is a weedy plant of moderate height, native to North America and now found throughout the world. The roots and aerial parts of the plant are used in medicine. The herb contains cineol, camphor, linalool, thujone, sesquiterpene lactones, flavonoids, and hydroxycoumarins.

Use
The drug is used as a tonic, sedative, and digestive. Psychophysiologic activity has never been evaluated in scientific studies. It is reputed to be a vermifuge, but this use has not been evaluated. In Chinese medicine, mugwort is used in moxibustion. It is sold as a tincture and dried herb used for tea.

Cautions
Mugwort is not safe for use in pregnancy due to its abortifacient actions.

Withania somnifera *(Ashwagandha)*

Biology
Ashwagandha is an adaptogenic herb popular in Ayurvedic medicine. The name comes from Sanskrit and is a combination of *ashva* meaning "horse" and *ghadha* meaning "smell" because the root has a strong, horse-like smell. The primary chemical constituents are alkaloids and steroidal lactones, which are believed to have anxiolytic properties (Dar et al., 2016).

Uses
Ashwagandha has been found to produce an anxiolytic effect comparable to lorazepam in rats. A review of five research studies showed improvements in measures of anxiety and stress. However, it is not clear whether Ashwagandha provides improvements in patients with generalized anxiety disorder or whether it performs better than placebo. Future studies will be needed to clarify its use in psychiatric patients.

Cautions
There is some evidence that Ashwagandha might reduce blood sugar levels, reduce blood pressure, increase thyroid hormone levels, and cause stomach irritation. Also, Ashwagandha should not be used in pregnancy as there is some suggestion that it might cause miscarriages.

Eleutherococcus senticosus *(Siberian Ginseng)*

Biology
Siberian Ginseng is often confused with, and sold as, *Panax ginseng*. Despite some common effects, the plants are different and have different components. It is a shrub native to Northeast Asia. The roots are dried and used for tea. The herb contains a complex mixture of lignans, sterols, steroid glycosides, coumarins, saponins, phenypropanols, and several provitamins. Various components have been noted to stimulate the immune system, inhibit platelet aggregation, and stimulate the pituitary adrenal axis. There may also be anti-inflammatory, sedative, anabolic, gonadotropic, and antiviral properties; however, these have not been demonstrated by careful clinical trials.

Use
Commission E recommends Siberian Ginseng for lack of stamina and tendency to infection. It has been used to increase resistance to stress and infections and to improve memory and concentration, but these have not been proven (Deyama, Nishibe, & Nakazawa, 2001). Siberian Ginseng has not been as well studied as Panax.

Cautions
The drug is contraindicated in patients with hypertension. Possible drug interactions include digoxin, antidiabetic agents, and anticoagulants. Its safety in pregnancy has not been documented.

Leonurus cardiaca *(Motherwort)*

Biology
Motherwort is a shrub with bright red flowers and an unpleasant odor. It is native to northern Europe but is now established in the wild in North America. The aerial portions of the plant are dried and prepared as tinctures and fluid

extracts. Compounds include stachydrine, leocardin, leonuride, flavonoids, leonurinine, bufenolide, betonicine, ursolic acid, and others. The herb has a mild sedative effect. Its glycocodes act to inhibit cardiac activity, stimulate uterine smooth muscle, and inhibit coagulation. Motherwort stimulates the release of oxytocin, and one of its components, ursolic acid, has been shown to inhibit tumor growth.

Use
Motherwort is available in extracts and tinctures. Tea made by infusion of 3 g of dried herb in 250 mL of boiling water. In folk medicine, motherwort was used to decrease the anxiety often experienced by mothers (Wojtyniak, Szymański, & Matławska, 2013). It is approved by Commission E for nervous heart complaints. It has a chronotropic effect, slowing the heart rate.

Cautions
No serious side effects have been noted at ordinary doses. Excess of 3 g per day has been known to cause diarrhea and uterine bleeding. Motherwort may increase the effect of sedatives and herbs containing cardiac glycosides. It is not recommended in pregnancy.

Melissa officinalis *(Lemon Balm)*

Biology
Lemon balm is a small perennial plant of the mint family native to the Mediterranean but cultivated throughout the world. The leaves are dried and used as tea. Distillation provides an essential oil. The herb contains a complex mixture of volatile substances including geranial (citral A), neral (citral B), citronellal, linalool, geraniol, rosmaric acid, eugenol glycoside, and many other compounds. These act as sedative and calming agents. The herb is most effective when used within a few months of harvest. The source of the sedative effects has not been determined.

Use
Commission E approves lemon balm for nervousnous and insomnia. The herb also has been studied in small trials for its benefit with anxiety, depression, and as a neuroprotectant, but more studies are required to confirm these findings (Shakeri, Sahebkar, & Javadi, 2016). The herb is used as a culinary flavoring agent. It may be taken as a tea made by infusion of 3 g of leaves in 250 mL of water. It is also sold in capsule form.

Cautions
The herb is relatively benign. It may potentiate sedatives and interfere with thyroid replacement therapy.

Papaver Species: Papaver rhoeas *(Corn Poppy)* and Eschscholzia californica *(California Poppy)*

Biology
Papaver somniferum, the opium poppy, has been thoroughly treated in standard textbooks of pharmacology. Its two cousins—one a native of Europe, the other of North America—may be considered together. Both are annual plants with bright attractive yellow to red flowers. Flower heads and aerial parts are dried. Both herbs have a variety of alkaloids but relatively sparse content of the alkaloid opium. The alkaloids of corn poppy include rhoeadine, isorhoeadine, rheoagenine, and others. The California poppy contains the alkaloids californidine, eschscholzine, protopine, cyptopine, and others. Alkaloids of the California poppy have been shown to bind to benzodiazepine receptors. Californidine has been shown to promote sleep and decrease anxiety in animals; however, there have been no controlled human trials with either herb to confirm sedative and calming effects, and Commission E withholds support for the use of these poppy products.

Use
The dried flowers and petals are used in teas prepared by steeping 1 to 3 g of dried herb in 250 mL of water for 15 minutes. Infusions and extracts may be found. The indications reported are primarily for insomnia and anxiety.

Cautions
Poppy may potentiate the effects of sedatives. These herbs have not been evaluated for safety in pregnancy.

Scutellaria *(Scullcap)*

Botany
Skullcap is an attractive native American wildflower with a bitter taste. It is cultivated in other areas for its medicinal properties and as a ornamental. The aerial portions of the plant are dried and powdered. The plant contains a complex mixture of flavonoids and volatile oils, which have not been thoroughly explored. No studies have been performed to confirm its physiologic effects.

Use
Scullcap has been prescribed for hysteria, anxiety, and other nervous disorders. The herb has not been subjected to controlled evaluation of therapeutic efficacy (Brock et al., 2014). It is prepared as powder and as a fluid extract.

Cautions
No known adverse side effects are reported with moderate use of this medicine. Large amounts may cause vertigo, somnolence, and confusion. Scullcap may potentiate other sedative substances. Its safety in pregnancy has not been established.

BOTANICALS THAT ARE ILLEGAL OR HAVE TOXIC OR ADDICTIVE CHARACTERISTICS

Atropa belladonna *(Belladonna)*

Biology
Atropa belladonna is a European wildflower now cultivated throughout the world for the pharmacologic properties of its leaves and roots. It is a plant with three interesting features: it is poisonous; it has a fascinating history having been used to dilate the pupils of women in order to enhance their attractiveness, and drug manufacturers extract the active alkaloids for use as single agents. The active compounds include atropine, hyoscyamine, and scopolamine. These are powerful anticholinergic agents acting as antagonists at the peripheral muscarinic parasympathetic autonomic receptors and in the brain, where they produce a characteristic delirium with agitation, confusion, and hallucinations.

Use
Belladonna may be obtained as a powder or a liquid extract for gastrointestinal conditions. Commission E lists the leaf for liver and gall bladder complaints in dose of 50 to 100 mg of leaf. Commercially, atropine and scopolamine are extracted from the plant and prepared as an injection for use in anesthesia and other purposes. Capsules containing atropine, hyoscyamine, scopolamine and phenobarbital are available in most pharmacies with a prescription. Due to the variable amounts of alkaloid in the plants and their extreme toxicity, manufacturers carefully control the strength of alkaloids in the products. The direct use of the plant materials is dangerous.

The significance of belladonna for psychiatrists involves its recreational use to induce hallucinations. It should be noted that a number of other anticholinergic substances, such as *Hyoscyamus niger* (Henbane), *Mandragora* species (Mandrake), *Datura* species (Thorn Apple and Jimson Weed), *Solanum dulcamara* (Bittersweet nightshade), all contain tropane alkaloids and have similar effects. Even more ubiquitous deliriants are the leaves of solanaceous garden vegetables such as tomatoes, potatoes, and peppers. Recently, the recreational use of tropane alkaloids has declined with the increased illegal use of other psychotomimetic substances.

Cautions
Anticholinergic drugs increase heart rate, impair bodily temperature through inhibition of perspiration, and slow gastrointestinal motility. Hyperthermia and cardiac arrhythmias may be fatal. Toxic effects are increased in the elderly. *Atropa belladonna* and similar botanicals are contraindicated in fever, acute narrow angle glaucoma, and gastro-esophageal reflux disorder. The frenzy of delirium may threaten life. These agents should not be used for recreational purposes. Their use in pregnancy is limited.

Catha edulis *(Khat)*

Biology
Catha edulis is an evergreen tree native to East Africa; it is a prime recreational substance in Islamic countries, where the religion proscribes alcohol. The phenethylamine compounds cathine and cathinone are chief active agents. Norpseudoephedrine, norephedrine, and related compounds contribute to stimulating effects. The more volatile cathinone dissipates rapidly. The ingredients have a sympathomimetic and central stimulating action, which result in alertness, euphoria, and suppression of hunger.

Use
The fresh leaves may be chewed, made into paste, or taken as tea. The drug is said to increase self-regard and alertness and act as an aphrodisiac. Many countries attempt to restrict its recreational use. The WHO has declared it a drug of abuse. It is banned in many countries and is a schedule 1 controlled substance in the United States.

Cautions
Excitement, hypertension, and appetite suppression result from Khat use. Long-term use leads to apathy and anorexia. The drug may be habituating, and a withdrawal syndrome of depression and fatigue result from sudden cessation. The effects in pregnancy have not been documented.

Ephedra sinica *and Other Species*

Biology
Ephedra sinica is a botanical commonly used in Chinese medicine as Ma Huang. However, *Ephedra* species are widely distributed throughout temperate regions. The aerial portions of the plant are dried and used as tea. More commonly, a fluid extract is used as tincture or capsules. The active principles are the alkaloids ephedrine, pseudophedrine, norephedrine, and norpseudoephedrine. These are powerful peripheral sympathomimetic and central nervous system stimulants.

Use
Ephedrine and pseudoephedrine are extracted from the plant and used as decongestants in commercial cold medicine and nose drops. Ephedra root may be used as tea at 0.5 to 3 g per cup but more commonly as extracts. It is approved for treatment of cough and bronchitis by Commission E and the WHO. There is no evidence that it increases stamina in athletes. Ephedrine has been abused for its stimulant properties and is a raw material for illegal stimulants in the underground drug economy.

Cautions
Ephedrine products have been popular in pharmacies and health food stores; they are sold over the counter to control appetite and increase energy. Ephedrine is never used alone in Asian medicine but rather is combined with other botanicals that modify its effects. Its use in nose drops results in rebound nasal turgor. It can be habituating with chronic use. Ephedrine increases blood pressure and is contraindicated in hypertension. Other contraindications include thyrotoxicosis, pheochromocytoma, and lower urinary tract obstruction. It is contraindicated in pregnancy. Drug interactions, some potentially fatal, include MAOI, stimulants, and other sympathomimetic drugs.

Erythroxylum coca *(Cocaine)*

Botany
A shrubby tree native to the Andes mountains of South America, *Erythroxylum coca* is cultivated elsewhere in mountainous regions. The fibrous leaves are dried or chewed in their native environment. The chemical processing of

coca leaves is the basis of a large illegal enterprise. The plant contains a number of active substances, but the chief agent is the tropane alkaloid cocaine. Cocaine is a local anesthetic agent. It stimulates release of monoamine neurotransmitters and blocks their reuptake. Its strongest effect is on dopamine, which accounts for the prominent euphoria. Other effects—such as hypertension, irritability, restlessness, anxiety, and paranoia—may result from excess of other monoamines.

Use

It has been used as a local anesthetic. Leaves are chewed by Andean workers to increase stamina on long journeys. Cocaine's use is illegal in most countries.

Cautions

Use in pregnancy causes fetal abnormalities. Coca may be habituating. Adrenergic effects may lead to acute vascular events of cardiac and cerebral arteries, although such untoward effects are more common with the refined alkaloid, cocaine.

Conclusion

This chapter has attempted to summarize the current state of herbal pharmacopoeia in psychiatry. Table 7.1, which contains the most common herbal psychotropic medicines, may be helpful in prescribing. Doses are difficult to quantitate because of the variation of potency, so great care must be taken on the part of the physician to ensure the proper dose is used and will not interact with, alter, or be altered by other medications and supplements. Also, many of these medicines, particularly those used for insomnia and anxiety, are sold in combination. The growth of interest in this area has produced two contrasting effects. On a positive note, interest has insured increased funding for scientific exploration of botanicals and of the differences between herbal and ordinary medical practice. More disturbing developments are the uncontrolled proliferation of products, lack of standardization, and wide disparity in outlets selling herbal products. The enthusiasm of the consumer, who often feels that these products are healthy (and one can never have too much health) may lead to injudicious and excessive use of these products. Taking a complete history is important as the practitioner may uncover bizarre mixtures, contaminated, or unsanitary medicines, as well as ones that are carefully produced and used.

Table 7.1. Common Phytopsychopharmaceuticals

Herbal	Indications	Dose	Side Effects
Coffea	Somnolence, fatigue	90–100 mg	Anxiety, cardiac arrhythmia, gastric irritation
Ginkgo	Organic cognitive disfunction, memory impairment	120–240 mg	Potentiates anticoagulants
Hops	Insomnia, anxiety	1 g of strobile as tea, 1–2 mL tincture	Somnolence, potentiates depressants
Hypericum	Depressive disorder	900 mg daily	Photosensitivity, induces CYP450 enzymes, lowers levels of several medicines
Ginseng	Stress, fatigue, cognitive impairment	100–400 mg daily	Hypertension, mastalgia, interactions with a number of drugs
Rauwolfia	Schizophrenia, anxiety, insomnia	0.05–1 mg	Hypotension, nasal congestion, potentiates depressants, increased incidence of breast tumors with chronic use
Cannabis	Chronic pain, headache	Variable depending on concentration and route	Dry mouth, reduced motivation, and lung effects when inhaled
Valerian	Insomnia, anxiety	300–900 mg at bedtime. 300–450 three times/day	Potentiates depressants
Rhodiola rosea	Depression	Up to 1300 mg daily	Agitation, irritability, insomnia, brain fog, dry mouth
Chamomile	Anxiety	Up to 1500 mg per day	Sedation, anticoagulation

Acknowledgment

This chapter is a revised/updated chapter based on an earlier version written for the first edition by Dr. Howard L. Field.

REFERENCES

Akhondzadeh, S., Naghavi, H. R., Vazirian, M., Shayeganpour, A., Rashidi, H., & Khani, M. (2001). Passionflower in the treatment of generalized anxiety: A pilot double-blind randomized controlled trial with oxazepam. *Journal of Clinical Pharmacy and Therapeutics, 26*(5), 363–367.

Amsterdam, J. D., & Panossian, A. G. (2016). Rhodiola rosea L. as a putative botanical antidepressant. *Phytomedicine, 23*(7), 770–783.

Baek, J. H., Nierenberg, A. A., & Kinrys, G. (2014). Clinical applications of herbal medicines for anxiety and insomnia: Targeting patients with bipolar disorder. *The Australian and New Zealand Journal of Psychiatry, 48*(8), 705–715.

Baron, E. P. (2015). Comprehensive review of medicinal marijuana, cannabinoids, and therapeutic implications in medicine and headache: What a long strange trip it's been. *Headache, 55*(6), 885–916.

Beaubrin, G., & Gray, G. E. (2000). A review of herbal medicines for psychiatric disorders. *Psychiatric Services, 51*(9), 1130–1134.

Bhattacharyya, S., Atakan, Z., Martin-Santos, R., Crippa, J. A., & McGuire, P. K. (2012). Neural mechanisms for the cannabinoid modulation of cognition and affect in man: A critical review of neuroimaging studies. *Current Pharmaceutical Design, 18*(32), 5045–5054.

Blumenthal, M., & Busse, W. R. (1998). *Complete German Commission E monographs: Therapeutic guide to herbal medicines/developed by a special expert committee of the German Federal Institute for Drugs and Medical Devices.* Boston: Integrative Medicine Communications.

Blumenthal, M., Goldberg, A., & Brinkmann, J. (Eds.). (2000). *Herbal medicine: Expanded commission E monographs.* Newton, MA: Integrative Medicine Communications.

Brock, C., Whitehouse, J., Tewfik, I., & Towell, T. (2014). American skullcap (*Scutellaria lateriflora*): A randomised, double-blind placebo-controlled crossover study of its effects on mood in healthy volunteers. *Phytotherapy Research, 28*(5), 692–698.

Cappelletti, S., Piacentino, D., Sani, G., & Aromatario, M. (2015). Caffeine: Cognitive and physical performance enhancer or psychoactive drug? *Current Neuropharmacology, 13*(1), 71–88. doi:10.2174/1570159X13666141210215655

Dar, P. A., Singh, L. R., Kamal, M. A., & Dar, T. A. (2016). Unique medicinal properties of Withania somnifera: Phytochemical constituents and protein component. *Current Pharmaceutical Design, 22*(5), 535–540.

Davis, D. L. (1999). Opening comments from the Department of Health and Human Services. In D. Eskinazi (Ed.), *Botanical medicine*. Larchmont, NY: Mary Ann Liebert, Inc.

DeKosky, S. T., Williamson, J. D., Fitzpatrick, A. L., Kronmal, R. A., Ives, D. G., Saxton, J. A., et al. (2008). Ginkgo biloba for prevention of dementia: A randomized controlled trial. *Journal of the American Medical Association, 300*(19), 2253–2262.

DeSmet, P. A. G. M. (2005). Herbal medicine in Europe—relaxing regulatory standards. *New England Journal of Medicine, 352*(12), 1176–1178.

Deyama, T., Nishibe, S., & Nakazawa, Y. (2001). Constituents and pharmacological effects of Eucommia and Siberian ginseng. *Acta Pharmacologica Sinica, 22*(12), 1057–1070.

Ernst, E. (2007). Herbal medicine: Buy one get two free. *Postgraduate Medical Journal, 83*, 615–616.

Gage, S. H., Hickman, M., & Zammit, S. (2016). Association between cannabis and psychosis: Epidemiologic evidence. *Biological Psychiatry, 79*(7), 549–556.

Gagnier, J. J., DeMelo, J., Boon, H., Rochon, P., & Bombardier, C. (2006). Quality of reporting of randomized controlled trials of herbal medicine interventions. *American Journal of Medicine, 119*, 800.e1–800.e11.

Hypericum Depression Trial Study Group. (2002). The effect of *Hypricum perforatum* (St. John's wort) in major depressive disorder: A randomized controlled trial *Journal of the American Medical Association, 287*(10), 1807–1814.

Kachur, K., & Suntres, Z. E. (2016). The antimicrobial properties of ginseng and ginseng extracts. *Expert Review of Anti-Infective Therapy, 14*(1), 81–94.

Kasper, S., Gastpar, M., Müller, W. E., Volz, H. P., Möller, H. J., Dienel, A., & Schläfke, S. (2010). Silexan, an orally administered Lavandula oil preparation, is effective in the treatment of "subsyndromal" anxiety disorder: A randomized, double-blind, placebo controlled trial. *International Clinical Psychopharmacology, 25*(5), 277–287.

Kasper, S., Gastpar, M., Müller, W. E., Volz, H. P., Möller, H. J., Schläfke, S., & Dienel, A. (2014). Lavender oil preparation Silexan is effective in generalized anxiety disorder: A randomized, double-blind comparison to placebo and paroxetine. *International Journal of Neuropsychopharmacology, 17*(6), 859–869.

Keefe, J. R., Mao, J. J., Soeller, I., Li, Q. S., & Amsterdam, J. D. (2016). Short-term open-label chamomile (*Matricaria chamomilla L.*) therapy of moderate to severe generalized anxiety disorder. *Phytomedicine, 23*(14), 1699–1705.

Koetter, U., Schrader, E., Käufeler, R., & Brattström, A. (2007). A randomized, double blind, placebo-controlled, prospective clinical study to demonstrate clinical efficacy of a fixed valerian hops extract combination (Ze 91019) in patients suffering from non-organic sleep disorder. *Phytotherapy Research, 21*(9), 847–851.

Lachenmeier, D. W., Walch, S. G., Padosch, S. A., & Kröner, L. U. (2006). Absinthe—a review. *Critical Reviews in Food Science and Nutrition, 46*(5), 365–377.

Mao, J. J., Xie, S. X., Zee, J., Soeller, I., Li, Q. S., Rockwell, K., & Amsterdam, J. D. (2015). Rhodiola rosea versus sertraline for major depressive disorder: A randomized placebo-controlled trial. *Phytomedicine, 22*(3), 394–399.

Marcus, D. M., & Grollman, A. P. (2002). Botanical medicines—the need for new regulations. *New England Journal of Medicine, 347*(25), 2073–2076.

Miyasaka, L. S., Atallah, A. N., & Soares, B. G. (2006). Valerian for anxiety disorders. *Cochrane Database of Systematic Reviews, 4*, CD004515.

Mohanta, T. K., Tamboli, Y., & Zubaidha, P K. (2014). Phytochemical and medicinal importance of Ginkgo biloba L. *Natural Product Research, 28*(10), 746–752.

Movafegh, A., Alizadeh, R., Hajimohamadi, F., Esfehani, F., & Nejatfar, M. (2008). Preoperative oral Passiflora incarnata reduces anxiety in ambulatory surgery patients: A double-blind, placebo-controlled study. *Anesthesia and Analgesia, 106*(6), 1728–1732.

Ng, Q. X., Venkatanarayanan, N., & Ho, C. Y. (2017). Clinical use of *Hypericum perforatum* (St John's wort) in depression: A meta-analysis. *Journal of Affective Disorders, 210*, 211–221.

Nur, S., & Adams, C. E. (2016). Chlorpromazine versus reserpine for schizophrenia. *Cochrane Database of Systematic Reviews, 4*, CD012122. doi:10.1002/14651858.CD012122.pub2

Oliveira, A. I., Pinho, C., Sarmento, B., & Dias, A. C. (2016). Neuroprotective activity of *Hypericum perforatum* and its major components. *Frontiers in Plant Science, 7*, 1004. doi:10.3389/fpls.2016.01004

Oxman, A. D., Flottorp, S., Håvelsrud, K., Fretheim, A., Odgaard-Jensen, J., Austvoll-Dahlgren, A., et al. (2007). A televised, web-based randomised trial of an herbal remedy (valerian) for insomnia. *PLoS One, 2*(10), e1040.

Panossian, A., Wikman, G., & Sarris, J. (2010). Rosenroot (Rhodiola rosea): Traditional use, chemical composition, pharmacology and clinical efficacy. *Phytomedicine, 17*, 481–493.

Sarris, J., LaPorte, E., & Schweitzer, I. (2011). Kava: A comprehensive review of efficacy, safety, and psychopharmacology. *The Australian and New Zealand Journal of Psychiatry, 45*(1), 27–35.

Schrot, R. J., & Hubbard, J. R. (2016). Cannabinoids: Medical implications. *Annals of Medicine, 48*(3), 128–141.

Shakeri, A., Sahebkar, A., & Javadi, B. (2016). Melissa officinalis L.—A review of its traditional uses, phytochemistry and pharmacology. *Journal of Ethnopharmacology, 188*, 204–228.

Smith, I., Williamson, E. M., Putnam, S., Farrimond, J., & Whalley, B. J. (2014). Effects and mechanisms of ginseng and ginsenosides on cognition. *Nutrition Review, 72*(5), 319–333.

Straus, S. E. (2002). Herbal medicines—what's in the bottle? *New England Journal of Medicine, 347*(25), 1997–1998.

Thompson Health Care. (2007). *Physicians desk reference for herbal medicines* (4th ed.). Montvale, NJ: Author.

Thomson, P. D. R. (2003). *Natural medicines comprehensive database* (5th ed.). Stockton, CA: Therapeutic Research Faculty.

Weill, A. T. (1999). Botanical efficiency in the clinical setting. In D. Eskinazi (Ed.), *Botanical medicine* (pp. 43–44). Larchmont, NY: Mary Ann Liebert.

Wojtyniak, K., Szymański, M., & Matławska, I. (2013). Leonurus cardiaca L. (motherwort): A review of its phytochemistry and pharmacology. *Phytotherapy Research, 27*(8), 1115–1120.

World Health Organization. (1999). *Monographs on selected medicinal plants* (Vol. 1). Geneva: Author.

8

Acupuncture and Chinese Medicine

JINGDUAN YANG AND DANIEL A. MONTI

> **Key Points**
>
> - Chinese medicine is a complete system of healing that first appeared in written form around 100 BC. China, Japan, Korea, and Vietnam have since developed their own distinct versions of the original Chinese system.
> - Chinese medicine describes human physiology and psychology in term of *Qi*, a vital energy that circulates through energetic channels called *meridians*. Chinese medicine uniquely relates specific mental and physical functioning to corresponding meridians that are associated with internal organs.
> - Qi balance is described in terms of Yin and Yang, which represent opposing energetic qualities.
> - Human beings are considered healthy when the Qi circulating in each meridian is balanced in forces of Yin and Yang, sufficient in amount, and moving freely in the correct direction.
> - As one of the major treatment modalities of Chinese medicine, acupuncture is the oldest and most commonly used medical procedure in the world.
> - Acupuncture has been used alone or integrated with Western medicine to treat a variety of psychiatric conditions, such as depression, anxiety, insomnia, pain, and addiction.
> - The literature to support the use of acupuncture is encouraging for some psychiatric problems but too limited to draw definitive conclusions.

Introduction

Several practices that are considered part of complementary and alternative medicine in the United States are derived from traditional health systems from other cultures (National Institute of Health, 1998). One that has become particularly popular over the past several decades is Chinese medicine, which is an ancient medical system that originated over 4,000 years ago in China (Jeon, 1998; Ong, Bodeker, Grundy, Burford, & Shein, 2005; Rister, 1999), forms of which are widely practiced today in the United States (Barnes, Powell-Griner, McFann, & Nahin, 2004). This chapter reviews some fundamental concepts of Chinese medicine with an emphasis on applications of acupuncture, particularly in regard to treatment of psychiatric problems.

Chinese medicine maintained a relatively complete body of knowledge at the time it was first documented in book form between 100 and 200 BC (Unschuld, 2003). However, over the centuries, practitioners have amassed much additional information about the formulation and clinical indications of individual herbs and clinical applications of acupuncture (Hsu, 2007). Today, this ancient medical system is the major component of what is known as traditional Chinese medicine (TCM) in China (Scheid, 2002), Kempo in Japan (Rister, 1999; Tsumura, 1991), and traditional Korean medicine in Korea (Jeon, 1998).

The theoretic foundations of TCM, such as theories of Qi, meridians, Yin and Yang, internal organ function, five elements, and the relationship of human beings with nature, provide a unique system of understanding the internal and external factors that comprise human existence (Kaptchuck, 2000). In that context, Chinese medical interventions, such as acupuncture and herbal remedies, are considered to influence the mind, body, and spirit at the same time (Hammer, 1991).

Clinical reports and reviews of the literature have suggested that Chinese medicine could potentially be useful in treating conditions that are similar to *Diagnostic and Statistical Manual of Mental Disorders* (fifth edition; American Psychiatric Association, 2013) diagnoses such as depressive disorders (Gallagher, Allen, & Hitt, 2001; Luo, Meng, Jia, & Zhao, 1998; Manber, Schnyer, Allen, Rush, & Blasey, 2004; Yang, Liu, Luo, & Jia, 1994; Yu et al., 2007), anxiety disorders (Eich, Agelink, Lehmann, Lemmer, & Klieser, 2000; Gibson, Bruton, Lewith, & Mullee, 2007; Pilkington, Kirkwood, Rampes, Cummings, & Richardson, 2007), schizophrenia (Rathbone et al., 2007; Rathbone & Xia, 2005), pain disorders (Facco et al., 2007; Haake et al., 2007; Usichenko et al., 2007), insomnia (Kalavapalli & Singareddy, 2007), and addiction (He, Medbø, & Høstmark, 2001; Zhang, Gu, Wang, & Zahng, 2004).

However, there are considerable limitations to this data set, which are discussed in this chapter, making definitive conclusions impossible at this time.

This chapter reviews theoretical constructs of classic Chinese medicine and available evidence for its effectiveness, with an emphasis on acupuncture and mental health. The goal of this chapter is to provide a basic understanding of the system and how it is applied in daily practice and to review available data regarding treatment of specific psychiatric problems.

Theoretical Framework of Chinese Medicine

Since Chinese medicine is inherited from an ancient civilization, our knowledge of the original system is incomplete. First, we do not know how Chinese medicine originated or how its creators came to conceptualize the energetic aspects of the human body, which is a significant component of the system (Li, 2006). Second, some valuable information may no longer be available due to the loss of ancient volumes (Chan & Lee, 2001). Third, texts were written in an ancient Chinese language and interpreted by different scholars and practitioners at different times. Therefore, the incarnations of translated texts may have resulted in lost information (Galambos, 1996). The best-known resource for the basic concepts of the original Chinese medicine system are described in a Chinese version of the *Yellow Emperor's Internal Classics*, the first book to systematically describe Chinese medicine in 100 BCE (Huangdi Neijing Suwen, 1956). The concepts described in this chapter are based on the overall model of Chinese medicine. Many of these concepts do not have clear correlates in standard Western model of human physiology and health. Thus the concepts described relate only to how they are characterized within the TCM system.

CONCEPT OF *QI*

Qi (also spelled "Chi") is the essential concept in Chinese medicine. Much like the Chinese written characters, Qi has a variety of meanings and is used in different contexts. In the broadest sense, Qi means a form of energy that exists both inside and outside the human body. It can be further defined and classified according to the characteristics and constituents to which it is attached. For example, common terms describing human physiology such as blood Qi (Xue Qi, 血气), defending Qi (Wei Qi, 卫气), organ Qi (Qi of Zang Fu, 脏腑之气), meridian Qi (Qi of Jing Luo, 经络之气), nutritional Qi (Ying Qi, 营气) (Chen & Deng, 2005), and those describing pathogenic energy from outside such as Qi for wind, dampness, heat, cold, and dryness reflect that Qi is the energy behind every aspect or function of ourselves and the universe around us. In keeping with this concept, Qi also is part of the description of mental functions and emotions. In the Chinese language, emotions are followed by the word Qi; for example, anger is called "anger Qi" (Nu Qi, 怒气) and joy is called "joyful Qi" (Xi Qi, 喜气) (Hanyu da zidian, 1995).

Qi is believed to come from two sources. The first is called "prenatal Qi," which is inherited from parents in a predetermined quantity; this kind of Qi does not increase and only decreases over time. Prenatal Qi resides in the kidney meridian and is distributed to other meridians in the course of development. It determines basic mental and physical constitution. Another kind of Qi is derived from environmental sources, such as air, food, and water. It is therefore called "postnatal Qi." The postnatal energies are mostly obtained through the lung and spleen meridians and then dispersed to every other meridian. Postnatal Qi is important to provide the energy for the body to function on a daily basis and also to replenish to a certain degree the prenatal Qi that decreases over time. Lack of postnatal Qi is the focus of most medicinal interventions, and its imbalance causes most of the difficulties with illnesses that people encounter (Holland, 2000).

Qi flows in networks of channels called meridians. Sufficient and free flow of Qi is a necessity for mental and physical health. Direction of Qi flow is important. For example, stomach Qi ideally moves downward to facilitate food to be digested; when it moves upward it will cause nausea and vomiting. Spleen Qi ideally moves upward and buoys internal organs in their places; when it moves downward it causes diarrhea and heavy menstruation and prolapsed organs ensue. Lung Qi normally moves downward to disperse the Qi to the rest of the body; when it moves upward it causes wheezing and coughing. These energy pathways are intended to balance one another. For example, heart Qi moves down to warm the entire body by circulating the blood; kidney Qi moves up to balance the heat of the heart Qi and to nourish the brain. Within this model, when the heart Qi and kidney Qi are disconnected, which often is due to deficiency of kidney Qi, anxiety, panic attacks, and insomnia can occur. Liver Qi is dispersing in nature and facilitates directional free flow of Qi in the entire body; when it is stagnated, it causes pain in the entire body, particularly in the areas the liver meridians reach, such as neck and shoulder, and in deep connective tissues, and it causes depression (Chen & Deng, 2005).

YIN AND YANG

The quality of Qi is categorized into two major groups, Yin and Yang. Yin Qi manifests as the material foundation of the meridians, stillness, and the energies of dampness and coldness (Maciocia, 1989). Yang Qi is manifested as the function of the meridians themselves, movements, the energies of heat and wind, and dryness.

Yin and Yang are opposite energies but exist interdependently. Yang Qi needs Yin Qi's nourishment in order to function, and Yin Qi needs Yang Qi's function in order to be produced and utilized. The opposite nature of the two energies balances the other to have coordinated movement of all Qi and to regulate temperature and metabolism (Weyer, 1997). Similar regulatory mechanisms of opposite forces creating homeostasis are seen on the physical level in the human nervous, immune, and hormonal systems (Chan & Halpern, 2007).

As illustrated in the tai chi emblem, there is Yin Qi inside the Yang Qi and there is Yang Qi inside Yin Qi; the extreme of Yin energy is the beginning of Yang energy and vice versa. In a healthy state, the Yin Qi and Yang Qi have a circadian rhythm and are balanced by each other.

When Yin Qi is deficient, Yang Qi will be relatively excessive. This pattern can manifest in symptoms like hot flashes, night sweats, anxiety, restlessness, elevated blood pressure, and constipation. When Yang Qi is deficient, Yin Qi is relatively excessive, which can manifest in increasing feelings of coldness, fatigue, diarrhea, and slowed metabolism, with water retention, lower blood pressure, and psychomotor retardation.

When Yin Qi is excessive itself, Yang Qi is relatively deficient. Major depression is considered the extreme psychiatric manifestation of this imbalance; mania is the opposite, with extreme manifestation of excessive Yang Qi and deficiency of Yin Qi. The abnormal transition between extreme Yin and extreme Yang is similar to the pattern of cycling in bipolar disorders (Flaws & Lake, 2001).

A primary treatment goal of physicians of Chinese medicine is to balance Yin Qi and Yang Qi. When Yin is sufficient and Yang is balanced, both mental and physical health ensues.

MERIDIANS

Meridians are the main channels in which Qi circulates. Since meridians are energetic conduits, they are not observable with conventional scientific tools, though some feel they eventually may be visualized by new technology (Schlebusch, Maric-Oehler, & Popp, 2005). The 12 principal meridians (Table 8.1) are named after the organ in which Qi is centered. For instance, the liver meridian includes the Qi centered in the liver and channels that connect the Qi at the liver to the parts of the body that are functionally dependent on the Qi at the liver, such as part of the brain, gall bladder,

Table 8.1. Twelve Main Meridians

Meridian	Points	Location	Partner
Lung	11	Begins in the upper chest below the clavicle and ends at the corner of the thumbnail	Large intestine
Large intenstine	20	Begins at the index fingernail and ends at the side of the nostril	Lung
Stomach	45	Begins at the face under the eye, moving down to the front side of body along center of foot, and ends outside the second toenail	Spleen
Spleen	21	Begins at the big toe onto calf and thigh, groin, abdomen, medial chest and axilla, and ends at the fifth intercostal space of the chest	Stomach
Heart	9	Begins under armpit onto inner surface of arm and ends at the cornr of the fifth fingernail	Small intestine
Small intestine	19	Begins at the fifth finger, moving up to the side of hand, back of arm, shoulder, neck, and face, and ends in the front of the ear	Heart
Urinary bladder	67	Begins at the inner corner of eye, moving over the head, down to the neck and back, and ends at the edge of the fifth toenail	Kidney
Kidney	27	Begins at bottom of foot, moving up to the inside ankle, calf and thigh up center of body to chest along sternum, and ends beneath the clavicle	Urinary bladder
Pericardium	9	Begins at the lateral to the nipple, moving along the inside of the arm down to the middle of the forearm, and ends by the nail of the middle finger	Triple burner
Triple burner	23	Begins by the nail of fourth finger, moving up along the back of the hand and the arm, and ends at the point just lateral to the eyebrow	Pericardium

Table 8.1. Continued

Meridian	Points	Location	Partner
Gall bladder	44	Begins at outer corner of eye, moving around lateral side of the head, then down to the side of body and leg, and ends at the fourth toenail	Liver
Liver	14	Begins at the edge of big toenail, moving up inside the leg, groin area, and ends just under the rib cage at the tip of the ninth rib	Gall bladder
Ren (conception vessel	24	Begins below the navel on the midline, moving up along the chest, and ends at the lower lip	Du
Du (Governor vessel)	28	Begins at the tailbone, moving up to the back, then over the head, and ends at the upper lip	Ren

uterus, esophagus, spleen, stomach, eyes, genital area, breast, connective tissues, and so on (Figure 8.1).

Therefore, in Chinese medicine, "the liver" really means the liver meridian, an energetic network rather than just an anatomic organ. In biomedicine, the body is connected by nerves, blood vessels, muscles, and ligaments. In Chinese medicine, the body is connected by the meridians, and the pattern of connection does not correspond to the pathways of nerves and vessels (Li, 2006).

In addition to the 12 principal meridians, there are some meridians that are connected to the principal meridians but have a special area or functional focus; these include eight extra meridians (Qi Jing Ba Mai, 奇經八脈), which are at the same level as the principal meridians (Table 8.2); the 12 associated meridians (Jing Bia, 經別) for connecting Yin meridians and Yang meridians interiorly around the chest, abdomen, and head (Figure 8.2); 15 connecting meridians (Luo Mai, 絡脈) for connecting Yin meridians with Yang meridians exteriorly in the extremities; 12 peripheral meridians (Jin Jin, 筋經) for connecting muscular with skeletal functions; and meridians of the skin area (Pi Bu, 皮部), which connects to the surface of the skin and is the first defense of the body (Figures 8.3). Due to the complex web-like meridian connections, it can be difficult to find a point or technique for so-called sham acupuncture, because stimulation on any part of the body at any level could potentially affect a main meridian response. People tend to mistake the artificial lines that connect acupuncture points on the surface of the body as meridians (Figure 8.4).

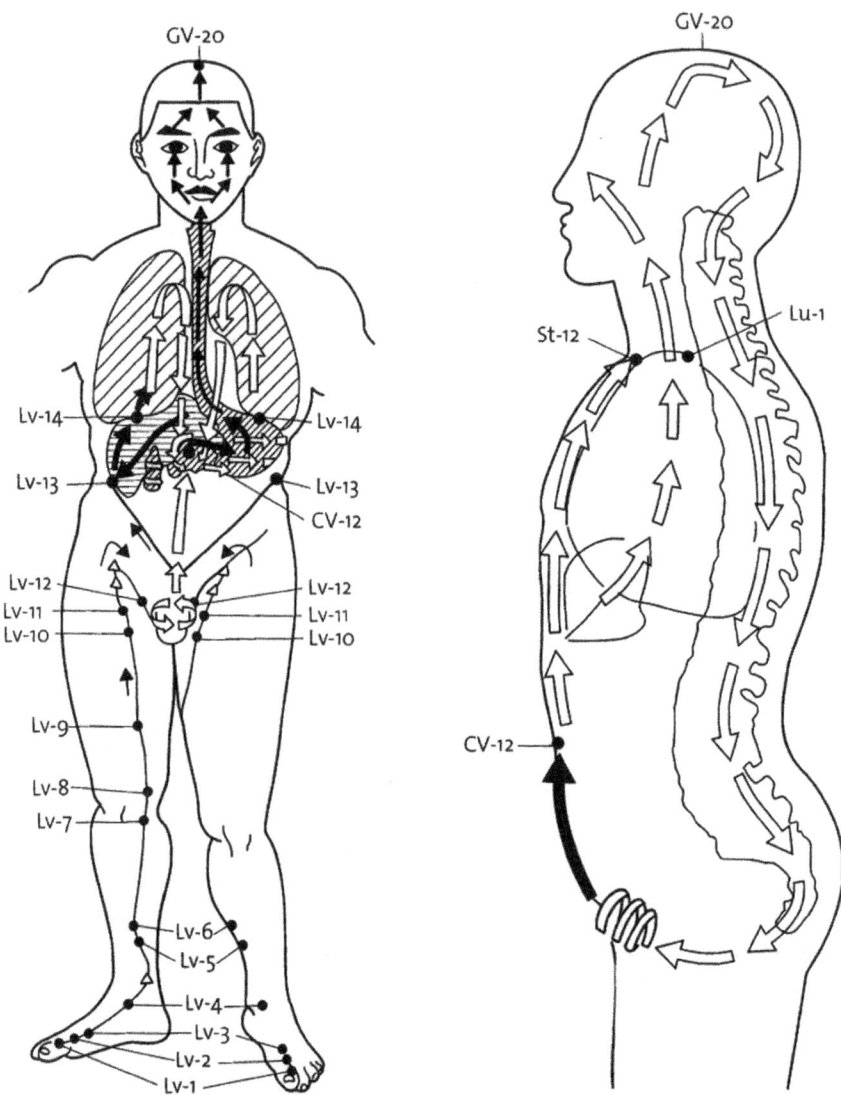

FIGURE 8.1. Liver meridian.
(A) The internal and external Qi flow of the internal liver (Lv) channels. (B) Side view of the liver channels' flow of energy.

Function of the Principal Meridians

Due to the inclusive, interrelated, web-like nature of the meridian system model in Chinese medicine, specific connections between each meridian and physical and emotional functions are available, making it a rather complete

Table 8.2. Eight Extra Meridians

Meridian	Area Supplies	Connecting Meridian	Function
Du Vessel	Posterior midline	Foot-Yang Ming and Ren	Governing channel of Yang meridians and reservoir of Yang Qi of entire body
Ren Vessel	Anterior midline	Foot-Yang Ming and Du	Governing channel of Ying meridians and reservoir of Yying Qi of entire body. In charge of reproductivity
Chong Vessel	First lateral line of the abdomen	Foot-Shao Yin	Reservoir of Qi and blood in 12 main meridians, assiting Ren Mai in reproductivity
Dai Vessel	Lateral side of the lumbar region	Foot-Shao Yang	Regulates the function of all meridians, in particular, kidney meridian qi and essence
Yang Qiao Vessel	Lateral side of the lower extremities, shoulder, and head	Hand and Foot-Tai Yang, Hand and Foot-Yang Ming, and Foot-Shao Yang	Regulate motions in lower extremities
Yin Qiao Vessel	Medial aspect of the lower extremities and eye	Foot-Shao Yin and Foot-Tai Yang	Same as Yang qiao
Yang Wei Vessel	Lateral aspect of the lower extremities, shoulder, and vertex	Hand and Foot-Tai Yang, Du, Hand and Foot-Shao Yang, and Foot-Yang Ming	Regulates the flow of Qi in the Yin and Yang meridians and helps maintain coordination and equilibrium between Yin and Yang meridians
Yin Wei Vessel	Medial aspect of the lower extremities, third lateral line of the abdomen and neck	Foot-Shao Yin, Foot-Tai Yin, Foot-Jue Yin, and Ren	Same as Yang Wei

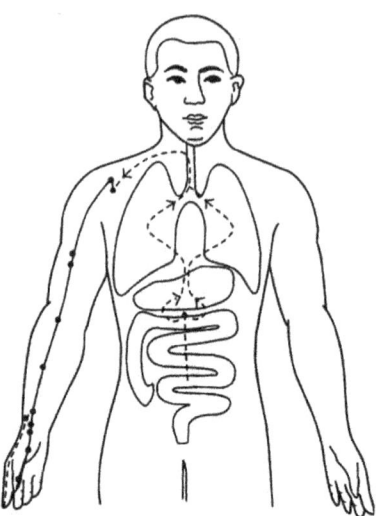

FIGURE 8.2. Jing Bia of the lung meridian.

paradigm for understanding physical and mental health (Chen & Deng, 2005). Cognitive and emotional expressions are viewed as components of Qi, and each meridian is responsible for specific mental functions and emotions (Flaws & Lake, 2001). For example, grief is expressed through the lung meridian, and people in a grieving process may be more susceptible to upper respiratory infections. While the biomedical model might explain such an association in terms of diminished immune responsiveness from the chronic stress of intense grief, Chinese medicine would characterize the problem in terms of the emotional stressor causing imbalance in the lung meridian (that governs grief), which becomes relatively Qi deficient.

In Chinese medicine, emotions and mental functions are not confined to the brain but are viewed more as the interaction between the brain and each individual meridian. Another way of looking at it is that the brain is part of each individual meridian. Each meridian's health affects the brain, a so-called extraordinary organ in Chinese medicine (Sakatani, 2007).

Understanding the connections is important for identifying meridians that are related to clinical symptoms so that a treatment plan can be formulated. Integrative mental health professionals who utilize this system aim to identify the meridians involved in an overall presentation, which leads to specific connections with specific emotional states and mental functions. Having additional ways of categorizing signs and symptoms may potentially expand the range of treatment options.

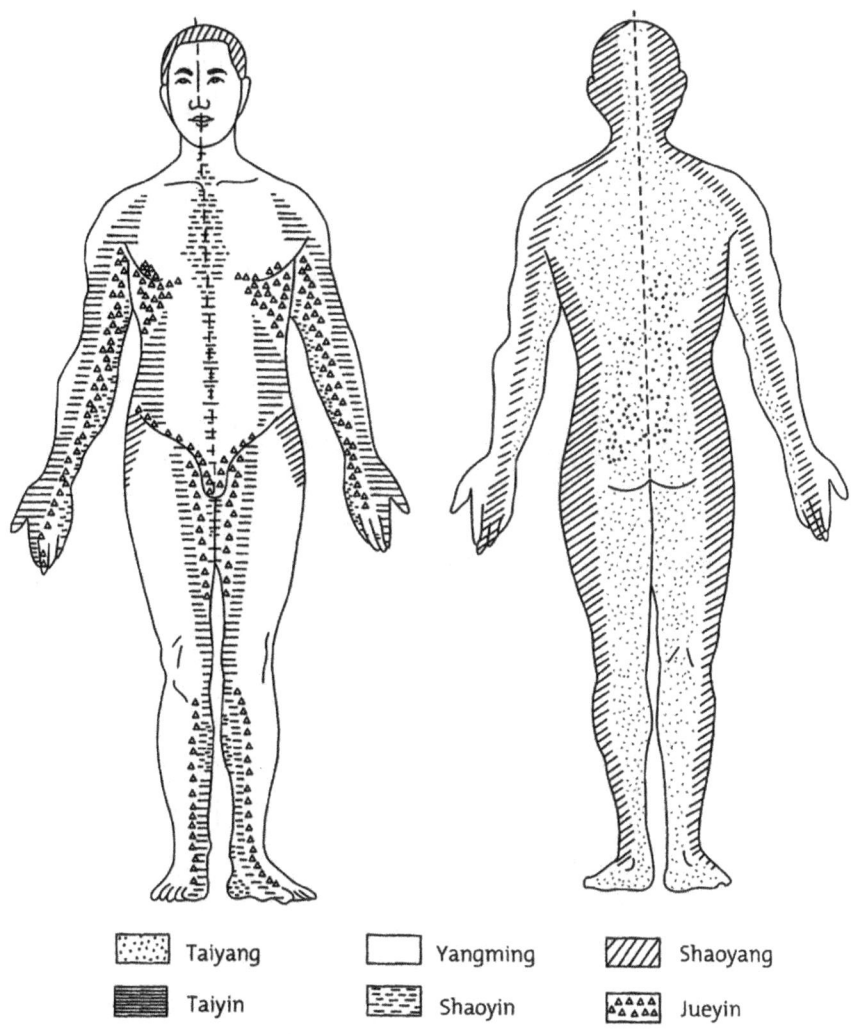

FIGURE 8.3. Pi Bu of 12 meridians.

Five Elements

In Chinese medicine, the human body is created as part of the natural universe and therefore shares the characteristics of nature. The five major pair of meridians share the nature of the five elements and energies and their relationship with each other (Table 8.3). The liver meridian shares the nature of wood and wind; the heart meridian, fire and heat; the spleen meridian, earth and

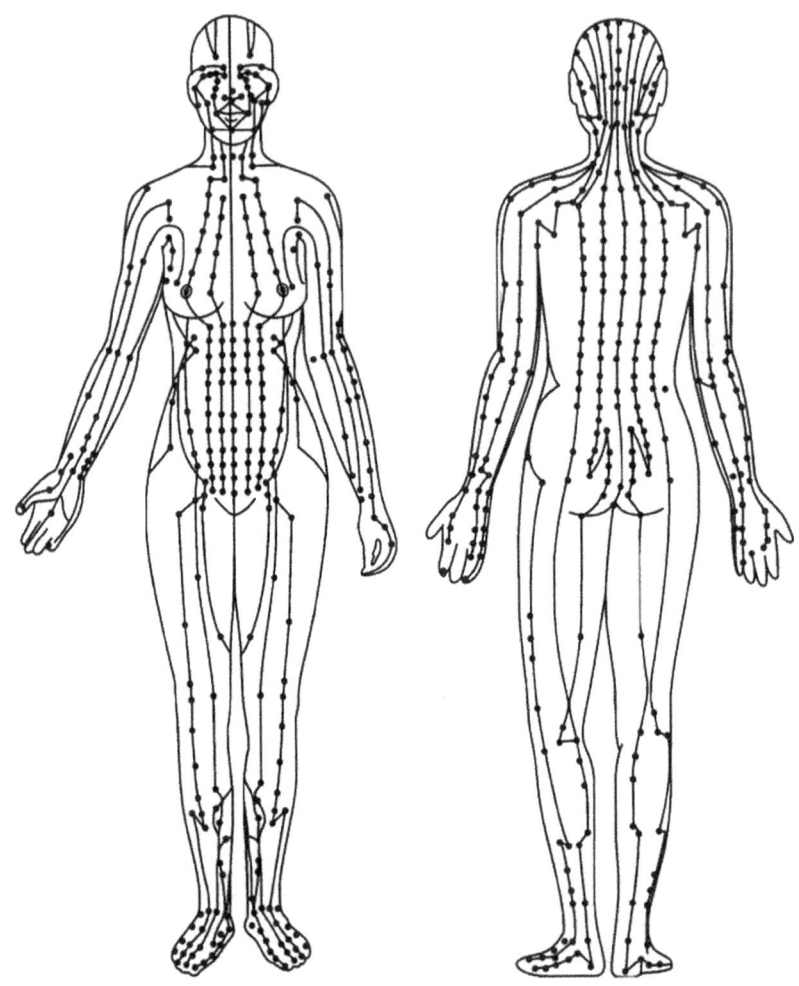

FIGURE 8.4. Artificial lines connecting acupuncture points.

dampness; the lung meridian, metal and dryness; and the kidney meridian, water and coldness.

There is also something called Shen and Ko cycles that explain the relationship of one element to another (Figure 8.5). The Shen cycle describes the generative relationship of the five elements: wood can generate fire; fire can contribute to earth; earth can provide metal; metal can be melted into water; and water can help the growth of wood. Therefore, the emotions of those elements have the same generative (Shen) relationship: fulfillment (liver) may generate joy (fire); the joy (heart) leads to self-confidence (earth); self-confidence to

Table 8.3. Five Elements

Element	Directions	Tastes	Colors	Environmental Factors	Seasons	Zang	Fu	Five Sensory Organs	Five Tissues	Emotions
Wood	East	Sour	Green	Wind	Spring	Liver	Gall-bladder	Eye	Tendon	Anger
Fire	South	Bitter	Red	Heat	Summer	Heart	Small Intestine	Tongue	Vessel	Joy
Earth	Middle	Sweet	Yellow	Dampness	Late summer	Spleen	Stomach	Mouth	Muscle	Worry
Metal	West	Pungent	White	Dryness	Autumn	Lung	Large Intenstine	Nose	Skin and body hair	Sadness
Water	North	Salty	Black	Cold	Winter	Kidney	Bladder	Ear	Bone and hair	Fear

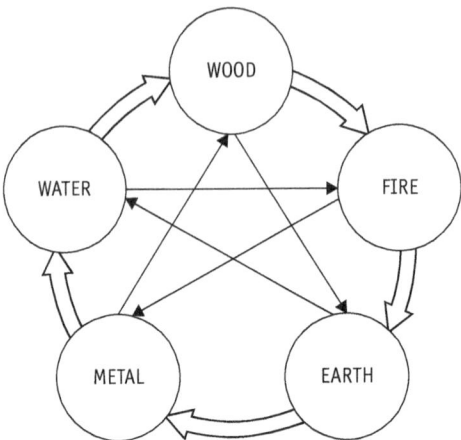

FIGURE 8.5. Shen/Ko relationship of five elements.

empowerment (metal), which leads to motivation (water); and the motivation may once again give the sense of fulfillment.

The Ko Cycle describes the degenerative relationship of the five elements: water extinguishes fire; fire melts metal; metal cuts wood; wood punctures earth; and earth blocks water (Connelly, 1994). Likewise, there is the same degeneration in the emotional aspect of these meridians: fear (kidney, water) can overshadow overexcitement (heart, fire); overexcitement can overshadow sadness (lung, metal); sadness can repress anger (liver, wood); anger can cover up worries (spleen, earth); and worry can overshadow fear (Huangdi Neijing Suwen, 1956). Sometimes correlations can be made between Chinese medicine and Western medicine. For example, a crying patient may be covering underlying anger; anger may manifest as being worried. Fear may be used to control impulses for excitement, and thrill-seeking behavior may be used to avoid grieving.

The homeostatic goal of a living system is for the five elements to be in balance. However, when one element is too excessive or deficient, it may affect that element's relationship among the other elements. An excessive wood energy, for example, may become rebellious for the control of the metal energy and overwhelm the earth energy. For example, when liver energy is stagnated with excessive anger and resentment, it can cause symptoms in the lung meridian, such as coughing, wheezing, and grief; as well as affect the spleen meridian, causing symptoms like indigestion, fatigue, and worrying. When one element is too deficient, it may fail to generate and control. For example, if kidney Qi is very deficient, because of its relationships in the Shen and Ko cycle, it may cause deficiency in the liver meridian, such as poor sleep, dizziness and vertigo, and depression, as well as relative excess in the heart meridians, such as heart palpitations, anxiety, and insomnia (Chen & Deng, 2005). Therefore, clinical symptoms of a particular meridian/element imbalance may be a primary issue to that meridian/element or secondary to another meridian/element that is having a downstream effect. The experienced Chinese medicine practitioner has ways of assessing these issues and determining primary and secondary dysfunctions.

The theoretical frameworks of Chinese medicine provide a unique and holistic view of mind–body medicine. Whether or not this approach is viable and testable according to Western scientific standards, it is, nevertheless, a complete system for diagnosing and treating problems that are often challenging for the biomedical model to conceptualize, such as psychosomatic conditions, cognitive deficits, sleep disorders, mood disorders, anxiety disorders, sexual dysfunction, chemical dependence, and pain disorders. A more comprehensive description of the theories and clinical application of Chinese medicine can be found in a recently compiled textbook (Yang & Monti, 2017).

Acupuncture

According to Chinese medicine theory, meridians have points on the surface of the body that are constantly communicating with the outside environment. These surface points, also called acupoints, can be used to manipulate the status of Qi via the meridians that reach far inside the body. This aspect of meridians is the foundation for acupuncture, moxabustion, Chinese herbal medicine, and Tui Na.

In the classic practice of Chinese medicine, the practitioner must evaluate a patient's Qi status in the involved meridians and decide a treatment strategy accordingly, then select and combine acupoints and manipulation techniques to restore the balance. This evaluation is done by well-trained practitioners who will make systematic inquiry to symptoms and examine signs, including use of a unique technique of tongue and pulse readings.

In modern times, acupuncture is not always practiced in accordance with the theoretical framework of classic Chinese medicine, such as when acupuncture is used as a biochemical tool to stimulate nerves and muscles (Wong, 1999). Some add electric stimulation with the needles to enhance their efficacy, or replace them with hand manipulations (Dang, 1999). Others develop a fixed treatment protocol for every patient with a given condition, without making differentiation of Qi status and meridians involved (Zhang & Lu, 2002). The inconsistency in how acupuncture is approached and utilized is reflected in the published research on acupuncture and may be partially responsible for the differences among the studies reviewed here. When done in accordance to the principles of Chinese medicine, acupuncture relies heavily on energetic evaluation that is dependent on the acupuncturist's clinical experience and training in conceptual and theoretical foundations of Chinese medicine (Liu, 2007). The individualized energy pattern differentiation and customized needling techniques make it difficult to create double-blinds and standardized experimental protocols (Paterson & Dieppe, 2005).

The efficacy of acupuncture and Chinese medicine in treating mental illness has been reported in studies of various types of design and quality. Although most of the studies from the People's Republic of China are case reports and nonrandomized controlled trial studies, they may have anecdotal value and, to some degree, inform future studies. Therefore, we focus our review of the literature on specific psychiatric diagnoses to selected studies that appear to have reasonably good design, and a few compelling case series, with the understanding that no conclusive recommendations can be made from this overall data set.

ANXIETY DISORDERS

A systematic review of the literature on the efficacy of acupuncture in the treatment of anxiety revealed promising but insufficient evidence, due to the poor quality of the design of most studies and lack of reliable assessments (Pilkington et al., 2007). However, a better randomized controlled trial (RCT) of auricular acupuncture (AA) on preoperative anxiety was more effective than acupuncture at a sham point. In a placebo-controlled, randomized, modified double-blind study, 43 patients with minor depression and 13 patients with generalized anxiety disorders received body needle acupuncture (Du.20, Ex.6, He.7, Pe.6, Bl.62) versus sham acupuncture and were assessed by the Clinical Global Impression Scale (CGI) before and after treatments. After completing a total of 10 acupuncture sessions, the experimental group (true acupuncture) group ($n = 28$) showed a significantly larger clinical improvement on the CGI, lower Hamilton Anxiety Rating Scale (HAM-A) scores as well as more responders (60.7% versus 21.4%; chi-square test, $p < 0.01$) as compared to the sham acupuncture group ($n = 28$; Eich et al., 2000). The total sum of acupuncture sessions seemed important in this study, because no differences in the response rates were evident between the two groups at the point of five sessions.

A single-blind crossover trial was carried out comparing the effects of four weeks of either acupuncture or breath training on patients with hyperventilation syndrome (HVS). Ten patients diagnosed with HVS were recruited to the trial and randomized into the two groups. Patients were crossed over from the treatment condition they were not assigned after a one-week washout period. The results showed statistically significant treatment differences between acupuncture and breathing retraining, in favor of acupuncture. Reductions were found in the Hamilton Anxiety Score (anxiety; $p = 0.02$) and Nijmegen (symptoms; $p = 0.03$) scores (Gibson et al., 2007), suggesting that acupuncture may be beneficial in the management of HVS, although a large-scale study is warranted.

In another study, 58 patients with generalized anxiety were randomly assigned to two groups, a medication group that used selective serotonin reuptake inhibitors and alprazolam and the acupuncture group (Li, Zeng, & Zhuang, 2006). Both groups received treatment for six weeks. In addition to the HAM-A, CGI, and Treatment Emergent Symptom Scale, the concentration of 5-hydroxytryptamine (5-HT) in platelets, and plasma levels of corticosterone and adrenocorticotropic hormone (ACTH) were measured before and after treatment. The results suggest that the clinical effects in the two groups were equivalent, while the adverse reaction found in the acupuncture group was less than that in the medication group ($p < 0.05$). The platelet concentration of 5-HT and plasma ACTH level decreased significantly in both groups after treatment with insignificant difference between the groups ($p < 0.05$; Luo, Liu, & Mei, 2007).

Another pilot study showed that acupuncture may help people with posttraumatic stress disorder (PTSD). The researchers analyzed depression, anxiety, and impairment in 73 people with a diagnosis of PTSD. The participants were assigned to receive either acupuncture or group cognitive-behavioral therapy over 12 weeks or were assigned to a wait-list control group. The people in the control group were offered treatment or referral for treatment at the end of their participation. The researchers found that acupuncture provided treatment effects similar to group cognitive-behavioral therapy; both interventions were superior to the control condition. Additionally, treatment effects of both the acupuncture and the group therapy were maintained for three months after the end of treatment (Hollifield, Sinclair-Lian, Warner, & Hammerschlag, 2007). In a case series, cancer patients with traumatic stress symptoms were treated with neuro-emotional technique, an intervention that links acupuncture points with psychological processing techniques. Pre- to postoutcome scores on psychological measures and autonomic reactivity to distressing cues showed marked improvement (Monti, Gomella, Peterson, & Kunkel, 2007).

A study examining immune variables in patients with anxiety indicated that acupuncture may positively impact immune functions such as chemotaxis, phagocytosis, lymphoproliferation, and natural killer activity and modulate superoxide anion levels and lymphoproliferation in women with anxiety.

Effects appeared as early as 72 hours after a single session (Arranz, Guayerbas, Siboni, & De la Fuente, 2007).

An RCT of 100 elderly patients who received auricular acupressure at specific relaxation points while being transported to the hospital were reported to be less anxious and anticipated less pain than the sham-treated group (Mora et al., 2007). AA was also reported to help anxiety induced by dental work in a study of 67 patients who were randomized to three groups of AA, placebo acupuncture, and intranasal midazolam and compared with a no-treatment group. The AA group and the midazolam group were significantly less anxious at 30 minutes as compared with patients in the placebo acupuncture group. In addition, patient compliance assessed by the dentist was significantly improved if AA or application of intranasal midazolam had been performed (Karst et al., 2007).

A combination of AA and body acupuncture is reported to be effective in reducing preoperative anxiety and intraprocedural analgesia in patients undergoing lithotripsy (Wang, Punjala, Weiss, Anderson, & Kain, 2007). The acupuncture group was less anxious prior to the procedure, used a lesser amount of alfentanil, and had lower pain scores on admission to the recovery room than those in the sham control group. Similar results were reported for patients who underwent cataract surgery in an RCT of 75 patients; the pre- and postprocedure anxiety were significantly less in the acupuncture group (Gioia et al., 2006). Another study suggested that acupuncture may also decrease the demand for sedative drugs and increase satisfactory sedation during colonoscopy (Fanti et al., 2004).

An animal study showed that acupuncture treatment reduced anxiety-like behavior in adult rats following maternal separation and modulated the neuropeptide Y immunohistochemistry in the basolateral amygdala. It was noted that only acupuncture on the Heart 7 (seventh point on the heart meridians, known to help anxiety) acupoint produced the result, not the Stomach 36 (Park, Chae, et al., 2005).

More recently, a study using electroacupuncture (EA) at acupoint, stomach 36 (EA St_{36}) examined if it is effective in preventing chronic cold stress-induced increased hormone levels in the rat. Three groups were exposed to cold, one of which was a nontreatment control group. Before exposure to the cold, two groups were treated with either EA St_{36}, or sham-EA, before 10 days of cold stress. The EA St_{36} animals demonstrated a significant decrease in peripheral HP hormones (ACTH and CORT) compared with stress animals ($p < 0.05$). Rats receiving sham-EA had elevation of these hormones, similar to the stress-only animals. Furthermore, corticotropin releasing hormone levels were significantly ($p < 0.05$) reduced in EA St_{36} animals compared with the other animals. EA St_{36} also was effective in preventing stress-induced elevation in the production of adrenal Npy mRNA. These results indicate that EA St$_{36}$ blocks the chronic stress-induced elevations in the hypothalamic–pituitary–adrenal axis (HPA)and the sympathetic neuropeptide Y pathway, which may be a mechanism for its specific stress-allaying effects (Eshkevari, Permaul, & Mulroney, 2013).

Twenty-one patients meeting International Classification of Diseases-10 diagnosis of obsessive-compulsive disorder who failed at least two years of adequate medication treatment were given, five times per week, EA at the point of GV20 (Bai Hui) and M-NH-1 (Yin Tang) for six weeks. The median Yale-Brown Obsessive Compulsive Scale scores and HAM-A score improved after treatment. Among them, five were claimed cured (23.8%), four were significantly improved, nine improved moderately, and three were nonresponsive (Zhang & Lu, 2002). These results should be considered within the context of the clear study limitations of a small sample size and a uncontrolled design. In addition, classic Chinese medicine pattern differentiation diagnosis was not used.

DEPRESSION

Depression is the most studied mental illness treated with acupuncture and herbal medicine. Results are promising, but again, there are clear methodological limitations in the majority of studies (Leo & Liqot, 2007). Recent efforts have been made to improve the quality of research, such as using needle manipulation according to classic Chinese medicine theory (MacPherson, Thorpe, Thomas, & Geddes, 2004; Manber et al., 2004). We review a few that have particular interest and/or merit.

A randomized controlled pilot study of 61 women with major depression during pregnancy, with a 17-item Hamilton Rating Scale for Depression score above 14, suggested that the active acupuncture group showed a significantly higher response rate (69%) than both the sham acupuncture group (47%) and the massage group (32%) (Manber et al., 2004). However, the same group then investigated acupuncture as monotherapy in 152 patients with major depressive disorder and failed to demonstrate efficacy (Allen et al., 2006).

A study on depression relapse rates at six months among women treated with acupuncture suggested that acupuncture designed in accordance with classic Chinese medicine produced results comparable to other validated treatments for depression such as psychotherapies and medications (Gallagher et al., 2001). However, in a small-size RCT of 33 women who completed eight weeks of acupuncture treatment, 4 (24%) out of 17 women who achieved full remission at the conclusion of treatment experienced a relapse six months later (Gallagher et al., 2001).

In a nonrandomized comparison of EA and maprotyline (Han, Li, & Luo, 2002), 30 depressed patients were treated with EA and had comparable score reduction on the Hamilton Depression Rating Scale (HAM-D) and Self-Rating Scale for Depression to the 31 patients treated with maprotyline. The same group (Han, Li, Luo, Zhao, & Li, 2004) replicated these findings and noted additionally that, after treatment, the plasma cortisol levels and the endothelin-1 levels of the two groups were decreased ($p < 0.01$), without significant between-group differences ($p > 0.05$). Two other small studies that compared acupuncture with amitriptyline reported similar positive efficacy between groups (Luo et al., 1998; Yang et al., 1994). A nonrandomized study comparing acupuncture with fluoxetine reported equal efficacy between two groups after six weeks of treatments (Lin, Li, Zhou, & Liu, 2005). An RCT compared 22 patients with EA combined with paroxetine to 20 patients treated with paroxetine alone for six weeks (Zhang et al., 2007). The significant improvement rate evaluated at the end of the six-week treatment was notably higher in the group with combined therapies than that in the paroxetine alone (72.7% vs. 40.0%). All of these studies are methodologically limited by small samples, nonblinding, nonrandomized design, and short duration of treatment.

Using a special group of acupoints (GV 24, 20, 14, 11, 9) and needling techniques called Governor Vessels Daoqi, a small RCT compared the efficacy of acupuncture combined with antidepressants or antidepressants alone in a small group of patients with depression and dyssomnia (Wang, Jiang, & Wang, 2006). HAM-D and Pittsburgh Sleep Quality Index scores were measured before and after four weeks of treatments for both groups. Combined therapy appeared superior to antidepressants alone. However, the short treatment duration and variety of antidepressants involved limit the value of the study.

The mechanisms by which acupuncture may have effects in depression is not clear, and more studies will be required. However, several studies have suggested possible mechanisms of action of acupuncture in depression.

A study measuring guanosine triphosphate-binding protein (G protein) in platelet membranes in patients with major depression revealed significantly increased G-alpha-i and G-alpha-q in depressed patients. Although EA and fluoxetine both produced similar clinical efficacy in patients with moderate depression, fluoxetine failed to reduce levels of G protein alpha subtypes in this small study (Song, Zhou, Fan, Luo, & Halbreich, 2007).

In a large RCT of 755 patients, acupuncture was shown to be as effective as counseling in treating depression. Patients were randomized to receive acupuncture, counseling, or usual care alone. Compared to usual care, there was a statistically significant reduction in epression scores at 3 and 12 months for the acupuncture and counseling groups (MacPherson et al., 2013).

Scalp acupuncture (SA) used to treat depression was shown to positively affect regulation of cortex-limbic circuitry dysfunction and increase glucose metabolism in various brain regions (Huang et al., 2005). In this study, 12 depressive patients were treated by scalp acupuncture on middle line of vertex (MS5), middle line of forehead (MS1), and bilateral lateral line 1 of forehead (MS2) once a day for six days per week and received positron emission tomography brain scans before and after the six-week acupuncture treatment protocol. SA increased glucose metabolism at bilateral frontal lobes, bilateral parietal lobes, right occipital lobe, right caudate nucleus, right cingulate gyrus, and left cerebellum and decreased metabolism at right temporal lobe and bilateral thalamus.

A recent functional magnetic resonance imaging (fMRI) study (Wang et al., 2017) showed that depressed patients receiving acupuncture plus fluoxetine had significantly increased resting state functional connectivity between the ventral striatum and medial prefrontal cortex, ventral rostral putamen and amygdala/parahippocampus, as well as the dorsal caudate and middle temporal gyrus, and significantly decreased functional connectivity between the right ventral putamen and right dorsolateral prefrontal cortex and right caudate and bilateral cerebellar tonsil. The areas of increased functional connectivity were positively associated with decreased clinical scores at the end of the eight-week treatment. The authors suggest that the fMRI findings show that acupuncture's mechanism of action may be related to corticostriatal reward/motivation circuitry in patients with major depressive disorder. A related study showed that acupuncture plus fluoxetine resulted in increased functional connectivity between the left amygdala and anterior cingulate cortex and between the right amygdala and left parahippocampus, which corresponded with improvements in depressive symptoms (Wang et al., 2016).

SCHIZOPHRENIA

There are very limited scientific data on the use of acupuncture for patients with schizophrenia. The Cochrane Schizophrenia Group (Rathbone & Xia, 2005) has analyzed five RCTs comparing acupuncture, EA, and laser acupuncture with antipsychotic alone and antipsychotic combined with acupuncture. Due to the problematic study designs and poor methodology, no conclusions could be drawn except for the possibility that acupuncture combined with antipsychotic medications may potentially produce fewer medication-related side effects. A recent meta-analysis by Cochran reviewed 30 randomized studies to see what acupuncture might do for patients with chronic schizophrenia. While it is equivocal if acupuncture has some antipsychotic effects, the results indicate acupuncture plus standard antipsychotic treatment may reduce side effects such as insomnia, dry mouth, akathisia, blurred vision, and tachycardia (Shen, Xia, & Adams, 2014).

INSOMNIA

A review of the effectiveness of AA on insomnia included six RCTs that cumulatively included 402 patients treated with AA among 673 participants. The improvement rates produced by AA were encouraging; however, given the overall poor quality of the studies, it was concluded that further clinical trials with higher design quality, longer duration of treatment, and longer follow-up were needed (Chen et al., 2007).

Another review considered RCTs of acupressure, AA, seed therapy (herbal or metal seed placed on the relevant meridian), and transcutaneous electrical acupoint stimulation (TEAS). Based on the findings from individual trials, the review suggested that acupuncture and acupressure may help to improve sleep quality scores when compared to sham acupuncture. TEAS also resulted in better sleep quality scores in one trial. Again, due to the great variability in acupuncture techniques and evaluative measurements, definitive conclusions or recommendations from this review cannot be made (Cheuk, Yeung, Chung, & Wong, 2008).

PAIN DISORDERS

There is some suggestion that meridian and acupuncture points may have chemical and physiological effects (Pearson, Colbert, McNames, Baumgartner, & Hammerschlag, 2007; Schlebusch et al., 2005; Shen et al., 2006; Usichenko, Lysenyuk, Groth, & Pavlovic, 2003; Wick, Wick, & Wick, 2007), and biological markers associated with acupuncture treatment include release of endorphins (Ulett, Han, & Han, 1998), changes in neurotransmitters and hormone levels (Ma, 2004), increased blood circulation (Sandberg, Lundeberg, Lindberg, & Gerdle, 2003; Tsuchiya, Sato, Inoue, & Asada, 2007), and effects on immune variables (Cabyoglu, Ergne, & Tan, 2006). Neuroimaging studies have shown that acupuncture affects brain regions involved with pain perception, emotions, and cognitive functioning (Dhond, Kettner, & Napadow, 2007; Lundeberg, Lund, & Näslund, 2007; Newberg et al., 2005; Yoo, Teh, Blinder, & Jolesz, 2004).

RCTs examining efficacy of acupuncture on migraine and tension headaches have revealed promising but mixed results (Linde et al., 2005, 2007; Vincent, 1989). A prospective RCT of 160 patients suffering from migraine without aura suggested that acupuncture plus Rizatriptan was more effective than the drug alone, and acupuncture seemed to decrease the amount of Rizatriptan needed to manage symptoms (Facco et al., 2007). This study had several merits. First, it used TCM diagnoses and selected acupuncture points and techniques accordingly; second, it used a needle with a blunt tip that did not penetrate the skin for the sham control; and third, it used an additional sham acupuncture group that did not follow TCM diagnoses and treatment.

A German acupuncture trial for chronic lower back pain showed both therapeutic and sham acupuncture was twice as effective as conventional therapies such as the combination of drugs, physical therapy, and exercise (Haake et al., 2007). This was a randomized, multicenter, blinded, parallel-group trial with three groups totaling 1,162 patients aged 18 to 86 years. It is unclear why the sham acupuncture group did so well, but possible explanations include placebo effects and the fact that in classic Chinese medical theory it is difficult to find a point on the body that will not affect meridians in some way because of the complexity of the meridian system. In 121 patients undergoing ambulatory arthroscopic knee surgery with standard general anesthesia, an RCT (Usichenko et al., 2007) with intention-to-treat analysis showed that patients from the control group ($n = 59$) required significantly more ibuprofen than patients from the AA group ($n = 61$).

A small RCT from China on EA in relieving labor pain (Qu & Zhou, 2007) studied 36 first-time pregnant women randomly divided into either the EA group or the control group. The EA group exhibited a lower pain intensity and better degree of relaxation ($p = 0.018$, $p = 0.031$) as well as increased release of β-endorphin and 5-HT in peripheral blood at the end of first stage ($p = 0.037$, $p = 0.030$).

A meta-analysis that used individual patient data from selected RCTs of acupuncture for chronic pain concluded that acupuncture is effective for the treatment of chronic pain and is therefore a reasonable referral option (Vickers et al., 2012). This analysis looked at a total of 17,922 patients analyzed in order to determine the effect size of acupuncture for four chronic pain conditions: back and neck pain, osteoarthritis, chronic headache, and shoulder pain. Patients receiving acupuncture had less pain, with scores that were 0.23, 0.16, and 0.15 standard deviations lower than sham controls for back and neck pain, osteoarthritis, and chronic headache, respectively. These results were robust to a variety of sensitivity analyses, including those related to publication bias.

Finally, the most recent recommendations from the American College of Physicians suggests acupuncture for the management of acute and particularly chronic low back pain (Qaseem et al., 2017). This recommendation was based on a review of over 100 articles of a variety of pharmacological and nonpharmacological interventions for acute and chronic low back pain (Chou et al., 2017).

ADDICTIONS

The Acupuncture Consensus Panel of the United States National Institutes of Health (National Institute of Health, 1998) stated that acupuncture "may be useful as a supportive treatment, or acceptable alternative, or part of a comprehensive program" in drug-addiction therapy, including nicotine dependency. However, despite success in several small studies, a RTC and review of studies of AA on cocaine dependence could not confirm that AA was effective as a sole treatment (D'Alberto, 2004; Gates, Smith, & Foxcroft, 2006; Kim, Schiff, Waalen, & Hovell, 2005; Margolin et al., 2002). Likewise, a large RCT of AA for alcohol dependence failed to show efficacy of auricular across 503 patients (Bullock et al., 2002). There is some suggestion that it may be useful as an adjunctive treatment for alcohol withdrawal symptoms (Karst et al., 2007) but that, too, has not been a consistent result (Kunz, Schulz, Lewitzky, Driessen, & Rau, 2007). A more recent systematic meta-analysis has failed to confirm that acupuncture is effective in treating psychological symptoms associated with opiate addiction (Lin, Chan, & Chen, 2012).

Smoking Cessation

Acupressure using beads on acupoints in the ears was used to treat patients on nicotine replacement therapies (NRT) for smoking cessation (White, Moody, & Campbell, 2007). This open-label, randomized pilot study was unable to detect any effects of acupressure on smoking withdrawal as an adjunct to the use of NRT. Of note, this study used only one or two points on the ear, instead of the standard five that normally are recommended.

Chinese investigators used a modified acupuncture technique called wrist ankle acupuncture (Zhang et al., 2004) in an RCT with a control group treated with traditional acupuncture points. Both groups used the "smoking cessation point" (an empirical point between L7 and LI5). In the experimental group, patients received additional needles implanted subcutaneously at points at the ankle and wrist for 24 hours every other day for four weeks of treatment. Out of 30 in each group, the experimental group had 28 subjects who were able to quit for more than one year in comparison with 14 in the other group.

Researchers in Taiwan combined auricular acupressure with an Internet-assisted smoking-cessation program (Chen, Yeh, & Chao, 2006) and found that it was more effective than using acupressure alone. An RCT examined the effectiveness of combining acupuncture and education for smoking cessation (Bier, Wilson, Studt, & Shakleton, 2002), showing acupuncture and education, alone and in combination, significantly reduced smoking; however, combined they show a significantly greater effect at 18-month follow-up, particularly in subjects with greater pack/year histories.

Korean investigators attempted to evaluate genetic determinants for responsiveness to acupuncture for smoking cessation (Park, Kim, et al., 2005). They found that people who responded favorably had a higher DRD2*A2 allele frequency than low responders, suggesting that DRD2 TaqI A polymorphism could be related to acupuncture responsiveness in smoking-cessation treatment.

Conceptual Integration of Biomedicine and Chinese Medicine

Some investigators who are familiar with both modern Western medicine and Chinese medicine have noticed conceptual similarities between the biomedical model of allostasis/altostatic load and the emotional motor system (EMS) with the ancient paradigm of Chinese medicine (Tan, Tillisch, & Mayer, 2004). Both systems stress the fundamental importance of homeostasis in the body. In the process of allostasis, Western medical homeostatic mechanisms involve ascending monoaminergic systems (including the serotonergic, noradrenergic, and cholinergic pathways), the HPA axis, endogenous pain modulation networks, and autonomic pathways (McEwen, 2003), while Chinese medicine involves balancing Yin and Yang, Qi, blood, and essence (which is the physical manifestation of Qi). The functional somatic syndromes described in modern medicine are comparable to patterns of energetic imbalance in Chinese medicine. Both systems explore the complicated interaction of physical and emotional stressors in the genesis of symptoms and diseases. The EMS is a parallel set of outputs from limbic and paralimbic circuits, which generate distinct patterns of body functions ("body map") associated with specific emotions (fear, anger, joy, etc.; Holstege, Bandler, & Saper, 1996). Similarly, Chinese medicine has long recognized that specific emotional stress produces imbalance of Qi in specific meridians and results in specific physical and mental dysfunctions (Maciocia, 1989).

CLINICAL CONSIDERATIONS

Overall, while the available evidence does not support the use of Chinese medicine/acupuncture as the sole therapy for psychiatric problems, there may be a role for this approach in an integrative model that is primarily guided by biomedicine with an integration of complementary therapy. It has been our clinical experience that Chinese medicine most often does not replace medication and conventional psychotherapies. Patients need to be screened for serious psychopathology and safety issues and carefully evaluated for the need for medication or the continued use of medication. If the acupuncturist is not a psychiatrist, then decisions about medication changes need to be deferred to the clinical judgment of the psychiatrist who is working with the patient. Finally, due to financial and logistical reasons, patients can rarely receive acupuncture on a daily basis, which is the ideal approach in the classic Chinese model and the typical treatment in China, even when Western medicine is also part of the treatment plan. Therefore, the Westernized treatment schedule for acupuncture that is common in the United States makes it difficult to predict how long a course of acupuncture will be needed to see a clinical effect.

Conclusion

Chinese medicine in general, and acupuncture in particular, for the treatment of psychiatric problems has more definite efficacy for some types of anxiety, postpartum depression, and chronic pain and modest supportive data as complementary therapy for depression and pain. Overall, the majority of studies in the field suffer from problematic methodological design and lack of standardized treatment approaches among studies, making definitive conclusions and recommendations impossible. Nonetheless, this system of health has a several-thousand-year history that has been developed and documented with countless case descriptions that could potentially provide a unique perspective when considering possible integrative approaches to enhance the treatment plan of complicated mind–body and psychiatric problems.

REFERENCES

Allen, J. J., Schnyer, R. N., Chambers, A. S., Hitt, S. K., Moreno, F. A., & Manber, R. (2006). Acupuncture for depression: A randomized controlled trial. *Journal of Clinical Psychiatry, 67*, 1665–1673.

American Psychiatric Association. (2013). *Diagnostic and statistical manual of mental disorders* (5th ed.). Washington, DC: American Psychiatric Publishing.

Arranz, L., Guayerbas, N., Siboni, L., & De la Fuente, M. (2007). Effect of acupuncture treatment on the immune function impairment found in anxious women. *American Journal of Chinese Medicine, 35*, 35–51.

Barnes, P. M., Powell-Griner, E., McFann, K., & Nahin, R. L. (2004). *Complementary and alternative medicine use among adults: United States (2002)* (CDC Advance Data Report #343). Atlanta, GA: Centers for Disease Control and Prevention.

Bier, I. D., Wilson, J., Studt, P., & Shakleton, M. (2002). Auricular acupuncture, education, and smoking cessation: A randomized, sham-controlled trial. *American Journal of Public Health, 92*, 1642–1647.

Bullock, M. L., Kiresuk, T. J., Sherman, R. E., Lenz, S. K., Culliton, P. D., Boucher, T. A., & Nolan, C. J. (2002). A large randomized placebo controlled study of auricular acupuncture for alcohol dependence. *Journal of Substance Abuse Treatment, 22*, 71–77.

Cabyoglu, M., Ergne, N., & Tan, U. (2006). The mechanism of acupuncture and clinical applications. *International Journal of Neuroscience, 116*, 115–125.

Chan, B., & Halpern, G. M. (2007). *The Yin and Yang of cancer: Breakthroughs from the East and the West*. Square One Publishers. Garden City Park, NY.

Chan, K., & Lee, H. (2001). *The way forward for Chinese medicine*. New York: CRC Press.

Chen, H. H., Yeh, M. L., & Chao, Y. H. (2006). Comparing effects of auricular acupressure with and without an Internet-assisted program on smoking cessation and self-efficacy of adolescents. *Journal of Alternative and Complementary Medicine, 12*, 147–152.

Chen, H. Y., Shi, Y., Ng, C. S., Chan, S. M., Yung, K. K. L., & Zhang, Q. L. (2007). Auricular acupuncture treatment for insomnia: a systematic review. *Journal of Alternative and Complementary Medicine, 13*(6), 669–676.

Chen, X., & Deng, L. (2005). *Chinese acupuncture and moxibustion* (2nd ed.). Beijing: Foreign Languages Press.

Cheuk, D. K. L., Yeung, W. F., Chung, K. F., & Wong, V. (2008). *Acupuncture for insomnia*. New York: Thieme.

Chou, R., Deyo, R., Friedly, J., Skelly, A., Hashimoto, R., Weimer, M., et al. (2017). Nonpharmacologic therapies for low back pain: A systematic review for an American College of Physicians clinical practice guideline. *Annals of Internal Medicine, 166*(7), 493–505.

Connelly, D. M. (1994). *Traditional acupuncture: The law of the five elements* (2nd ed.). Traditional Acupuncture Institute.

D'Alberto, A. (2004). Auricular acupuncture in the treatment of cocaine/crack abuse: A review of the efficacy, the use of the National Acupuncture Detoxification Association protocol, and the selection of sham points. *Journal of Alternative Complementary Medicine, 10*, 985–1000.

Dang, Y. (1999). *Acupuncture and moxibustion*. Beijing: Academy Press.

Dhond, R. P., Kettner, N. & Napadow, V. (2007). Do the neural correlates of acupuncture and placebo effects differ? *Pain, 128*, 8–12.

Eich, H., Agelink, M. W., Lehmann, E., Lemmer, W., & Klieser, E. (2000). Acupuncture in patients with minor depressive episodes and generalized anxiety: Results of an experimental study. *Fortschritte der Neurologie-Psychiatrie, 68*, 137–144.

Eshkevari, L., Permaul, E., & Mulroney, S. E. (2013). Acupuncture blocks cold stress-induced increases in the hypothalamus-pituitary-adrenal axis in the rat. *Journal of Endocrinology, 217*(1), 95–104. doi:10.1530/JOE-12-0404

Facco, E., Liguori, A., Petti, F., Zanette, G., Coluzzi, F., & Nardin, M. D. (2007). Traditional acupuncture in migraine: A controlled, randomized study. *Headache, 48*, 398–407.

Fanti, L., Gemma, M., Passaretti, S., Guslandi, M., Testoni, P. A., Casati, A., & Torri, G. (2004). Electroacupuncture analgesia for colonoscopy: A prospective, randomized, placebo-controlled study. *Gastroenterology, 126,* 355–356.

Flaws, B., & Lake, J. (2001). *Chinese medical psychiatry—a textbook and clinical manual.* Boulder, CO: Blue Poppy Press.

Galambos, I. (1996). The origins of Chinese medicine. The early development of medical literature in China. Retrieved from www.logoi.com

Gallagher, S. M., Allen., J. J. B., & Hitt, S. K. (2001). Six-month depression relapse rates among women treated with acupuncture. *Complementary Therapies in Medicine, 9,* 216–218.

Gates, S., Smith, L. A., & Foxcroft, D. R. (2006) Auricular acupuncture for cocaine dependence. *Cochrane Database of Systematic Reviews, 1,* CD005192.

Gibson, D., Bruton, A., Lewith, G. T., & Mullee, M. (2007). Effects of acupuncture as a treatment for hyperventilation syndrome: A pilot, randomized crossover trial. *Journal of Alternative and Complementary Medicine, 13,* 39–46.

Gioia, L., Cabrini, L., Gemma, M., Fiori, R., Fasce, F., Bolognesi, G., et al. (2006). Sedative effect of acupuncture during cataract surgery: Prospective randomized double-blind study. *Journal of Cataract & Refractive Surgery, 32,* 1951–1954.

Haake, M., Muller, H., Shade-Brittinger, C., Basler, H. D., Schafer, H., Maier, C., Endres, H. G., Trampisch, H. J., Molsberger, A., et al. (2007). German acupuncture trials for chronic lower back pain. *Archives of Internal Medicine, 167,* 1892–1898.

Hammer, L. (1991). *Dragon rises, red bird flies: Psychology, energy and Chinese medicine.* Station Hill Press: Barrytown, NY.

Han, C., Li, X. W., & Luo, H. C. (2002). Comparative study of electro-acupuncture and maprotiline in treating depression. *Zhonggu Zhong Xi Yi Jie He Za Zhi, 22,* 512–514, 521.

Han, C., Li, X., Luo, H., Zhao, X., & Li, X. (2004). Clinical study on electro-acupuncture treatment for 30 cases of mental depression. *Journal of Traditional Chinese Medicine, 24,* 172–176.

Hanyu da zidian weiyuanhui. (1995). *Hanyu da zidian* (Comprehensive Chinese Character Dictionary). Wuhan, China: Hubei cishu chubanshe and Sichuan cishu chubanshe.

He, D., Medbø, J. I., & Høstmark, A.T. (2001). Effect of acupuncture on smoking cessation or reduction: An 8-month and 5-year follow-up study. *Preventive Medicine, 33,* 364–372.

Holland, A. (2000). *Voices of Qi: An introductory guide to traditional Chinese medicine.* Berkeley, CA: North Atlantic Books.

Hollifield, M., Sinclair-Lian, N., Warner, T. D., & Hammerschlag, R. (2007). Acupuncture for posttraumatic stress disorder: A randomized controlled pilot trial. *Journal of Nervous and Mental Disease, 195,* 504–513.

Holstege, G., Bandler, R., & Saper, C. B. (1996). The emotional motor system. In G. Holstege, R. Bandler, & C. B. Saper (Eds.), *The emotional motor system* (pp. 3–6). Amsterdam: Elsevier.

Hsu, E. (2007). *Innovation in Chinese medicine* (Needham Research Institute Studies No. 3). Cambridge, UK: Cambridge University Press.

Huang, Y., Li, D. J., Tang, A. W., Li, Q. S., Xia, D. B., Xie, Y. N., et al. (2005). Effect of scalp acupuncture on glucose metabolism in brain of patients with depression. *Zhongguo Zhong Xi Yi Jie He Za Zhi, 25*, 119–122.

Huangdi Neijing Suwen. (1956). *People's health press*. Beijing. (Chinese)

Jeon, S.-W. (1998). *A history of science in Korea*. Seoul: Jimoondang International.

Kalavapalli, R., & Singareddy, R. (2007). Role of acupuncture in the treatment of insomnia: A comprehensive review. *Complementary Therapies in Clinical Practice, 13*, 184–193.

Kaptchuck, T. (2000). *The web that has no weaver*. New York: McGraw-Hill.

Karst, M., Winterhalter, M., Münte, S., Francki, B., Hondronikos, A., Eckardt, A., et al. (2007). Auricular acupuncture for dental anxiety: A randomized controlled trial. *Anesthesia and Analgesia, 104*, 295–300.

Kim, Y. H., Schiff, E. I., Waalen, J., & Hovell, M. (2005). Efficacy of acupuncture for treating cocaine addiction: A review paper. *Journal of Addictive Diseases, 24*, 115–132.

Kunz, S., Schulz, M., Lewitzky, M., Driessen, M., & Rau, H. (2007). Ear acupuncture for alcohol withdrawal in comparison with aromatherapy: A randomized-controlled trial. *Alcoholism, Clinical and Experimental Research, 31*, 436–442.

Leo, R. J., & Liqot, J. S. Jr. (2007). A systematic review of randomized controlled trials of acupuncture in the treatment of depression. *Journal of Affective Disorders, 97*, 13–22.

Li, X. D. (2006). *Who can invent Chinese medicine? Decoding Huang Di Nei Jing* (2nd ed.). Beijing: China Changan Press.

Li, Y. F., Zeng, D. Y., & Zhuang, L. X. (2006). Analysis on the composing law of Jin's 3-needle. *Journal of Clinical Acupuncture and Moxibustion, 22*, 35–36.

Lin, H., Li, G. Q., Zhou, Z. B., & Liu, J. X. (2005). Observation on therapeutic effect of combination of acupuncture with drug on depression. *Zhongguo Zhen Jiu, 25*, 27–29.

Lin, J., Chan, Y., & Chen, Y. (2012). Acupuncture for the treatment of opiate addiction. *Evidence-Based Complementary and Alternative Medicine, 2012*, 1–10. doi:10.1155/2012/739045

Linde, K., Streng, A., Hoppe, A., Weidenhammer, W., Wagenpfeil, S., & Melchart, D. (2007). Randomized trial vs. observational study of acupuncture for migraine found that patient characteristics differed but outcomes were similar. *Journal of Clinical Epidemiology, 60*, 280–287.

Linde, K., Streng, A., Jurgens, S., Hoppe, A., Brinkhaus, B., Witt, C., et al. (2005). Acupuncture for patients with migraine: A randomized controlled trial. *Journal of the American Medical Association, 293*, 2118–2125.

Luo, H., Meng, F., Jia, Y., & Zhao, X. (1998). Clinical research on the therapeutic effect of the electro-acupuncture treatment in patients with depression. *Psychiatry and Clinical Neurosciences, 52*(Suppl.), S338–S340.

Luo, W. Z., Liu, H. J., & Mei, S. Y. (2007). Clinical study on "Jin's three-needling" in treatment of generalized anxiety disorder. *Zhongguo Zhong Xi Yi Jie He Za Zhi, 27*, 201–203.

Liu, T. (2007). Role of acupuncturists in Acupuncture treatment. *Evidence-Based Complementary and Alternative Medicine, 4*, 3–6.

Lundeberg, T., Lund, I., & Näslund, J. (2007). Acupuncture—self-appraisal and the reward system. *Acupuncture in Medicine, 25*, 87–99.

Ma, X.-S. (2004). Neurobiology of acupuncture: Toward CAM. *Evidence-Based Complementary and Alternative Medicine, 1*, 41–47.

Maciocia, G. (1989). *The foundations of Chinese medicine: A comprehensive text for acupuncturists and herbalists.* New York: Churchill Livingstone.

MacPherson, H., Richmond, S., Bland, M., Brealey, S., Gabe, R., Hopton, A., et al. (2013) Acupuncture and counselling for depression in primary care: A randomized controlled trial. *PLoS Medicine, 10*(9), e1001518. doi:10.1371/journal.pmed.1001518

MacPherson, H., Thorpe, L., Thomas, K., & Geddes, D. (2004). Acupuncture for depression: First steps toward a clinical evaluation. *Journal of Alternative and Complementary Medicine, 10*, 1083–1091.

Manber, R., Schnyer, R., Allen, J., Rush, A., & Blasey, C. (2004). Acupuncture: A promising treatment for depression during pregnancy. *Journal of Affective Disorders, 83*, 89–95.

Margolin, A., Kleber, H. D., Avants, S. K., Konefal, J., Gawin, F., Stark, E., et al. (2002). The treatment of cocaine addiction: A randomized controlled trial. *Journal of the American Medical Association, 287*, 55–63.

McEwen, B. S. (2003). Interacting mediators of allostasis and allostatic load: Towards an understanding of resilience in aging. *Metabolism, 52*, 10–16.

Monti, D., Gomella, L., Peterson, C., & Kunkel, E. (February 2007). *Preliminary results from a novel psychosocial program for men with prostate cancer.* Paper presented at the 2007 Prostate Cancer Symposium, American Society of Clinical Oncology.

Mora, B., Iannuzzi, M., Lang, T., Steinlechner, B., Barker, R., Dobrovits, M., et al. (2007). Auricular acupressure as a treatment for anxiety before extracorporeal shock wave lithotripsy in the elderly. *Journal of Urology, 178*, 160–164.

National Institute of Health Consensus Conference. (1998). Acupuncture. *Journal of the American Medical Association, 280*, 1518–1524.

Newberg, A. B., Lariccia, P. J., Lee, B. Y., Farrar, J. T., Lee, L., & Alavi, A. (2005). Cerebral blood flow effects of pain and acupuncture: A preliminary single-photon emission computed tomography imaging study. *Journal of Neuroimaging, 15*(1), 43–49.

Ong, C. K., Bodeker, G., Grundy, C., Burford, G., & Shein, K. (2005). *WHO global atlas of traditional, complementary and alternative medicine.* Geneva: WHO Kobe Centre.

Park, H. J., Chae, Y., Jang, J., Shim, I., Lee, H., & Lim, S. (2005). The effect of acupuncture on anxiety and neuropeptide Y expression in the basolateral amygdala of maternally separated rats. *Neuroscience Letters, 4*(377), 179–184.

Park, H. J., Kim, S. T., Yoon, D. H., Jin, S. H., Lee, S. J., Lee, H. J., & Lim, S. (2005). The association between the DRD2 TaqI A polymorphism and smoking cessation in response to acupuncture in Koreans. *Journal of Alternative Complementary Medicine, 11*, 401–405.

Paterson, C., & Dieppe, P. (2005). Characteristic and incidental (placebo) effects in complex interventions such as acupuncture. *British Medical Journal, 330*, 1202–1205.

Pearson, S., Colbert, A. P., McNames, J., Baumgartner, M., & Hammerschlag, R. (2007). Electrical skin impedance at acupuncture points. *Journal of Alternative and Complementary Medicine, 13*, 409–418.

Pilkington, K., Kirkwood, G., Rampes, H., Cummings, M., & Richardson, J. (2007). Acupuncture for anxiety and anxiety disorders—a systematic literature review. *Acupuncture in Medicine, 25*, 1–10.

Qaseem, A., Wilt, T. J., McLean, R. M., Forciea, M. A., & Clinical Guidelines Committee of the American College of Physicians. (2017). Noninvasive treatments for acute, subacute, and chronic low back pain: A clinical practice guideline from the American College of Physicians. *Annals of Internal Medicine, 166*(7), 514–530.

Qu, F., & Zhou, J. (2007). Electro-acupuncture in relieving labor pain. *Evidence-Based Complementary and Alternative Medicine, 4*, 125–130.

Rathbone, J., & Xia, J. (2005). Acupuncture for schizophrenia. *Cochrane Database of Systematic Reviews, 4*, CD005475.

Rathbone, J., Zhang, L., Zhang, M., Xia, J., Liu, X., Yang, Y., & Adams, C. E. (2007). Chinese herbal medicine for schizophrenia—Cochrane systematic review of randomized trials. *British Journal of Psychiatry, 190*, 379–384.

Rister, R. (1999). *Japanese herbal medicine: The healing art of Kampo.* New York: Avery.

Sakatani, K. (2007). Concept of mind and brain in traditional Chinese medicine. *Data Science Journal, 6*(Suppl.), S220–S224.

Sandberg, M., Lundeberg, T., Lindberg, L. G., & Gerdle, B. (2003). Effects of acupuncture on skin and muscle blood flow in healthy subjects. *European Journal of Applied Physiology, 90*, 114–119.

Scheid, V. (2002). *Chinese medicine in contemporary China: Plurality and synthesis.* Durham, NC: Duke University Press.

Schlebusch, K., Maric-Oehler, W., & Popp, F.-A. (2005). Biophotonics in the infrared spectral range reveal acupuncture meridian structure of the body. *Journal of Alternative and Complementary Medicine, 11*, 171–173.

Shen, X. Y., Wei, J. Z., Zhang, Y. H., Ding, G. H., Wang, C. H., Zhang, H. M., et al. (2006). Study on volt–ampere (V-A) characteristics of human acupoints. *Zhongguo Zhen Jiu, 26*, 267–271.

Shen, X., Xia, J., & Adams, C. E. (2014). Acupuncture for schizophrenia. *Cochrane Database of Systematic Reviews, 10*, CD005475. doi:10.1002/14651858.CD005475.pub2

Song, Y., Zhou, D., Fan, J., Luo, H., & Halbreich, U. (2007). Effects of electroacupuncture and fluoxetine on the density of GTP-binding-proteins in platelet membrane in patients with major depressive disorder. *Journal of Affective Disorders, 98*, 253–257.

Tan, S., Tillisch, K., & Mayer, E. (2004). Functional somatic syndromes: Emerging biomedical models and traditional Chinese medicine. *Evidence-Based Complementary and Alternative Medicine, 1*, 35–40.

Tsuchiya, M., Sato, E. F., Inoue, M., & Asada, A. (2007). Acupuncture enhances generation of nitric oxide and increases local circulation. *Anesthesia and Analgesia, 104*, 301–307.

Tsumura, A. (1991). *Kampo: How the Japanese updated traditional herbal medicine.* Japan Publications.

Ulett, G. A., Han, S., & Han, J. S. (1998). Electro acupuncture: Mechanisms and clinical application. *Biological Psychiatry, 44,* 129–138.

Unschuld, P. U. (2003). *Huang di nei jing su wen: Nature, knowledge, imagery in an ancient Chinese medical text.* Berkeley and Los Angeles: University of California Press.

Usichenko, T. I., Kuchling, S., Witstruck, T., Pavlovic, D., Zach, M., Hofer, A., et al. (2007). Auricular acupuncture for pain relief after ambulatory knee surgery: A randomized trial. *Canadian Medical Association Journal, 176,* 179–183.

Usichenko, T. I., Lysenyuk, V. P., Groth, M. H., & Pavlovic, D. (2003). Detection of ear acupuncture points by measuring the electrical skin resistance in patients before, during and after orthopedic surgery performed under general anesthesia. *Acupuncture Electro-therapeutics Research, 28,* 167–173.

Vickers, A. J., Cronin, A., Maschino, A. C., Lewith, G., MacPherson, H., Foster, N. E., et al. (2012). Acupuncture for chronic pain: Individual patient data meta-analysis. *Archives of Internal Medicine, 172*(19), 1444–1453.

Vincent, C. A. (1989). A controlled trial of the treatment of migraine by acupuncture. *Clinical Journal of Pain, 5,* 305–312.

Wang, J., Jiang, J. F., & Wang, L. L. (2006). Clinical observation on governor vessel Daoqi method for treatment of dyssomnia in the patient of depression. *Zhongguo Zhen Jiu, 26,* 328–330.

Wang, S. M., Punjala, M., Weiss, D., Anderson, K., & Kain, Z. N. (2007). Acupuncture as an adjunct for sedation during lithotripsy. *Journal of Alternative and Complementary Medicine, 13,* 241–246.

Wang, X., Wang, Z., Liu, J., Chen, J., Liu, X., Nie, G., et al. (2016). Repeated acupuncture treatments modulate amygdala resting state functional connectivity of depressive patients. *NeuroImage: Clinical, 27*(12), 746–752.

Wang, Z., Wang, X., Liu, J., Chen, J., Liu, X., Nie, G., et al. (2017). Acupuncture treatment modulates the corticostriatal reward circuitry in major depressive disorder. *Journal of Psychiatric Research, 84,* 18–26.

Weyer, R. V. D. (1997). *Huang Di: The balance of Yin and Yang.* Tandem Library: Topeka, KS.

White, A. R., Moody, R. C., & Campbell, J. L. (2007). Acupressure for smoking cessation—a pilot study. *BMC Complementary and Alternative Medicine, 7,* 8.

Wick, F., Wick, N., & Wick, M. C. (2007). Morphological analysis of human acupuncture points through immunohistochemistry. *American Journal of Physical Medicine & Rehabilitation, 86,* 7–11.

Wong, J. Y. (1999). *A manual of neuro-anatomical acupuncture.* Vol. I: *Musculoskeletal disorders.* Toronto: Toronto Pain and Stress Clinic.

Yang, J. D., & Monti, A. D. (2017). *Clinical acupuncture and ancient Chinese medicine.* New York: Oxford University Press.

Yang, X., Liu, X., Luo, H., & Jia, Y. (1994). Clinical observation on needling extra-channel points in treating mental depression. *Journal of Traditional Chinese Medicine, 14,* 14–18.

Yoo, S. S., Teh, E. K., Blinder, R. A., & Jolesz, F. A. (2004). Modulation of cerebellar activities by acupuncture stimulation: Evidence from fMRI study. *NeuroImage, 22,* 932–940.

Yu, J., Liu, Q., Wang, Y. Q., Wang, J., Li, X. Y., Cao, X. D., & Wu, G. C. (2007). Electroacupuncture combined with clomipramine enhances antidepressant effect in rodents. *Neuroscience Letters, 421,* 5–9.

Zhang, G. J., Shi, Z. Y., Liu, S., Gong, S. H., Liu, J. Q., & Liu, J. S. (2007). Clinical observation. *Chinese Journal of Integrative Medicine, 13,* 228–230.

Zhang, Q. G., Gu, K. W., Wang, D., & Zahng, H. J. (2004). Treatment of tobacco dependence with wrist-ankle acupuncture: A report of 30 cases. *Chinese Journal of Integrative Medicine, 2,* 444, 480.

Zhang, Z., & Lu, W. (2002), A clinical analysis on treatment of depression by electroacupuncture combined with paroxetine of the electroacupuncture treatment of obsessive compulsive disorders. *Si Chuan Zhong Yi (The Journal of Si Chuan Chinese Medicine), 1,* 75–76.

9

The Role of Chiropractic in Mind–Body Health

GEORGE ZABRECKY

Key Points

- Chiropractic is based on the principles that disease is caused by disturbances in the nervous system and that such disturbances are often related to musculoskeletal problems.
- Chiropractic therapies utilize an integrative approach to health and well-being.
- Chiropractic therapies are most well known for the management of chronic and acute pain.
- At the present time, there is little direct evidence that chiropractic care improves mental health outside of the benefits related to pain alleviation.
- Based on the overall chiropractic model, there is reason to believe that chiropractic therapy can potentially benefit a wide variety of psychological symptoms, but more research is needed.

Introduction

Chiropractic is a healing art that is concerned with a holistic but mechanistic approach to human health and disease processes. Doctors of chiropractic are physicians who consider the patient as an integrated being but give special attention to spinal mechanics and neurological, muscular, and vascular relationships (Chapman-Smith, 2000).

Scientific Theories and Principles of Chiropractic

Chiropractic is built on three scientific theories and principles.

1. Disease may be caused by disturbances in the nervous system. While many factors impair human health, the most important component of disease pathophysiology involves disturbances in the nervous system. The nervous system normally coordinates basic inter and extracellular activities to help the body adapt to external and internal environmental changes in a balanced manner, also called *homeostasis*. Environmental agents and conditions that interfere with or disturb the nervous system, and to which the body cannot successfully adapt, alter the pattern of neuronal coordination resulting in a deviation from the normal body balance, also called *homeostenosis*. When the body cannot adapt effectively, many diseases may arise.
2. Many diseases arise from disturbances in the nervous system ultimately caused by derangement in the musculoskeletal structures of the neck and body. Malalignments of the vertebral and pelvic segments are common mechanical clinical findings in human beings in large part due to our bipedal walking. Extended abnormal involvement of the nervous system may result in disturbances, strains, sprains, and stresses arising within the musculoskeletal system due to the person's attempt to maintain this erect posture. The mechanical lesion, or subluxation, is a common result of gravitational strains and asymmetrical activities and efforts. In addition, developmental defects or other mechanical, chemical, or psychological irritations of the nervous system can result in alterations in the musculoskeletal system.
3. Disturbances in the nervous system may cause or aggravate diseases afflicting various structures or functions of the body. Vertebral and pelvic subluxations may be associated with common functional disorders of a visceral and/or vasomotor nature. Such disorders may eventually cause problems in the major organs. And almost any function of the nervous system may directly or indirectly cause reactions within any other body structure by means of reflex mediation.

The Practice and History of Chiropractic

Manipulation of the spine and extremities predates modern medicine by almost a millennium. Historically, the initiation of contemporary chiropractic is attributed to Daniel David Palmer. The science, art, and philosophy of chiropractic originally developed out of Palmer's extensive independent research and analysis of human health and disease. His model was based on three determining causes of health and disease: mental or cognitive issues, biological issues, and environmental issues (Palmer, 1910). Following the successful application of his approach to initial patients in 1895, he began teaching others in Davenport, Iowa. The record indicates that he adjusted the spine of a deaf individual, William Harvey Lillard, and he regained his hearing. D. D. Palmer was the inventor of chiropractic, and later his son, Bartlett Joshua Palmer, elaborated upon his father's hypotheses.

An important component of the chiropractic model that is relevant specifically to psychiatry is the relationship between mental and cognitive issues and overall health. Other developers of the chiropractic technique have noted the relationship between concepts such as temperament and physiological processes. Bartlett Palmer suggested that mental illness could be caused by vertebral subluxations (Stephenson, 1948). While the original concepts relating mental state with illness in the development of chiropractic were limited by current scientific knowledge, current data strongly supports this overall link. It is known that depression is associated with poorer overall health outcomes while positive emotions and optimism are associated with improved health outcomes (Kim et al., 2017). Thus the ability of chiropractic care to embrace the importance of psychology, and perhaps even assist in the evaluation and management of psychological problems, seems reasonable.

The National Institutes of Health classifies chiropractic as a manipulation and body-based form of complementary and alternative medicine (CAM), although chiropractors, mindful of the major strides they have made toward mainstream status, more often prefer to be known as "integrative" rather than CAM practitioners (Redwood, Hawk, Cambron, Vinjamury, & Bedard, 2008).

Chiropractic as a healing art was born in the United States in the late 19th century. The United States is home to approximately 70,000 doctors of chiropractic, and worldwide there are over 75,000 (Chapman-Smith, 2000). The chiropractic profession is currently the third largest independent health profession in developed countries after medicine and dentistry.

Doctors of chiropractic are licensed throughout the English-speaking world. In many countries, chiropractors function as primary-care providers who are licensed for both diagnosis and treatment of patients without medical referral. In 2005, the World Health Organization (WHO) published the *WHO Guidelines on Basic Training and Safety in Chiropractic*. These guidelines attempted to formalize chiropractic education and practice worldwide. The goal of these guidelines was to ensure high standards particularly in nations where chiropractic was in the early stages of development (WHO, 2005).

The 1970s was the breakthrough decade for chiropractic field. During this time, the US federal government included chiropractic services in Medicare and federal workers' compensation coverage. The Council on Chiropractic

Education was approved as the accrediting body for chiropractic colleges and also sponsored an National Institutes of Health conference on the state of the science for spinal manipulation. Since that time, the chiropractic profession has grown and matured into an important part of the US healthcare system.

The basic philosophy that underlies chiropractic care emphasizes the inherent recuperative and self-healing abilities of the human body by promoting the balance of body and mind through natural methods of prevention and treatment. Chiropractic is currently the only CAM approach covered by Medicare and also a substantial majority of health insurance policies.

Since the 1970s, research on the effectiveness of chiropractic care and the manual methods described as spinal manipulation or adjustment has greatly expanded (Shekelle et al., 1991). There are hundreds of randomized clinical trials on spinal manipulation for various disorders. Most of these studies explore the effects of chiropractic techniques on back pain, neck pain, and headaches. However, a growing number of studies have evaluated other targets of chiropractic practice, including extremity (leg and arm) problems and nonmusculoskeletal conditions such as infantile colic, hypertension, and epilepsy. In many of these studies, spinal manipulation and other chiropractic techniques outperformed comparison therapies or placebo.

To increase the peer-reviewed, science-based research database, the US Health Resources and Services Administration (HRSA) funded for 12 years (1995–2006) an annual chiropractic Research Agenda Conference (RAC), where researchers and practitioners met to discuss outcomes of completed investigations, create and implement new research projects, develop strategies for interdisciplinary collaboration, and advance overall chiropractic research. Since completion of funding from the US HRSA, the profession has self-funded continued annual RAC meetings in conjunction with the annual meeting of the Association of Chiropractic Colleges (Redwood, 2010).

Most research on chiropractic techniques focuses on the effectiveness of manual adjustments of the spine and other musculoskeletal structures as a way of reducing various symptoms, particularly pain. While this is the chiropractor's primary area of specialty, the care delivered by chiropractors includes much more and provides expertise in diagnosis, radiological evaluation, rehabilitation, physiotherapy, non-force-related manual therapies, nutrition, disease prevention, and health promotion.

The purpose of this chapter is to focus on the research supporting the clinical application of chiropractic to improve brain health with a focus on selected disorders, some commonly associated with chiropractic treatment and others for which chiropractic would not often be considered.

Mechanism of Chiropractic on Innate Wellness and Recovery

Medical authors of the mid- to late 19th century referred to the entire separation of joint surfaces as a "luxation." If a partial or incomplete separation, it was called a "subluxation," hence the term *subluxation*, used by chiropractors to describe a misalignment of articulating surfaces (Lantz, 1995). In bipedal humans, the anatomical relationship between spinal vertebrae and their associated spinal nerves is intricate. Any displacement of these articulations will produce pressure on nerves, producing neurological dysfunction and inflammation.

> Doctors of Chiropractic have been teaching patients and the medical community for over 100 years that spinal mis-alignments (subluxations) produce nervous system dysfunctions, which have negative effects on the function of the peripheral nervous system (PNS), autonomic nervous system (ANS), central nervous system (CNS), and the patient's overall ability to maintain homeostasis. Essentially, they go into a state of disease, or homeostenosis. (Studin & Owens, 2015)

Several authors have suggested that muscle tension is correlated with changes in brain areas such as the reticular activating system that regulate overall arousal. Theoretically, muscle tension could produce a state of chronic arousal via the RAS. If this were the case, then chiropractic approaches to managing subluxations in the spine might reduce muscle tension and, hence, reduce psychological arousal (Haldeman, 1971).

Early informal surveys by the International Chiropractic Association suggested that as many as one-half of patients presenting to chiropractors have psychological illness. Such a finding further suggests the importance of considering mental health in conjunction with the chiropractic model. In fact, Quigley (1973) suggested that chiropractic might even represent a form of psychotherapy.

The past 20 years have brought significant advances in understanding the fundamentals of how chiropractic works and shown that the Palmers were essentially correct, while clarifying the specific physiological mechanisms related to chiropractic's ability to alleviate pain. Through early studies on pain mechanisms, contemporary research has begun to allow us to understand how chiropractic works with systemic and autonomic dysfunction and potential disease treatment through the chiropractic adjustment affecting CNS interactions (Studin & Owens, 2015).

Current technology has allowed an ever-expanding armamentarium of research tools, which has significantly increased our scientific knowledge. The quest to understand the mechanism behind the power of a chiropractic adjustment has been daunting. Before we focus on a few of the illnesses benefited by chiropractic, it is worthwhile to explain the science regarding the effect of spinal manipulation on body and brain physiology.

Research on Chiropractic Adjustment Modulation of Pain Mechanisms and Brain Function

Research has furthered our understanding of how chiropractic works. Recent investigations on CNS processing of pain reduction by Coronado et al. (2012) reported that "Reductions in pain sensitivity, or hypoalgesia, following spinal manipulative therapy or chiropractic adjustment (SMT) may be indicative of a mechanism related to the modulation of afferent input or CNS processing of pain" (p. 752). The authors theorized that the improvement in clinical pain was related to changes within the lumbar innervated areas and not the cervical areas. Furthermore, the findings suggested that the mechanism was related to a reduction in dorsal horn excitability as opposed to a generalized change in pain sensitivity. These findings indicate that chiropractic spinal adjustment most likely works by affecting the dorsal horns at the root levels located in CNS. Furthermore, the mechanisms of SMT are theorized to result from both spinal cord–mediated mechanisms as well as supraspinal-mediated mechanisms.

Reed, Pickar, Sozio, and Long (2014) reported that specific forms of manual therapy have been shown to increase mechanical pressure pain thresholds (i.e., decrease sensitivity) in both symptomatic and asymptomatic subjects. In particular, cervical spine manipulation produced unilateral and bilateral mechanical hypoalgesia. In addition, the hypoalgesia associated with manual therapy treatments occurs quickly and has been associated with activation of descending pain inhibitory systems and also alterations in peripheral and central pain processing.

Reed and colleagues (2014) also reported that only higher intensity levels of manipulative stimuli (i.e., 85% body weight vs. 55% body weight or control) resulted in a decrease in mechanical sensitivity of lateral thalamic neurons. This critical parameter coincides with other reports relating graded mechanical or electrical stimulus intensity to the magnitude of central inhibition of pain in the brain.

This is very significant as it indicates that chiropractic adjustments with higher intensity thrusts produce central decreases in pain, whereas spinal mobilization (low intensity) does not have the central pain-inhibiting benefits. The studies by Reed et al. (2014), Coronado et al. (2012), and many others have determined the effects of chiropractic adjustments on modulation through the CNS.

The next important finding regarding chiropractic effects relates to changes in the thalamus, a key structure in the brain's pain pathways. The thalamus is a large mass of gray matter in the dorsal part of the diencephalon of the brain. The thalamus has many functions with a variety of neuronal inputs and outputs. It acts as a critical relay between subcortical areas and the cerebral cortex. Every sensory system (with the exception of the olfactory system) connects through a thalamic nucleus that receives original sensory signals and sends them to the associated primary cortical areas. For example, inputs from the retina are sent to the lateral geniculate nucleus of the thalamus, which in turn projects to the visual cortex in the occipital lobe. Similarly, the medial geniculate nucleus acts as a key auditory relay between the inferior colliculus of the midbrain and the primary auditory cortex. The ventral posterior nucleus, a key somatosensory relay, sends touch and proprioceptive neuronal information to the primary somatosensory cortex. The thalamus is connected to the cerebral cortex via the thalamocortical radiations and, importantly, is believed to regulate consciousness, sleep, and alertness (Bickford, 2016).

Mohammadian, Gonsalves, Tsai, Hummel, and Carpenter (2004) investigated the effects of a single SMT on acute inflammatory reactions. Their results clearly demonstrated hypoalgesic effects from SMT but not from non-spinal manipulative therapy. They also reported that their findings confirmed the view that the hypoalgesic effects of a single SMT might be due to central modulation of pain. Spinal manipulation (chiropractic spinal adjustments) stimulates mechanoreceptors of the spinal joints, resulting in afferent discharges and subsequently causing inhibitory reactions at the dorsal horn neurons. Their study suggested that chiropractic spinal adjustment affects the nocioceptors and mechanoreceptors at the joint level, causing central modulation of an effect at the cord and/or the brain levels and pain reductions in multiple areas as a result.

Other researchers came to the same conclusion: that SMT (chiropractic adjustment) produced neurophysiological effects through higher brain centers (Daligadu, Haavik, Yielder, Baarbe, & Murphy, 2013; Gay, Robinson, George, Perstein, & Bishop, 2014; Souvlis, Vicenzino, & Wright, 2004). The study by Gay et al. utilizing functional magnetic resonance imaging (fMRI), revealed immediate changes in resting-state functional connectivity in the brain following chiropractic adjustments. The regions of the brain that are activated following chiropractic manipulation and their functions are summarized in Table 9.1.

Table 9.1. Regions of the Brain That Might Be Associated With Effects of Chiropractic Manipulation

Brain Region	Function
Cingulate cortex	Regulation of emotions, motivation
Insular cortex	Homeostasis, emotional awareness, perception, motor xontrol
Motor cortex	Voluntary movements
Amygdala cortex	Emotional reactions, memory
Somatosensory cortex	Proprio- and mechano-reception, touch, temperature, pain
Periaqueductal gray	Ascending and descending spinothalamic tracts for carrying pain and temperature fibers

The efforts of Gay et al. (2014) were to answer the question "Can the processing of pain be modulated or regulated from an external force without the use of pharmacy or surgery?" The authors indicated that, within the brain, pain perception results from activity within a network of brain regions including the thalamus, primary and secondary somatosensory, cingulate, and insular cortices. This network of structures is also referred to as the *pain processing network* (PPN). This PPN is involved with all aspects of the pain experience, including the basic sensory perception of pain, as well as the cognitive and emotional components of pain. The perception of pain also requires the interaction between the PPN and other brain structures, particularly the descending pain modulatory system. It is for this reason that each patient may experience pain differently. Gay et al. note that some patients can function well with anxiety and depression while others have substantial difficulty functioning normally. Chiropractors are believed to be able to help influence higher centers of the brain that contribute to these symptoms with little or no side effects. Gay et al. (2014) went on to argue that their results were consistent with other studies that found changes using alternative neurophysiologic outcomes such as the Hoffman-reflex and motor-neuron excitability, changes in electroencephalogram with somatosensory-evoked potentials, effects of transcranial magnetic stimulation, and task-based fMRI responses.

Effect of Chiropractic Care on Psychiatric Conditions

There is little systematic data regarding the use of chiropractic techniques for psychiatric conditions. Most of the available data is based on case reports or case series. We present some of that information here. However, traditional randomized placebo-controlled trials will be necessary before any of these approaches can be considered beneficial in the mental health setting.

In one early report by Schwartz and Harmann (1949), of 350 patients with various types of nervous or mental disorder, the majority demonstrated improvement in their symptoms with chiropractic care. With regard to depression and anxiety, there are no randomized controlled trials (RCTs) on the beneficial effect of chiropractic care in patients specifically expressing such symptoms. Most of the data available show that improving chronic pain symptoms is associated with a concomitant reduction in depression and anxiety symptoms. For example, one study evaluated 192 patients with two to six weeks of low back pain receiving chiropractic care, muscle relaxants, or placebo (Hoiriis et al., 2004). As an entire group, the patients had significantly reduced depression symptoms with chiropractic, but there were no significant differences when chiropractic care was compared to either the muscle relaxant or even the placebo group.

In a small, uncontrolled study of 19 women with chronic pelvic pain, six weeks of chiropractic therapy was associated with significant reductions in pain and also depressive symptoms as measured using the Beck Depression Index (Hawk, Long, & Azad, 1997). Similarly, a series of 15 patients with a history of depression demonstrated significant improvements in depression symptoms based on the Beck Depression Inventory following orthospinology care (Genthner, Friedman, & Studley, 2005). Again, though, there were no control groups for a more rigorous evaluation in these studies.

One large retrospective survey study of 2,818 patients receiving Network Spinal Analysis chiropractic care indicated that up to three-quarters of patients reported substantial improvements in their physical state, mental/emotional state, stress state, and quality of life (Blanks, Schuster, & Dobson, 1997). One case series of six adults with anxiety and depression symptoms, as well as the presence of upper cervical subluxation, showed that after 12 sessions of adjustments there were significant reductions in anxiety and depressive symptoms as measured by the Generalized Anxiety Disorder–7 and Patient History Questionnaire–9 (Roth, Zelman, Clum, & Roth, 2013). However, a small randomized study of 21 hypertensive patients showed that while hypertension was reduced, there were no changes in state anxiety in the chiropractic group when compared to the control group (Yates, Lamping, Abram, & Wright, 1988).

A systematic review of the literature revealed only five articles that included three case reports, one cohort series, and one randomized trial (Alcantara, 2011). The results suggest that chiropractic therapy might be beneficial for improving sensorimotor integration, which is a common element of autistic spectrum disorders. A small randomized clinical trial compared full-spine, high-velocity, low-amplitude spinal manipulation to upper cervical adjustments in 14 autistic children and found both forms of manual therapy resulted in improvements in approximately 75% of patients as measured by the Autism Treatment Evaluation Checklist (Khorshid, Sweat, Zemba, & Zemba, 2006). However, much more research will be needed to determine if chiropractic care can be recommended in patients with autism.

Chiropractic Care in Neurological Conditions

CHRONIC PAIN

The use of chiropractic techniques for patients with chronic pain is the most widely studied and accepted application. A large number of studies have demonstrated the benefits of chiropractic techniques for the management of chronic pain conditions, specifically those related to the back, neck, and spine. While the data of chiropractic care in various pain conditions is too extensive to review thoroughly in this chapter, we present a brief overview of the research and clinical findings. Additionally, while pain is not specifically a psychiatric condition, there is a well-known relationship between pain and mental health. Psychological problems can result in patients being more sensitive and affected by pain and, hence, less responsive to therapy (Ailliet, Rubinstein, Knol, van Tulder, & de Vet, 2016; Kongsted, Aambakk, Bossen, & Hestbaek, 2014). The reciprocal relationship has also been observed such that patients with chronic pain symptoms frequently report depression and anxiety in the face of dealing with the chronic pain (Fernandez et al., 2017). It has even been shown that emotional pain activates the same neurological pathways as physical pain (Kross, Berman, Mischel, Smith, & Wager, 2011). Such findings further support the chiropractic model relating the psychological and physical aspects of health and well-being.

With respect to pain conditions, chiropractic care is best studied for patients with back pain. In fact, the most recent guidelines from the American College of Physicians lists chiropractic care as a well-developed, well-tested, first-line therapy in patients with low back pain (Qaseem, Wilt, McLean, & Forciea, 2017). The data on chiropractic techniques in low back pain is relatively strong, with a number of RCTs demonstrating a benefit for both acute and chronic low back pain (Chou et al., 2017).

Chiropractic care has also been shown to be of benefit to patients with neck and back pain. Extensive reviews have indicated the potential benefit of chiropractic therapy in patients with neck and back pain, especially when they have actual musculoskeletal components associated with that pain (Plastaras,

Schran, Kim, Darr, & Chen, 2013). For example, a report designed to provide guidelines for chiropractic treatment of neck pain reviewed 41 RCTs (Bryans et al., 2014). This report indicated that manipulation and mobilization in combination with other modalities was beneficial in patients with acute and chronic neck pain. Thoracic manipulation was not recommended for the treatment of acute neck pain along with modalities such as transcutaneous nerve stimulation, thoracic manipulation, laser therapy, and traction.

A summary of the guidelines published by the Danish Health Authority suggested that, based on low- to moderate-quality evidence, patients with low back pain or lumbar radiculopathy benefitted from patient education, supervised exercise, and manual therapies (Stochkendahl et al., 2017). These particular guidelines recommend against the use of acupuncture, extraforaminal glucocorticoid injection, paracetamol, nonsteroidal anti-inflammatory drugs, and/or opioids.

However, other analyses suggest that the strength of the data supporting chiropractic therapy is not as strong, such as a Cochrane review of 27 trials that indicated low-quality support for the benefit of spinal manipulation in patients with neck pain (Gross et al., 2010). A more recent analysis had a similar conclusion in that there was evidence that chiropractic therapy was beneficial, but the data was too weak to make any strong recommendations (Yeganeh, Baradaran, Qorbani, Moradi, & Dastgiri, 2017).

In addition to back and neck pain, chiropractic therapy has also been evaluated for use in other pain syndromes such as fibromyalgia. Common therapy for fibromyalgia includes aerobic exercise and cognitive-behavioral therapy, massage, muscle strength training, and acupuncture (Schneider, Vernon, Ko, Lawson, & Perera, 2009). Several small studies and case series have suggested that chiropractic therapy might be beneficial in patients with fibromyalgia; however, most systematic reviews indicate that there is insufficient data to make any definite conclusions (Ernst, 2009; Terhorst, Schneider, Kim, Goozdich, & Stilley, 2011).

CHIROPRACTIC IN VERTIGO

Vertigo is a form of dizziness that gives the individual the illusion of movement. Vertiginous symptoms suggest one of two underlying disorders: an inner ear problem or a CNS problem. The inner ear is a collection of organs responsible for transforming vibrations in the air into signals that travel directly to the brain, which are then processed as sound. The inner ear also contains organs that coordinate with the brain to help with balancing the body as it moves. The CNS (the brain and spinal cord) is responsible for controlling thoughts, muscle movement, and the transportation of sensory stimuli into the brain.

If the source of vertigo is caused from the inner ear, the condition caused is peripheral vertigo. The following are some subtypes of peripheral vertigo.

Meniere's disease: An abnormal fluid level inside the inner ear, causing pressure and overstimulation, resulting in vertigo and, not uncommonly, hearing loss.

Benign paroxysmal positional vertigo (BPPV): One of the most common forms of peripheral vertigo, BPPV occurs when crystal deposits in the inner ear and become dislodged, ending up in the canals. As the patient moves, the crystals disrupt the flow of the fluid in the inner ear, confusing his or her balance organs, resulting in dizziness.

Labyrinthitis: This condition is brought on by inflammation in the inner ear's labyrinth. The labyrinth contains both the balance and hearing organs, thus it produces not only vertigo but hearing loss as well.

When the CNS is a source of disorder, it is known as central vertigo. Diseases that have been linked with this condition include the following.

Multiple sclerosis (MS): MS is a condition caused by inflammation and injury to the myelin coating of nerve fibers. This causes muscle weakness, coordination difficulties, visual problems, and vertigo.

Migraines: Migraines are specific types of headaches, more painful than common headaches. The pain can cause vertigo, often accompanied with nausea and vomiting.

Acoustic neuritis: Acoustic neuritis occurs when a benign tumor grows in the cranial nerve of the inner ear. Expansion of the tumor compresses adjacent nerves, causing vertigo, hearing loss, headaches, and facial numbness.

All the types of vertigo mentioned are associated with disorders of the brain, its associated organs such as the inner ear, or blood vessels. With regard to the application of chiropractic techniques, we can focus on the peripheral vertigo conditions: Meniere's disease, BPPV, and labyrinthitis, caused by excess fluid in the inner ear, crystals in the inner ear, and inflammation of the inner ear, respectively. Although the difference in pathophysiology is distinct, all are the manifestation of local disorders in homeostasis.

Meniere's Disease

The National Institute on Deafness and Other Communications Disorders estimates that 615,000 people in the United States have Meniere's disease. It is most likely to occur in people in their 40s and 50s. It is commonly a chronic, long-term disorder, but many with Meniere's will go into remission within a few years of their diagnosis. No medical cure is known. Symptoms of Meniere's disease are often episodic and come on as "attacks." Most people with Meniere's disease do not experience symptoms between episodes. Symptoms of Meniere's disease include vertigo, hearing loss, tinnitus, feeling of fullness in the ear, loss of balance, headaches, and nausea or vomiting.

To be accurate in the diagnosis, specific tests may be performed to rule out other causes of the symptoms. This may include audiometric studies to evaluate the type and level of hearing loss. Testing for balance is often used to confirm the presence of vertigo associated with Meniere's disease. Other than a neurological examination, specific balance testing may include the following.

- Rotational test
- Sharpened Romberg test
- Dix-Hallpike maneuver
- Sermont diagnositic maneuver

Brain positron-emission tomography (PET)/magnetic resonance
Brain computerized axial tomography (CT) scan
Magnetic resonance angiography
Electronystagmogram

Treatment for Meniere's disease is not often successful. Although there are no RCTs, one case report indicated that a 40-year-old woman with vertigo, tinnitus, hearing loss, and headaches experienced an almost complete resolution after three months of chiropractic treatment (Emary, 2010). Specifically, she was found to have left-sided upper cervical joint dysfunction and myofascial trigger points in the middle and upper trapezius muscle. She remained substantially improved even up to 2½ years of follow-up after upper cervical manipulation.

Benign Paroxysmal Positional Vertigo

BPPV is the most common cause of recurrent vertigo (Fife et al., 2008). It is estimated that between 17% and 42% of patients presenting with vertigo have BPPV (Devaiah & Andreoli, 2010). It is predominantly believed that the cause of BPPV is canalithiasis, where otoliths of calcium carbonate crystals become lodged within one of the semicircular canals (canalithiasis). Alteration in endolymph currents produce abnormal stimulation of the inner ear with head motion, resulting in subsequent vertigo and nystagmus (Bhattacharyya et al., 2008).

The application of the Dix-Hallpike maneuver will confirm the diagnosis of BPPV. Although we present a brief description of the Dix-Hallpike maneuver for conceptual purposes here, some formal training with an experienced practitioner is recommended to fully understand how to apply this manipulative technique.

A combination of two steps is required to properly perform the Dix-Hallpike maneuver: First, the patient is seated and his or her head is rotated 45 degrees to the side to be evaluated, which aligns the ipsilateral posterior semicircular canal with the sagittal plane of the body. Second, the patient is quickly brought into a supine position with the neck slightly extended to approximately 20 degrees. A positive test will reproduce the vertigo and will also bring on upbeating rotatory nystagmus toward the downside ear after a brief latency period (Evren, Demirbilek, Elbistanl, Köktürk, & Çelik, 2017; Zuma e Maia, Albernaz, & Cal, 2016). The vertiginous symptoms and nystagmus brought on by the maneuver commonly dissipates within one minute, and it is important to note that the nystagmus is fatigable, meaning that repeated attempts of the maneuver will produce a diminished response (Lantz, 1995).

Treatment is then provided by the Epley maneuver. It is the most commonly applied procedure (canalith repositioning) for BPPV and was first described by J. M. Epley in 1980 (Studin & Owens, 2015). Initially, the patient is seated and the head is rotated 45 degrees toward the side of the vertigo. The patient is then brought into a supine position and the head is extended approximately 20 degrees and held in this position for 20 to 30 seconds, while the head is still in rotation. The head is then rotated 90 degrees toward the unaffected side and held in this position for 20 to 30 seconds. The patient's body is then turned 90 degrees (lateral decubitus) and held in this position for another 20 to 30 seconds before being brought up into a seated position, at which point the head is flexed and held in this position for a final 20 to 30 seconds. Both the initial results of this technique and duration of improvement are typically quite significant.

As previously mentioned, there are contraindications to the Dix- Hallpike and Epley maneuver. Patients with cervical pathology including a history of head or neck surgery, metabolic diseases, active CNS disorder, otitis media, cardiovascular diseases (transient ischemic attacks, angina, hypertension), otosclerosis, as well as other red flags should be noted in the patient's medical screening questionnaires (Nørregaard, Lauridsen, & Hartvigsen, 2009).

Recovery of BPPV via the application of the Epley maneuver is good, but it does not occur in every case. Published clinical outcomes give a sensitivity of the Dix-Hallpike test of posterior semicircular BPPV at 79% and specificity at 75%. Also, the recurrence rate is high, with approximately 35% to 50% recurrence within the first two years (Hilton & Pinder, 2014).

Epilepsy

Epilepsy is the fourth most common neurologic disorder in the United States behind migraine, stroke, and Alzheimer's disease (Hirtz et al., 2007). Seizures are thought to occur when nerve cells in the brain fire at abnormally high rates. Seizures may result in impaired movements, actions, and/or levels of consciousness. A patient that suffers two or more unprovoked seizures is considered to have epilepsy. Epilepsy is estimated to affect up to 2.2 million people in the United States and 65 million people worldwide (Epilepsy Foundation, n.d.).

Several studies discussing the application of chiropractic in the treatment of epilepsy have been published. Many are case studies, and some present a comprehensive review of other reported outcomes (Elster, 2004; Hooper & Manis, 2011; Hubbard, Crisp, & Vowles, 2010; Pistolese, 2001). Specifically, these case reports document that patients with seizures, and particularly those with vertebral subluxations, seem to have improvements in the frequency of their seizures. These improvements appear to last up to a year or more in duration. Unfortunately, it is not clear from these case reports whether chiropractic care was the causal factor in reducing seizures. However, the reports suggest the possibility of future clinical trials with the goal of better assessing if chiropractic care can be used as an adjunct intervention for the management of seizures.

Risks of Chiropractic Care

The risks of chiropractic therapy are general low, and thus it is a relatively well-tolerated intervention. The most common side effects include local discomfort, headaches, or fatigue, which usually resolve within the first 24 hours (Senstad, Leboeuf-Yde, & Borchgrevink, 1997). The most severe reported complication is a vertebrobasilar artery stroke, which occurs in about one in 1 million manipulations, although the actual range varies considerably (Cassidy et al., 2008; Haldeman, Kohlbeck, & McGregor, 2002). Certainly, when done by well-qualified chiropractors who perform an appropriate physical and history on the patient, the risk of such severe events is very low. This might also be compared to the risk of chronic use of nonsteroidal anti-inflammatory medications, which result in side effects of 1% to 2% and several thousand deaths per year (Cryer, 2005).

Conclusion

Overall, chiropractic care has generally been shown to be effective in chronic and acute pain management as well as in vertigo and several other neurological disorders. There is still limited data showing how chiropractic care can reduce depression or anxiety symptoms, specifically in patients with mood or anxiety disorders. The best data at the present time supports the notion that chiropractic care reduces pain, particularly in patients with chronic pain, and that by alleviating pain, patients have reduced stress and anxiety. However, in this context, the reduction in depression and anxiety is a secondary effect related to pain relief. There is some data to support that chiropractic therapy might directly reduce anxiety and depression symptoms; however, more studies, including larger RCTs, will be required to make such therapy a primary intervention in patients with psychiatric disorders.

REFERENCES

Ailliet, L., Rubinstein, S. M., Knol, D., van Tulder, M. W., & de Vet, H C W. (2016). Somatization is associated with worse outcome in a chiropractic patient population with neck pain and low back pain. *Manual Therapy, 21*, 170–176.

Alcantara, J. D. (2011). A systematic review of the literature on the chiropractic care of patients with autism spectrum disorder. *Explore, 7*(6), 384–390.

Bhattacharyya, N., Baugh, R. F., Orvidas, L., Barrs, D., Bronston, L. J., Cass, S., et al. (2008). Clinical practice guideline: Benign paroxysmal positional vertigo. *Otolaryngology—Head and Neck Surgery, 139*(5), S47–S81.

Bickford, M. E. (2016). Thalamic circuit diversity: Modulation of the driver/modulator framework. *Frontiers in Neural Circuits, 9*, 86.

Blanks, R. H., Schuster, T. L., & Dobson, M. (1997). A retrospective assessment of network care using a survey of self rated health, wellness and quality of life. *Journal of Vertebral Subluxation Research, 1*, 11–27.

Bryans, R., Decina, P., Descarreaux, M., Duranleau, M., Marcoux, H., Potter, B., et al. (2014). Evidence-based guidelines for the chiropractic treatment of adults with neck pain. *Journal of Manipulative and Physiological Therapeutics, 37*(1), 42–63.

Cassidy, J. D., Boyle, E., Côté, P., He, Y., Hogg-Johnson, S., Silver, F. L., & Bondy, S. J. (2008). Risk of vertebrobasilar stroke and chiropractic care: Results of a population-based case-control and case-crossover study. *Spine, 33*(4 Suppl.), S176–S183.

Chapman-Smith, D. A. (2000). *The chiropractic profession*. Des Moines, IA: NCMIC Group.

Chou, R., Deyo, R., Friedly, J., Skelly, A., Hashimoto, R., Weimer, M., et al. (2017). Nonpharmacologic therapies for low back pain: A systematic review for an American College of Physicians clinical practice guideline. *Annals of Internal Medicine, 166*(7), 493–505.

Coronado, R. A., Gay, C. W., Bialosky, J. E., Carnaby, G. D., Bishop, M. D., & George, S. Z. (2012). Changes in pain sensitivity following spinal manipulation: A systematic review and meta-analysis. *Journal of Electromyography and Kinesiology, 22*(5), 752–767.

Cryer, B. (2005). NSAID-associated deaths: The rise and fall of NSAID-associated GI mortality. *The American Journal of Gastroenterology, 100*(8), 1694–1695.

Daligadu, J., Haavik, H., Yielder, P. C., Baarbe, J., & Murphy, B. (2013). Alterations in cortical and cerebellar motor processing in subclinical neck pain patients following spinal manipulation. *Journal of Manipulative and Physiological Therapeutics, 36*(8), 527–537.

Devaiah, A. K., & Andreoli, S. (2010). Postmaneuver restrictions in benign paroxysmal positional vertigo: An individual patient data meta-analysis. *Otolaryngology—Head and Neck Surgery, 142*(2), 155–159.

Elster, E. L. (2004). Treatment of bipolar, seizure, and sleep disorders and migraine headaches utilizing a chiropractic technique. *Journal of Manipulative and Physiological Therapeutics, 27*(3), 217.

Epilepsy Foundation. (n.d.). About epilepsy: The basics. Retrieved from http://www.epilepsy.com/

Emary, P. C. (2010). Chiropractic management of a 40-year-old female patient with Ménière disease. *Journal of Chiropractic Medicine, 9*, 22–27.

Ernst, E. (2009). Chiropractic treatment for fibromyalgia: A systematic review. *Clinical Rheumatology, 28*(10), 1175–1178.

Evren, C., Demirbilek, N., Elbistanl, M. S., Köktürk, F., & Çelik, M. (2017). Diagnostic value of repeated Dix-Hallpike and roll maneuvers in benign paroxysmal positional vertigo. *Brazilian Journal of Otorhinolaryngolgy, 83*(3), 243–248.

Fernandez, M., Colodro-Conde, L., Hartvigsen, J., Ferreira, M. L., Refshauge, K. M., Pinheiro, M. B., et al. (2017). Chronic low back pain and the risk of depression or anxiety symptoms: Insights from a longitudinal twin study. *The Spine Journal, 17*(7), 905–912.

Fife, T. D., Iverson, D. J., Lempert, T., Furman, J. M., Baloh, R. W., Tusa, R. J., et al. (2008). Practice parameter: Therapies for benign paroxysmal vertigo (an evidenced-based review): Report of the Quality Standards Subcommittee on the American Academy of Neurology. *Neurology, 70*, 2067–2074.

Gay, C. W., Robinson, M. E., George, S. Z., Perstein, W. M., & Bishop, M. D. (2014). Immediate changes after manual therapy in resting-state functional connectivity as measured by functional magnetic resonance imaging in participants with induced low back pain. *Journal of Manipulative and Physiological Therapeutics, 37*(9), 614–627.

Genthner, G. C., Friedman, H. L., & Studley, C. F. (2005). Improvement in depression following reduction of upper cervical vertebral subluxation using orthospinology technique. *Journal of Vertebral Subluxation Research*, 1–4.

Gross, A., Miller, J., D'Sylva, J., Burnie, S. J., Goldsmith, C. H., Graham, N., et al. (2010). Manipulation or mobilisation for neck pain: A Cochrane review. *Manual Therapy*, 15(4), 315–333.

Haldeman, S., Kohlbeck, F. J., & McGregor, M. (2002). Stroke, cerebral artery dissection, and cervical spine manipulation therapy. *Journal of Neurology*, 249(8), 1098–1104.

Hawk, C., Long, C., & Azad, A. (1997). Chiropractic care for women with chronic pelvic pain: A prospective single-group intervention study. *Journal of Manipulative and Physiological Therapeutics*, 20(2), 73–79.

Hilton, M. P., & Pinder, D. K. (2014). The Epley (canalith repositioning) manoeuvre for benign paroxysmal positional vertigo. *Cochrane Database of Systematic Reviews*, 8(12), CD003162. doi:10.1002/14651858.CD003162.pub3

Hirtz, D., Thurman, D. J., Gwinn-Hardy, K., Mohamed, M., Chaudhuri, A. R., Zalutsky, R. (2007). How common are the "common" neurologic disorders? *Neurology*, 68(5), 326–337.

Hoiriis, K. T., Pfleger, B., McDuffie, F. C., Cotsonis, G., Elsangak, O., Hinson, R., & Verzosa, G. T. (2004). A randomized clinical trial comparing chiropractic adjustments to muscle relaxants for subacute low back pain. *Journal of Manipulative and Physiological Therapeutics*, 27(6), 388–398.

Hooper, S., & Manis, A. (2011). Upper cervical care in a nine-year-old female with occipital lobe epilepsy: A case study. *Journal of Upper Cervical Chiropractic Research*, 10–17.

Hubbard, T. A., Crisp, C. A., & Vowles, B. (2010). Upper cervical chiropractic care for a 25-year-old woman with myoclonic seizures. *Journal of Chiropractic Medicine*, 9(2), 90–94.

Khorshid, K. A., Sweat, R. W., Zemba, D. A., & Zemba, B. N. (2006). Clinical efficacy of upper cervical versus full pine chiropractic care on children with autism: A randomized clinical trial. *Journal of Vertebral Subluxation Research*, 1–7.

Kim, E. S., Hagan, K. A., Grodstein, F., DeMeo, D. L., De Vivo, I., & Kubzansky, L. D. (2017). Optimism and cause-specific mortality: A prospective cohort study. *American Journal of Epidemiology*, 185(1), 21–29.

Kongsted, A., Aambakk, B., Bossen, S., & Hestbaek, L. (2014). Brief screening questions for depression in chiropractic patients with low back pain: Identification of potentially useful questions and test of their predictive capacity. *Chiropractic & Manual Therapies*, 22(1), 4.

Kross, E., Berman, M. G., Mischel, W., Smith, E. E., & Wager, T. D. (2011). Social rejection shares somatosensory representations with physical pain. *Proceedings of the National Academy of Sciences of the United States of America*, 108(15), 6270–6275.

Lantz, C. A. (1995). A review of the evolution of chiropractic concepts of subluxation. *Topics in Clinical Chiropractic*, 2(2).

Mohammadian, P., Gonsalves, A., Tsai, C., Hummel, T., & Carpenter, T. (2004). Areas of capsaicin-induced secondary hyperalgesia and allodynia are reduced by a single chiropractic adjustment: A preliminary study. *Journal of Manipulative and Physiological Therapeutics, 27*(6), 381–387.

Nørregaard, A. R., Lauridsen, H. H., & Hartvigsen, J. (2009). Chiropractic management of a patient with benign paroxysmal positional vertigo: A case report. *Journal of Manipulative and Physiological Therapeutics, 32*(5), 387–390.

Palmer, D. D. (1910). *The science, art and philosophy of chiropractic.* Portland, OR: Portland Printing House.

Pistolese, R. A. (2001). Epilepsy and seizure disorders: A review of literature relative to chiropractic care of children. *Journal of Manipulative and Physiological Therapeutics, 24*(3), 199–205.

Plastaras, C., Schran, S., Kim, N., Darr, D., & Chen, M. S. (2013). Manipulative therapy (Feldenkrais, massage, chiropractic manipulation) for neck pain. *Current Rheumatology Reports, 15*(7), 339.

Qaseem, A., Wilt, T. J., McLean, R. M., & Forciea, M. A. (2017). Noninvasive treatments for acute, subacute, and chronic low back pain: A clinical practice guideline from the American College of Physicians. *Annals of Internal Medicine, 166*(7), 514–530.

Redwood, D. (2010). *Chiropractic research and practice—state of the art.* Cleveland: Cleveland Chiropractic College.

Redwood, D., Hawk, C., Cambron, J., Vinjamury, S. P., & Bedard, J. (2008). Do chiropractors identify with complementary and alternative medicine? Results of a survey. *Journal of Alternative and Complementary Medicine, 14*(4), 361–368.

Reed, W. R., Pickar, J. G., Sozio, R. S., & Long, C. R. (2014). Effect of spinal manipulation thrust magnitude on trunk mechanical activation thresholds of lateral thalamic neurons. *Journal of Manipulative and Physiological Therapeutics, 37*(5), 277–286.

Roth, L., Zelman, D., Clum, L., & Roth, J. (2013). Upper cervical chiropractic care as a complementary strategy for depression and anxiety: A prospective case series analysis. *Journal of Upper Cervical Chiropractic Research*, 49–59.

Schneider, M., Vernon, H., Ko, G., Lawson, G., & Perera, J. (2009). Chiropractic management of fibromyalgia syndrome: A systematic review of the literature. *Journal of Manipulative and Physiological Therapeutics, 32*(1), 25–40.

Schwartz, H. S., & Harmann, G. W. (1949). Preliminary analysis of 350 mental patients' records treated by chiropractors. *Journal of National Chiropractic Association, 19*, 12–15.

Senstad, O., Leboeuf-Yde, C., & Borchgrevink, C. (1997). Frequency and characteristics of side effects of spinal manipulative therapy. *Spine, 22*(4), 435–440.

Shekelle, P. G., Adams, A. H., Chassin, M. R., Hurwitz, E. L., Park, R. E., Phillips, R. B., Brook, R. H. (1991). *The appropriateness of spinal manipulation for low-back pain: Indications and ratings by a multidisciplinary expert panel.* Santa Monica, CA: RAND.

Souvlis, T., Vicenzino, B., & Wright, A. (2004). Neurophysiological effects of spinal manual therapy. In J. D. Boyling & G. A. Jull (Eds.), *Grieve's modern manual therapy: The vertebral column* (pp. 367–380). Edinburgh, UK: Churchill Livingstone.

Stevenson, R. W. (1948). *Chiropractic Text Book*. The Palmer School of Chiropractic: Davenport, IA.

Stochkendahl, M. J., Kjaer, P., Hartvigsen, J., Kongsted, A., Aaboe, J., Andersen, M., et al. (2017). National clinical guidelines for non-surgical treatment of patients with recent onset low back pain or lumbar radiculopathy. *European Spine Journal*. 2017 Apr 20. doi: 10.1007/s00586-017-5099-2.

Studin, M., & Owens, W. (2015). How does the chiropractic adjustment work? A literature review of pain mechanisms and brain function alteration. *The American Chiropractor, 37*(8), 30, 33–34, 36–38, 40, 42–43.

Terhorst, L., Schneider, M. J., Kim, K. H., Goozdich, L. M., & Stilley, C. S. (2011). Complementary and alternative medicine in the treatment of pain in fibromyalgia: A systematic review of randomized controlled trials. *Journal of Manipulative and Physiological Therapeutics, 34*(7), 483–496.

World Health Organization. (2005). *WHO guidelines on basic training and safety in chiropractic*. Geneva: Author.

Yates, R. G., Lamping, D. L., Abram, N. L., & Wright, C. (1988). Effects of chiropractic treatment on blood pressure and anxiety: A randomized, controlled trial. *Journal of Manipulative and Physiological Therapeutics, 11*(6), 484–488.

Yeganeh, M., Baradaran, H. R., Qorbani, M., Moradi, Y., & Dastgiri, S. (2017). The effectiveness of acupuncture, acupressure and chiropractic interventions on treatment of chronic nonspecific low back pain in Iran: A systematic review and meta-analysis. *Complementary Therapies in Clinical Practice, 27*, 11–18.

Zuma e Maia, F. C., Albernaz, P. L., & Cal, R. V. (2016). Behavior of the posterior semicircular canal after Dix-Hallpike maneuver. *Audiology Research, 6*(1), 140. doi:10.4081/audiores.2016.140

10

Homeopathy and Psychiatry

BERNARDO A. MERIZALDE

Key Points

- Homeopathy is based primarily on the notion of using different preparations of substances that induce or inhibit various symptoms and illnesses.
- Although a controversial therapy, there is a substantial literature base that supports the potential benefits of homeopathy in psychiatric illness.
- Much of the data on homeopathy is not based on randomized controlled trials.
- Homeopathy is believed to work best when it is individualized to the specific patient.
- The placebo effect plays an important role in the patient's response to homeopathic medicines.
- Multiple homeopathic medicines are often required for optimum treatment response.
- The individualized homeopathic consultation can have an important therapeutic effect.
- The constitution of the person is believed to help determine responsiveness to particular remedies.

Introduction

Homeopathy is a controversial complementary and alternative medicine (CAM) system of treatment that prevails despite serious challenges to its theories and application. During the 19th century, it was favored in the United States among prominent individuals, such as major leaders of industry; political figures, including a couple of presidents; and distinguished scientists and physicians (Davidson, 2014; Ullman, 2007). It began its decline after publication of the Flexner report, which criticized medical education and training in many medical schools, many of which were homeopathic (King, 1984). Yet homeopathic training and investigation continues, outside the dominant health system. Currently a substantial subset of health professionals practice homeopathy and large numbers of patients throughout the world use it. It is estimated that homeopathy rose 500% between 1996 and 2003, and sales of homeopathic medicines grew 39.5% between 2003 and 2005 (Jonas, Kaptchuk, & Linde, 2003; SPINS, 2006). The growth then decreased to about a 3% annual growth between 2008 and 2013 (Hanson, 2013).

The literature base on homeopathy is immense, with thousands of publications in many languages, spanning over two centuries; however, its premodern scientific framework with wide variations in study designs and results leave as many questions as answers. Regardless, since the popularity of homeopathy continues to grow, and one of the uses is in the treatment of psychiatric conditions among patients and its practitioners, it is a subject worth probing. This chapter reviews a condensed history of homeopathy and the philosophical constructs of this system as it has been applied to healthcare, as well as the available data on its use in psychiatric care.

Brief History of Homeopathy

Samuel Hahnemann (1755–1843) was a German physician who, dissatisfied with the medical practices of his time, which included bloodletting, purging, vomiting, and the corporal punishment of persons with mental illness, turned to translating medical texts for income, which inadvertently led to his developing homeopathy. While translating Cullen's *Materia Medica* section on Cinchona (Peruvian Bark), which was used to treat malaria, he noticed that Cinchona's secondary effects resembled the symptoms of malaria itself. This led to Hahneman's concept of treating diseases with substances capable of producing pathological conditions similar to the patient's complaints.

He tested approximately 99 other substances, across the domains of mineral, vegetable, and animal kingdoms. Hippocrates had previously postulated this therapeutic approach (Haehl, 1922). Hahneman referred to his testing process as "proving" (the testing of the substance to find out the effects of substances on the organism), which he did initially in substantial doses of one to four grains (a grain equals approximately 62 mg). Hahnemann changed the particulars of the practical application of his theory several times during his career. At some point he prepared the medicines by serially diluting the solutions in flasks that were forcefully shaken and struck against a hard surface; the dilutions could go up to one part in 100^{-30}, a quinquillionth. This dilution was labeled "30C." This process is called potentization, through which the medicinal substance is supposed to maintain biological activity in spite of such high dilution. Although these dilutions are well beyond Avogadro's number and are expected to have no atoms of the original substance, Hahnemann postulated that some essence of the substance remained. Dilution of a given remedy can vary widely. Some are in ratios of 1/10, labeled as "X" (e.g., 3X, 6X, 12X); others are dilutions of 1/100, labeled as "C" (e.g., 3C, 6C, 12C); others are 1/50,000 and labelled LM (e.g., 1LM, 2LM, 3LM; Homœopathic Pharmacopœia of the United States, 2016).

Using these highly diluted substances as medicine is the most controversial aspect of the theory, and this is not the space to delve into those particulars. However, it is important to clarify that homeopathy is also applied in concentrations that are within material and measurable concentrations, in spite of critiques within the homeopathy community that only the use of ultradiluted preparations is appropriate. Nevertheless, the phenomenon of a dose–response phenomenon characterized by low-dose stimulation and high-dose inhibition has been observed in pharmacology in both in vitro and in vivo experiments and is referred to as hormesis. In the nonhomeopathic literature, the phenomenon describes the reactions of organisms to substances at measurable amount. For example, low dosages of antipsychotic drugs can treat hallucinations, but higher dosages may produce them. Research on hormesis is relatable to homeopathy (Boericke, 1965; Calabrese, 2013; Calabrese & Blain, 2004; Calabrese & Jonas, 2010; Merizalde, 2005).

In Hahneman's early investigations, preparations were ingested by "healthy" individuals in a semicontrolled manner, with close observation and recording of the symptoms elicited. To participate in a proving, an individual had to be free from any evident pathology, so that the symptoms could be most reliable. The *materia medica* is the reference database, with an alphabetical inclusion of the medicinal substances including all symptoms elicited in the provings, categorized and listed by organ system. In therapy, homeopaths decide dilution strengths based on numerous variables, such as recurrence of disease, chemical sensitivities, allergies, or untoward reactions to medicines in general, and are related to the examination of the patient and the nature of symptoms presented (Dunham, 1984).

Although the philosophical concepts that define homeopathy are often challenging, and at times anachronistic, there are interesting parallel concepts in conventional biomedical science. For example, sleep deprivation or insomnia (a symptom of depression), taken to the extreme, can be a treatment for depression (Post & Weiss, 1992). Likewise, the model of time-dependent sensitization indicates that exposure to a strong compound sensitizes an organism to a smaller dose of the same compound, which results in an amplified response. This type of effect has relevance to kindling phenomena and also overlaps conceptually with hormesis (Antelman, 1988).

Like several other CAM modalities, there are no "one-size-fits-all" homeopathic treatment protocols for a given diagnosis or set of symptoms, such as generalized anxiety; medicines need to be individualized according to the uniqueness of the patient's condition. This can make doing and interpreting homoepathic research a challenge. Some investigators have chosen to use a set number of different remedies (four to eight) that may suit a majority of patients with a diagnosis, but this may leave out the actual medicine that could be effective for a particular individual when considering his or her unique syndromatic characteristics. There are also consistency issues with potencies chosen and dosages of the remedies given from one trial to another, making comparisons virtually impossible.

Research in Homeopathy

Even though it is often postulated that homeopathy has no evidence, when the data is looked at closely, there is a significant amount of it even if it does not meet the highest criteria according to the modern framework of evidence-based medicine (National Institute for Health and Care Excellence, 2016). According to such criteria, the highest degree of acceptable scientific evidence methodologies are systematic reviews and meta-analysis of randomized controlled trials (RCTs). Nevertheless, other data, even if not as reliable, can come from nonrandomized intervention studies, such as cohort studies, and noneexperimental studies, such as meaningful and significant case reports. The later set of data can be used as pilot material for the design of a higher quality research protocol. Even though expert opinions are at the lowest level of reliable, they should always be dismissed beforehand (Harbour & Miller, 2001).

Although there are substantial numbers of documented homeopathic provings, they are essentially case reports with the inherent limitations thereof, unclear sources of the therapeutic compound, unclear parameters for the proving, and small numbers of provers. Numerous objective studies have been attempted, but most are wrought with methodological limitations with wide variations in results. One extensive review of the homeopathic literature concluded that, in spite of a great deal of experimental and clinical work, there is only a little scientific evidence to suggest that homeopathy could be effective. This is largely because of poor design, execution, or reporting or failure to repeat experimental work. The authors did conclude that there was sufficient evidence to warrant the execution of well-designed, carefully controlled experiments. Sadly, this conclusion has been repeated in almost all meta-analysis done up to date, 32 years after this author published one of the first reviews (Scofield, 1984).

A well-known study by Linde et al. (1997) reviewed the available literature and concluded that homeopathy seemed to have a therapeutic effect in conditions such as allergic rhinitis and asthma, dermatitis, diarrhea, gastritis, irritable bowel syndrome, sprains, cramps, headaches, seasickness, premenstrual syndrome, and cystitis, despite its implausibility. Another study, sponsored by the European Commission Homeopathic Medicine Research Advisory Group, came to similar conclusions, using only randomized controlled studies with concrete, predefined outcome measures. However, they concluded that use of the meta analysis method does not provide conclusions regarding which homeopathic treatment is effective for which diagnosis or set of symptoms. (Cucherat, Haugh, Gooch, & Boissel, 2000). In another comparative review of homeopathic, controlled, clinical trials, the authors concluded that the clinical effects of homoeopathy are placebo effects (Shang et al., 2005). It has been counterargued that the methodology of this review was flawed and unfairly biased against homeopathy (Fisher, 2006).

Comissioned by the Swiss health authorities, a full report was published by the Health Technology Assessment (HTA) on the effectiveness, appropriateness, safety, and costs of homeopathy in healthcare. Prior to this report, some studies carried by the Swiss Complementary Medicine Evaluation Programme were leaked prior to official publication, which resulted in some data being used out of context or reported with significant bias toward reporting negative outcomes for homeopathy. The HTA report, in contrast, presented a more comprehensive evaluation of the research and practice of homeopathy, confirming that homeopathy is a valuable addition to the conventional medical model, offering effectiveness, safety, and cost savings (Bornhoft & Mathiessen, 2011).

In March, 2015, the Australian National Health and Medical Research Council (NHMRC) published an information paper on homeopathy concluding there was no reliable data that homeopathy was effective in the treatment of any medical condition. However, the review does state that there is research showing homeopathy is more effective than placebo, as reported in some of the original published reports, and that such research needs to be replicated with larger, well-designed studies. However, the statement is made to seem insignificant beside the main conclusion of the article (NHMRC, 2015).

The Homeopathy Research Institute, based in London, UK, reviewed the NHMRC report in detail and noted that no member in the committee had any expertise in homeopathy and this could be the cause for some of the serious errors made in the evaluation of the evidence. One such error was that the results of the trials were analyzed together as a whole, with large and heterogenous sets mixed in together and with negative trials cancelling out positive ones, even though they were testing completely different treatments—a totally invalid analytical method. Another mistake was to confuse the use of a combination homeopathic medicine—manufactured with several medicines at an arbitrary potency/strength—with the need to individualize the single indicated medicine, which is a basic tenet in classical homeopathy; therefore, to conclude that a combination medicine does not work in a particular clinical condition is not an indictment on homeopathy at large but only on the use of a combination medicine for that particular condition treated in the study (infantile diarrhea in that case).

The NHMRC study only included controlled, prospective studies, leaving out actual observational studies, which, though not from the highest rung in the evidence ladder, are still valid under certain terms, such as reliable cohort studies and case series. The review also did not include positive and high-quality studies that were not published in English, nor did it include articles if they did not meet the Council's apparent idiosyncratic and inconsistent criteria. Therefore, the NHMRC's conclusions that homeopathy is not effective for any medical condition is invalid (Homeopathy Research Institute, 2015).

There is some evidence that homeopathy can be effective in the relief of symptoms in the treatment of several different conditions including allergic rhinitis, anxiety, arthritis, asthma, depression, dermatitis, fibromyalgia, headaches/migraines, infantile diarrhea, otitis media, and vertigo (American Institute of Homeopathy, 2016). Unfortunately, such evidence is very small, as noted previously, mostly due to the low quality of the executed trials and the lack of sufficient replication.

An important question to ask is whether conventional research methodology can accomodate the particulars of research in homeopathy, considering the greater number of variables involved in homeopathic therapeutics (i.e., the need to individualize not just the medicine but also the potency and the dosage). Some people will respond to high potencies (30C, 200C, and above) and others to low potencies (6X, 6C, 12C), and even others will require the LM potency range, which are much more diluted medicines.

Unfortunately, the subset of literature that is psychiatrically based is no less ambiguous. All of the research studies showing effectiveness of homeopathy in mental health conditions need to be replicated. The following is a discussion of some history of homeopathy in mental health and relevant studies that focus on mental illness. Although definitive conclusions cannot be drawn, it is hoped that this review will inform the practicing psychiatrist sufficiently to discuss with interested patients what is and is not known about the subject matter.

Homeopathy and Psychiatry

The first homeopathic hospital for the mentally ill was founded in Middletown, New York, in May 1874. One prominent physician who used homeopathy at the time to treat the mentally ill was Charles Frederick Menninger, founder of the notable Menninger Clinic, which is still in operation but no longer uses homeopathy. Menninger was an active member of the American Institute of Homeopathy and is quoted as saying,

> Homeopathy is wholly capable of satisfying the therapeutic demands of this age better than any other system or school of medicine . . . it is imperative that we exhaust the homeopathic healing art before resorting to any other mode of treatment, if we wish to accomplish the greatest success possible. (Menninger, 1897)

Few studies on the use of homeopathy in mental health have been published that follow current standards of scientific methodology, though some meta-analyses of the studies that exist have suggested overall positive effects that warrant further investigation. In one review, 8 of 10 reasonably high-quality studies on the treatment of mental or psychological problems, including depression, insomnia, nervous tension, agitation, aphasia, and behavior problems in children, showed positive effects from homeopathic treatment. Although none of those studies has been replicated, they cumulatively suggest potential value and the need for further exploration of homeopathic treatments (Kleijnen, Knipschild, & terRiet, 1991; Linde et al., 1997).

Some other interesting studies worthy of mention have been published. One suggested that homeopathy may be useful in the treatment of some patients with anxiety or depression, either as an adjunctive or sole treatment, in patients who specifically request it. In this case series, 12 patients with depression and/or anxiety were treated homeopathically. Six of these patients were taking conventional medicines for anxiety and/or depression and had been at a stable dose for 4 to 12 months. Clinical response was determined through the Clinical Global Improvement scale; in addition, the Symptom Checklist–Revised-90 or the Brief Social Phobia Scale was used. Improvement was considered significant at a 50% reduction in either measure used. Such criteria is often used in studies of this kind (Davidson, Morrison, Shore, Davidson, & Bedayn, 1997).

Of course, when patients choose the intervention, a selection bias toward such intervention can influence the placebo effect—people who believe in the treatment tend to respond better to it. In addition, the authors noted several limitations to this study, concluding that only larger, double-blind, controlled trials can provide answers to the questions that arise when using homeopathy in the treatment of disease in general and in psychiatry in particular.

Chapman, Weintraub, Milburn, Pirozzi, and Woo (1999) performed a randomized, double-blind, placebo-controlled study on 60 patients with persistent mild traumatic brain injury (MTBI). Their results suggested that homeopathy alone, or used concurrently with conventional pharmacological and rehabilitation therapies, may be effective in treating patients with persistent MTBI, a condition for which there are limited treatment options. The patients were recruited with symptoms that had lasted a minimum of two years (mean 2.93) posttrauma, and treatment efficacy was measured by a statistically significant improvement in 10 of the most common symptoms in MTBI related to social and cognitive dysfunctions (i.e., reading, writing, scheduling, shopping, socializing; Chapman et al., 1999).

Lamont (1997) performed a double-blind, placebo-controlled study on the treatment of 43 children with a diagnosis of attention deficit hyperactivity disorder (ADHD), showing statistically significant improvement in the homeopathy group as compared to the control, supporting the notion that homeopathic treatment is superior to placebo. Improvement was measured by statistically significant change in a 5-point scale measure of hyperactivity based on diagnostic criteria in the *Diagnostic and Statistical Manual of Mental Disorders* (fourth edition), as measured by the children's caretakers (Lamont, 1997).

Another set of studies also addresses the treatment of ADHD. One double-blind, placebo-controlled study of 115 children in Switzerland found positive results from a course of homeopathic treatment over a period of three months. These children were treated according to a more classical homeopathic approach, in which the remedy selection was individualized to the particular patient's symptoms (Frei & Thurneysen, 2001). This same research group decided to do a "crossover" phase of the study and stopped the remedies. They found that the children who had improved with homeopathy deteriorated when the placebo was given and then responded again when the remedy was reinstated, indicating a likely effect of the homeopathic medicine (Frei et al., 2005).

However, one of the challenges in designing these types of studies is that some people can respond to one or two doses of the homeopathic medicine and not need a repetition for months, so there can be a carry-over effect. These prolonged medicinal responses are not uncommon in homeopathic therapeutics, and if the treatment is only placebo, it makes it a very efficient one. Also, because the homeopathic medicines are stopped when a clinical effect is achieved, there is the possibility that the medicine may have to be restarted when the symptoms return, if there was an initial positive effect. Conversely, if the medicine is used too long, the symptoms can return or get worse, or other symptoms could appear that could be considered a proving on the part of the patient. These could be considered adverse events and, though often minor, are not discussed in the homeopathic literature as such.

The same group, Frei and colleagues (2007), published a retrospective analysis of their work and noted some of the difficulties in performing research in homeopathy such as the need to individualize the medicine and determining appropriate placebo conditions. For these and other reasons, studies purporting to determine the clinical efficacy of one or even several homeopathic medicines will easily miss the therapeutic agent for a particular individual. Frei et al. found that a median of three homeopathic medicines (range one to nine) are often tried before finding a positive clinical response, something that is also not unusual in conventional medicine. The researchers identified patients who were responsive to their individualized homeopathic medicine during the pretrial treatment and used this as criteria for eligibility into the study. It took an average of five months to meet the response criteria to be included in the randomized controlled, cross-over phase of the trial. Eighty-four percent of the subjects (70 patients) were included in the study. They concluded that before comparing these patients with a placebo group in a RCT, an optimal homeopathic medication must be identified in order for the trial to be reliable (Frei et al., 2007).

In a systematic review of homeopathic treatments in psychiatry (25 eligible studies out of 1,431), Davidson, Crawford, Ives, and Jonas (2011) found that homeopathy showed efficacy in the treatment of functional somatic syndromes, such as fibromyalgia and chronic fatigue syndrome. From the studies they selected they could not find evidence for effectiveness in anxiety, and they found mixed results in other disorders. They did not find placebo-controlled studies on depression that met their criteria. The same issue continues to plague the homeopathic field: the number of studies is limited, and many trials are underpowered and of low quality, though some of the data indicates it is worthy of replication. There is some indication that homeopathy could be helpful in ADHD, fibromyalgia and chronic fatigue syndrome, premenstrual syndrome, sleep disorders, and traumatic brain injury. It is possible that homeopathy could be helpful in relieving anxiety and depression symptoms as well, but the lack of evidence of effect could be due to the high placebo response in these conditions, spontaneous recovery, or other factors, including methodological issues, such as the length of the consultations and enhanced rapport with the practitioner (Davidson et al., 2011).

In general, Davidson et al. (2011) found that homeopathic medicines did not show any significant adverse effects, compared to placebo, and the drop-out rates were significantly lower than those normally seen in conventional studies. This supports the likely safety of homeopathic treatment. However, they point out the possible "harm" that could occur when patients are not offered an effective medically established treatment for a condition that could lead to disability or morbidity and instead are given only a yet unproven homeopathic treatment by conventional standards without confirmed efficacy.

A multiple RCT of depression is being carried out in England, considering that there is a lack of good quality trials in this area. Nonetheless, in observational studies, 50% to 80% of patients receiving treatment from homeopaths for depression report at least moderate improvement. For this study, the researchers are using a cohort multiple RCT with over 27,000 patient recruited from 451 general practice practices in the South Yorkshire area. Nine percent (2,000) of the participants self-report long-standing depression. To this group, there will be additional patients added, estimating the total number to about 5,700 (Viksveen & Relton, 2014).

Hundreds of case reports have been published in homeopathic journals since the 19th century about patients suffering from mental disorders who were treated with homeopathy. Even though some of them refer to the diagnosis of the cases inadequately according to modern standards, many of these patients would have met criteria for a mental disorder according to the *Diagnostic and Statistical Manual of Mental Disorders* (fifth edition) and would have been candidates for conventional pharmacotherapy in the present day.

The following is a brief overview of some case reports that have relatively clear and thorough descriptions of the disorders and treatment effect. They are mainly provided as a reference for those who would like more in-depth examples of the homeopathic process. Although case reports are not the gold standard of investigational inquiry in conventional biomedicine, some CAM modalities such as homeopathy consider case descriptions and outcomes crucial because of the individualized treatment approach of the intervention. Also, some feel that detailed case reports in the homeopathic literature are important and relevant to establishing its evidence base (Slonim & White, 1983).

Detinis (1994) presented six interesting cases of patients suffering from depression with suicidal ideation, chronic pain, sleep disorder, premenstrual syndrome, and anxiety disorder treated homeopathically. The patients were interviewed by the author as part of a practitioner training seminar, and the process of case taking and analysis was done with the group. Only three cases are reported as having a follow-up review. One patient, a 22-year-old male with suicidal depression of several years' duration also suffered with histrionic symptoms and intrusive persecutory thoughts, and conventional medications had not been helpful. After seven months, having received one dose of a high dynamization of his symptomatically correspondent medicine, he was no longer depressed.

A second patient, a 42-year-old woman, consulted for severe drawing and burning back pain radiating to the legs of several years' duration; the pain had gotten worse through the course of 17 months after a second back surgery. She received one dose of the corresponding homeopathic medicine, in her case Lachesis 1M, At the follow-up two months later, she reported having had a symptomatic aggravation for one week (not uncommon in homeopathic treatments) and then progressively felt better with complete resolution of the pain. She also noticed an increase in strength in her legs and was now able to walk four to five blocks without problems. Her family was astounded at her recovery (Detinis, 1994).

A third patient, a 49-year-old female patient with arthritis of the spine and hips, migraines, menopausal symptoms, and generalized anxiety, after several years of unsuccessful treatment with conventional modalities, reported a complete resolution of her pain, migraines, anxiety, and menopausal symptoms, with a restart of her menses, within seven months after the consultation. She continued well at a subsequent follow-up two years later, during which time she continued the homeopathic treatment (Detinis, 1994).

Bodman (1990) presents a series of cases of depression, anxiety, sleep disorder, phobias, neurosis, cerebral sequelae from a stroke, Meniere's disease, migraines, and other conditions treated successfully with homeopathy. One of the cases presented was a 14-year-old girl with a highly superior intelligence assessed by psychological testing. She was referred because of alarming temper outbursts, which were terrifying to her mother and siblings. She was a middle child and was jealous of her older sister and younger brother. Between the outbursts she was a shy, reserved girl with a demure expression. She was attending a good school, but, due to the severity of her tantrums, she was going to be expelled. An electroencephalogram performed showed a nonspecific abnormality. She received one dose of Hepar Sulphuris 30C. After that one dose, the family and the school reported she was a different girl; she was more willing and helpful around the house, was on better terms with her brother, and showed proper behavioral control. Ten months later she had another tantrum, but it was milder; she received another dose of Hepar Sulphuris 30C. Several months later, her improvement continued (Bodman, 1990).

Boltz (1968) presented six cases of patients with acute psychosis, treated primarily with homeopathy, in the Binghampton State Hospital in Binghampton, New York. In this article he reports that most of his patients, beyond the cases he presents, remained recovered for 17 to 30 years, which contrasts with what was generally seen clinically at that time. For these types of results he recommends using a "constitutional" (medicines that cover the totality of the case, including the patient's temperament and susceptibilities) plus an "organ" medicine (that address the acute symptoms of the patient). He postulates that the symptomatology of psychosis corresponds to disorders of the diencephalon and that the most frequently used medicines for psychosis—hyosciamus, stramonium, and belladonna—have toxicological clinical pictures that correspond to diencephalic dysfunction, which is why they can be helpful. An example of the cases presented was a 20-year-old man with no family history of mental illness who was sickly as a child and had few close friends; he was "not a good mixer" and had no interest in the opposite sex. Six months before his admission he had gone to visit a male cousin 13 years his senior in a nearby city. He stayed for about one month. When he returned he appeared overactive and silly, his conversation was irrelevant, and he had periods of aimless excitement. He became careless about his personal appearance, interrupted conversations, displayed involuntary silly laughter, and would lie on the floor. He also expressed persecutory ideation: "two men are on my trail; I am doubtful about the reality of my mother; strangers call me bastard, crazy, etc; I hear whispers; the moon draws me and makes my feet feel like kicking someone; I receive messages by telepathy; many people call me names, both good and bad." In the ward he appeared aimlessly overactive and silly; he would jump over tables, unscrew electric bulbs, and push chairs over, and he was not interested in therapeutic activities. He identified himself as the reincarnation of Christ, displayed mannerisms, spit constantly, and kept shaking his legs. At times he would bark like a dog and tear up objects. His condition did not change until he was given Stramonium 200X, five drops once per week. Three months into his hospitalization he started showing improvement. At six months into his stay his symptoms were reassessed, including a thyroid adenoma, skipped heart beats, salt cravings, and increased thirst. He received six pellets of Natrum Muriaticum (Nat. Mur.) 200X. One month later he received a second dose of Nat. Mur 200X. On the next day he requested to be transferred to the open ward for less disturbed patients, he started participating in therapeutic activities, and all his physical symptoms disappeared. Soon after, he was transferred to the surgical ward to have the adenoma removed. He was discharged a few days after. The patient was treated for a year and a half, during which time he was given several doses of Nat. Mur, about every 14 to 15 days. The patient continued doing well; he got married and raised several children, who were in their 20s when the patient was contacted to check how he was doing. The other cases discussed in the paper are similar syndromatically, as well as in treatment and follow-up. All patients also received hydrotherapy, massage, physical exercise, electric cabinet baths (a sort of sauna), and other herbal treatments to treat dysmenorrhea in the female patients (Boltz, 1968).

Saine (1997) presented a series of cases of patients with psychosis, manic-depressive disorder, obsessions, and neurosis. One of the patients was a man with of acute episodes of mania with generalized hypersensitivity. The patient was 43 years old when first seen. He complained of extreme sensitivity to molds, pollen, air-pollution, fruits, and chemicals, all since childhood. The patient was aggravated between November 15 to December 31, when the cold arctic air would come in. The attacks were worse between the evening and early morning, and the duration and intensity of the episodes were longer, lasting up to five days at a time. Recently they were lasting three to four weeks. He reported having psychotic symptoms, and he was diagnosed with schizophrenia. He was afraid of going out and of looking people in the eye; he had visual distortions, extreme exhaustion, and had feelings of being frantic and excited. He would feel bursts of energy with strong and fast heart beats, severe wandering pains through his body, throbbing headaches, weakness in the limbs, with cramps in the calves, and cold hands and feet. His body would break out in a cold sweat, and he would have loss of appetite and thirst. He was also sleepless through the night and felt restless. He would drink hard liquor to the point of passing out to end the attack. He had also experienced tunnel vision for 20 0years. He reported that as an infant he cried constantly and slept only two hours at night and two in the morning. He used as alpha wave audio track to help him go to sleep, and he had had night sweats all of his life.

He received one dose of Sulphur 6C, considering his clinical picture and particular symptoms, especially his hypersensitivity. Five and a half weeks later, he reported a severe aggravation of symptoms, the worst in three years, but it lasted only one day instead of the usual five. Afterwards he felt a 30% to 40% improvement overall. His tunnel vision disappeared completely; his mind felt clearer, and he felt like exercising, which he not done in two years. Three weeks later he reported that he had continued improving, up to 60% to 70% but in the last two days he had felt a return of his typical acute attacks, and the repetition of the Sulphur had not helped.

He received Belladona 30C, and two days later he reported having felt improvement promptly after the medicine. He then received one dose of Sulphur 12C, since he had responded to Sulphur earlier and not responded to the lower (6C) dynamization given previously. Belladona is not a deep-acting constitutional medicine for this patient's symptomatic picture, but it could be used for the acute episodes, based on the presenting symptoms.

Two weeks after the Sulphur 12C he reported having had an aggravation followed by improvement but felt only slightly better than with the Sulphur 6C. This means that Sulphur is only a similar medicine and not the "simillimum" (the closest medicine picture to the patient's global clinical picture). Nevertheless, he felt mentally clearer than in 30 years. His stamina improved to the point he could run three miles in 24 minutes. At this point, it was noted that the patient had suffered from tuberculosis years ago.

For several months, he was treated with Tuberculinum 6C, and the dynamization was increased progressively for about six months. He then received one dose of Tuberculinum 30C, and three weeks later he reported a great aggravation with it but after that felt much clearer, and his energy was much better. He was now experiencing a new acute episode.

He received single doses of Belladona 30C, and 200c without improvement. He received Hyosciamuc 30C and 200C, but that did not help either. He went back to the Tuberculinum, at a much lower dynamization, and the medicine was dissolved in water to minimize the dosage and prevent aggravations. After that, his allergies to weeds and molds disappeared. However, his acute states were still occurring.

With a more direct observation of an attack, a detailed picture was gathered. His face and ears would turn bright red; his eyes were glazed and pupils dilated; and his pulse was full, strong, and fast. He was abusive verbally and cursed constantly. He was sarcastic, aggressive, and arrogant; he would also have hysterical fits of laughter. He was paranoid and forbid his wife from going out, afraid something terrible would happen to her. When he did not curse, he would moan and grimace. He was extremely restless and walked around with closed fists and violently pounded on the walls and furniture. When he was too weak to stand, he rolled on the floor, twisting and turning, while flailing his arms. He was give Melilotus 30C, which fit best the current picture, and he improved dramatically. Within 30 minutes he fell asleep until the following morning and was completely recovered on waking.

He did not have any attacks for three months, and when one happened he took Melilotus 1M and felt better immediately; the acute attack melted away as soon as he took the medicine. A few days later, the patient reported having felt acute feelings of rage, which he had suppressed since childhood. He then mentioned that his father and brother had been abusive and violent toward him when he was a child.

He continued having sporadic, brief attacks that always responded to Melilotus 30C. The dynamization was increased progressively through three years of treatment. At that point, his picture changed and he no longer responded to Melilotus. The new picture involved the medicine Tuberculium Aviare, which was similar to the Tuberculinum he had taken earlier in the treatment. His clinical picture improved 85% to 90% to what it had been from the beginning of the treatment. He used a dose of Melilotus every several months when he felt the symptoms starting; all other organic functions were normal. He received only homeopathic medicines in his treatment (Saine, 1997).

Shevin (1989) has presented several cases of patients with dissociative disorders, character pathology, and posttraumatic stress disorder treated homeopathically. One of the cases, a 41-year-old woman who had been assaulted by a psychotic neighbor received a concussion, a back injury resulting in neuropathic pain, and a diagnosis of posttraumatic stress disorder. After four years of conventional treatment, which included two surgical procedures, she had experienced no relief. She received one dose of Bryonia 200C and was encouraged to start psychotherapy. Two months later she received Sepia, based on the remaining symptoms. She had significant improvement of physical and emotional symptoms. Six months later, her symptoms recurred and she received a second dose of Sepia 200C. Several months later, some symptoms returned and she received Sepia 1M—a higher dynamization—with no response. She then received Calcarea Carbonica 1M, and she again felt well, with no more neuropathic pain or emotional reactivity. Though the psychotherapeutic treatment was important to help her process the emotional trauma, how promptly and extensively this patient recovered cannot be solely attributed to the psychotherapy, particularly since she had relapses that responded to the indicated homeopathic medicine (Shevin, 1989).

Gallavardin (1960/1990) published a series of cases of patients treated for alcoholism, among others with other significant psychological and physical pathology with virtually no chance of spontaneous remission. An example of such cases was a man of a wicked, sullen, and jealous character who had been drinking for three years, neglecting his family and business. He was given (November 19, 1879) one dose of Lachesis 200C. One month later, the wife reported he was no longer jealous and was less sullen and wicked but was still drinking. He received one dose of Lachesis 1M. One year later, the wife said he had only gotten drunk five times instead of 30 times per month. He had become more responsible with his family and business; he received a placebo, since he was improving. Six months later, he came in for a tubercular fever; he had not been drunk in six months. He received Sulphur 5M, which improved the fever. A month later, it was reported he had become intoxicated twice and had tubercular pneumonia in the right lung. He received one dose of Phosphorus 200C. Three months later, he was better from his pneumonia but had been drunk five times. He received Lachesis 2M. Two months later, the spouse reported he was drinking six to seven times per week but now, instead of doing it with people, he was doing it alone. Considering the Lachesis did not work as it had before and his characteristics had changed, he received a single dose of Sulphur 5M. A year later, the patient had again stopped drinking even when he was with people who were drinking; he just drank water with his meals and was fully recovered, having received as treatment only six doses of the indicated homeopathic in the course of two years of healing, including an episode of tubercular pneumonia. His character changed to a man who was strong, active, alert, and responsible, without the aid of any other therapeutic intervention. The book contains many similar cases and worse cases, with delirium tremens and seizures (Gallavardin, 1960/1990).

Grazyna and Trzebiatowska-Trzeciak (1993), from Poland, presented a series of 30 men (ages 32–61) treated for alcohol withdrawal, five of whom had delirium tremens (DTs). All patients engaged in binge drinking at least once a week, but most had been drinking for several years (range = 6 months to 25 years). The patients were treated with Sulphur 30x, at least once per week; the DTs were treated with Sulphur 30X and 200C at frequent intervals, Belladona 30X, twice daily, and Phosphorus 30X or 200X, once daily. Each case of DT lasted no longer than 48 hours. Thirty percent of patients continued treatment for 12 to 18 months, and, if they lapsed, they reported not having a positive from alcohol and did not relapse. The patients were followed for up to seven years (Grazyna & Trzebiatowska-Trzeciak, 1993).

Haidvogl, Lehner, and Resch (1993), from Austria, treated 40 children with various cognitive handicaps, including traumatic brain injury. The children were selected from a group attending a special nursery and school for children with handicaps. The staff of the facility requested the intervention due to difficulty managing them due to the intensity of the symptoms presented by the children. Eighteen of the children responded extremely well in all target symptoms. Each had a combination of two or more symptoms such as irritability, anger, restlessness, sleep disorders, enuresis, encopresis, autistic behaviors, mental retardation, apathy, tantrums, and hypersexual behavior, among others. Eleven children responded extremely well to some but not all target symptoms; seven did not respond at all, and four had outcomes that could not be assessed due to difficult social backgrounds with lack of adequate parental participation to determine treatment effect. The homeopathic medicines used were chosen according to the classical homeopathic treatment approach (see later discussion) and single doses of medicines from the LM30, 30X, to the 200C were used (Haidvogl et al., 1993).

Amy Lansky (2003), a former computer science researcher with NASA, published her journey from a skeptic to a believer after her son was diagnosed with severe autism with poor prognosis. She researched homeopathy as a therapy, applied them to her son, and found the results "miraculous." Her son went from being withdrawn and asocial at 2½ years of age to being more verbal and sociable, and his hyperactivity symptoms become moderate. He no longer fit the diagnosis of autism; he was cured in less than one year, though he still needed nonpharmacological clinical support for sensory integration and residual cognitive challenges for a few more years (Lansky, 2003).

M. A. Rajalakshmi (2015) has also reported successful results of the treatment of autistic children, with features that would not be expected to improve significantly with just standard therapies; some of them also had mental retardation. Six children, between 2½ and 11 years of age, were treated homeopathically. An 11-year-old boy with autism, mental retardation, and a seizure disorder, treated with medication, responded to treatment within three months, with a decrease in temper tantrums, phobias, and crying spells. The episodes went from an almost daily occurrence to twice a month. A 5½-year-old boy with obsessive-compulsive behavior and malicious aggression responded promptly with a significant decrease of symptoms, which returned after a period of time, but again showed improvement when the medicine was restarted. The child imroved to the point he was able to "function at an optimal level in a regular school." A five-year-old boy with self-injurious biting, sleeplessness, mood swings, and mental dullness improved to the point he no longer hurt himself, was able to sleep, had regulated moods, and was able to learn and integrate instructions for self-care, which previously had to be repeated, step by step, every day. An eight-year-boy with autism and mental retardation with extreme sensory sensitivity, gross and fine motor disturbances, enuresis, and encopresis, who would just recoil to a corner to be left alone, responded within six months to homeopathic treatment with development of normal sensitivity and improvement in comprehension, going from being unresponsive to being interactive with others and even acquiring some musical skills. Finally, a seven-year-old girl with autism had extreme oral sensitivity and an aversion to multiple foods. She also had sleeplessness and continuous self-talk. After a few months she was calmer, she slept, and her food sensitivities improved. She also stopped having frequent upper respiratory infections, which were the norm before (Rajalakshmi, 2015).

This case series is significant, since all of these children received the homeopathic intervention after they had passed the time when early intervention for autism and mental retardation would have been most effective; the results to the treatment appeared pretty quickly, to a degree usually not seen with other conventional interventions, and without corresponding side effects.

One case series of 20 children with enuresis and behavioral problems reported 50% improvement in both symptoms. Unfortunately, this investigation was not done as a controlled study, making it difficult to evaluate (Cortina, 1994).

Boericke (1965) reported an interesting case of a patient suffering from dementia with psychosis treated with a homeopathic preparation of Chlorpromazine after the patient had gotten worse at usual dosages of this drug. This corresponds well to the phenomenon of hormesis referred to previously.

What is remarkable about these case series is that these are conditions that do not tend to respond well to conventional pharmacological treatment, and psychological treatments have shown limited success and require longer periods of time to manifest the degree of improvement. Though these are not results from randomized, double-blind, placebo-controlled studies, they still fit within the evidenciary pyramid, as case series and case reports with intrinsic validity and external validity, since these are experiences reported by thousands of practitioners from around the world. Ignoring such facts is unscientific and irrational.

Placebo as Therapy

It is ironic that while detractors of homeopathy affirm that homeopathic treatment is just placebo, a number of articles have concluded that the effect of antidepressants in the treatment of depression is almost all placebo effect. Starting in 1998, Kirsch and Saperstein began evaluating the data from antidepressant trials and determined that the effect of this class of drugs is mostly placebo. The reason for that is that one of the main characteristics of depression is hopelessness, and what makes patients most depressed is to be depressed. Therefore, the promise of an effective treatment replaces hopelessness with the hopefulness of recovery.

When the researchers analyzed the data they found up to a 75% percent improvement in patients who were given placebo. They also found that the effect of the medications on depression was very small over that of placebo (Kirsch & Saperstein, 1998).

Because of the tremendous controversy they raised, these authors decided to replicate the study, this time including all of the data sent by pharmaceutical companies to the Food and Drug Administration, a necessary step for the drug approval process, though only about half of such data is published. It has been shown that most of it shows a failure to find significant benefit of the drug over placebo (Turner, Mathews, Linardatos, Tell, & Rosenthal, 2008). In a second review article, Kirsch, Moore, and Scoboria (2002) found that only 43% of trials showed a statistical benefit of the drug over placebo. The remaining 57% were failed or negative trials. The placebo response to these antidepressants was 82%, a result that has appeared in other studies.

In a follow-up article, Kirsch et al. (2008) reported that

> Drug-placebo differences in antidepressant efficacy increase as a function of baseline severity, but are relatively small even for severely depressed patients. The relationship between initial severity and antidepressant efficacy is attributable to decreased responsiveness to placebo among very severely depressed patients, rather than to increased responsiveness to medication.

The placebo effect has been shown to be very powerful in the treatment of many medical conditions. The effect can vary between 30% and 60% or more, as noted previously, of the clinical effect of an intervention, particularly when associated with a compassionate and caring interaction with the treating practitioner or researcher (Harvard Health Letter, 2012).

One of the components of the homeopathic treatment, besides the actual medicines, the effect of which is still questioned, is the homeopathic interview. The homeopathic consultation involves a complete exploration of all the patient's complaints and concerns, as well as his or her constitutional, temperamental, and emotional makeup, their beliefs and concepts, particularly about the causes of their disease and suffering, including religious-spiritual constructs and perspectives. Such an approach leads the patient to feel understood and validated. It is common for the patient to express thoughts and feelings that have been dismissed outright by others, even well -intended practitioners (Mercer, 2005).

This therapeutic framework provides the patient the feeling of empathy, empowerment, and acknowledgement, which enhances the therapeutic relationship and is therapeutic in itself. It also provides the opportunity for the patient to acquire insight into his or her illness, sensations and reactions, and the adequacy of his or her coping mechanisms. Recovery is often accompanied by an intense process of self-discovery and an experience of change and transformation (Koithan, Embrey, & Bell, 2015).

In an RCT, a group of patients with rheumatoid arthritis were divided into five groups that received classical homeopathic consultation with individualized homeopathy, complex homeopathic compound for rheumatism or placebo, or a regular medical consultation with complex homeopathic compound for rheumatism or placebo. An individualized homeopathic medicine can only be selected through the classical homeopathic consultation. Nevertheless, both homeopathic approaches were compared to placebo. Though there was no significant effect noted in any of the treatment groups for the primary outcomes, which is determined by a specified degree of improvement in rheumatism according to conventional measures of clinical improvement, there were significant differences in the groups that received a homeopathic consultation with both individualized medicine and placebo in the measures of joint swelling and pain, which were part of the secondary outcome measures. It was not possible to see any difference in effect between the individualized medicine versus the complex medicine or the placebo. The conclusion is that the benefits of homeopathy in this research is attributable to the homeopathic consultation. This confirms previous demonstrations that therapeutic effects and benefits ensue as a result of the enhanced communication and narrative, empathy, hope, and enablement the patient experiences during the homeopathic consultation. Unfortunately, the adequacy of the individualized homeopathic medicine selection and prescription is not published in this study and has not been analyzed to check for internal and external validity of this component of the treatment (Brien, Lachance, Prescott, McDermott, & Lewith, 2011).

Others have found a relationship between the individualized homeopathic consultation (IHC) and other forms of psychotherapy, particularly humanistic and narrative approaches, as healing interventions per se. Beyond the common factors with psychotherapeutic approaches, IHCs involve, in addition, specific processes that emerge from the way the encounter is framed, organized, and delivered (Davidson & Jonas, 2016).

The framing comes from the concept that the person is seen as a whole entity, not just body, mind, and spirit but also one who extends through time, from birth until the present, through which prior conditions are antecedents of the present complaint, even if they are from other organ systems. Evolutionarily, the whole organism develops from one single and is interconnected through life. From this broad view, a truly integrative perspective, the treatment sets an expectation for improvement that extends beyond symptomatic relief, or cure of the complaint, to achieve healing when, as Hahnemann (1842/1996) noted: "our indwelling, rational spirit can freely avail itself of this living, healthy instrument for the higher purposes of our existence."

This means not only to be free of physical disease for the patient but to be able to experience fully the quality of life, including happiness, creativity, productivity, and the ability to be of service to others. Rarely does conventional medicine conceive of healing in this broader context.

The narrative exploration engaged in with the patient provides an empathic and open space, akin to humanistic psychology, that can lead to insight about illness and the self. The whole history gathered will then be put into a framework that corresponds to a specific homeopathic medicine picture analogous to the syndromatic picture of the patient. The homeopathic medicine becomes a "transactional symbol" that will embody and convey meaning and hope for healing to the patient (Thompson & Weiss, 2006).

Besides the individualized homeopathic consultation and its own therapeutic effect, there is the yet unanswered question of whether the homeopathic medicine itself has a biological effect. Ironically, if we take the homeopathic medicines being just placebo "sugar pills" or "alcoholic solutions," there is an argument supporting the contention that they can be therapeutic as placebos, in and by themselves.

In reality "placebos" are inert; they usually do not have a biological activity; so it is not what they are but what they represent. They stand for something; they mean something to each person and to each culture, with greater or lesser applicability across the world. For example, the color red is usually associated with activation, with stimulation, whereas blue is usually associated with calmness, like the blue sky or the blue sea, and sedation (except in Italy, where it is associated with the "Azzurro" soccer shirt color of the National Team, and Italian males, in particular, get activated by that particular shade of blue). Placebos are symbolic, and the meaning they may have is what has been called the "meaning response," in correspondence with Herbert Benson's "relaxation response." The meaning response is activated by the particular significance of signs, symbols, and metaphors that are culturally enforced. It is this learned process and context that gives placebos, or other factors, their significance and potential effect (Moerman & Jonas, 2002).

Placebos work by a process that activates opioid and endocannabinoid systems, and probably other circuits, and the associated organic changes have been shown through evident and quantifiable physiological changes in specific brain areas by functional magnetic resonance imagery. Their activity is based on expectation and the clinical response can be learned (Marchant, 2016).

Furthermore, for the last half of a decade, researchers have been carrying out "open-label" research on placebos, proving that patients can respond to knowingly taking a placebo with a significant decrease of symptomatology in conditions such as irritable bowel syndrome, depression, and low back pain. Even so, the placebo cannot change organic pathology, and it is likely not going to shrink a tumor or reverse an ulcer. From a procedural perspective, it is no longer true that giving placebos has to be deceptive and perhaps unethical (Carvalho et al., 2016).

The way placebos may work is because of the activation of hope and expectation, in association with the behaviors that may have been associated in the past with the intake of therapeutic compounds, such as the experience of opening the medicine bottle, pouring the medicine, swallowing, and so on, as these may have become conditioned behaviors associated with symptomatic relief in the past. These can be nonconscious processes that actively contribute to the placebo response.

The use of placebo in homeopathic therapeutics dates as far back to Hahnemann, who initially suggested the use of placebo to satisfy the patient's desire to take something even if it was not indicated to repeat the active homeopathic medicine while it was still acting, in order not to disturb its beneficial effect. However, on August 5, 1830, in a letter to his disciple Stapf, he wrote: "The homeopathic physician must come to a point when he refuses to give placebos and will only give the helpful remedy when and where it is required." However, the use of placebos by homeopathic practitioners continues until today, and often, the patients know they are receiving them and why—to not interfere with a medicine that is acting (Haehl, 1922, p. 327).

The Process of Homeopathic Treatment

After the homeopath takes a complete case history, a meaningful and comprehensive set of symptoms is selected based on their importance, severity, and the predominant characteristics and peculiarities that are unusual or out of the ordinary; for example, preferring cold wraps for headaches, while being chilly in the rest of the body. Such peculiarities help with the choice of one remedy over another for a patient with a particular illness. For example, if the aaforementioned chilly patient also has depression, he or she may need phosphorus, while a depressed patient who tends to be hot may need a different remedy such as pulsatilla. These are examples of the particular features elicited through the provings of each of the homeopathic compounds, which have been corroborated by generations of homeopathic practitioners from around the world in day-to-day clinical practice. They could be considered just anecdotal, if they were reported by only a few individuals.

Hahnemann (1842/1996) used the term "constitution" to refer to those distinguishing characteristics of an individual present at birth, along with such intrinsic factors as climate, education, diet, morals, customs, and habits that contribute to the manifestation of chronic diseases. He advised that physicians have to consider a patient's physical constitution, as well as his or her affective and intellectual character, lifestyle, social position, family relations, age, sexual life, and so on in order to determine the best treatment for the patient.

Assessment of constitution continues to be an important part of the homeopathic evaluation. Within this context, it is the person's particular constitution with its corresponding susceptibilities that will determine responsiveness to particular remedies. By identifying a person's constitutional makeup, the homeopath identifies the best-suited remedies for that patient.

Homeopathic researchers have developed the Constitutional Type Questionaire (CTQ), which tests the validity and reliability of 20 common homeopathic constitutional, broad-spectrum-acting remedies in a patient population with various diagnosis. The goal of this instrument is to help the homeopath screen individuals for provings, as well as to help select remedies for patients (Davidson, Fisher, Van Haselen, Woodbury, & Connor, 2001; Van Haselen, Cinar, Fisher, & Davidson, 2001).

One study (Bell, Baldwin, Schwartz, & Davidson, 2002) examined the association between the CTQ and scores on standardized psychological and medical measures. Patients were recruited from 15 outpatient clinics in the UK, and 447 patients provided useful data through questionaires. The scales included were the chemical intolerance index for environmental sensitivity, the Neuroticism-Extraversion-Openness (NEO) personality inventory, the

Marlowe-Crowne Social Desirability Scale (MCSD) for defensiveness, the Harvard Parental Caring Scale for perceived mother and father traits, the Profile of Mood State (POMS) scale, the Pannebaker Symptom Checklist, and a global health rating scale.

The majority of CTQ constitutional-type scores correlated significantly with greater neuroticism, lower MCSD defensiveness, and greater psychological distress on the POMS subscales. NEO Extraversion and Openness subscales correlated with specific CTQ scores in directions consistent with clinical remedy pictures. They also found confirmation of traditional homeopathic views for specific remedies with scores from standardized conventional scales. Some of these constitutional types in homeopathy are exemplified by the medicines exiguously described in Table 10.1.

Homeopathic remedies are generally safe and nontoxic. Lower potency remedies commonly are found in health food stores, usually in dilutions of 6X, 6C, 12C, and 30C. Recommended frequency of the dosage varies depending on the acuity of the symptoms: if they are acute, the remedy can be repeated every two to four hours; if they are moderate, every six to eight hours; and if they are mild, once per day.

A remedy is considered effective if the patient improves after three to four dosages. If there is no improvement, it is an indication that a different remedy or potency may be needed.

Homeopathic training is rather involved, and it can take several years to learn the nuances of remedy selection and follow-up, as well as gain the knowledge of the homeopathic materia medica and the repertory—the dictionary of symptoms with the corresponding remedies. Homeopaths use various remedies with apparently different biological actions. Some induce symptoms acutely, such as Belladona, Hyosciamus, Stramonium, and Veratrum album. Other, so-called slow-acting remedies, like Natrum Muriaticum (sodium chloride), silica, phosphorus, or sepia (Cuttlefish tincture), take a longer time and repeated dosages to manifest their particular symptom picture. The selection of the remedies is always based on the totality of symptoms of the patient and considering his or her peculiar and characteristic qualities (Hahnemann, 1842/1996).

There are about 39 remedies cited by Guernsey (1866), with their characteristic symptoms for the treatment of mental illness. Besides the mental symptoms, the characteristics of local (in what segment of the body), organic (which particular organ), and pathology are matched with the clinical pictures observed during the proving in order to select the correct remedy (Boericke, 1927; Guernsey, 1866).

The clinical picture, supposedly elicited in some published proving, is described in such a way as to resemble clinical syndromes found in

Table 10.1. Homeopathic Remedies in Psychiatry

Remedy	Indications	Characteristic Symptoms
Aconite	Anxiety, apprehension, palpitations	Pulsations, fear of death, ailments from fright and shock, flushing
Arnica	Traumas, concussions, post-surgical recovery	Sore, achy pain; sore muscles and soft tissues from contusive/concussive trauma, traumatic extravasations
Coffea	Sleep disorders	Hyperactive mind, sleepless from overactivation and thinking
Ignatia	Grief, loss, mortification	Shortness of breath, constriction of the throat, sensation of a ball rising from the stomach to the esophagus
Natrum Muriaticum	Chronic grief; coryza; rhinitis	Persistent thoughts, stoicism, reserved character, dislikes consolation; sad but unable to cry
Nux Vomica	Irritability, grouchiness, substance abuse withdrawal, cramps	Hurried, rushing, contrary, quarrelsome, twitching, craving for stimulants
Phosphoric Acid	Fatigue, physical and mental	Ailments from overwork, physical and/or mental
Staphysagria	Ailments from abuse, suppressed anger from mortification, neonuptial cystitis	Recurrent urinary tract infections, styes

conventional nosology. For example: the narrative of the proving of Aurum Metallicum (gold) reports: "hopeless, despondent and great desire to commit suicide, disgust of life, feeling of self-condemnation and utter worthlessness" (Guernsey, 1866). For more information about specific remedies, the largest reservoir of data and the main tools of any practicing homeopath are the homeopathic materia medica and the homeopathic repertory (see Table No. 9.1; Neatby & Stonham, 1948/1987; Schroyens, 2004).

Conclusion

Homeopathy is an alternative system of health that at one time was in high favor among physicians but is no longer part of mainstream Western medicine. Several of the premises behind homeopathy are uncorroborated by modern research and statistical methods, which may have some limitations in this case. Nevertheless, there are some homeopathic principles that have interesting correspondences with accepted scientific theories. The available data on the treatment effectiveness for homeopathy is inadequate, inconsistent, and controversial, and it is particularly limited in the mental health arena. The current evidence is insufficient to support the use of homeopathy as a primary psychiatric treatment, but there is sufficient data for its possible positive effect as an adjuvant to conventional psychiatric treatment, though more research is needed to identify its usefulness. While the biological effect of homeopathic medicines themselves has not been proven, their effect as meaningful and symbolic representations that elicit a legitimate placebo response is evident. A new area of research is to determine how the individualized homeopathic interview, with its comprehensiveness and detail, may be a particular type of therapeutic model, akin to psychotherapy, and have clinical efficacy in itself.

Despite the challenges, there continues to be significant interest in homeopathy among clinicians and patients throughout the world, likely because of the wide breadth of positive anecdotal accounts. Many cases are scattered around the literature, often without following a methodology that withstands the scrutiny for modern scientific evidence. However, it is possible that with modern software development, it will become possible to gather hundreds of cases of medical conditions not amenable, or not responsive, to conventional medicines and treated successfully with homeopathy as a means toward better demonstrating the efficacy of homeopathy, once and for all.

REFERENCES

American Institute of Homeopathy. (2016). Research on specific medical conditions. Retrieved from http://www.homeopathyusa.org/

Antelman, S. M. (1988). Time-dependent sensitisation as the cornerstone for a new approach to pharmacotherapy: Drug as a foreign/stressful stimuli. *Drug Development Research*, 14, 1–30.

Bell, I. R., Baldwin, C. M., Schwartz, G. E., & Davidson, J. R. T. (2002). Homeopathic constitutional type questionnaire correlates of conventional psychological and physical health scales: Individual difference characteristics of young adults. *Homeopathy*, 91, 53–74.

Bodman, F. (1990). *Insights into homeopathy*. London: Beaconsfield Press.

Boericke, W. (1927). *Materia medica and repertory* (9th ed.). Philadelphia, PA: Boericke and Runyon.

Boltz, O. (1968). Some original investigations on the treatment of schizophrenia and associated symptoms due to a functional disturbance of integration in the diencephalon using the principle of similia similibus curantur. *Journal of the American Institute of Homeopathy*, 61(4), 219–234.

Boericke, G. (1965). Tranquilizing drugs used homeopathically and homeopathic tranquilizers. *Journal of the American Institute of Homeopathy, 58,* 20–23.

Bornhoft, G., & Mathiessen, P. F. (2011). *Homeopathy in healthcare: Effectiveness, appropriateness, safety, costs.* Berlin, Heidelberg, Germany: Springer Verlag.

Brien, S., Lachance, L., Prescott, P., McDermott, C., & Lewith, G. (2011). Homeopathy has clinical benefits in rheumatoid arthritis patients that are attributable to the consultation process but not the homeopathic remedy: A randomized controlled clinical trial. *Rheumatology, 50,* 1070–1082.

Calabrese, E. (2013). Hormetic mechanisms—review. *Critical Reviews in Pharmacology, 43*(7), 580–606.

Calabrese, E. J., & Blain, R. (2004). The hormesis database: An overview. *Toxicology and Applied Pharmacology, 202*(3), 289–300.

Calabrese, E., & Jonas, W. (2010). Hormesis and homeopathy. *Biological Effects of Low Level Exposures Newsletter, 16*(1), 1–55.

Carvalho, C., Machado, J., Cunha, L., Rebouta, P., Kaptchuk, T. J., & Kirsch, I. (2016). Open-label placebo treatment in chronic low back pain: A randomized controlled trial. *Pain, 157*(12), 2766–2772.

Chapman, E. H., Weintraub, R. J., Milburn, M. A., Pirozzi, T. O., & Woo, E (1999). Homeopathic treatment of mild traumatic brain injury: A randomized, double-blind, placebo-controlled clinical trial. *Journal of Head Trauma Rehabilitation, 14*(6), 521–542.

Cortina, J. (1994). Enuresis and its homeopathic treatment: Study of 20 cases treated with Ilex Paraguenses. *British Homeopathic Journal, 83*(4), 220–222.

Cucherat, M., Haugh, M. C., Gooch, M., & Boissel, J. P. (2000). Evidence of clinical efficacy of homeopathy: A meta-analysis of clinical trials. *European Journal of Clinical Pharmacology, 56,* 27–33.

Davidson, J. (2014). *A century of homeopaths: Their influence on medicine and health.* New York: Springer.

Davidson, J., Crawford, C., Ives, J., & Jonas, W. (2011). Homeopathic treatments in psychiatry: A systematic review of randomized placebo-controlled studies. *Journal of Clinical Psychiatry, 72*(6), 795–805.

Davidson, J., Fisher, R., Van Haselen, R., Woodbury, M., & Connor, K. (2001). Do constitutional types exist? A further study using grade of membership analysis. *British Homoepathic Journal, 90,* 138–147.

Davidson, J., & Jonas, W. (2016). Individualized homeopathy: A consideration of its relationship to psychotherapy. *Journal of Alternative and Complementary Medicine, 22*(8), 594–598.

Davidson, J., Morrison, R., Shore, J., Davidson, R. T., & Bedayn, G. (1997). Homeopathic treatment of depression and anxiety. *Alternative Therapies, 3*(1), 46–49.

Detinis, L. (1994). *Mental symptoms in homeopathy.* London: Beaconsfield.

Dunham, C. (1984). *Homeopathy: The science of therapeutics.* New Delhi: Jain Publishers.

Fisher, P. (2006). Scientific research on homeopathic medicine, proving and improving the efficacy. 1st Joint American Homeopathic Conference. NCH26-320. Retrieved from www.conferencerecordings.com

Frei, H., Everts, R., von Ammon, K., Kaufmann, F., Walther, D., Hsu-Schmitz, S. F., et al. (2005). Homeopathic treatment of children with attention deficit hyperactivity disorder: A randomised, double blind, placebo controlled crossover trial. *European Journal of Pediatrics, 164,* 758–767.

Frei, H., Everts, R., von Ammon, K., Kaufmann, F., Walther, D., Hsu, S. F., et al. (2007). Ransomised controlled trials of homeopathy in hyperactive children: Treatment procedure leads to an unconventional study design. *Homeopathy, 96,* 35–41.

Frei, H., & Thurneysen, A. (2001). Treatment for hyperactive children: Homeopathy and methylphenidate compared in a family setting. *British Homeopathic Journal, 90,* 183–188.

Gallavardin, J. (1990). *Psychism and homeopathy.* New Delhi: B. Jain Publishers. (Original work published 1960)

Grazyna, M., & Trzebiatowska-Trzeciak, O. (1993). Homeopathic treatment of alcohol withdrawal. *British Homeopathic Journal with Simile, 82*(4), 249–251.

Guernsey, H. (1866). Hysteria. *Hahnemanian Monthly, 1*(11), 387–404.

Haehl, R. (1922). *Hahnemann, his life and work.* London: London Homeopathic Publishing Company.

Hahnemann, S. (1996). *Organon of medicine* (6th ed.). Trans. W. Brewster-O'Reilly. Redmond, WA: Birdcage Books. (Original work published 1842)

Haidvogl, M., Lehner, E., & Resch, D. (1993). Homeopathic treatment of handicapped children. *British Homeopathic Journal, 82*(4), 227–236.

Hanson, R. J. (2013). Homeopathic products: A growing segment in OTC? Retrieved from http://www.pharmacytimes.com/publications/issue/2013/september2013/homeopathic-products-a-growing-segment-in-otc

Harbour, R., & Miller, J. (2001). A new system for grading recommendations inevidence based guidelines. *British Medical Journal, 323,* 334–336.

Harvard Health Letter. (2012, April). Putting the placebo effect to work. Retrieved from http://www.health.harvard.edu/mind-and-mood/putting-the-placebo-effect-to-work

Homœopathic Pharmacopœia of the United States. (2016). The Homœopathic Pharmacopœia of the United States. Retrieved from http://www.hpus.com/index-of-the-hpus.php

Homeopathy Research Institute. (2015). Australian NHMRC review in detail. Retrieved from https://www.hri-research.org/resources/homeopathy-the-debate/the-australian-report-on-homeopathy/australian-nhmrc-report-in-detail/

Jonas, W. B., Kaptchuk, T. J., & Linde, K. (2003). A critical overview of homeopathy. *Annals of Internal Medicine, 138*(5), 393–399.

King, L. S. (1984). The Flexner report of 1910. *Journal of the American Medical Association, 251*(8), 1079–1086.

Kirsch, I., Deacon, B., Huedo-Medina, T., Scoboria, A., Moore, T. J., & Johnson, B. T. (2008). Initial severity and antidepressant benefits: A meta-analysis of data submitted to the Food & Drug Administration. *PLoS Medicine, 5,* e45. doi:10.1371/journal.pmed.0050045

Kirsch, I., Moore, T., & Scoboria, A. N. (2002). the emperor's new drugs: An analysis of antidepressant medication data submitted to the US Food and Drug Administration. *Prevention & Treatment, 5*, 23. doi:10.1037/1522-3736.5.1.523a

Kirsch, I., & Saperstein, G. (1998). Listening to Prozac but hearing placebo. *Prevention & Treatment, 1*, 2a. doi:10.1037/1522-3736.1.1.12a

Kleijnen, J., Knipschild, P., & terRiet, G. (1991). Clinical trials of homeopathy. *British Medical Journal, 302*(6782), 316–323.

Koithan, M., Embrey, M., & Bell, I. (2015). Qualitative evaluation of successful homeopathic treatment of individuals with chronic diseases: Descriptive phenomenology of patients' experiences. *Journal of Medicine and the Person, 12*, 23–35.

Lamont, J. (1997). Homeopathic treatment of attention deficit hyperactivity disorder—a controlled study. *British Homeopathic Journal, 86*, 196–200.

Lansky, A. (2003). *Impossible cure: The promise of homeopathy*. Portola Beach, CA: R. L. Ranch Press.

Linde, K., Clausius, N., Ramirez, G., Melchart, D., Eitel, F., Hedges, L. V., & Jonas, W. B. (1997). Are the clinical effects of homeopathy placebo effects? A meta-analysis of placebo-controlled trials. *The Lancet, 359*(9081), 834–843.

Marchant, J. (2016). Honest fakery. *Nature, 535*, S14–S15.

Menninger, C. (1897). Some reflections relative to the symptomatology and materia medica of typhoid fever. *Transactions of the American Institute of Homeopathy*, 430.

Mercer, S. (2005). Practitioner empathy, patient enablement and health outcomes of patients attending the Glasgow Homeopathic Hospital: A retrospective and prospective comparison. *Wiener medizinische Wochenschrift, 155*, 498–501.

Merizalde, B. (2005). Samuel Hahnemann: Hormesis and a probable mechanism of action of homeopathic remedies. *American Journal of Homeopathic Medicine, 98*(4), 249–254.

Moerman, D., & Jonas, W. (2002). Deconstructing the placebo effect and finding the meaning response. *Annals of Internal Medicine, 136*, 471–476.

Neatby, E., & Stonham, T. (1987). *Manual of homeo-therapeutics* (Indian edition). New Delhi: Jain Publishers. (Original work published 1948)

National Health and Medical Research Council. (2015). NHMRC information paper: Evidence on the effectiveness of homeopathy for treating health conditions. Canberra, Australia: Author. Retrieved from https://www.nhmrc.gov.au/health-topics/complementary-medicines/homeopathy-review

National Institute for Health and Care Excellence. (2016). Improving health and social care through evidence-based guidance. Retrieved from https://www.nice.org.uk/

Post, R. M., & Weiss, S. R. B. (1992). Endogenous biochemical abnormalities in affective illness: Therapeutic versus pathogenic. *Biological Psychiatry, 32*, 469–484.

Rajalakshmi, M. A. (2015) Homeopathic treatment as adjunct to neuropsychological therapies in children with autism spectrum disorders. *International Journal of Public Mental Health and Neurosciences, 2*(3), 13–18.

Saine, A. (1997). *Psychiatric patients: Back to the roots: Steps in case taking*. Eindhoven, The Netherlands: Lutra Services.

Schroyens, F. (2004). *Synthesis repertory* (Synthesis Repertorium Homeopathicum Syntheticum) (9.1 ed.). London: Homeopathic Book Publishers.

Scofield, A. M. (1984). Experimental research in homeopathy—a critical review. *British Homeopathic Journal, 73*(3–4), 161–180, 211–226.

Shang, A., Huwiler-Müntener, K., Nartey, L., Jüni, P., Dörig, S., Sterne, J. A., et al. (2005). Are the clinical effects of homeopathy placebo effects? Comparative study of placebo-controlled trials of homeopathy and allopathy. *The Lancet, 366*, 726–32.

Shevin, W. (1989). Case presentations. *Journal of the American Institute of Homeopathy, 77*(2), 59–66.

Slonim, D., & White, K. (1983). Homeopathy and psychiatry. *Journal of Mind and Behavior, 4*(3), 401–410.

SPINS. (2006). Homeopathic medicines are growing at double-digit rates, A. C. Nielsen ScanTrack, 52 W ending 12/31/2005.

Thompson, T., & Weiss, M. (2006). Homeopathy: What are the active ingredients? An exploratory study using the UK Medical Research Council's Framework for the Evaluation of Complex Interventions. *BMC Complementary and Alternative Medicine, 6*(37). doi:10.1186/1472-6882-6-37

Turner, E., Mathews, A., Linardatos, E., Tell, R., & Rosenthal, R. (2008). Selective publication of antidepressant trials and its influence on apparent efficacy. *New England Journal of Medicine, 358*, 252–260.

Ullman, D. (2007). *The homeopathic revolution: Why famous people and cultural heroes choose homeopathy*. Berkeley, CA: North Atlantic Books.

Van Haselen, R. A., Cinar, S., Fisher, P., & Davidson, J. R. T. (2001). The constitutional type questionaire: Validation in a patient population of the Royal Homeopathic Hospital. *British Homeopathic Journal, 90*, 131–137.

Viksveen, P., & Relton, C. (2014). Depression treated by homeopaths: A study protocol for a pragmatic cohort multiple randomised trial. *Homeopathy, 103*, 147–152.

11

Hypnosis and Biofeedback as Prototypes of Mind–Body Medicine

MARIE STONER

> ## Key Points
>
> - Hypnotizability is a strong moderator for treatment outcome.
> - Biofeedback has Level I, Grade A support for use with migraine headaches.
> - Hypnosis is able to reduce distress and pain in short procedures and has been particularly useful in cancer procedures.
> - Gut-directed hypnotherapy for irritable bowel syndrome has shown substantial results for structured short-term scripted treatment.
> - Biofeedback for hypertension is successful when clinical practice guidelines identifying patient characteristics are followed.
> - Heart rate variability biofeedback shows promise as a technique to directly target self-regulatory mechanisms.
> - Innovative use of real-time functional magnetic resonance imaging neurofeedback is showing promise for altering neural patterns underlying diverse disorders such as clinical depression and chronic pain.
> - Obsessive-compulsive disorder and eating disorder patients may be selectively responsive to hypnotic suggestion.

Introduction to Mind–Body Medicine

Mind–body medicine is one of four major domains of complementary and alternative medicine (CAM) designated by the National Center for Complementary and Alternative Medicine (National Center for Complementary and Integrative Health, 2007). Within this category are those interventions that emphasize the interactions among the brain, mind, body, and spirit. The interest in techniques such as relaxation, hypnosis, visual imagery, meditation, yoga, biofeedback, tai chi, qi gong, autogenic training, and spirituality share the common goals of actively training the mind to positively affect physiology, modulate behavior, and enhance wellness.

Mind–body interventions constitute a major portion of CAM patient visits. In the latest National Health Interview Survey gathered in 2012, 37% of US adults surveyed reported visiting a CAM practitioner in the past year (Frass et al, 2012). The mind–body techniques most frequently endorsed were yoga and a category called "deep breathing" that includes hypnosis, biofeedback, and meditation (Clarke, Black, Stussman, Barnes, & Nahin, 2015).

Hypnosis and biofeedback are two well-established mind–body medicine techniques that can be integrated with biomedicine to further the biopsychosocial model of health and illness. This paradigm was introduced by Engel (1977) to broaden the biological disease model to include psychological and social determinants of illness. Contemporaneous to this shift, hypnosis and biofeedback were being increasingly studied and used in clinical practice.

There are methodological limitations to much of the mind–body research literature. The gold standard of traditional medical research has been that neither the subject nor the researcher knows whether an active standardized treatment or a placebo is being assigned to a subject. This concept is difficult to apply to the mind–body techniques of biofeedback and hypnosis because their success is dependent upon the patient's interactive participation in the treatment. For example, the most potent hypnotic suggestions are elicited from the subject's internal experience, not from a standard protocol. In biofeedback training (BFB), accurate information about physiology precludes double- or even single-blind procedures. The use of sham feedback or placebo (inactive) conditions dependent on the subject's lack of awareness of the intervention is an inappropriate and contradictory concept for these techniques (Yucha & Gilbert, 2004).

Another problem confronting research in this area is the question of which patients are most likely to respond to a specific mind–body intervention. Failure to understand and consider moderators of response can lead to poor research design and meaningless results (Nicholson, Hursey, & Nash, 2005). In fact, individual response sets in behavioral treatments will create more variability than in pharmaceutical research because these treatments require patients to make complex behavioral changes over time (Nielson & Weir, 2001). With the growing importance of personalized medicine, moderators of response are increasingly relevant.

Introduction to Hypnosis

In 2014, the American Psychiatric Association Division 30 clarified competing definitions of hypnosis with the following: "A state of consciousness involving focused attention and reduced peripheral awareness characterized by an enhanced capacity for response to suggestion" (Elkins, Barabasz, Council, & Spiegel, 2015). This definition allows for differing theoretical orientations about the mechanisms of hypnosis.

The clinician typically uses an induction technique that may incorporate focus on the breath, relaxation, directing attention, confusion, and/or imagery that evokes memories of previous dissociative experience. Some researchers have achieved comparable responsiveness using an induction in which relaxation was prevented (Banyai & Hilgard, 1976), suggesting that patients in awkward circumstances can be hypnotized.

The first use of hypnosis in medicine was by Franz Mesmer (1734–1815), a French physician, who is considered to be the father of hypnosis (Gauld, 1992). Interest in hypnosis increased in the United States after World War II, when Weitzenhofer and Hilgarde founded a laboratory to study hypnosis at Stanford University where they developed the Stanford Hypnotic Susceptibility Scale (Weitzenhofer & Hilgard, 1959). Hypnotizability is measured by this scale, and later the Harvard scale of Hypnotic Susceptibility (Shor & Orne, 1963) was developed for group administration. Box 11.1 lists some common hypnotic phenomena tested with these scales and associated

---

Box 11.1 Examples of Hypnotic Phenomena Tested with Stanford and Harvard Scales

- Amnesia
- Catalepsy
- Hypermnesia
- Ideomotor movement
- Posthypnotic suggestion
- Analgesia and anaesthesia
- Time distortion
- Dissociation
- Age regression
- Positive hallucination
- Future progression
- Negative hallucination

Table 11.1. Characteristics of Highly Hypnotizable People

Factor	Example	Reference
Age	Between ages 8 and 10 maximum susceptibility	Hilgard (1967)
	Children show higher amounts of amnesia and hallucination	
IQ	Slight positive correlation	Udolf (1987)
Absorptive capacity	Positive-constructive daydreaming	Brown (1991)
	Use of vivid imagery; greater intensity of affect	
EEG findings	Longer alpha durations	London et al. (1967)

Note: EEG = electroencephalography.

with hypnotizability. With these research tools, hypnosis could be studied scientifically and began to be integrated into conventional medical and psychological treatment.

Hypnotizability is a stable trait (Piccione, Hilgard, & Zimbardo, 1989). Within a random population there is evidence that 15% to 20% will demonstrate a high level of hypnotic propensity, 70% to 75% score in the intermediate range, and the remaining have low hypnotizability (Sacerdote, 1982). Hypnotizability seems to be affected by childhood experiences of normal dissociation, and the trait seems relatively stable through adulthood (Hilgard, 1970). Table 11.1 provides some characteristics of the highly hypnotizable population including those related to their Intelligence Quotient (IQ) as well as brain electroencephalography (EEG) findings.

As a stable characteristic, hypnotizability is an example of the class of research and treatment variables known as moderators, which are variables that can predict the level of impact a treatment will have. Barabasz and Perez (2007) review evidence for hypnotizability as a moderating core construct. Three well-controlled studies with large samples established that hypnotizability is an outcome predictor that is significantly stronger than expectations and context (Benham, Woody, Wilson, & Nash, 2006; Liossi & Hatira, 2003; Milling, Reardon, & Carosella, 2006). Milling et al. demonstrated the importance of hypnotizability as a trait for response to hypnotic suggestion for pain treatments, even when participants were not told that they were being hypnotized. Finally, in a study of pediatric cancer patients undergoing lumbar puncture, Liossi et al. (2006) concluded that baseline hypnotizability was significantly and strongly associated with the magnitude of the therapeutic benefit for the hypnosis intervention group only.

MECHANISMS OF HYPNOSIS

Genetic and neuroimaging data have contributed to understanding hypnotizabilty. Genetic determinants were explored by Morgan (1973) in a comparison of monozyotic and dizygotic twins. She computed a heritability index of .64, strongly suggestive of a genetic contribution. Lichtenberg, Bachner-Melman, Gritsenko, and Ebstein (2000) traced individual differences in DNA (polymorphism of the catechol O-methyltransferase gene) to hypnotizability, more significantly in males than females and Bryant, Hung, Dobson-Stone, and Schofield (2013) found an association between the oxytocin receptor gene and the capacity to respond to hypnotic suggestion.

Investigations using neuroimaging techniques have focused on the process of hypnosis. Horton, Crawford, Harrington, and Downs (2004) in an functional magnetic resonance imaging (fMRI) comparison of high and low hypnotizable normal subjects found that high hypnotizables show a significantly ($p < 0.003$) larger (31.8%) rostrum area. This is the area of the brain involved in allocation of attention and transfer of information between the two prefrontal cortices, suggesting that high hypnotizables possibly have more efficient frontal attention systems that allow them to inhibit stimuli in a trance state. Hoeft et al. (2012) reported greater functional connectivity between the left dorsolateral prefrontal cortex (part of executive control region) and the salience network (involved in detecting and integrating relevant somatic, autonomic, and emotional information) in high hypnotizables. Cojan, Piguet, and Vuilleumier (2015) compared selective attention engagement in high versus low hypnotizables outside of hypnosis and also found differences in attention. High hypnotizables appear to have greater attentional flexibility that they posit as underlying the increased dissociation characteristic of hypnosis. In a comprehensive discussion of the literature, Raz (2005) concludes that results from neuroimaging studies support a potential common mechanism of dopaminergic modulation affecting both attentional and hypnotic performance and that these mechanisms operate differently in high and low hypnotizables.

Although some describe hypnosis in terms of behavior that is elicited by cues and context, it is clearly a phenomenon of body and mind that at least involves a complex interplay of genetics, brain structure, imagination, and patterns of neural networking. Further research is needed to understand the dynamic interaction of all these variables.

Introduction to Biofeedback

BFB is a technique in which an individual learns to consciously control involuntary responses, such as heart rate, brain waves, and muscle contractions.

Information about a normally unconscious physiologic process is electronically monitored and relayed back to the patient as part of a program to enact change, initially with the support of the reinforcing properties of the computerized signal and the biofeedback therapist, then generalized to self-regulation in everyday life.

Miniaturization of electronics after World War II, combined with research documenting the ability to train normal subjects to isolate separate motor units within a muscle and to activate them consciously, helped to launch the field of biofeedback (Basmajian, 1963). Early BFB applications in the 1960s were neuromuscular (electromyogram [EMG]) and included protocols for stroke (Andrews, 1964; Marinacci & Horande, 1960) and tension headaches (Budzynski, Stoyva, Adler, & Mullaney, 1973).

Subsequently, biofeedback procedures were applied to clinical problems associated with the autonomic nervous system (ANS), building on the work of researchers such as Miller (1969) with animals and Kimmel (1974) with humans that demonstrated that the ANS could be modified through operant conditioning. Researchers at the Menninger Foundation developed a clinical protocol for migraines with a 74% improvement in subjects treated with thermal (bloodflow) biofeedback (Sargent, Green, & Walters, 1972). This work led to the establishment of the Menninger Voluntary Controls Program for research and clinical applications in biofeedback and the first National Institutes for Health (NIH) grant for the study of biofeedback in 1967 (Green, Ferguson, Green, & Walters, 1970).

MECHANISMS OF BIOFEEDBACK

The psychophysiological pathways of biofeedback are complex and at least involve several levels of the central nervous system that interact with the ANS. A number of techniques can be used to evaluate the physiological processes associated with biofeedback treatment effects (Table 11.2). A simple example of a pathway is neuromuscular feedback. A sensor is placed on a muscle area of interest, and the patient, through trial and error, learns to either recruit or inhibit the electrical activity under the sensor.

Work with elimination disorders over the past 30 years has validated the surface EMG modality for these conditions. A 2015 ANMS-ESNM Task Force strongly supported biofeedback therapy for short- and long-term treatment of constipation with dyssynergic defecation (Level I, Grade A) and fecal incontinence (Level II, Grade B) (Satish et al., 2015). Biofeedback training was found to be specifically efficacious in females for training of pelvic floor musculature in incontinence (Glazer & Laine, 2006). A systematic review of nonsurgical

Table 11.2. Sensors and Physiology Measured in Biofeedback Treatment

Sensor	Measures
EMG	Surface muscle tension
ECG	Heart rate
EEG	Brain electrical activity
fMRI	Brain blood flow activity
Skin conductivity	Electrical activity of skin
Peripheral temperature	Vasocontriction/vasodilation
Respiration	Breath pace and depth

Note: EMG = electromyogram; ECG = electrocardiogram; EEG = electroencephalography; fMRI = functional magnetic resonance imaging.

treatment for stress urinary incontinence (Imamura, 2010) found clear evidence that pelvic floor muscle training plus biofeedback was more effective than basic pelvic floor muscle training.

As the technique of biofeedback moved into disorders of the ANS, the main system of interest was the sympathetic branch of the ANS and the "fight-flight response" first discussed by Cannon (1929). Prolonged and repeated activation of the hypothalamic-pituitary-adrenal axis triggered by this response is posited to underlie stress-related disorders. More recently, some physiologists have shown interest in the influence of the vagal withdrawal of the parasympathetic branch of the ANS in response to stress (Porges, 1995; Porges, 2007). Self-regulation of the ANS with biofeedback is accomplished via monitoring and training of the parameters of vasoconstriction (hand-cooling), heart rate, electrodermal activity, muscle tension, and breathing, all potential indicators of stress reactivity. Repeated conditioning of lower arousal states leads to less reactivity and lowered baselines within the ANS. With the help of the biofeedback therapist, patients learn to recognize stress cues and practice their conditioned response.

Advances in EEG technology have supported the clinical use of neurofeedback (EEG biofeedback), which is the retraining of brainwave patterns through operant conditioning. Three decades of case studies and controlled group studies using neurofeedback to treat attention deficit hyperactivity disorder have been reviewed by Monastra et al. (2005) with a report of significant clinical improvement in approximately 75% of patients in each of the studies, and a meta-analysis by Micouland-Franchigh et al. (2014) found significant changes in both parent and teacher rating scores.

Best Evidence for Common Disorders Treated by Hypnosis and Biofeedback

BIOFEEDBACK FOR HEADACHES

Four decades after work at the Menninger Clinic demonstrated that thermal BFB was an effective treatment for migraine headaches, BFB continues to hold a prominent place in headache management. The treatment of migraine and tension-type headaches utilizes a range of physiological feedback: temperature, blood volume pulse, EMG, brain waves (EEG), and any of these modalities in combination to achieve improvement through BFB-assisted relaxation or BFB more specifically targeting the underlying physiology of headache (Andrasik, 2010).

The most recent meta-analysis found that all of these forms of biofeedback produced significant medium to large effect sizes for migraine treatment compared to wait-list and at least equally effective to relaxation and pharmacotherapy (Nestoriuc & Martin, 2007). In a review of 55 studies, biofeedback resulted in symptom reduction of over half a standard deviation and treatment effects remained stable at follow-up of over one year on average. Symptoms of depression and anxiety were also reduced in the BFB group, thought to be associated with improved self-efficacy scores and the continued practice and application of BFB at home.

Nestoriuc, Rief, and Martin (2008) also reviewed 53 studies of BFB for tension-type headache with less robust findings. Patients treated with BFB experienced significant relief compared to pretreatment but not significantly more than drug therapy, physical therapy, or cognitive-behavioral therapy (CBT). Within BFB treatment modalities, EMG feedback with relaxation was the most effective. In a multivariate analysis of children and adolescents, the ability to raise hand temperature by 3 degrees F at the end of treatment was associated with a positive response to biofeedback (Blume, Brockman, & Breuner, 2012).

This body of evidence brought mind–body practices to the attention of a number of expert panels, including the multidisciplinary US Headache Consortium (Campbell, Penzien, & Wall, 2000). Table 11.3 presents guidelines for migraine prevention and treatment based on review of evidence.

Table 11.3. Evidence-Based Guidelines for Migraine Headaches, US Headache Consortium[a]

Grade A For prevention of migraine	1. Relaxation training 2. Thermal biofeedback combined with relaxation training 3. EMG biofeedback 4. Cognitive-behavioral therapy
Grade B Behavior therapy combined with drug for prevention of migraine	1. Thermal biofeedback plus relaxation plus cognitive-behavioral therapy 2. Thermal biofeedback plus relaxation 3. EMG biofeedback

Note: Grade A = multiple well-designed randomized clinical trials. Grade B = some evidence from randomized clinical trials. EMG = electromyogram.

[a] Campbell et al. (2000).

HYPNOSIS AND BIOFEEDBACK FOR ACUTE AND CHRONIC PAIN

The variable experience of pain prompted Melzack and Wall's (1965) gate control theory, which recognized many factors, including psychological, that can modulate pain. This theory, even with subsequent modifications and exceptions, makes the treatment of pain conditions very amenable to the biopsychosocial model and multimodal treatment approaches involving mind–body techniques. Painful conditions are the most common reasons why American adults use CAM techniques, spending more than $30 billion yearly (Nahin, Boineau, Khalsa, Stussman, & Weber, 2016). A 1996 NIH Technology Assessment Panel found strong evidence for the use of relaxation in reducing chronic pain and hypnosis for pain associated with cancer. Moderate evidence was cited for the effectiveness of biofeedback in relieving chronic pain (National Institutes of Health Technology Assessment Panel on Integration of Behavioral and Relaxation Approaches into the Treatment of Chronic Pain and Insomnia, 1996).

A hypnotic trance state, with the ability to alter sensory experience, has shown promise in alleviating the experience of pain and distress during invasive procedures and surgery. Even before the development of modern anesthesiology, Esdaile pioneered the use of hypnosis in surgery in 1845. He was surprised to notice that the mortality rate in surgery patients went from

50% before the use of hypnosis to 5% among the patients who had hypnosis (Mutter, 1998).

More recently the increase in short procedures and procedures for which the patient is awake has highlighted the effects of anxiety and distress as variables in outcome. Schupp, Berbaum, Berbaum, and Lang (2005) found a significant correlation between patients' baseline anxiety prior to the procedures and the amount of anxiety and pain during the procedure. Further, the amount of medication needed, and the duration of the procedure, were also predicted by baseline anxiety (Lang & Rosen, 2002).

Lang et al. (1999, 2006) conducted two large randomized prospective trials of 241 patients undergoing radiological intervention in the kidneys and vascular system and 236 women undergoing large-core breast biopsies in outpatient surgery. All received local anesthesia. In both studies the self-hypnosis relaxation condition reported significantly less distress than the control conditions. In Lang et al.'s radiological group, the self-hypnosis group had a procedure time averaging 17 minutes shorter and fewer complications, resulting in a savings of $330 per procedure.

A meta-analysis of 26 trials (2,342 participants) of hypnosis used in medical procedures found an overall large effect size of 0.88 in the reduction of anxiety and distress compared to patients in a control group (Schnur, Kafer, Marcus, & Montgomery, 2008). Effect size was highest for children and when the intervention was delivered prior to the medical procedure using a live rather than audio recording.

Hypnosis has been studied specifically for its use with cancer populations. Potie et al. (2016) reviewed the role of hypnosis during the entire perioperative period for cancer patients. Hypnosis preoperatively reduces distress, self-reported postoperative pain, and postoperative nausea, vomiting, and analgesic requirements. The review discussed evidence that hypnosis during surgery can modulate the immune system through reduction of the general stress response. Postoperative hypnosis is discussed for its ability to manage nausea, vomiting, pain, and fatigue, with some evidence on positive effects on wound healing.

In pediatric populations hypnosis has a beneficial effect on anxiety and pain associated with bone marrow aspiration (Liossi & Hatira, 1999) and lumbar puncture (Liossi & Hatira, 2003). Montgomery et al. (2002) reached similar conclusions with a randomized group of breast biopsy patients assigned to a brief presurgery hypnosis intervention. Hypnosis treatment has also been associated with less nausea and vomiting for chemotherapy patients (Jacknow, Tschann, Link, & Boyce, 1994), and there is some evidence for use with pain in terminally ill patients (Iglexias, 2004).

Biofeedback has demonstrated efficacy for specific chronic pain disorders and for patients with certain characteristics, often as part of a multimodal package. Flor and Birbaumer (1993) compared the efficacy of EMG biofeedback, CBT, and conservative medical treatment in two patient populations: chronic back pain and chronic temporomandibular pain. The biofeedback group (trained in muscle relaxation at the site of pain) obtained the most substantial improvement and was the only group to maintain improvement at the 6- and 24-month follow-up. There has been a resurgence of interest in EMG biofeedback due to inexpensive portable equipment that allows for real-time home monitoring. As an example, Ma et al. (2011) compared a group using equipment daily to monitor muscle tension while using a computer to active exercise, passive treatment, and control groups. Average pain and neck disability indices were significantly reduced, more in the biofeedback group than other treatment conditions, and this was maintained at six months.

In one study, the use of a real-time fMRI to provide feedback about brain areas involved in pain perception and regulation generated media attention in 2005. Working with an image of a flame reflecting activation of the rostral anterior cingulate cortex, normal subjects were able to increase and decrease perception of pain caused by a noxious stimulus. This research was extended to chronic pain patients who were able to significantly decrease pain perception in comparison to traditional autonomic feedback methods (deCharms et al., 2005).

HYPNOSIS AND IBS

Hypnosis has established efficacy in the treatment of irritable bowel symdrome (IBS) symptoms. In a comprehensive review of 30 years of investigation into hypnosis as a treatment for gastrointestinal disorders, Palsson (2015) concludes that all IBS hypnotherapy studies report significant improvement in symptoms, and a substantial number of the randomized controlled trials found superior outcomes for hypnosis compared to control groups. Work by Palsson and others over 20 years using scripted hypnotic protocols in a two- to three-month protocol led to response rates in clinical trials ranging from 53% to 94% with gains maintained up to 12 months in follow-ups (Palsson & Van Tilburg, 2015). This gut-directed hypnotherapy was pioneered in the 1980s within the University Hospital of South Manchester, UK, and is known as the Manchester Approach (Gonsalkorale, 2006). Box 11.2 provides an overview of the protocol that is tailored for individual characteristics and also recorded for daily home practice (Gonsalkorale, 2006).

> **Box 11.2 The Manchester Approach for Treatment of Irritable Bowel Syndrome**
>
> Consultation and Patient Education
>   Explanation of IBS symptoms and rationale for hypnosis
>
> Treatment Sessions: up to 12 sessions, usually weekly
> Sessions 2 (3)
>   Hypnotic induction, relaxation
>   Relevant ego-strengthening
> Sessions 3–12: Introduction of gut-directed suggestions
>   Control and normalization
>   *Imagine a surge of control from your mind over your gut*
>   Imagery
>   *Popular image is of river that can go from rushing (diarrhea) or slow and sluggish (constipation) to steady and smooth*
>   Direct Suggestion
>   *Place hand on abdomen and increase feeling of warmth*
>   *Lining of the gut is becoming less sensitive*
>   *Posthypnotic suggestion that use of word "calm" will induce relaxation*

BIOFEEDBACK AND HYPERTENSION

The most extensively researched mind–body cardiac disorder is hypertension. After positive findings by Blanchard et al. (1986) and McGrady, Yonker, Tan, Fine, and Woerner (1981) for EMG and thermal biofeedback interventions on systolic and diastolic blood pressure, subsequent research did not replicate these findings (Blanchard et al., 1993). A 2003 meta-analysis (Nakao, Yano, Nomura, & Kuboki, 2003) of 22 randomized, controlled studies with 905 essential hypertensive subjects found biofeedback to be superior to no treatment but only better than a sham treatment or nonspecific behavioral treatment when the biofeedback was combined with relaxation, leaving doubt as to the antihypertensive effect of biofeedback as separate from effects of the general relaxation response.

A review of more than 100 randomized controlled trials testing efficacy of all behavioral treatments for hypertension (Linden & Moseley, 2006) found a modest decrease in blood pressure in those treated with BFB over wait-list or other inactive controls. Noted in this review are the variable effect sizes and difficulty reaching conclusions based on many different selection criteria, trial designs, and measurement choices. The recommendation for clinical practice guidelines that match behavioral treatments for hypertension with patient

Table 11.4. Prediction Models for Response to Biofeedback and Behavioral Treatment for Essential Hypertension

Based on McGrady (1996)	
Who Responds?	*How Much Will BP Decrease?*
Patients with:	**Factors are:**
High heart rate	High heart rate
Cool hands	Cool hands
High EMG	High anxiety
High PRA	High-normal cortisol

Based on Yuccha et al. (2005)

Factors predicting outcome of 5 mmHg or more decrease in SBP
- Not taking hypertensive medicine
- Lowest starting finger temperature
- Smallest standard deviation in daytime mean arterial pressure
- Lowest score on Multidimensional Health Locus of Control–Internal scale

Note: BP = blood pressure; EMG = electromyogram; PRA = Plasma Renin Activity; SBP = Systolic Blood Pressure.

characteristics has been addressed by two studies (McGrady, 1996; Yucha, Tsai, Calderon, & Tian, 2005) and is outlined in Table 11.4. Matching patient characteristics with disease management is an important challenge for mind–body research and treatment.

HEART RATE VARIABILITY BIOFEEDBACK FOR ANS DISORDERS

The expanding knowledge base regarding mechanisms of mind–body interaction and increasingly sophisticated technology to measure and monitor those interactions are leading to biofeedback treatments that target complex homeostatic mechanisms in the body, rather than end-organ symptoms. A new biofeedback approach that uses breathing as a pacemaker for oscillatory variability in heart rate is an example of this approach.

Heart rate variability (HRV) refers to the beat-to-beat alterations in heart rate and has historically been associated with cardiovascular health. Low HRV is the best predictor for nonsurvival in severe cardiovascular disease (La Rovere et al., 1998) and is also associated with hypertension (Mancia, Ludbrook, Ferrari, Gregorini, & Zanchetti, 1978), presence and severity of ischemic heart disease (Huikuri & Makikallio, 2001), and rejection risk after heart transplant (Izrailtyan et al., 2000). Disorders of autonomic dysregulation such as asthma (Kazuma, Otsuka, Matsuoka, & Murata, 1997) and depression (Agelink, Boz, Ulrich, & Andrich, 2002) also show decreased amplitude and complexity of HRV.

The broad range of disorders that can be tracked by this physiological marker has led some to suggest that HRV is a measure of general adaptability and diminished HRV a sign of vulnerability to stress of any type. Biofeedback training to increase HRV is conceptualized as directly targeting the complex self-regulatory reflexes of the body (Lehrer, 2007). Pilot studies with fibromyalgia (Hassett et al., 2007) and major depression (Katsamanis et al., 2007) report positive outcomes correlated with practicing breathing to increase amplitude of HRV. A more controlled study taught this paced breathing to a group of patients with coronary artery disease, a population with diminished HRV known to be a risk factor. In comparison to a control group, the subjects were able to increase HRV over a six-week period, and these changes were maintained at three-month follow-up (Del Pozo, Gevirtz, Scher, & Guarneri, 2004).

HYPNOSIS AND BIOFEEDBACK FOR PSYCHIATRIC POPULATIONS

In a survey of over 2,000 respondents that was representative of the US population, Kessler et.al (2001) reported on use of 24 complementary and alternative treatments, including hypnosis and biofeedback. CAM therapies were used more frequently by people with psychiatric disorders, particularly anxiety and depression, than those without mental health diagnoses. In this survey, CAM therapies were used more than conventional therapies by people with self-defined anxiety attacks and severe depression. Additionally, most patients visiting conventional mental health providers for these problems also used complementary and alternative therapies in the 12-month period surveyed. These results suggest that the majority of people in the United States with self-defined anxiety or severe depression use CAM therapies.

BIOFEEDBACK FOR ANXIETY DISORDERS

The most common psychiatric disorders treated with biofeedback are the anxiety disorders (Schoenberg & David, 2014). Schoenberg and David reviewed several decades of BFB research and concluded that the self-control of physiology learned as part of the BFB experience may be particularly helpful to anxiety disorders where ANS arousal can heighten symptoms. Treatment protocols have used all modalities and multimodal approaches. Table 11.5 lists some successful uses of biofeedback for anxiety.

Table 11.5. Biofeedback for Anxiety Disorders

Modality	Patient Group	Results
EEG	GAD	Significant results in both theta and alpha training groups (Vanathy, 1998)
EMG	GAD and panic disorder	Both patient groups improved significantly, continued at follow-up (Barlow et al., 1984)
HRV	GAD, phobia, OCD	Significant decrease in anxiety scores, improved sleep and positive emotions (Reiner, 2008)

Note: EEG = electroencephalography; EMG = electromyogram; HRV = heart rate variability; GAD = generalized anxiety disorder; OCD = obsessive-compulsive disorder.

Two randomized trials treating generalized anxiety disorder (GAD) showed greater efficacy for EEG BFB in comparison to EMG BFB, suggesting a difference in the relaxation states trained (Micoulaud-Franchi et al., 2015). The authors of this review propose that EEG BFB may be indicated for those GAD patients who find it difficult to relax with other techniques and recommend further research into the neuroplasticity effects of EEG BFB for anxiety disorders, in particular posttraumatic stress disorder.

BIOFEEDBACK FOR MAJOR DEPRESSION

Clinicians and researchers have been exploring the use of neurofeedback to treat clinical depression. Early clinical work and research focused on normalizing hemispheric asymmetry using surface EEG sensors over the frontal lobes (Kumano et al., 1996; Rosenfeld, 2000) and a pilot study (Waldkoetter & Sanders, 1997). Criticisms of methodological shortcomings in these early studies were addressed in a nine participant pilot (Peeters, Oehlen, Ronner, van Os, & Lousberg, 2014) with the finding of decreased mean frontal alpha asymmetry over a 10-week treatment period that was associated with a clinical response in one and remission in four of the participants. These positive results were noted with no changes in the use of antidepressants.

Linden (2014) reviews the therapeutic applications of real-time fMRI-based neurofeedback, which has the advantage of access to deep brain structures. Yuan et al. (2004) used fMRI neurofeedback to target and measure neuroplastic changes in subjects who were rewarded for upregulation of the left amygdala during recall of positive autobiographical memories and observed reversal of the abnormal amygdala hypo-activity seen in major depression. Increased connectivity with temporal cortical regions, including the hippocampus, was found only in the active treatment group, and this correlated with larger decreases of depression compared to a group of depressed subjects targeting a brain area not associated with emotional processing. Young et al. (2014) used this same technique to train upregulation of the left amygdala resulting in improved mood.

COGNITIVE HYPNOTHERAPY FOR MENTAL HEALTH POPULATIONS

Although there are mixed findings for hypnosis and psychiatric disorders, conceptual work by Alladin (2012) laid the framework for cognitive hypnotherapy (CH), which combines hypnosis with CBT. In a meta-analysis of 18 studies in which CBT was compared with the same therapy plus hypnosis, treatment outcome was substantially enhanced by the addition (Kirsch, Montgomery, & Sapirstein, 1995). Combining this finding with evidence of higher hypnotizability for certain disorders provides a promising avenue for the use of CH. Representative diagnoses in these studies included obsessive compulsive disorder (OCD) and eating disorders.

HYPNOSIS-FACILITATED CBT FOR OCD

Behavioral and cognitive therapies combined with psychopharmacology are the treatment of choice for Axis I OCD. Unfortunately, up to 25% of patients do not respond to this treatment combination (Bjorgvinsson, Hart, & Heffelinger, 2007). Frederick (2007) presents an argument that the strong link between dissociation and OCD reported in three studies by Watson, Wu, and Cutshall (2004) strengthens Shusta's (1999) recommendation that all OCD refractory patients be screened for dissociation. She further presents case material in which hypnotically facilitated treatment of refractory OCD had good results.

HYPNOSIS-FACILITATED CBT FOR EATING DISORDERS

Bulimic patients have been shown to be significantly more hypnotizable than a control group and scored higher on a self-report of dissociative experiences (Covino, Jimerson, Wolfe, Franko, & Frankel, 1994). Barabasz (2012) reviews several studies of treatments combining CBT and hypnosis using a standardized manual detailing both behavior modification and hypnotic suggestions provided from a script (Griffiths, 1995; Griffiths, Hadzi-Pavlovic,

& Channon-Little, 1996). To address methodological issues, Barabasz reports on a more recent study by Barga and Barabasz (in press) that compares CBT alone to CH, also in a highly scripted protocol. Results included significantly lower binge frequency for the CH group at posttreatment; and within-treatment measures for this group indicated statistically significant improvement on all measures from pretreatment to posttreatment to three-month follow-up.

Even though anorexic patients show similar levels of hypnotizability, the control issues central to this disorder necessitate a more permissive and individualized approach. Baker and Nash (1987) treated 36 women within this paradigm of hypnosis for self-control with 76% showing remission of symptoms at 5 and 12 months, compared to 53% for a group who did not receive hypnosis as part of their psychotherapy treatment. Pop-Jordanova (2000) found that anorexic patients responded better to electrodermal biofeedback than a bulimic group. The contrast of the methods used for these two highly hypnotizable populations (bulimia and anorexia) highlights the necessity of choosing an approach that will allow the patient to activate potential for change.

Conclusion

Consumers of health services are increasingly utilizing mind–body medicine techniques, and there is a substantive evidence-base for some modalities, particularly hypnosis and biofeedback. There are research challenges to find more sophisticated models to assess mediators and moderators of treatment effect, overcome limitations of blinded controls, and better determine which populations are most responsive to given techniques.

Hypnosis and biofeedback are good representatives of the transition from the biomedicine to biopsychosocial model. Hypnosis appears to be best for alterations of thought and sensation. This can be an especially powerful treatment for the subgroup of the population that is highly hypnotizable. More research is needed to elucidate this important moderating variable. CH shows promise as a way to conceptualize and develop treatments for the unique characteristics of differing psychiatric populations.

Biofeedback engages mental activities to create objective physiological changes and has an impact on the way in which it can lead to healthier and more balanced self-regulatory patterns. Like hypnosis, there is much to understand about mechanisms of action, and, also like hypnosis, there are problems and illnesses that are more responsive to treatment. Research in this area can explore the fluid boundaries of mind–body distinctions.

REFERENCES

Agelink, M. W., Boz, C., Ulrich, H., & Andrich, J. (2002). Relationship between major depression and heart rate variability. Clinical consequences and implications for antidepressive treatment. *Psychiatry Research, 113*, 139–149.

Alladin, A. (2012). Cognitive hypnotherapy for major depressive disorder. *American Journal of Clinical Hypnosis, 54*(4), 275–293.

Andrasik, F. (2010). Biofeedback in headache: An overview of approaches and evidence. *Cleveland Clinic Journal of Medicine, 77*, 72–76.

Andrews, J. M. (1964). Neuromuscular re-education of hemiplegic with aid of electromyography. *Archives of Physical Medicine and Rehabilitation, 45*, 530–532.

Baker, E. L., & Nash, M. R. (1987). Applications of hypnosis in the treatment of anorexia nervosa. *American Journal of Clinical Hypnosis, 29*, 185–193.

Banyai, E. I., & Hilgard, E. R. (1976). A comparison of active-alert hypnotic induction with traditional relaxation induction. *Journal of Abnormal Psychology, 85*(2), 218–224.

Barabasz, A., & Perez, N. (2007) Salient findings: Hypnotizability as core construct and the utility of hypnosis. *International Journal of Clinical and Experimental Hypnosis, 55*, 372–379.

Barabasz, M. (2012). Cognitive hypnotherapy with bulimia. *American Journal of Clinical Hypnosis, 54*, 353–364.

Barga, J., & Barabasz, M. (in press). The effects of cognitive behavior therapy plus hypnosis in the treatment of bulimia. *International Journal of Clinical and Experimental Hypnosis.*

Barlow, D. H., Cohen, A. S., Waddell, M. T., Vermilyea, J. A., Klosko, J. S., Blanchard, E. B., et al. (1984). Panic and generalized anxiety disorders: Nature and treatment. *Behavior Therapy, 15*, 431–449.

Basmajian, J. V. (1963). Control and training of individual motor units. *Science, 141*, 440–441.

Benham, G., Woody, E. Z., Wilson, K. S., & Nash, M. R. (2006). Expect the unexpected: Ability, attitude, and responsiveness to hypnosis. *Journal of Personality and Social Psychology, 91*, 342–350.

Bjorgvinsson, T., Hart, J., & Heffelinger, S. (2007). Obsessive-compulsive disorder: Update on assessment and treatment. *Journal of Psychiatric Practice, 13*, 362–372.

Blanchard, E. B., McCoy, C. C., Musso, A., Gerardi, M. A., Pallmeyer, T. P., Gerardi, R. J., et al. (1986). A controlled comparison of thermal biofeedback and relaxation training in the treatment of essential hypertension: I. Short-term and long-term outcome. *Behavior Therapy, 17*, 563–579.

Blanchard, E. B., Eisele, G., Gordon, M. A., Cornish, P. J., Wittrock, D. A., Gillmore, L., et al. (1993). Thermal biofeedback as an effective substitute for sympatholytic medication in moderate hypertension: A failure to replicate. *Biofeedback and Self Regulation, 18*, 237–253.

Blume, H., Brockman, L., & Breuner, C. (2012). Biofeedback therapy for pediatric headache: Factors associated with response. *Headache, 52*, 1377–1386.

Brown, P. (1991). *The hypnotic brain.* New Haven, CT: Yale University Press.

Bryant, R., Hung, L., Dobson-Stone, C., & Schofield, P. (2013). The association between the oxytocin receptor gene (OXTR) and hypnotizability. *Psychoneuroendocrinology, 38,* 1979–1984.

Budzynski, T. H., Stoyva, J. M., Adler, C. S., & Mullaney, D. J. (1973). EMG biofeedback and tension headache: A controlled outcome study. *Psychosomatic Medicine, 35,* 484–496.

Campbell, J. K., Penzien, D. B., & Wall, E. M. (2000). Evidence-based guidelines for migraine headaches: Behavioral and physical treatments. Retrieved from http://www.aan.com/

Cannon, W. B. (1929). Organization for physiological homeostasis. *Physiological Reviews, 9,* 399–431.

Clarke, T. C., Black, L. I., Stussman, B., Barnes, P., & Nahin, R. (2015). Trends in the use of complementary health approaches among adults. *National Health Statistics Reports, 79.*

Cojan, Y., Piguet, C., & Vuilleumier, P. (2015). What makes your brain suggestible? Hypnotizability is associated with differential brain activity during attention outside hypnosis. *NeuroImage, 117,* 367–374.

Covino, N. A., Jimerson, D. C., Wolfe, B. E., Franko, D. C., & Frankel, F. H. (1994). Hypnotizability, dissociation, and bulimia nervosa. *Journal of Abnormal Psychology, 103,* 455–459.

deCharms, R. C., Maeda, F., Glover, G. H., Ludlow, D., Pauly, J. M., Soneji, D., et al. (2005). Control over brain activation and pain learned by using real-time functional MRI. *Proceedings of the National Academy of Sciences of the United States of America, 102,* 18626–18631.

Del Pozo, J. M., Gevirtz, R. N., Scher, B., & Guarneri, E. (2004). Biofeedback treatment increases heart rate variability in patients with known coronary artery disease. *American Heart Journal, 147,* G1–G1.

Elkins, G., Barabasz, A., Council, J., & Spiegel, D. (2015). Advancing research and practice: The revised APA Division 30 definition of hypnosis. *American Journal of Clinical Hypnosis, 57*(4).

Engel, G. L. (1977). The need for a new medical model: A challenge for biomedical science. *Science, 196,* 129–136.

Flor, H., & Birbaumer, N. (1993). Comparison of the efficacy of electromyographic biofeedback, cognitive-behavioral therapy and conservative medical interventions in the treatment of chronic musculoskeletal pain. *Journal of Consulting and Clinical Psychology, 61,* 653–658.

Frass, M., Strassi, R., Friehs, H., Mullner, M., Kundi, M., & Kaye, A. (2012). Use and acceptance of complementary and alternative medicine among the general population and medical personnel: A systematic review. *The Ochsner Journal, 12,* 45–56.

Frederick, C. (2007). Hypnotically facilitated treatment of obsessive-compulsive disorder: Can it be evidence-based? *International Journal of Clinical and Experimental Hypnosis, 55,* 189–206.

Gauld, A. (1992). *A history of hypnotism*. New York: Cambridge University Press.

Glazer, H. I., & Laine, C. D. (2006). Pelvic floor muscle biofeedback in the treatment of urinary incontinence: A literature review. *Applied Psychophysiology and Biofeedback, 31*, 187–201.

Gonsalkorale, W. (2006). Gut-directed hypnotherapy: The Manchester Approach for treatment of irritable bowel syndrome. *International Journal of Clinical and Experiemental Hypnosis, 54*(1), 27–50.

Green, E. E., Ferguson, D. W., Green, A. M., & Walters, E. D. (1970). Preliminary report on the voluntary controls project: Swami Rama. Voluntary Controls Project: Menninger Foundation. Topeka, KS (Mimeograph).

Griffiths, R. (1995). Hypnobehavioural treatment for bulimia nervosa: A treatment manual. *Australian Journal of Clinical and Experimental Hypnosis, 21*(1), 25–46.

Griffiths, R. A., Hadzi-Pavlovic, D., & Channon-Little, L. (1996). The short-term follow-up effects of hypnobehavioural and cognitive behavioural treatment for bulimia nervosa. *European Eating Disorders Review, 4*, 12–31.

Hassett, A. L., Radvanski, D. C., Vaschillo, E. G., Vaschillo, B., Sigal, L. H., Karavidas, M. K., et al. (2007). A pilot study of the efficacy of heart rate variability (HRV) biofeedback in patients with fibromyalgia. *Applied Psychophysiology and Biofeedback, 32*, 1–10.

Hilgard, E. R. (1967). Individual differences in hypnotizability. In J. E. Gordon (Ed.), *Handbook of clinical and experimental hypnosis* (pp. 391–443). New York: Macmillan.

Hilgard, J. R. (1970). *Personality and hypnosis: A study of imaginative involvement*. Chicago: University of Chicago Press.

Hoeft, F., Gabrieli, J., Whitfield-Gabrieli, S., Hass, B., Bammer, R., Menon, V., & Spiegel, D. (2012). Functional brain basis of hypnotizability. *Archives of General Psychiatry, 69*(10), 1064–1072.

Horton, J. E., Crawford, H. J., Harrington, G., & Downs, J. H. (2004). Increased corpus callosum size associated with hypnotizability and the ability to control pain. *Brain, 127*, 1741–1747.

Huikuri, H. V., & Makikallio, T. H. (2001). Heart rate variability in ischemic heart disease. *Autonomic Neuroscience: Basic and Clinical, 90*, 95–101.

Iglexias, A. (2004). Hypnosis and existential psychotherapy with end-stage terminally ill patients. *American Journal of Clinical Hypnosis, 46*, 201–213.

Imamura, M., Abrams, P., Bain, C., Buckley, B., Cardozo, L., Cody. J., et.al. (2010). Systematic review and economic modelling of the effectiveness and cost-effectiveness of non-surgical treatments for women with stress urinary incontinence. *Health Technology Assessment, 14*(40).

Izrailtyan, I., Kresh, J. Y., Morris, R. J., Brozena, S. C., Kutalik, S. P., & Wechsler, A. S. (2000). Early detection of acute allograft rejection by linear and nonlinear analysis of heart rate variability. *Journal of Thoracic and Cardiovascular Surgery, 120*, 737–745.

Jacknow, D. S., Tschann, J. M., Link, M. P., & Boyce, W. T. (1994). Hypnosis in the prevention of chemotherapy-related nausea and vomiting in children: A prospective study. *Journal of Developmental and Behavior Pediatrics, 15*, 258–264.

Katsamanis Karavidas, M, Lehrer, P. M., Vaschillo, E., Vaschillo, B., Marin, H., Buyske, S., et al. (2007). Preliminary results of an open label study of heart rate variability biofeedback for the treatment of major depression. *Applied Psychophysiology and Biofeedback, 32*, 19–30.

Kazuma, N., Otsuka, K., Matsuoka, I., & Murata, M. (1997). Heart rate variability during 24 hours in asthmatic children. *Chronobiology International, 14*, 597–606.

Kessler, R., Soukup, J., Davis, R. B., Foster, D. F., Wilkey, S. A., Van Rompay, M. I., & Eisenberg, D. M. (2001). The use of complementary and alternative therapies to treat anxiety and depression in the United States. *American Journal of Psychiatry, 158*, 289-294.

Kimmel, H. (1974). Instrumental conditioning of autonomically mediated responses in human beings. *American Journal of Psychology, 29*, 325.

Kirsch, I., Montgomery, G., & Sapirstein, G. L. (1995). Hypnosis as an adjunct to cognitive-behavioral psychotherapy: A meta-analysis. *Journal of Consulting and Clinical Psychology, 63*, 214–220.

Kumano, H., Horie, H., Shidara, T., Kuboki, T., Suematsu, H., & Yasushi, M. (1996). Treatment of a depressive disorder patient with EEG-driven photic stimulation. *Biofeedback and Self Regulation, 21*, 323–334.

Lang, E. V., Berbaum, K. S., Faintuch, S., Hatsiopoulou, O., Halsey, N., Li, X., et al. (2006). Adjunctive self-hypnotic relaxation for outpatient medical procedures: A prospective randomized trial with women undergoing large core breast biopsy. *Pain, 126*(1–3), 3–4.

Lang, E. V., Lutgendorf, S., Logan, H., Benotsc, E., Laser, E., & Spiegel, D. (1999). Nonpharmacologic analgesia and anxiolysis for interventional radiological procedures. *Seminars in Interventional Radiology, 16*, 113–123.

Lang, E. V., & Rosen, M. (2002). Cost analysis of adjunct hypnosis for sedation during outpatient interventional procedures. *Radiology, 222*, 375–382.

La Rovere, M. T., Bigger, J. T. J., Marcus, F. I., Mortara, A., & Schwartz, P. J. (1998). Baroreflex sensitivity and heart-rate variability in predictions of total cardiac mortality after myocardial infarction. *Lancet, 351*, 478–484.

Lehrer, P. M. (2007). Biofeedback training to increase heart rate variability. In P. M. Lehrer, R. L. Woolfolk, & W. E. Sime (Eds.), *Principles and practice of stress management* (3rd ed., pp. 227–248). New York: Guilford Press.

Lichtenberg, P., Bachner-Melman, R., Gritsenko, I., & Ebstein, R. P. (2000). Exploratory association between catechol-O-methyltransferase (COMT) high/low enzyme activity polymorphism and hypnotizability. *American Journal of Medical Genetics, 96*, 771–774.

Linden, D. (2014). Neurofeedback and networks of depression. *Dialogues in Clinical Neuroscience, 16*(1),103–112.

Linden, W., & Moseley, J. V. (2006). The efficacy of behavioral treatment for hypertension. *Applied Psychophysiology and Biofeedback, 31*, 51–63.

Liossi, C., & Hatira, P. (1999). Clinical hypnosis versus cognitive behavioral training for pain management with pediatric cancer patients undergoing bone marrow aspirations. *International Journal of Clinical and Experimental Hypnosis, 47*, 104–116.

Liossi, C., & Hatira, P. (2003). Clinical hypnosis in the alleviation of procedure-related pain in pediatric oncology patients. *International Journal of Clinical and Experimental Hypnosis, 51,* 4–28.

Liossi, C., White, P., & Hatira, P. (2006). Randomized clinical trial of local anesthetic versus a combination of local anesthetic with self-hypnosis in the management of pediatric procedure-related pain. *Health Psychology, 25,* 307–315.

London, P., Hart, J. T., Leibovitz, M. P., & McDevitt, P. A. (1967). The psychophysiology of hypnotic susceptibility. In L. Chertok (Ed.), *Psychophysiological mechanisms of hypnosis* (pp. 151–172). Berlin: Springer-Verlag.

Ma, C., Szeto, G., Yan, T., Wu, S., Lin, C., & Li, L. (2011). Comparing biofeedback with active exercise and passive treatment for the management of work-related neck and shoulder pain: A randomized controlled trial. *Archives of Physical and Medicine Rehabilitation, 92,* 849–858.

Mancia, G., Ludbrook, J., Ferrari, A., Gregorini, L., & Zanchetti, A. (1978). Baroreceptor reflexes in human hypertension. *Circulation Research, 43,* 170–177.

Marinacci, A. A., & Horande, M. (1960). Electromyogram in neuromuscular re-education. *Bulletin of the Los Angeles Neurological Society, 25,* 57–71.

McGrady, A. (1996). Good news—bad press: Applied psychophysiology in cardiovascular disorders. *Biofeedback and Self-Regulation, 21,* 335–346.

McGrady, A. V., Yonker, R., Tan, S. Y., Fine, T. H., & Woerner, M. (1981). The effect of biofeedback-assisted relaxation training on blood pressure and selected biochemical parameters in patients with essential hypertension. *Biofeedback and Self-Regulation, 6,* 343–353.

Melzack, R., & Wall, P. D. (1965). Pain mechanisms: A new theory. *Science, 150,* 171–179.

Micoulaud-Franchi, J. A., Geoffroy, P. A., Fond, G., Lopez, R., Bioulac, S., & Philip, P. (2014). EEG neurofeedback treatments in children with ADHD: An updated meta-analysis of randomized controlled trials. *Frontiers in Human Neuroscience, 8,* 1–7.

Micoulaud-Franchi, J. A., McGonigal, A., Lopex, R., Daudet, C., Kotwas, I., & Bartolomei, F. (2015). Electroencephalographic neurofeedback: Level of evidence in mental and brain disorders and suggestions for good clinical practice. *Neurophysiologie Clinique/Clinical Neurophysiology, 45,* 423–433.

Miller, N. (1969). Learning of visceral and glandular responses. *Science, 163,* 434–445.

Milling, L. S., Reardon, J. M., & Carosella, G. M. (2006). Mediation and moderation of psychological pain treatments: Response expectancies and hypnotic suggestibility. *Journal of Consulting and Clinical Psychology, 74,* 253–262.

Monastra, V. J., Lynn, S., Linden, M., Lubar, J. E., Gruzelier, J., & LaVaque, T. J. (2005). Electroencephalographic biofeedback in the treatment of attention-deficit/hyperactivity disorder. *Applied Psychophysiology and Biofeedback, 30,* 95–114.

Montgomery, G. H., Welta, C. R., Selta, M., & Bovberg, D. H. (2002). Brief presurgery hypnosis reduces distress and pain in excisional breast biopsy patients. *International Journal of Clinical and Experimental Hypnosis, 50,* 17–32.

Morgan, A. H. (1973). The heritability of hypnotic susceptibility in twins. *Journal of Abnormal Psychology, 82,* 55–61.

Mutter, C. B. (1998). History of hypnosis. In C. D. Hammond (Ed.), *Hypnotic induction & suggestion* (pp. 10–12). Chicago: American Society of Clinical Hypnosis.

Nahin, R., Boineau, R., Khalsa, P., Stussman, B., & Weber, W. (2016). Evidence-based evaluation of complementary health approaches for pain management in the United States. *Mayo Clinical Proceedings, 91*(9), 1292–1306.

Nakao, M., Yano, E., Nomura, S., & Kuboki, T. (2003). Blood pressure-lowering effects of biofeedback treatment in hypertension: A meta-analysis of randomized controlled trials. *Hypertension Research, 26*, 37–46.

National Center for Complementary and Integrative Health. (2007). What is CAM? Retrieved from http://nccam.nih.gov/health/backgrounds/mindbody.htm

National Institutes of Health Technology Assessment Panel on Integration of Behavioral and Relaxation Approaches into the Treatment of Chronic Pain and Insomnia. (1996). *Journal of the American Medical Association, 276*, 313–318.

Nestoriuc, Y., & Martin, A. (2007). Efficacy of biofeedback for migraine: A meta-analysis. *Pain, 128*, 111–127.

Nestoriuc, Y., Rief, W., & Martin, A. (2008). Meta-analysis of biofeedback for tension-type headache: Efficacy, specificity, and treatment moderators. *Journal of Consulting and Clinical Psychology, 76*(3), 379–396.

Nicholson, R. A., Hursey, K., & Nash, J. M. (2005). Moderators and mediators of behavioral treatment for headache. *Headache, 45*, 513–519.

Nielson, W. R., & Weir, R. (2001). Biopsychosocial approaches to the treatment of chronic pain. *Clinical Journal of Pain, 17*, S114–S127.

Palsson, O. (2015). Hypnosis treatment of gastrointestinal disorders: A comprehensive review of the empirical evidence. *American Journal of Clinical Hypnosis, 58*(2), 134–158.

Palsson, O., & vanTilburg, M. (2015). Hypnosis and guided imagery treatment for gastrointestinal disorders: Experience with scripted protocols developed at the University of North Carolina. *American Journal of Clinical Hypnosis, 58*, 5–21.

Peeters F., Oehlen, M., Ronner, J., van Os, J., & Lousberg, R. (2014). Neurofeedback as a treatment for major depressive disorder—a pilot study. *PLoS One, 9*(3), e91837.

Piccione, C., Hilgard, E. R., & Zimbardo, P. G. (1989). On the degree of stability of measured hypnotizability over a 25-year period. *Journal of Personality and Social Psychology, 56*, 289–295.

Pop-Jordanova, N. (2000). Psychological characteristics and biofeedback mitigation in preadolescents with eating disorders. *Pediatrics International, 42*, 76–81.

Potie, A., Roelants, F., Pospiech, A., Momeni, M., & Watremez, C. (2016). Hypnosis in the perioperative management of breast cancer surgery: Clinical benefits and potential implication. *Anesthesiology Research and Practice, 2016*, 1–8.

Porges, S. W. (1995). Cardiac vagal tone: A physiological index of stress. *Neuroscience and Biobehavioral Reviews, 19*, 225–233.

Porges, S. W. (2007). A phylogenetic journey through the vague and ambiguous Xth cranial nerve: A commentary on contemporary heart rate variability research. *Biological Psychology, 74*(2), 301–307.

Raz, A. (2005). Attention and hypnosis: Neural substrates and genetic associations of two converging processes. *International Journal of Clinical and Experimental Hypnosis, 53*, 237–258.

Reiner, R. (2008). Integrating a portable biofeedback device into clinical practise for patients with anxiety disorders: Results of a pilot study. *Applied Psychophysiology and Biofeedback, 33*, 55–61.

Rosenfeld, J. P. (2000). An EEG biofeedback for affective disorders. *Clinical Electroencephalography, 31*, 7–12.

Sacerdote, P. (1982). Why is hypnosis effective in pain control? In D. Waxman, P. Misra, M. Gibson, & M. A. Basker (Eds.), *Modern trends in hypnosis* (pp. 249–258). New York: Plenum Press.

Sargent, J. D., Green, E. E., & Walters, E. D. (1972). The use of autogenic feedback in a pilot study of migraine and tension headaches. *Headache, 12*, 120–125.

Satish, R., Benninga, M., Bharucha, A., Chiarioni, G., Di Lorenzo, C., & Whitehead, W. (2015). ANMS-ESNM position paper and consensus guidelines on biofeedback therapy for anorectal disorders. *Neurogastroenterol Motility, 27*(5), 594–609.

Schnur, J., Kafer, I., Marcus, C., & Montgomery, G. (2008). Hypnosis to manage distress related to medical procedures: A meta-analysis. *Contemporary Hypnosis, 25*(3–4), 114–128.

Schoenberg, P., & David, A. (2014). Biofeedback for psychiatric disorders: A systemic review. *Applied Psychophysiological Biofeedback, 39*, 109–135.

Schupp, C., Berbaum, D., Berbaum, M., & Lang, E. V. (2005). Pain and anxiety during interventional radiological procedures: Effect of patients' state anxiety at baseline and modulation by nonpharmacologic analgesia adjuncts. *Journal of Vascular & Interventional Radiology, 16*, 1585–1592.

Shor, R. E., & Orne, E. C. (1963). Norms on the Harvard Group Scale of Hypnotic Susceptibility. *International Journal of Clinical Experimental Hypnosis, 11*, 39–47.

Shusta, S. R. (1999). Successful treatment of refractory obsessive-compulsive disorder. *American Journal of Psychotherapy, 53*, 377–391.

Udolf, R. (1987). *Handbook of hypnosis for professionals* (2nd ed.). New York: Van Nostrand Reinhold.

Vanathy, S., Sharma, P. S. V. N., & Kumar, K. B. (1998). The efficacy of alpha and theta neurofeedback training in treatment of generalized anxiety disorder. Indian *Journal of Clinical Psychology, 25*(2), 136–143.

Waldkoetter, R. O., & Sanders, G. O. (1997). Auditory brainwave stimulation in treating alcoholic depression. *Perceptual and Motor Skills, 84*, 226.

Watson, D., Wu, K., & Cutshall, C. (2004). Symptom subtypes of obsessive-compulsive disorder and their relation to dissociation. *Journal of Anxiety Disorders, 18*, 435–458.

Weitzenhofer, A. M., & Hilgard, E. R. (1959). *Stanford Hypnotic Susceptibility Scale, Form A*. Palo Alto, CA: Consulting Psychologist Press.

Young, K., Zotev, V., Phillips, R., Misaki. M., Yuan, H., Drevets, W. C., et al. (2014). Real-time fMRI neurofeedback training of amygdala activity in patients with major depressive disorder. *PLoS One, 9*(2), 1–13.

Yuan, H., Kymberly, D., Young, R., Zotev, V., Misaki, M., & Bodurka, J. (2014). Resting-state functional connectivity modulation and sustained changes after real-time functional magnetic resonance imaging neurofeedback training in depression. *Brain Connectivity, 4*(9), 690–701.

Yucha, C., & Gilbert, C. (2004). *Evidence-based practice in biofeedback and neurofeedback*. Wheat Ridge, CO: AAPB.

Yucha, C. B., Tsai, P. S., Calderon, K. S., & Tian, L. (2005). Biofeedback-assisted relaxation training for essential hypertension: Who is most likely to benefit? *Cardiovascular Nursing, 20*, 198–205.

12

Mindfulness-Based Interventions for Psychiatric Disorders

ALEEZE MOSS AND DIANE REIBEL

Key Points

- Mindfulness-Based Interventions (MBIs) are nonpharmacological interventions that show promise for the treatment of a number of mental health conditions.
- There are many types of MBIs including the formal Mindfulness-Based Stress Reduction (MBSR) program and Mindfulness-Based Cognitive Therapy (MBCT) program.
- MBSR and MBCT have been shown to be effective in the treatment of anxiety and depression.
- Dialectical Behavior Therapy (DBT) has been shown to be effective in the treatment of borderline personality disorder and Acceptance and Commitment Therapy (ACT) effective in the treatment of obsessive-compulsive disorder.
- MBIs have also been developed to work specifically with populations suffering with posttraumatic stress disorder, eating disorders, addictions and attention deficit hyperactivity disorder.
- Current research on neural mechanisms associated with mindfulness training and its benefits are demonstrating specific structural and functional changes in the brain.

Introduction

According to a recent World Health Organization (2012) report, 450 million people worldwide suffer from some form of psychiatric disorder. In the United Sates, a national survey estimated that 43.6 million adults were diagnosed with mental illness in 2014 (National Institute of Mental

Health, n.d.). Mental illness includes diagnoses of anxiety disorders, mood disorders, major depression, bipolar disorder, schizophrenia, posttraumatic stress disorders, and attention deficit disorders. Major depression is one of the most common mental disorders in the United States and carries the heaviest burden of disability (National Institute of Mental Health, n.d.).

Given the staggering numbers of people affected by psychiatric disorders and the significant public health burden on individuals and society, there has been a growing interest in treatment options, including the use of nonpharmacological treatments as adjuncts to conventional treatment approaches. Mindfulness-Based Interventions (MBIs) are effective and relatively inexpensive nonpharmacological interventions for the treatment of a number of mental health conditions. This chapter begins with descriptions of several MBIs, specifically Mindfulness-Based Stress Reduction (MBSR), Mindfulness-Based Cognitive Therapy (MBCT), Dialectical Behavior Therapy (DBT) and Acceptance and Commitment Therapy (ACT), followed by a review of the research that supports the efficacy of these interventions in the treatment of psychiatric disorders.

Mindfulness-Based Stress Reduction

MBSR was founded by Jon Kabat-Zinn in 1979 and designed to teach patients with chronic medical conditions how to live fuller, healthier, more adaptive lives. MBSR is a formalized and well-structured group intervention that is patient-centered, experiential, and educational. The core of the eight-week program involves intensive training in mindfulness meditation and its applications for daily living and coping with stress, pain, and illness. Mindfulness meditation is moment-to-moment awareness that is intentionally nonreactive and nonjudgmental.

Kabat-Zinn (1990) defines mindfulness operationally "as the awareness that arises by paying attention on purpose, in the present moment and nonjudgmentally" (p. 4). This operational definition has been further expounded by Shapiro, Carlson, Astin, and Freedman (2006) who posit that mindfulness contains three axioms: intention, attention, and attitude. These three axioms are not sequential but engaged simultaneously throughout the process of cultivating mindfulness. The *intention*—what motivates the participant to engage in the program and the practices—has been shown to shift along a continuum "from self-regulation, to self-exploration, and finally to self-liberation." The *attention* is trained in two capacities: sustained focus and flexibility of focus. The *attitude* is one of nonjudgment and of having an accepting, open, and kind curiosity toward one's experience. In elaborating these three axioms of mindfulness, Shapiro and colleagues suggest a meta-mechanism that they call "reperceiving," which they define as a switch in a person's consciousness in which what was previously perceived as the 'subject' now becomes 'object.' They suggest that mindfulness training strengthens and accelerates the growth of this capacity to move from a position in which one is completely identified with one's experience to a position in which one's experience becomes available for observation. It is important to clarify that this reperceiving does not create distance and disconnection but rather enables one to look and know more deeply and allows for the possibility of making conscious choices, responding to rather than reacting to emergent situations (McCown, Reibel, & Micozzi, 2010). Reperceiving's nonreactive character gives one space and time to encounter formerly disturbing emotions, thoughts, and body sensations, which reduces their capacity for disruption.

MBSR is an eight-week program with participants attending 2½-hour sessions once a week and one full-day (seven-hours) class between the sixth and seventh sessions. Class time each week is divided between formal meditation practice, small and large group discussions, didactic presentations (including on stress physiology and the role that perception plays in the shaping of one's experience), and inquiry with individuals into their present-moment experiences. The standard MBSR program has an orientation process whereby prospective participants fill out intake forms and meet with teachers to determine the appropriateness of the program for their needs. While MBSR has been shown to be effective for a variety of physical and mental disorders, it is important to note that there are certain precautions when referring or enrolling individuals in the program. For example, the standard MBSR program is not currently considered to be suitable for individuals with active substance abuse, psychosis, suicidal ideation, schizophrenia, or uncontrolled bipolar disorder (Britton, 2016). There are some MBIs that are specifically designed to work with some of these populations.

The standard eight-week MBSR program teaches formal practices including body scan meditation, sitting meditation (with focus on the breath), mindful hatha yoga, sitting meditation (moving from focus on the breath to an expanded awareness of other objects of attention, i.e., body sensations, hearing, thoughts, emotions, and eventually with an open awareness of all that is arising in the present moment), walking meditation, and eating meditation. Class discussions focus on group members' experiences in the formal meditation practices and the application of mindfulness in day-to-day life. Home practice is an integral part of MBSR (Kabat-Zinn, 1990). In Kabat-Zinn's original program, participants are asked to commit to formal practice, supported by audio recordings of guided meditations, for 45 minutes a day, six days per week.

The curriculum begins with the body scan meditation to cultivate mindfulness of the body. In this practice participants are guided to bring attention to different areas of the body sequentially, learning to be with direct sensory experience with an attitude of nonjudgment and curiosity. Through this initial focus of attention on body sensations, participants often come to realize that their thoughts and judgments about sensory experience can be untangled from the direct experience of sensations arising in the present moment. This cultivates their ability to have some degree of freedom from thoughts and beliefs about difficult sensations that can often produce or exacerbate stress and anxiety.

The curriculum also teaches participants mindfulness of "feeling tone." Here feeling tone refers not so much to mood states but rather to whether experiences are perceived as pleasant, unpleasant, or neutral. Through reflection at home and discussion in class, participants become more aware of their reactivity to pleasant and unpleasant experiences and come to understand how their reactions (grasping/pushing away) can cause more stress and suffering. Formal practices help participants learn to pause and respond more consciously in ways that are more skillful and can bring ease even in the midst of difficult circumstances. The ability to respond skillfully to mental processes that contribute to emotional distress and maladaptive behavior has been shown to be of great benefit for people with anxiety and mood disorders (Hoffman, Sawyer, Witt, & Oh, 2010; Kabat-Zinn et al., 1992).

Researchers who have reviewed the literature on the possible mechanisms of action through which mindfulness meditation may work suggest that mindfulness meditation exerts its effects through attention regulation, body awareness, emotion regulation, and a change in perspective on the self. These practices work synergistically to establish enhanced self-regulation (Farb, Anderson, & Segal, 2012; Farb et al., 2010; Gonzales-Garcia, Borras, Lopez, & McNeil, 2016; Hölzel, Lazar, Gard, Schuman-Olivier, & Ott, 2011; Vago & Silbersweig, 2012). The changes in attention and emotion regulation after participating in an eight-week MBSR program have been shown to be associated with demonstrable functional and structural changes in the brain (Davidson et al., 2003; Lazar et al., 2005).

Mindfulness-Based Cognitive Therapy

Around the time that some of the initial findings of the benefits of MBSR for the treatment of mental illness were being disseminated, Segal, Williams, and Teasdale (2002) were working together to develop a program that could tackle one of the biggest problems of major depression—its tendency to recur in people who had suffered from depression previously. Influenced by the academic literature and their own research findings and understanding of recurrent depression, they eventually created the MBCT program.

Initially, Segal et al. (2002) came together in an attempt to understand the mechanisms that produce depression, particularly the changes in thinking and feeling. By the late 1980s there were already a number of psychological treatments for depression whose effects were on par with that found for pharmacological medication. One of these was cognitive-behavioral therapy (CBT; Beck, 1976; Beck, Rush, Shaw, & Emery, 1979). The problem remained, however, that some patients were more likely to relapse into depression again once they had recovered from an episode of depression. Segal et al. began to work on a project to create a "maintenance" version of cognitive therapy that could help prevent this relapse.

Originally it was thought that cognitive therapy, which targets changing belief in depressive thoughts and dysfunctional attitudes, had its effects through changes in the content of depressive thinking. The explicit emphasis in cognitive therapy had been in changing thought content. Segal et al. (2002) came to believe that patients could make a more general shift in their perspective on negative thoughts and feelings through the process of "decentering." Decentering is seeing thoughts in a wider perspective, seeing them as "just thoughts" and not necessarily as reflecting reality. They came to see decentering as not just one of a number of things going on in cognitive therapy but rather as a core component. They believed that mindfulness could help with the "decentering" process that they considered to be critical to the relapse prevention (RP) effects of cognitive therapy. In the early 1990s, they met with Jon Kabat-Zinn and colleagues at the Stress Reduction Clinic at the University of Massachusetts (UMASS) Medical Center. After they sat in on the first session of an MBSR class, they felt that they could incorporate mindfulness skills into cognitive therapy. What they found remarkable was the emphasis placed within MBSR on being able to see that "thoughts are just thoughts and that they are not 'you' or 'reality.'" As they quote from Kabat-Zinn (1990), "the simple act of recognizing your thoughts as thoughts can free you from the distorted reality they often create and allow for more clear-sightedness and a greater sense of manageability in your life" (p. 67).

Segal et al. (2002) initially called their program "Attentional Control Training." They used the eight-week group structure of MBSR (shortening each weekly session to 2 hours from 2½ hours) and piloted the program. They taught mindfulness skills by having the class listen to a 20-minute audiotape of mindfulness instructions led by Jon Kabat-Zinn (that they had shortened) and asked participants to listen to the tape daily as home practice. At the end of the program, they found that while some patients appeared to do well, others had considerable difficulty in applying the skills of attentional control and observation to their emotional upheaval.

They subsequently went back to the Stress Reduction clinic at UMASS and discovered important differences between attentional control training, as they had designed it, and the approach in MBSR that they had not understood before. In particular, they saw that the experienced MBSR teachers did not try to fix or give solutions to problems raised by participants but rather they encouraged participants to bring their difficulties (e.g., challenging moods and thoughts) into awareness and simply be with them and breathe with them. Participants were learning how to "allow" their experience, even the difficult thoughts and emotions, and to welcome all of experience with an awareness that was gentle, kind, and curious. As they write in their book *Mindfulness-Based Cognitive Therapy for Depression*, they understood the importance of MBSR instructors themselves practicing mindfulness meditation:

> We thought again about the fact that all of the MBSR instructors were themselves practicing mindfulness meditation, and that they seemed able to embody the same gentle approach to patients' difficulties that the patients themselves were being encouraged to take. The stance of the instructor was itself "invitational." In addition there was always the assumption of "continuity" between the experiences of the instructor and the participants. If class members described becoming aware of how they had been criticizing themselves, for example, the experience of dealing with self-critical thoughts was something the instructor had in common with others in the class. (Segal et al., 2013, p. 53)

There are two essential aspects that are highlighted in this passage that were incorporated into the MBCT curriculum. The first is the nonpathologizing nature of the MBSR curriculum; the second is the teacher's embodiment of mindfulness including the attitudinal foundations of mindfulness (McCown et al., 2010). Segal et al. (2002) realized that clinicians needed to develop their own mindfulness practice and experience it from the inside if they were to effectively teach it to their patients. They also came to understand that patients have within themselves the resources they need in order to learn to handle their problems. More than being taught a set of skills or techniques to be used to deal with stress, MBSR participants were learning a more general mode of being that could be enormously helpful in relating to difficult experience. Another shift that Segal and colleagues came to see as critical from their original treatment program was the role of the facilitator—they had to shift from being therapists, who felt responsible to help patients solve their problems, to being instructors, who left the responsibility with the patients themselves and saw their role as empowering patients to relate mindfully to their experience on a moment-by-moment basis. With these significant changes they were able to revise the Attentional Control Training program into what became the MBCT program.

MBCT, developed specifically to teach patients in remission from recurrent major depression to become aware of and relate differently to bodily sensations, thoughts, and mood states, integrates aspects of CBT for acute depression with key components of MBSR. It is different from basic CBT in that there is little explicit emphasis in MBCT in changing the content or changing the meaning of thoughts (Baer, 2006). Rather, MBCT helps participants relate to thoughts in a different way, as "mental events" rather than particular aspects of the self or as true reflections of reality (Teasdale et al., 2000). The core skill that is taught in MBCT is mindfulness, which translates into an ability, at times of potential relapse, to recognize and disengage from mind states characterized by self-perpetuating patterns of ruminative, negative thought (Davidson et al., 2003). While MBCT was originally designed to prevent relapse in people who had recovered from unipolar depression, it is now being used in the treatment of mood disorders in general, including populations with bipolar disorder and treatment-resistant depression (Baer, 2006).

Like MBSR, MBCT is designed as an eight-week group program, but whereas MBSR usually accommodates larger groups of 20 to 40 participants, ideally for MBCT there are 8 to 15 patients per group. The sessions include guided mindfulness practices (such as body scan, sitting meditation, yoga), inquiry into the patients' experience of these practices, as well as teaching/discussion of cognitive-behavioral skills. As in MBSR, home practice with guided audio recordings is an integral part of the program, and participants are asked to practice for 45 minutes daily. MBCT program participants learn to recognize habitual and unhelpful reactivity to difficult experiences and learn instead to bring an interested, accepting, and nonjudgmental attitude to all experience, including difficult sensations, emotions, thoughts, and behavior.

MBCT varies from MBSR in significant ways. In contrast to MBSR, there is a more specific emphasis in MBCT on depression and the particular patterns of negative thinking that affect people with depression. There is also an explicit focus on turning toward low mood and negative thoughts early in the program so that participants are able to gain experience with recognizing these symptoms and confidence in their ability to respond skillfully (Davidson et al., 2003). Participants also work on developing RP action plans. Another difference between MBSR and MBCT is that the MBCT instructor is required to be a trained psychotherapist.

Dialectical Behavior Therapy

DBT evolved out of Linehan's (1993) efforts to create a treatment for suicidal women with borderline personality disorders. Initially, Linehan was interested in investigating whether CBT could prove helpful for individuals whose suicidality was in response to extremely painful problems. Linehan and her research team encountered problems with the use of CBT in this population, including clients feeling invalidated with CBT's focus on changing and clients becoming angry and dropping out. They also found that the volume and severity of the problems presented by these women made the standard CBT format impossible to use. Linehan and her colleagues (1999) made significant changes to the standard CBT by incorporating mindfulness and an acceptance-based strategy into the change-based strategies of CBT. The dialectical strategy allowed the weaving together of acceptance and change.

DBT is a yearlong multimodal program that includes weekly individual therapy and skills training group sessions. The skills training group sessions include four modules: core mindfulness, interpersonal effectiveness, emotion regulation, and distress tolerance skills. In individual therapy sessions, clients work on applying skills learned in the group to their daily lives (Baer, 2006). In DBT mindfulness is taught through shorter, less formal mindfulness exercises rather than the extended meditations used in MBSR and MBCT. Also in contrast to MBSR and MBCT, DBT therapists do not necessarily have to have an ongoing mindfulness practice. However, the therapists do need to have a clear understanding of the mindfulness exercises they teach. As in MBSR and MBCT, group discussion immediately after the mindfulness exercises provide the opportunity to address obstacles and problems and further clarify what mindfulness is and how it can be of benefit. The development of mindfulness and awareness are crucial to the next modules of the DBT skills training. Observing, identifying, and labeling emotions are essential components of emotion regulation. Clients are taught how to experience emotions as they occur without judging them or trying to suppress or change them. The distress tolerance module emphasizes acceptance of reality, even when it is unpleasant and difficult, and willingness to experience life as it is in each moment.

Acceptance and Commitment Therapy

ACT is another intervention that uses mindfulness and acceptance strategies along with commitment and behavior change strategies to increase psychological flexibility to treat a wide range of conditions including anxiety, depression, obsessive-compulsive disorder (OCD), and chronic pain. ACT was founded by Hayes, Strosahl, and Wilson (1999) and is a particular orientation to individual psychotherapy rather than a group intervention. The goal of ACT therapy is psychological flexibility, defined as the capacity to accept whatever each situation or moment brings and, when possible, to choose to work toward change in the direction of one's closely held beliefs. A central concept of ACT is experiential avoidance, defined as the unwillingness to experience negative internal phenomena. According to the theoretical tenets of ACT, psychopathology is related to the counterproductive attempts to avoid negative internal experiences by engaging in behaviors such as substance abuse, binge eating, or avoidance of people, places, and things (Beck, 1976). ACT teaches patients psychological flexibility, which includes willingness to experience the present moment and to act in accordance with one's values. In order to teach this psychological flexibility ACT incorporates a number of different mindfulness exercises (Hayes et al., 1999). As in DBT, the mindfulness exercises are shorter and less formal than the practices taught in MBSR and MBCT. There are no specific recommendations that therapists using ACT need to have an ongoing mindfulness practice.

Other Mindfulness Programs Adapted for Specific Disorders

Other MBIs have been developed for working with specific populations. For instance, Mindfulness-Based Relapse Prevention (MBRP), created for populations with substance abuse disorders, is a group-based psychosocial program that integrates evidence-based practices from MBIs and cognitive-behavioral RP approaches (Bowen, Chawla, & Marlatt, 2011). Mindfulness-Based Eating Awareness Training (MB-EAT) developed for use with populations with a range of eating disorders, is a group program that is structured to introduce elements of mindfulness meditation practice, mindful eating, self-awareness, and self-acceptance (Kristeller & Wolever, 2010). Mindfulness-Based Art Therapy (MBAT) is another psychosocial group intervention that integrates mindfulness meditation skills and aspects of art therapy in order to reduce psychological distress in cancer patients (Monti et al., 2013). A program has been developed for working with people with attention deficit hyperactivity disorder, the Mindful Awareness Program (MAP for ADHD) that includes mindfulness practices tailored for this population (Zylowska, 2012). A trauma-informed MBSR program has been developed for working with people with posttraumatic stress disorder (PTSD.; Kelly & Garland, 2016; Magyari, 2016). All of these adapted MBIs include as core components a range of meditation practices including breath awareness and body-centered practices found in both MBSR and MBCT with the addition of specific practices geared for the target population. Clinicians teaching mindfulness to people with the specific disorders need to have expertise in their respective fields as well as training in mindfulness.

Research Evidence of the Efficacy of MBIs

One of the first studies published on MBSR by Kabat-Zinn and colleagues (1992) demonstrated that participants with generalized anxiety or panic disorders experienced clinically and statistically significant improvements in symptoms of anxiety and panic after completing an eight-week MBSR program. There were significant reductions in Hamilton and Beck Anxiety and Depression scores postintervention and at three-month follow-up. A three-year follow-up study of the same group of participants showed maintenance of the gains obtained in the original study on the Hamilton and Beck Anxiety scales as well as on their respective Depression scales (Miller, Fletcher, & Kabat-Zinn, 1995).

Other studies also demonstrate that participating in an eight-week MBSR program leads to statistically significant improvements in mental health for people with various medical illnesses as well as for those specifically with anxiety and mood disorders (Bohlmeijer, Prenger, Taal, & Cuijpers, 2010; Grossman, Niemann, Schmidt, & Walach, 2004; Hazlett-Stevens, 2012; Hoffman et al., 2010; Vøllestad, Sivertsen, & Nielsen, 2011). A study of MBSR for veterans with PTSD used a randomized control design with an active control condition of the same time duration. Participants were randomized to MBSR or present-centered group therapy and completed pre–post measures of PTSD symptom severity, depressive symptoms, health-related quality of life (HRQOL), and mindfulness. Study results demonstrate that participants in the MBSR group experienced a greater decrease in PTSD symptom severity than those in the active control group. Participants in the MBSR group also had clinically meaningful changes in mental component of HRQOL (Kearney, McDermott, Malte, Martinez, & Simpson, 2013).

A study investigated the effects of MBSR training on emotional reactivity and regulation of negative self-beliefs among adults with social anxiety disorder (Goldin & Gross, 2010). Participants completed two attention tasks before and after participating in an eight-week MBSR program. After the program, participants displayed lower levels of negative emotion, decreased amygdala activity, and increased levels of activity in areas of the brain associated with attentional deployment. Another study demonstrated that MBSR helps individuals reduce cognitive rumination in patients with depression (Ramel, Goldin, Carmona, & McQuaid, 2004).

A recent systematic review of studies assessing the effects of participating in MBSR on brain function and structure demonstrates that there are functional and structural changes in the brain that are consistent with improved attentional skills and emotion regulation (Gotink, Meijboom, Vernooij, Smits, & Hunink, 2016). The prefrontal cortex, the cingulate cortex, the insula, and the hippocampus show increased activity, connectivity, and volume. Additionally, the amygdala shows decreased functional activity, improved functional connectivity with the prefrontal cortex, and earlier deactivation after exposure to emotional stimuli (Holzel et al., 2010).

A multicenter, randomized control trial of MBCT with 145 participants found that MBCT significantly reduced the risk of relapse/recurrence in patients with three or more episodes of depression (Teasdale et al., 2000). Other studies also replicated these findings (Galante, Iribarren, & Pearce, 2013; Ma & Teasdale, 2004; Piet & Hougaard, 2011). While MBCT was originally designed for patients with recurrent major depressions who were in remission, there is some data that demonstrates its efficacy for other populations. One study that examined MBCT in patients with treatment-resistant depression found that even patients who were currently in a depressive phase were able to complete and benefit from the program (Kenny & Williams, 2007). This analysis was only conducted on patients who were symptomatic at the start of the MBCT program with a Beck Depression Inventory score greater than 10 and met *Diagnostic and Statistical Manual of Mental Disorders* (fourth edition) criteria for either major depressive disorder or bipolar affective disorder in the depressed phase. MBCT was effective in significantly reducing levels of depression, even in those who started with a more severe pattern, including suicidal depression.

A study of MBCT for people with bipolar disorder that used a randomized control trial design found that while MBCT did not lead to significant reductions in time to depressive or hypo/manic relapse, total number of episodes, or mood symptom severity at 12-month follow-up, there was some evidence for an effect on anxiety symptoms. This finding suggests a potential role of MBCT in reducing anxiety comorbid with bipolar disorder (Perich, Manicavasagar, Mitchell, Ball, & Hadzi-Pavlovic, 2013).

Studies have demonstrated the efficacy of DBT in reducing severe depressive symptoms, suicidal or self-harming behaviors, and hospitalizations compared to treatment as usual for patients with borderline personality disorder (Carter, Willcox, Lewin, Conrad, & Bendit, 2010; Linehan et al., 1999; Linehan, McDavid, Brown, Sayrs, & Gallop, 2008; Turner, Austin, & Chapman, 2014). There is also empirical support for the use of ACT for certain psychiatric disorders, including serious mental illness. Bach and Hayes found that a four-session ACT intervention with treatment as usual with inpatients reporting hallucinations or delusional beliefs was associated with decreased probability of rehospitalization at follow-up compared to the rehospitalization rates of patients who only received treatment as usual (Bach & Hayes, 2002). ACT has also been shown to be effective in the treatment of OCD (Twohig et al., 2010). Eight sessions of ACT resulted in clinically significant reductions in OCD severity and reduced depression and led to improvements in quality of life.

With respect to other MBIs, there have been fewer research studies but the evidence is encouraging. For instance, MBRP appears to provide long-term positive outcomes for participants with substance abuse disorders. In one study that compared MBRP to cognitive-based RP and treatment as usual, both MBRP and RP participants reported significantly lower risk of substance abuse or heavy drinking and, for those who used substances, significantly fewer days of substance use and heavy drinking at the six-month follow-up, compared to treatment as usual. At 12-month follow-up, MBRP offered added benefit over RP and treatment and usual in reducing drug use and heavy drinking (Bowen et al., 2014).

MB-EAT has been shown to be effective in treating compulsive eating patterns associated with binge eating disorders. In a clinical trial, participants were randomized to MB-EAT, a psychoeducation treatment (PE) or a wait-list group. Participants in the MB-EAT and PE group saw improvements in binge eating behavior and depression compared to the wait-list group (Kristeller & Wolever, 2010).

Research on MBAT has shown that participating in an eight-week program demonstrated significant decreases in psychological distress compared to an active control group in women with cancer (Monti et al., 2013). An magnetic resonance imaging study of a subset of women from the same MBAT study showed that the MBAT program was associated with significant changes in cerebral blood flow, which correlated with decreased anxiety after the program (Monti et al., 2012).

Research on Trauma Informed-MBSR demonstrated that participating in an eight-week program was associated with statistically and clinically significant decreases in PTSD and depressive symptoms in female survivors of interpersonal violence (Kelly & Garland, 2016).

The evidence base for MBIs also includes several recent meta-analytic reviews. One meta-analysis of 39 studies totaling 1,140 participants receiving MBIs for a range of conditions, including both psychiatric and medical conditions, examined treatment effect sizes. The majority of the interventions were MBSR or MBCT; however, there were a few studies with other MBIs included (DBT and MAPs for ADHD; Grossman et al., 2004). The meta-analysis found that MBIs were moderately effective for improving anxiety (Hedges's g = 0.63) and mood symptoms (Hedges's g = 0.59) from pre- to-posttreatment in the overall sample. In patients with anxiety and mood disorders, the interventions were associated with effect sizes (Hedges's g) of 0.97 and 0.95 for improving anxiety and mood symptoms, respectively. The authors conclude that these effect sizes were robust, were unrelated to publication year or number of treatment sessions, and were maintained over follow-up.

Another meta-analysis identified eight systematic reviews focusing specifically on the use of MBIs for depression (Klainin-Yobas, Cho, & Creedy, 2012). This meta-analysis found a positive pooled effect of MBIs (MBSR, MBCT, or DBT) either alone or in combination with usual care or medication, primarily compared to treatment as usual. The review concluded that MBIs are efficacious for alleviating depressive symptoms in adults with mental disorders.

Another comprehensive meta-analysis reviewed 209 studies (with a total of 12,145 participants) of MBIs, including MBSR and MBCT (Khoury et al., 2013). The authors used meta-analytic validity measures in order to clarify some inconsistencies concerning the therapeutic value and effect sizes of MBIs. They divided studies according to the methodological design. Within each of the groups, studies were then sorted in an ascending manner: according to the target population (i.e., type of participants), according to the implemented intervention, and according to the comparison group. The meta-analysis found that when investigating pre–post and wait-list controlled studies separately, effect sizes associated with MBIs were larger when treating psychological disorders and smaller when treating physical or medical conditions. More specifically, mindfulness-based training showed large and clinically significant effects in treating anxiety and depression, and the gains were maintained at follow-up. Among psychological disorders, anxiety disorders showed the largest effect sizes, followed by depression. These effects were even larger when only measures corresponding to the target disorder were included (e.g., only anxiety measures when the treatment targeted an anxiety disorder). Regarding study design and effect sizes, the results showed that mindfulness training is moderately effective in pre–post studies. When compared to some other active treatments (including psychoeducation, supportive therapy, relaxation, imagery, and art therapy), the effect sizes were small to moderate, suggesting the superiority of mindfulness training.

Conclusion

MBIs show promise in the treatment of a number of psychiatric disorders. MBSR and MBCT have been shown to be effective in the treatment of anxiety and depression. DBT has been shown to be effective in the treatment of borderline personality disorder and ACT effective in the treatment of OCD. New MBIs are being developed to work specifically with populations suffering with PTSD, eating disorders, addictions, and ADHD. While research in the field of MBIs is promising, more randomized studies with active controls are required to examine the specific effects of mindfulness training and potential mechanisms involved. Future research holds tremendous potential for uncovering more about the neurophysiological processes of mindfulness meditation and the benefits of mindfulness practice on the brain and on health.

REFERENCES

Baer, R. (Ed.). (2006). *Mindfulness-based treatment approaches: Clinician's guide to evidence base and applications.* Amsterdam: Elsevier.

Bach, P., & Hayes, S. C. (2002). The use of acceptance and commitment therapy to prevent the rehospitalization of psychotic patients: a randomized controlled trial. *Journal of Consultative and Clinical Psychology, 70*(5), 1129–1139.

Beck, A. T. (1976). *Cognitive therapy and the emotional disorders.* New York: International Universities Press.

Beck, A. T., Rush, A. J., Shaw, B. F., & Emery, G. (1979). *Cognitive therapy for depression.* New York: Guilford Press.

Bohlmeijer, E., Prenger, R., Taal, E., & Cuijpers, P. (2010). The effects of Mindfulness-Based Stress Reduction therapy on mental health of adults with a chronic medical disease: A meta-analysis. *Journal of Psychosomatic Research, 68*(6), 539–544.

Bowen, S., Chawla, N., & Marlatt, A. (2011). *Mindfulness-based relapse prevention for addictive behaviors: A clinician's guide.* New York: Guilford Press.

Bowen, S., Witkiewitz, K., Clifasefi, S. L., Grow, J., Chawla, N., Hsu, et al. (2014). Relative efficacy of mindfulness-based relapse prevention, standard relapse prevention, and treatment as usual for substance use disorders: A randomized trial. *JAMA Psychiatry, 71*(5), 547–556.

Britton, W. (2016). Scientific literacy as a foundational competency for teachers of mindfulness-based interventions. In D. McCown, D. Reibel, & M. Micozzi (Eds.), *Resources for teaching mindfulness: An international handbook* (pp. 93–120). New York: Springer.

Carter, G. L., Willcox, C. H., Lewin, T. J., Conrad, A. M., & Bendit, N. (2010). Hunter DBT project: Randomized controlled trial of dialectical behavior therapy in women with borderline personality disorder. *The Australian and New Zealand Journal of Psychiatry, 44*(2), 162–173.

Davidson, R. J., Kabat-Zinn, J., Schumacher, J., Rosenkranz, M., Muller, D., Santorelli, S. F., et al. (2003). Alterations in brain and immune function produced by mindfulness meditation. *Psychosomatic Medicine, 65*(4), 564–570.

Farb, N. A., Anderson, A. K., Mayberg, H., Bean, J., McKeon, D., & Segal, Z. V. (2010). Minding one's emotions: Mindfulness training alters the neural expression of sadness. *Emotion, 10*(1), 25–33.

Farb, N. A., Anderson, A. K., & Segal, Z. V. (2012). The mindfulness brain and emotion regulation in mood disorder. *Canadian Journal of Psychiatry, 57*(2), 70–77.

Galante, J., Iribarren, S. J., & Pearce, P. F. (2013). Effects of Mindfulness-Based Cognitive Therapy on mental disorders: A systematic review and meta-analysis of randomised controlled trials. *Journal of Research in Nursing, 18*(2), 133–155.

Goldin, P. R., & Gross, J. J. (2010). Effects of Mindfulness-Based Stress Reduction (MBSR) on emotion regulation in social anxiety disorder. *Emotion, 10*(1), 83–91.

Gonzales-Garcia, M., Borras, X., Lopez, J., & McNeil, K. (2016). Mindfulness-Based Cognitive Therapy application for people living with chronic disease: The case of HIV. In S. Eisendrath (Ed.), *Mindfulness-Based Cognitive Therapy* (pp. 83–103). New York: Springer International.

Gotink, R., Meijboom, R., Vernooij, M., Smits, M., & Hunink, M. (2016). 8-week Mindfulness-Based Stress Reduction induces brain changes similar to traditional long-term meditation practice—a systematic review. *Brain and Cognition, 108*, 32–41.

Grossman, P., Niemann, L., Schmidt, S., & Walach, H. (2004). Mindfulness-Based Stress Reduction and health benefits: A meta-analysis. *Journal of Psychosomatic Research, 57*(1), 35–43.

Hayes, S. C., Strosahl, K. D., & Wilson, K. G. (1999). *Acceptance and Commitment Therapy: An experiential approach to behavior change.* New York: Guilford Press.

Hazlett-Stevens, H. (2012). Mindfulness-Based Stress Reduction for comorbid anxiety and depression: Case report and clinical considerations. *Journal of Nervous and Mental Disorders, 200*(11), 999–1003.

Hoffman, S., Sawyer, T., Witt, A., & Oh, D. (2010). The effect of mindfulness-based therapy on anxiety and depression: A meta-analytic review. *Journal of Consulting and Clinical Psychology, 78*(2), 169–183.

Holzel, B., Carmody, J., Evans, K., Hoge, E. A., Dusek, J. A., Morgan, L., et al. (2010). Stress reduction correlates with structural changes in the amygdala. *Social Cognitive and Affective Neuroscience, 5*, 11–17.

Hölzel, B. K., Lazar, S. W., Gard, T., Schuman-Olivier, Z., & Ott, U. (2011). How does mindfulness meditation work? Proposing mechanisms of action from a conceptual and neural perspective. *Perspectives on Psychological Science, 6*(6), 537–559.

Kabat-Zinn, J. (1990). *Full catastrophe living.* New York: Dell.

Kabat-Zinn, J., Massion, A., Kristeller, J., Peterson, L. G., Fletcher, K. E., Pbert, L., et al. (1992). Effectiveness of a Meditation-Based Stress Reduction program in the treatment of anxiety disorders. *American Journal of Psychology, 149*, 936–943.

Kearney, D. J., McDermott, K., Malte, C., Martinez, M., & Simpson, T. L. (2013). Effects of participation in a mindfulness program for veterans with posttraumatic stress disorder: A randomized controlled pilot study. *Journal of Clinical Psychology, 69*, 14–27.

Kelly, A., & Garland, E. L. (2016). Trauma-informed Mindfulness-Based Stress Reduction for female survivors of interpersonal violence: Results from a stage I RCT. *Journal of Clinical Psychology, 72*, 311–328. doi:10.1002/jclp.22273

Kenny, M. A., & Williams, J. M. (2007). Treatment-resistant depressed patients show a good response to Mindfulness-Based Cognitive Therapy. *Behaviour Research and Therapy, 45*(3), 617–625.

Khoury, B., Lecomta, T., Fortina, G., Masse, M., Therien, P., & Bouchard, V. (2013). Mindfulness-based therapy: A comprehensive meta-analysis. *Clinical Psychology Review, 33*(6), 763–771.

Klainin-Yobas, P., Cho, M. A., & Creedy, D. (2012). Efficacy of mindfulness-based interventions on depressive symptoms among people with mental disorders: A meta-analysis. *International Journal of Nursing Studies, 49*(1), 109–121.

Kristeller, J., & Wolever, R. (2010). Mindfulness-based eating awareness training for treating binge eating disorder: The conceptual foundation. *Eating Disorders, 19*(1), 49–61.

Lazar, S. W., Kerr, C. E., Wasserman, R. H., Gray, J. R., Greve, D. N., Treadway, M. T., et al. (2005). Meditation experience is associated with increased cortical thickness. *NeuroReport, 16*(17), 1893–1897.

Linehan, M. M. (1993). *Cognitive-behavioral treatment of borderline personality disorder*. New York: Guilford Press.

Linehan, M., McDavid, J. D., Brown, M. Z., Sayrs, J. H., & Gallop, R. J. (2008). Olanzapine plus dialectical behavior therapy for women with high irritability who meet criteria for borderline personality disorder: A double-blind, placebo-controlled pilot study. *Journal of Clinical Psychiatry, 69*(6), 999–1005.

Linehan, M., Schmidt, H., Dimeff, L. A., Kanter, J. W., Craft, J. C., Comtois, K., & Recknor, K. L. (1999). Dialectical Behavior Therapy for patients with borderline personality disorder and drug-dependence. *American Journal of Addiction, 8*, 279–292.

Ma, S. H., & Teasdale, J. D. (2004). Mindfulness-Based Cognitive Therapy for depression: Replication and exploration of differential relapse prevention effects. *Journal of Consulting and Clinical Psychology, 72*, 31–40.

Magyari, T. (2016). Teaching individuals with traumatic stress. In D. McCown, D. Reibel, & M. Micozzi (Eds.), *Resources for teaching mindfulness: An international handbook* (pp. 339–358). New York: Springer.

McCown, D., Reibel, D., & Micozzi, M. (2010). *Teaching mindfulness: A practical guide for clinicians and educators*. New York: Springer.

Miller, J., Fletcher, K., & Kabat-Zinn, K. (1995). Three-year follow-up and clinical implications of a Mindfulness Meditation-Based Stress Reduction intervention in the treatment of anxiety disorders. *General Hospital Psychiatry, 17*(3), 192–200.

Monti, D. A., Kash, K. M., Kunkel, E. J., Brainard, G., Wintering, N., Moss, A. S., et al. (2012). Changes in cerebral blood flow and anxiety associated with an 8-week mindfulness programme in women with breast cancer. *Stress and Health, 28*(5), 397–407.

Monti, D. A., Kash, K. M., Kunkel, E. J., Moss, A., Mathews, M., Brainard, G., et al. (2013). Psychosocial benefits of a novel mindfulness intervention versus standard support in distressed women with breast cancer. *Psycho-Oncology, 22*(11), 2565–2575.

National Institute of Mental Health. (n.d.). Transforming and understanding the treatment of mental illness. Retrieved from https://www.nimh.nih.gov/health/statistics/prevalence/any-mental-illness-ami-among-us-adults.shtml

Perich, T., Manicavasagar, V., Mitchell, P. B., Ball. J. R., & Hadzi-Pavlovic, D. (2013). A randomized controlled trial of Mindfulness-Based Cognitive Therapy for bipolar disorder. *Acta Psychiatrica Scandinavica, 127*(5), 333–343.

Piet, J., & Hougaard, E. (2011). The effect of Mindfulness-Based Cognitive Therapy for prevention of relapse in recurrent major depressive disorder: A systematic review and meta-analysis. *Clinical Psychology Review, 31*(6), 1032–1040.

Ramel, W., Goldin, P. R., Carmona, P. E., & McQuaid, J. R. (2004). The effects of mindfulness meditation on cognitive processes and affect in patients with past depression. *Cognitive Therapy and Research, 28*, 433–455.

Segal, Z. V., Williams, J. M. G., & Teasdale, J. D. (2013). *Mindfulness-Based Cognitive Therapy for depression: Second Edition.* New York: Guilford Press.

Shapiro, S., Carlson, L., Astin, J., & Freedman, B. (2006). Mechanisms of mindfulness. *Journal of Clinical Psychology, 62*, 373–386.

Teasdale, J. D., Segal, Z. V., & Williams, J. M. G., Ridgeway, V. A., Soulsby, J. M., & Lau, M. A. (2000). Prevention of relapse/recurrence in major depression by Mindfulness-Based Cognitive Therapy. *Journal of Consulting and Clinical Psychology, 68*(4), 615–623.

Turner, B. J., Austin, S. B., & Chapman, A. L. (2014). Treating nonsuicidal self-injury: A systematic review of psychological and pharmacological interventions. *Canadian Journal of Psychiatry, 59*(11), 576–585.

Twohig, M. P., Hayes, S. C., Plub, J. C., Pruitt, L. D., Collins, A. B., Hazlett-Stevents, H., & Woidneck, M. R. (2010). A randomized clinical trial of Acceptance and Commitment Therapy versus progressive relaxation training for obsessive-compulsive disorder. *Journal of Consulting and Clinical Psychology, 78*(5), 705–716.

Vago, D. R., & Silbersweig, D. A. (2012). Self-awareness, self-regulation, and self-transcendence (S-ART): A framework for understanding the neurobiological mechanisms of mindfulness. *Frontiers in Human Neuroscience, 2012. 6*, 296. doi:10.3389/fnhum.2012.00296

Vøllestad, J., Sivertsen, B., & Nielsen, G. H. (2011). Mindfulness-Based Stress Reduction for patients with anxiety disorders: Evaluation in a randomized controlled trial. *Behaviour Research and Therapy, 49*(4), 281–288.

World Health Organization. (2012). Depression fact sheet. Retrieved from http://www.who.int/mediacentre/factsheets/fs369/

Zylowska, L. (2012). *Mindfulness prescriptions for adult ADHD.* Boston: Trumpeter.

13

Neuromodulation in Psychiatric Disorders

CHRISTINA HERRING

> **Key Points**
>
> - Neuromodulation refers to the science of electrical, chemical, and mechanical interventions changing the nervous system.
> - Quantitative electroencephalogram (qEEG) is the transformation of the EEG by spectral analysis in which the amount of electrical activity at a particular frequency is determined and compared against a normative data base.
> - Repetitive transcranial magnetic stimulation (rTMS) is a system of delivering multiple pulses within a short time period that induce changes that outlast the stimulation period.
> - Operant conditioning involves providing a reward to increase the probability of a certain behavior.
> - Neurofeedback involves recording, analyzing, and presenting results of qEEG analyses in near real time to patients in order to promote changes in brain electrical activity.

Introduction

Neuromodulation has been succinctly defined by Krames, Peckham, Rezai, and Aboelsaad (2009) as "technology impacting on the neural interface." It is the science of how electrical, chemical, and mechanical interventions can change the nervous system. The treatment of psychiatric disorders has been dominated by psychopharmacology for the past 50 years. The use of chemical substances began in 1840 with the discovery of general anesthesia (nitrous oxide, ether, and chloroform). Freud (1884) was aware of the stimulating effects of cocaine on the nervous system and wrote about its antidepressant effects. He later abandoned its use because of addicting properties. Freud mistrusted psychoactive drugs but predicted that many of the psychological symptoms he treated with psychoanalysis would someday be treated with chemical substances (Jones, 1953).

The chemical treatment of psychiatric disorders, especially depression, has been based on the monoamine theory, which suggests that disturbances in serotonin, norepinephrine, and dopamine transmission in the central nervous system cause psychiatric symptoms. In the treatment of depression, certain antidepressant drugs target symptom-specific neurotransmitters (Kropotov, 2009). In the same vein, it is postulated that children with attention deficit hyperactivity disorder (ADHD) have too much or too little of certain neurotransmitters so that treating with stimulant medications can normalize the neurotransmitters and change their behaviors (Kropotov, 2009).

Although antidepressant medication has revolutionized the treatment of depression, in the STAR*D study of over 3,000 patients with untreated depression, remission rates were 36.8% per single treatment step (selective serotonin reuptake inhibitor [SSRI]) and 33% treatment-resistance rate after four cumulative steps (Rush et al., 2006). A similar study investigating the effects of conventional treatment in ADHD (the NIMH-MFA trial) showed a lack of long-term effects for stimulant medication, multicomponent behavior therapy, and combined treatment beyond two years (Molina et al., 2009). These two studies demonstrate that current conventional treatment with its emphasis on psychopharmacology for both disorders is limited and there is a need for a more personalized approach. Personalized medicine, which is defined as prescribing the right treatment for the right person at the right time, has its roots in current immunotherapy in cancer treatment. Personalized medicine in psychiatry is in its infancy.

Mapping the Brain: qEEG

There has been knowledge about the electrical activity of the brain since 1928 when Hans Berger (Berger, 1929) first measured the human EEG and found it was composed of two fundamental wave forms: the larger 100 msec alpha waves that were correlated with mental activity and the smaller 35 msec beta waves that were associated with the metabolic activities of cortical tissue. Edgar Douglas Adrian, an English neurophysiologist, confirmed Berger's findings (Adrian & Yamagiwa, 1935) and was able to map sensory areas of the cerebral cortex, which was named the homunculus; his presentation is still considered an accurate depiction of the sensory areas of the cortex. Little use was made of these discoveries except as a diagnostic tool, since the central nervous system was regarded as unchangeable except through chemical intervention. The EEG is defined as the difference between two different recording locations plotted over time; it is generated by the synchronous activity of postsynaptic inhibitory and excitatory potentials. The EEG measures waveforms that are recorded along the scalp and therefore represent summed activity from large populations of neurons. This is because the electric field of each active source of the brain spreads in all directions and is registered in every electrode. Although Berger only described alpha and beta waves, five major brain waves have been distinguished by their frequency ranges: delta (.5–4 Hz), theta (4–7 Hz), alpha (8–12 Hz), beta (13–30 Hz), and gamma (above 30 Hz). Delta waves are primarily associated with deep sleep. Theta waves appear when wakefulness slips into drowsiness and is related to level of arousal. In older children and adults, large amounts of theta are associated with depression. Alpha waves indicate wakeful relaxation with closed eyes but are suppressed in eye opening. Beta waves are detected mostly over the frontal and central regions and are associated with active thinking and attention. Gamma waves are related to sensory processing and long-term memory (Thompson & Thompson, 2003). The EEG has limited anatomical specificity when compared with other functional brain imaging techniques such as functional magnetic resonance imaging (fMRI) but its time resolution is much higher than fMRI or positron emission tomography (PET). Although the EEG is a personalized recording of a subject's brain activity, the interpretation has been quite subjective and its use limited.

Not until the EEG was digitized by Ross Adey and his colleagues at the University of California in Los Angeles (UCLA) in the 1960s did the EEG become a tool for assessing brain function beyond its use for epilepsy and level of consciousness (Arns, de Ridder, Strehl, Breteler, & Coenen, 2009). The conventional EEG was submitted to a spectral analysis in which the amount of electrical activity occurring at a particular frequency could be determined and compared against a normative data base. The development of the quantitative (q) EEG has created a tool for neuromodulation techniques. The transformation of the EEG to the qEEG allows precise measurement of frequencies, amplitudes, and locations and then permits comparisons between an individual patient and a reference group (Thompson & Thompson, 2003). The qEEG has provided psychiatry with its first inroad into personalized medicine.

The qEEG and Depression

A key problem in the diagnosis of depression is that existing classification systems are solely based on the subjective descriptions of symptoms, and most clinicians use the *Diagnostic and Statistical Manual of Mental Disorders* (fifth edition [DSM-V]; American Psychiatric Association, 2013) as a resource for categorizing these symptoms. No biological feature separates one subtype from another, and there is no sure way to predict which antidepressant will produce remission. Early studies examined resting cerebral glucose metabolism and blood flow with PET scans in patients with depression and found decreased prefrontal activity. The decreased activity was correlated with severity of depression and was reversed with the remission of depressive symptoms (Pizzagalli, Oakes, & Davidson, 2003). Researchers also found increased alpha power (a marker that is that is inversely related to neural activity) in the left frontal regions of patients who report depression (Davidson, 1998). Since then there have been numerous neuroimaging studies that have shown that depressed mood is associated with abnormal neuronal activation in the medial prefrontal cortex. This area receives input through the anterior nucleus of the thalamus from the hippocampus, amygdala, and mammillary bodies of the hypothalamus. The activity in these areas is mediated mostly by serotonergic innervation from the midbrain raphe nucleus and partly by noradrenergic innervation from the locus ceruleus. It has been further elucidated that depression includes both mood symptoms and elements of the executive functioning system. Therefore the elements of the affective system involved include the orbito-frontal and medial cortical areas and the deficits in the executive system include the anterior cingulate cortex and the corresponding basal ganglia thalamo-cortical loop (Kropotov, 2009).

It has been argued that the use of a combination of indicators such as neuroimaging and qEEG may provide a more reliable diagnosis than observation of clinical symptoms and may have more potential in establishing treatment predictors and indeed selection of treatment. In 1983, a group led by Davidson (Tomarken & Davidson 1994) started publishing pioneering work on frontal alpha asymmetry in depression. The alpha wave is a symmetrical rhythm that originates in the thalamus and is between 8 to 12 Hz (frequency per second). These symmetrical waves are seen in about 90% of people when they close their eyes and are the dominant frequency of the EEG in adulthood. The alpha frequency is thought of as a resting state. The group headed by Davidson found a relative hyperactivation of the right frontal cortex that was not found for the parietal cortex. In 1990 Henriques and Davidson laid a further foundation for the concept of frontal asymmetry in depression in which they considered "approach" and "withdrawal" as the essential basis of asymmetry. The approach system facilitates appetitive behavior and generates a form of positive affect. The withdrawal system facilitates withdrawal from sources of aversive stimulation and generates negative affect. They interpreted the decreased left-sided frontal activation as a deficit in the approach system and thought those patients were more prone to depression given a certain amount of stress. They further suggested that right-sided frontal activation is related to withdrawal-related emotion and psychopathology such as anxiety disorders. The work by Henriques and Davidson thus provides the first qEEG evidence for differences between depressed individuals and the normative data bases.

Neuromodulation and Depression

The first use of neuromodulation was by an Italian neurologist Ugo Cerletti who in 1938 used a device to produce a seizure in subjects suffering from schizophrenia (Endler, 1988). The results were dramatic, and the treatment was extended to patients with depression where the effects were equally dramatic but the side effect was memory loss. Although the use of electroconvulsive therapy has been the gold standard for the treatment of refractory depression, the dramatic effects dissipate within six months. The second attempt at a device used for the treatment of depression occurred at the University of Sheffield in Great Britain in 1985. Barker, Jalinous, and Freeston (1985) developed a transcranial magnetic stimulation (TMS) device and used it to induce a motor-evoked potential by means of applying a TMS pulse over the motor cortex. TMS was used initially in studies on motor conductivity through investigating the temporal aspects and amplitude of the evoked motor responses after stimulating the motor cortex. With the developmental of multiple pulses, researchers were able to induce changes that outlasted the stimulation period. Serendipitously it was found that changes occurred in the mood of several volunteers who were undergoing motor conductivity studies (Wasserman & Lisanby, 2001).

TMS involves the application of short magnetic pulses over the scalp of a patient with the aim of inducing electrical currents in the neurons of the cortex (Spronk et al., 2010). A typical TMS device consists of a stimulator that can generate a strong electrical current and a coil in which the fluctuating electrical current generates magnetic pulses. If the magnetic pulses are delivered in the proximity of a conductive medium (the brain), a secondary current is generated in the conductive material (i.e., a current in the neurons is induced). For TMS to be effective, the magnetic field has to induce currents in the neurons of the cortex. The intensity of the magnetic field that induces this current is referred to as stimulation intensity. This is usually expressed as a percentage of the motor threshold. The minimal output intensity that yields a motor response (moving of the thumb) in at least half of the applied trials is determined to be the motor threshold (MT). In depression protocols, the lowest stimulation intensity used is 80% MT and maximal intensity is 120% MT.

In most TMS protocols, the stimulation is delivered in pulse trains. Trains are delivered in bursts and separated by certain time intervals. This is done for two reasons. First, the effect of TMS pulses is cumulative in the brain and this summation causes an increase in the likelihood of a seizure. Second, the repetitive release of strong electrical pulses causes heating of the electric coil in the TMS device. The intertrain interval allows the device to partially cool.

Once the MT is determined, then the next step is to localize the dorsolateral prefrontal cortex (DLPFC), which is the area determined as the site of abnormal neural circuitry. The motivation behind choosing this brain area stems from studies that have indicated depression is associated with regional brain dysfunction as well as the work of Henriques and Davidson. In most studies, localizing this area has been performed by means of the 5 centimeter rule. From the establishment of the MT, the coil is moved 5 centimeters anteriorly in a sagittal direction (Fitzgerald et al., 2009). This method is somewhat crude because of differences in head size and shape. The most common protocol for the treatment of depression using TMS is 15 sessions (performed five days per week) targeting the left dorsolateral prefrontal cortex. The most common stimulation frequency is 10 Hz. This refers to the number of pulses delivered per second. The 10 Hz pulse is delivered for 4 seconds followed by 26 second of rest until 3,000 pulses are delivered, which occurs in 37½ minutes. Only the Neurostar rTMS device is covered by health insurance in the United States, and all of these treatment parameters are programmed in the Neurostar software.

The precise mechanism for the remission of symptoms using TMS remains unknown, but there are a number of clues. As noted earlier, depressed patients have been shown to have decreased blood flow in certain regions (DLPFC) of the brain. Several neuroimaging studies have demonstrated changes induced by TMS. High-frequency TMS over the left DLPFC of depressed patients induces a local increase in regional cerebral blood flow as indicated by SPECT and fMRI blood-oxygen-level dependent response (Strafella, Paus, Barrett, & Dagher, 2001). Other brain regions have been reported to show a change in regional cerebral blood flow after TMS; these are the ventrolateral prefrontal cortex, right-dominant orbitofrontal cortex, anterior cingulate, left subgenual cingulate, anterior insula, and right putamen (Kito, Fukita, & Koga, 2008). These findings demonstrate specific alterations induced by TMS that are different from those induced by other antidepressant treatments. The TMS-induced effects on neuroanatomical functions are commensurate with known abnormalities in depression. Therefore, one postulated effect of TMS is to change regional blood flow in areas known to be involved in symptoms of depression.

Besides changes in regional blood flow, TMS has been associated with changes in neurotransmitters. As noted earlier, the use of antidepressants in the past 50 years has been based on the monoamine theory of depression; that is, three neurotransmitter systems—serotonin, norepinephrine, and dopamine—are involved in producing depressive symptoms and antidepressant medication is thought to act through enhancement of monoamines. TMS has been investigated as inducing changes in dopamine. Strafella et al. (2001) found an increased dopamine release after high-frequency TMS over the left DLPFC in the ipsilateral nucleus accumbens of healthy subjects by use of PET imaging. This finding suggests that the increased release was exerted through corticostriatal projections from the targeted DLPFC. In a study by Keck and colleagues (2000) a TMS-induced effect on dopamine was found by using intracerebral microdialysis. Here again there were no changes in serotonin or norepinephrine. These two studies would suggest that TMS targets mainly the dopamine system. No antidepressant works directly on the dopamine system. Another mechanism through which TMS targets depressive symptoms might be the modulation of gamma amino butyric acid (GABA) and glutamate. GABA is the main inhibitory transmitter whereas glutamate is the main excitatory transmitter. In a study of depressed patients with a specific focus on the nucleus accumbens (Zangen & Hyodo, 2002), changes in glutamate level were observed after successful treatment of 10 high-frequency TMS sessions. The pretreatment baseline level was related to treatment effects. Those who responded showed lower pretreatment levels of glutamate and higher levels of glutamate after successful treatment. TMS is also known to exert changes in excitability on a neuronal level. High-frequency TMS induces an increase in motor cortex excitability, which is thought to be maintained by a balance of levels of GABA and glutamate (Pascual-Leone et al., 1999). Thus it might be hypothesized that excitability of the motor cortex indirectly affects levels of GABA and glutamate.

Another possible mechanism for the TMS treatment effect in depression is the modulation and release of neurotrophins. Brain-derived neurotropic factor (BDNF) plays a part in the survival of neuronal cells and in synaptic plasticity and connectivity (Bath & Lee, 2006). Abnormal levels of BDNF have been shown in patients with depression, and successful treatment with antidepressants has produced increased levels of BDNF. In a study by Yukimasa (2006), TMS increased levels of BDNF in patients who were successfully treated.

If TMS is a more specific treatment for depression, then is the rate of remission for depression higher than that reported in the STAR*D study? The STAR*D study was conducted on patients who were depressed and had never been treated; studies using TMS for depression are normally conducted on patients with treatment-resistant depression. The definition of treatment-resistant depression has been that a patient has failed to achieve remission using two different antidepressants at therapeutic levels. Therefore, one would expect that remission rates for treatment using TMS might be decreased given the population that is inherent. Further, patients in both kinds of studies include those who have characterological problems such as borderline personality where it is doubtful that antidepressants or TMS would be helpful. Most TMS studies show a remission rate of about 40% in patients who have been termed treatment-resistant. Although this rate is not dramatic, still it presents hope to patients who have been unable to achieve remission by usual treatment.

In studying the patients who do not respond to TMS, we might discover some parameters to consider. Since we are attempting to change brain connectivity, it might be prudent to measure qEEG before prescribing TMS. If we know that alpha asymmetry is a good target for left-sided DLPFC TMS, then obtaining a qEEG would be helpful. Further, in looking at qEEGs of patients who did not respond to TMS, nonresponders showed a slowed alpha peak frequency and increased theta waves (Arns et al., 2009). Another finding was decreased prefrontal cordance in the delta and beta band, which is indicative of a less concordant EEG state possibly reflective of a lower relative perfusion in the underlying cortex. Cordance is a qEEG method that is a measure of regional brain activity. Lower concordance of frontal areas can be a predictor for non-response. Therefore, having a prior qEEG would be a method for screening patients for the appropriateness of TMS as a treatment. Another way to increase the efficacy of TMS would be to use neuro-navigation to determine the target point. Herwig, Padberg, Unger, Spitzer, and Schonfeldt-Lecuona (2001) compared the target area defined by the 5 cm rule with the target defined by DLPFC neuro-navigation. Of the 22 subjects, the targets were the same in only 7. Another study done by Fitzgerald in 2009 separated 52 patients having TMS for those where the target was found using the 5 cm rule and those where the target was found using neuro-navigation, and the result was a significantly higher remission rate in patients whose target was determined by neuro-navigation using fMRI.

All of this research in neuromodulation suggests that TMS as a treatment for depression is effective but would be more effective if other markers were employed in selecting the appropriate candidates for treatment. Since we have knowledge of appropriate markers from the qEEG, it would be imperative that this procedure be done before assigning patients to TMS treatment. Further, the 5 cm rule is quite approximate and does not take into account the shape of the skull. If neuro-navigation was employed to determine the DLPFC, remission rates would increase. The third suggestion would be to think of TMS as a first line rather than a last line of treatment for patients with depression since there are no side effects other than mild headache during treatment, which is easily treated with Tylenol. In areas where TMS is offered as a first line of treatment (the Netherlands, England) remission rates are around 80%.

ADHD and Neurofeedback

ADHD is the most common childhood mental health disorder with an estimated prevalence of 7% to 10% in boys and 3% in girls ages 4 to 11 (DeBeus, Ball, DeBeus, & Harrington, 2004). The causal theory of ADHD involves dopamine transmission. It is hypothesized that there is reduced dopamine in the fronto-meso-limbic system of the left hemisphere, which controls executive functioning (Kropotov, 2009). The core symptoms of ADHD consist of inattention, impulsivity, and hyperactivity, and, according to the DSM-V, there are three primary subtypes: predominantly hyperactive-impulsive type, predominantly inattentive type, and combined type. Methylphenidate blocks the reuptake of the dopamine and amphetamines stabilize dopamine and norepinephrine transporters. Currently, both stimulant medication and behavior therapy are the most often applied and accepted treatments for ADHD but, as noted earlier, the effects of combined treatment with stimulants plus behavior therapy do not endure beyond six months after cessation of medication and therapy. Further, 30% of children either do not respond to stimulant medication or cannot tolerate the side effects (Molina et al., 2009). Therefore, alternative treatment could address both the nonresponse and the limited effects of current treatment.

The evolution of an effective alternative treatment has been dependent on three developments: (a) operant conditioning, (b) qEEG, and (c) the realization of the plasticity of the central nervous system. Thorndike in 1905 was the first to conceptualize operant conditioning by proposing the "Law of Effect," which stated that responses that produce a satisfying effect in a particular situation become more likely to recur while responses that produce discomfort are less likely to recur. B. F. Skinner in 1948 then refined operant condition by stating that providing a reward will increase a behavior while a punishment will decrease a behavior. A reward is defined as any event that follows a specified response that is considered to be desirable and is intended to promote the specified response to occur again under the same conditions. If the consequence of the reward or punishment increases or decreases the probability of the response, the response becomes reinforced. If the reward or punishment achieves the goal, it is called a reinforcer. The timing of the reinforcement of a behavior is crucial to learning because delays as small as a fraction of a second can decrease the strength of the conditioning. The contingent relationship between the behavior and the reinforcement must be evident to the learner.

Neurofeedback, which is a behavior therapy technique to teach self-regulation of brain activity, can be traced back to the 1930s. Early studies demonstrated that the principles of classical conditioning could be applied to EEG parameters. The first successful application of EEG conditioning for clinical effects (i.e., anticonvulsant) was performed by Barry Sterman in the late 1960's and early 1970's (Sterman, Howe, & Macdonald, 1970; Sterman, Macdonald, & Stone, 1974). His work involved training of a certain wave form called sensori-motor rhythm (SMR) in cats. The SMR rhythm is between 12 and 15 Hz and is associated with being attentive but relaxed. Sterman is a sleep researcher who devised the following experiment: he placed 30 cats in cages and connected them to EEG machines. He deprived them of food and then placed them in an experimental chamber that had a lever and an empty bowl. Every time the cat would press the lever, the bowl would fill with milk and chicken broth. The cats began to be conditioned to press the lever when they wanted food. Sterman then introduced the tone. If the cat pressed the lever when the tone was on, no food would be delivered. The cat had to wait until the tone stopped to get the reward. Sterman saw that while the cat was waiting for the tone to stop, it entered a unique state of consciousness: it remained still but alert. Accompanying this state was an EEG reading of 12 to 15 Hz, which he called SMR. Then Sterman took the lever out of the cage and if the cat produced SMR, the cat was fed. By using food as a reward, the cats were trained to produce SMR. The training improved sleep quality in cats, but then Dr. Sterman did something that researchers did not approve of. NASA was testing a rocket fuel called monomethylhydrazine, which caused seizures in astronauts. Sterman decided to use cats to develop a model for inhibiting seizures. He used some of the cats that he had trained to produce SMR and found that those cats did not have seizures when exposed to the rocket fuel while other cats did have seizures. He hypothesized that training astronauts to produce SMR would prevent seizures, which indeed was the first time that neurofeedback was used in humans to prevent seizures.

This training of SMR to prevent seizures was then extended to other disorders. In 1976, Joel Lubar described the application of SMR neurofeedback in a child diagnosed with ADHD and found improvements in hyperactivity and distractibility. SMR rhythm of high alpha occurs most often at Cz (the area on the top of the head localized by measuring the distance between the tragi of the ears). During the same time period Ross Adey and his group at UCLA collected a normative database and transformed EEG data using Fast-Fourier Transform into the qEEG. Subsequently Lubar began using the qEEG as a way to diagnose ADHD and proposed that children with ADHD had an excess of theta waves and decreased beta waves and the Theta-Beta Ratio could differentiate ADHD patients from healthy children. This measure was then applied as a target for neurofeedback where children were taught to decrease the excess theta and increase beta EEG activity at fronto-central locations.

Neurofeedback provides a tool for treating ADHD and is based on three scientific facts (Kropotov, 2009):

1. EEG parameters reflect brain dysfunction in ADHD.
2. Subjects can voluntarily change the state of his or her brain so that changes can be associated with increasing or decreasing a certain parameter.
3. The brain can memorize this new state and hold on to it outside of the place where it was trained.

Neurofeedback is based on protocols derived from the qEEG assessment. Placement of at least 19 electrodes is required, and spectral characteristics of the EEG with eyes open and eyes closed are compared statistically to a normative data base. The statistically significant deviations from normality at spectral or coherence difference curves then define the parameters of the neurofeedback protocol such as the position of the electrodes and the neurofeedback parameter. Coherence is a measure of shared activity at two different locations (Kropotov, 2009). Although the DSM-V describes three groups of patients with ADHD, these groups do not hold up as distinct entities when comparing qEEG profiles. Arns, Gunkelman, Bretteler, and Spronk (2008) have described four subtypes of qEEG deviations in ADHD:

1. Abnormal increase of slow activity centrally or centrally frontally
2. Abnormal increase of frontal midline theta rhythm generated with maximum at Fz within the frequency range of 5.5 to 8 Hz in long bursts (more than 1 second) and increased with task load
3. Abnormal increase of beta activity within 13 to 30 Hz frontally
4. Excess of alpha at posterior, central, or frontal (rare) leads such as abnormal mu-rhythms at C3. Mu is a rhythm similar in waveform to alpha but does not attenuate with eyes open.

These subgroups are some of the first examples of an EEG phenotype in ADHD. The underlying idea is that neuroimaging data such as EEG, fMRI, and PET scans can be considered stable phenotypes that incorporate nature and nurture. The use of phenotypes can predict treatment outcome for medication and/or neurofeedback (Johnstone & Lunt, 2010). This is important in disorders where there is no Mendelian pattern of inheritance and is a step toward personalized medicine in the treatment of ADHD.

Depending on the qEEG findings, neurofeedback protocols are set to reward certain parameters and to inhibit others. For example, we need to define a neurofeedback parameter that we want to train. If the patient had a great deal of slow activity (theta) and not enough fast activity (beta), our task would be to enhance high-frequency and suppress low-frequency activity. The position of the electrodes would be determined by the qEEG, and a ground electrode would be placed on one of the earlobes. The electrodes simply measure the ongoing brain EEG while the computer regularly calculates the neurofeedback parameter and depicts it in some way to the patient. When the parameter is achieved (e.g., increased beta at a certain position), a reward is presented. Usually there are several simultaneous rewards such as visual and auditory and a system of reward points. Depending on the age of the subject, the visual presentation may be moving Pac-man around the board by virtue of producing the right brainwave or changing pictures of the Seven Wonders of the World. Simultaneously auditory rewards are given via headphones of music becoming audible when the correct brainwave occurs. These rewards can be modified for personal taste, but the visual should be interesting but not too interesting. Some practitioners have used movies as a visual reward and found that it is too stimulating. The aim of neurofeedback is to learn, not to entertain.

During the first session, the parameters are placed on automatic to gain an idea of how much of each brainwave is being produced. During the session, which can be 5 minutes with very young children or 10 minutes with adults, the parameters are changed to manual and the conditions for a reward are made more stringent as the training progresses. The second step in the neurofeedback procedure presumes that after each session the results of training are checked by the practitioner. To assess how well the patient controls the parameter, the software company supplies tools for computing "training curves." The training curve is a smoothed dynamic of the parameter during a single session. If the parameter during the training period is statistically different at $p < .05$ from the resting period, then the session is successful. The third step includes the assessment of improvements produced by sequential sessions. Usually around five sessions are required to learn to change the neurofeedback parameter in the desired direction while 20 to 35 additional sessions are required to practice this ability in order to consolidate the skill (Kropotov, 2009). There are a variety of instruments that can be used to assess change in behavior—for example, reports by parents and teachers and school grades.

Since neurofeedback is not the usual treatment for ADHD, the question is whether it is an effective treatment. Currently there are eight published randomized controlled trials that have investigated neurofeedback (Drechsler et al., 2007; Fuchs, Birbaumer, Lutzenberger, Gruzelier, & Kaiser, 2003; Gevensleben et al., 2009; Heinrich, Gevensleben, Freisleder, Moll, & Rothenberger, 2004; Heinrich, Gevensleben, & Strehl et al., 2007; Monastra, Monastra, & George,

2002; Strehl et al., 2006). Seven of the eight demonstrated significant improvements on measures of inattention, hyperactivity, or impulsivity compared to control groups. Meta-analysis in 2009 by Arns et al. incorporated 15 studies ($n = 1,194$) where it was concluded that neurofeedback resulted in large and clinically relevant effect sizes for inattention and impulsivity and a low to medium effect size for hyperactivity. The current controversy regarding the efficacy of neurofeedback in ADHD is centered on the appropriate design standards. Given the fact that neurofeedback is based on operant conditioning principles, it is crucial that the active treatment and planned control condition be in line with principles of learning theory and conditioning principles. It is difficult to design an appropriate control. The advantages of neurofeedback are obvious: it is relatively inexpensive and there are no side effects, but the most important advantage is that changes that occur to normalize the EEG remain. The therapy can be stopped but the skill will remain.

In the Monastra et al. (2002) study, all 100 ADHD children were medicated and 51 children also received neurofeedback. When medication was removed, only the patients who had neurofeedback were able to sustain their improvements. Strehl and colleagues (2006) showed that six-month follow-up scores in impulsivity, inattention, and hyperactivity were improved even further than at the end of treatment. Not only is neurofeedback an effective treatment for ADHD, but the skills learned in neurofeedback remain years after the therapy has ended. Recent research has included fMRI indices of change resulting from neurofeedback. Levesque, Beauregard, and Mensour (2006) demonstrated a normalization of key neural substrates of selective attention and response inhibition as noted in changes in the anterior cingulate cortex, caudate, and substantia nigra as a result of neurofeedback.

Conclusion

The treatment of depression and ADHD has been dominated by the use of psychotropic medication and psychotherapy despite the fact that recent large-scale studies have indicated that one-third of patients are treatment-resistant. The innovation of the qEEG has opened up new possibilities in determining EEG phenotypes that can aid in diagnosis and predict treatment outcome. TMS is an effective treatment for depression and may become more effective with the use of the qEEG to predict which patients will benefit, and the use of neuro-navigation will increase the likelihood of targeting the precise area. Neurofeedback is an effective treatment for ADHD and the effects remain years after the treatment has ended. Overall, these approaches have given psychiatry an inroad into personalized medicine, directing therapies for specific patients and making use of researchers' physiological and psychological findings.

References

Adrian, E. D., & Yamagiwa, D. (1935). The origin of the Berger rhythm. *Brain, 58*, 323–351.

American Psychiatric Association. (2013). *Diagnostic and statistical manual of mental disorders* (5th ed.). Washington, DC: American Psychiatric Publishing.

Arns, M., de Ridder, S., Strehl, U., Breteler, M., & Coenen, A. (2009). Efficacy of neurofeedback treatment in ADHD: The effects on inattention, impulsivity and hyperactivity: A meta-analysis. *Clinical EEG and Neuroscience, 40*(3), 180–189.

Arns, M., Gunkelman, J., Breteler, M., & Spronk, D. (2008). EEG phenotypes predict treatment outcome to stimulants in children with ADHD. *Journal of Integrative Neuroscience, 7*(3), 421–438.

Barker, A.T., Jalinous, R., & Freeston, I. L. (1985). Non-invasive magnetic stimulation of human motor cortex. *The Lancet, 1*(8437), 1106–1107.

Bath, K. G., & Lee, F. S. (2006). Variant BDNF impact on brain structure and function. *Cognitive and Affective Behavioral Neuroscience, 6*(1), 79–85.

Berger, H. (1929). Uber das elektrenkephalogramm des menschen. *Archiv für Psychiatrie und Nervenkrankheiten, 87*, 527–570.

Davidson, R. J. (1998). Anterior electrophysiological asymmetries, emotion, and depression: Conceptual and methodological conundrums. *Psychophysiology, 35*(5), 607–614.

DeBeus, R., Ball, J. D., DeBeus, M. E., & Harrington, R. (2004). Attention training with ADHD children: Preliminary findings in a double-blind placebo-controlled study. *Journal of Neurotherapy, 8*, 145–148.

Drechsler, R., Straub, D., Doehnert, M., Heinrich, H., Steinhausen, H., & Brandeis, D. (2007). Controlled evaluation of a neurofeedback training of slow cortical potentials in children with ADHD. *Behavioral and Brain Functions, 3*, 35.

Endler, N. (1988). The origins of electroconvulsive therapy (ECT). *Convulsive Therapy, 4*(1), 5–23.

Fitzgerald, P. B., Hoy, K., McQueen, S., Maller, J. J., Herring, S., Segrave, R., et al. (2009). A randomized trial of rTMS targeted with MRI based neuro-navigation in treatment-resistant depression. *Neuropsychopharmacology, 34*, 1255–1262.

Freud, S. (1884). Uber coca. *St. Louis Medical Surgery Journal, 47*, 502.

Fuchs, T., Birbaumer, N. Lutzenberger, W., Gruzelier, J. H., & Kaiser, J. (2003). Neurofeedback treatment for attention-deficit/hyperactivity disorder in children: A comparison with methylphenidate. *Applied Psychophysiology and Biofeedback, 28*(1), 1–12.

Gevensleben, H., Holl, B., Albrecht, B., Vogel, C., Schlamp, D., Kratz, O., et al. (2009). Is neurofeedback an efficacious treatment for ADHD? A randomized controlled clinical trial. *Journal of Child Psychology and Psychiatry and Allied Disciplines, 50*(7), 780–789.

Heinrich, H., Gevensleben, H., Freisleder, F. J., Moll, G. H., & Rothenberger, A. (2004). Training of slow cortical potentials in attention-deficit/hyperactivity disorder: Evidence for positive behavioral and neurophysiological effects. *Biological Psychiatry, 55*(7), 772-775.

Heinrich, H., Gevensleben, H., & Strehl, U. (2007). Annotation: Neurofeedback—train your brain to train behavior. *Journal of Child Psychology and Psychiatry, 48,* 3-16.

Henriques, J. B., & Davidson, R. J. (1990). Regional brain electrical asymmetries discriminate between previously depressed and healthy controls. *Journal of Abnormal Psychology, 99*(1), 22-31.

Herwig, U., Padberg, F., Unger, J., Spitzer, M., & Schonfeldt-Lecuona, C. (2001). Transcranial magnetic stimulation in therapy studies: Examination of the reliability of "standard" coil positioning by neuronavigation. *Biological Psychiatry, 50*(1), 58-61.

Johnstone, J., & Lunt, J. (2010). Use of quantitative EEG to predict therapeutic outcome in neuropsychiatric disorders. In R. Coben & J. R. Evans (Eds.), *Neurofeedback and neuromodulation techniques and applications* (pp. 3-23). London: Elsevier.

Jones, E. (1953). *Sigmund Freud: Life and works,* Vol. I. Chapter 6, 250. Basic Books, Inc.: New York.

Krames, E., Peckham, P. H., Rezai, A., & Aboelsaad, F. (2009). That is neuromodulation? In E. Krames, P. H. Peckham, & A. Rezai (Eds.), *Neuromodulation* (Vol. 1, pp. 3-8). London: Elsevier.

Keck, M. E., Sillaber, I., Ebner, K., Welt, T., Toschi, N., Kaehler, S. T., et al. (2000). Repetitive transcranial magnetic stimulation increases the release of dopamine in the mesolimbic and mesostriatal system. *Neuropharmacology, 43*(1), 101-109.

Kito, S., Fukita, K., & Koga, Y. (2008). Changes in regional cerebral blood flow after repetitive transcranial magnetic stimulation of the left dorsolateral prefrontal cortex in treatment-resistant depression. *Journal of Neuropsychiatry and Clinical Neurosciences, 20*(1), 74-80.

Kropotov, Y. (2009). In J. D. Kropotov (Ed.), *Quantitative EEG, event-related potentials and neurotherapy.* London: Elsevier, 450-462, 469-505.

Levesque, J., Beauregard, M., & Mensour, B. (2006). Effects of neurofeedback training on the neural substrates of selective attention in children with attention-deficit/hyperactivity disorder: A functional magnetic resonance imaging study. *Neuroscience Letters, 394,* 216-221.

Molina, B. S., Hinshaw, S. P., Swanson, J. M., Arnold, L. E., Vitiello, B., Jensen, P. S., et al. (2009). The MTA at 8 years: Prospective follow-up of children treated for combined-type ADHD in a multisite study. *Journal of the American Academy of Child and Adolescent Psychiatry, 48*(5), 484-5000.

Monastra, V. J., Monastra, D. M., & George, S. (2002). The effects of stimulant therapy, EEG biofeedback and parenting style on the primary symptoms of attention deficit/hyperactivity disorder. *Applied Psychophysiology and Biofeedback, 27*(4), 231-249.

Pascual-Leone, A., Tarazona, F., Keenan, J., Tormos, J. M., Hamilton, R., & Catala, M. D. (1999). Transcranial magnetic stimulation and neuroplasticity. *Neuropsychologia, 37*(2), 207-217.

Pizzagalli, D. A., Oakes, T. R., & Davidson, R. J. (2003). Coupling of theta activity and glucose metabolism in the human rostral anterior cingulate cortex: An EEG/PET study of normal and depressed subjects. *Psychophysiology, 40,* 939–949.

Rush, A. J., Trivedi, M. H., Wisniewski, S. R., Nierenberg, A. A., Stewart, J. W., Warden, D., et al. (2006). Acute and longer-term outcomes in depressed outpatients requiring one or several treatment steps: A STAR*D report. *American Journal of Psychiatry, 163,* 1905–1917.

Skinner, B. F. (1948). Superstition in the pigeon. *Journal of Experimental Analysis of Behavior, 47,* 261–271.

Spronk, D., Arns, M., & Fitzgerald, P. B. (2010). Repetitive transcranial magnetic stimulation in depression: Protocols, mechanisms and new developments. In R. Coben & J. R. Evans (Eds.), *Neurofeedback and neuromodulation techniques and applications* (pp. 257–318). London: Elsevier.

Sterman, M. B., Howe, R. C., & Macdonald, L. R. (1970). Facilitation of spindle-burst sleep by conditioning of electroencephalographic activity while awake. *Science, 167*(921), 1146–1148.

Sterman, M. B., Macdonald, L. R., & Stone, R. K. (1974). Biofeedback training of the sensorimotor electroencephalogram rhythm in man: Effects on epilepsy. *Epilepsia, 15*(3), 395–416.

Strafella, A. P., Paus, T., Barrett, J., & Dagher, A. (2001). Repetitive transcranial magnetic stimulation of the human prefrontal cortex induces dopamine release in the caudate nucleus. *Journal of Neuroscience, 21*(15), RC157.

Strehl, U., Leins, U., Goth, G., Klinger, C., Hinterberger, T., & Birbaumer, N. (2006). Self-regulation of slow cortical potentials: A new treatment for children with attention-deficit/hyperactivity disorder. *Pediatrics, 118,* 1530–1540.

Thompson, M., & Thompson, L. (2003). *The neurofeedback book: An introduction to basic concepts in applied psychophysiology.* Wheat Ridge, CO: Association for Applied Psychophysiology and Biofeedback.

Thorndike, E. L. (1905). *The elements of psychology.* New York: A. G. Seiler.

Tomarken, A. J., & Davidson, R. J. (1994). Frontal brain activation in repressors and nonrepressors. *Journal of Abnormal Psychology, 103*(2), 339–349.

Wasserman, E. M., & Lisanby, S. H. (2001) Therapeutic application of repetitive transcranial magnetic stimulation: A review. *Clinical Neurophysiology, 112*(8), 1367–1377.

Yukimasa, T., Yoshimura, R. Tamagawa, A., Uozumi, T., Shinkai, K., Ueda, N., et al. (2006). High-frequency repetitive transcranial magnetic stimulation improves refractory depression by influencing catecholamine and brain-derived neurotropic factors. *Pharmacopsychiatry, 39*(2), 52–59.

Zangen, A., & Hyodo, K. (2002). Transcranial magnetic stimulation induces increases in extracellular levels of dopamine and glutamate in the nucleus accumbens. *Neuroreport, 13*(18), 2401–2405.

SECTION 3

Integrative Psychiatry in Practice

14

Functional Neuroimaging: A Transformative Tool for Integrative Psychiatry

ABASS ALAVI AND ANDREW B. NEWBERG

Key Points

- Functional neuroimaging with positron emission tomography (PET), single photon emission computed tomography (SPECT), and functional magnetic resonance imaging (fMRI) can be highly useful in the evaluation and management of patients with psychiatric disorders.
- PET and SPECT imaging typically evaluate cerebral metabolism and blood flow, respectively, and can determine patterns associated with different disorders.
- PET and SPECT imaging can also evaluate neurotransmitter changes associated with different psychiatric disorders.
- fMRI is an excellent tool for studying the effects of psychiatric disorders on specific brain processes related to cognition and mood.
- fMRI activations studies allow researchers to present various stimuli to a subject in order to determine how the brain reacts and whether psychiatric disorders are associated with different brain reactivity patterns.
- Functional neuroimaging with PET, SPECT, and fMRI can be highly useful in the investigation of the mechanism of action of integrative therapies for psychiatric disorders.

Introduction

Functional brain imaging has provided an enormous amount of information regarding the pathophysiology, diagnosis, and treatment of neurological and psychiatric conditions. From cerebral blood flow (CBF) and metabolism to an array of neurotransmitters tracers, studies of the brain with positron emission tomography (PET), single photon emission computed tomography (SPECT), and functional magnetic resonance imaging (fMRI) have continued to advance our knowledge of these disorders. Functional neuroimaging might also be useful for evaluating therapeutic approaches for different disorders and may play a particularly important role for evaluating patients and research in the integrative medicine setting. Specifically, neuroimaging helps to determine the individualized nature of various disorders showing which specific brain structures and functions are affected. The ability to determine individual differences in the brain of people with different disorders will hopefully allow for a more individualized approach to treatment. Perhaps more important, neuroimaging might be useful for evaluating the mechanism of action of various integrative approaches to the management of neurological and psychiatric disorders. For example, neuroimaging studies can evaluate the effects of acupuncture or meditation in specific settings. Determining the mechanism of action is crucial for brining integrative medicine techniques into the mainstream.

PET and SPECT imaging involves the injection of a radioactively labeled molecule that follows some physiological processes in the brain. The commercially available tracers for brain PET are fluorodeoxyglucose (FDG), which measures cerebral glucose metabolism and several different amyloid probes for the detection of Alzheimer's disease. For SPECT imaging, there are two tracers (Neurolite and Ceretec) that measure CBF and Datscan (ioflupane) that measures dopamine transporter binding for the diagnosis of Parkinson's disease. In addition, there are a number of research-related tracers designed to measure changes for virtually every neurotransmitter system or disease process, as we consider in more detail later in the chapter. MRI does not require a tracer, although some studies are performed using contrast agents. But much of fMRI utilizes various sequences that can detect changes in CBF, functional connectivity, structural connectivity, and the concentration of specific molecules. Each of these fMRI techniques can lend itself to clinical and research applications in the context of integrative medicine.

The most common studies with PET and SPECT look at either cerebral metabolism or CBF, respectively. The result is a detailed evaluation of the pattern of cerebral activity for a given patient (see Figure 14.1). Other experimental tracers involve the injection of radioactively labeled molecules that bind to a wide variety of neurotransmitter receptors such as dopamine or gamma amino butyric acid. These tracers are particularly useful for the evaluation of various psychiatric disorders including depression, anxiety, posttraumatic stress disorder (PTSD), schizophrenia, and a variety of neurological disorders such as Parkinson's disease or seizures.

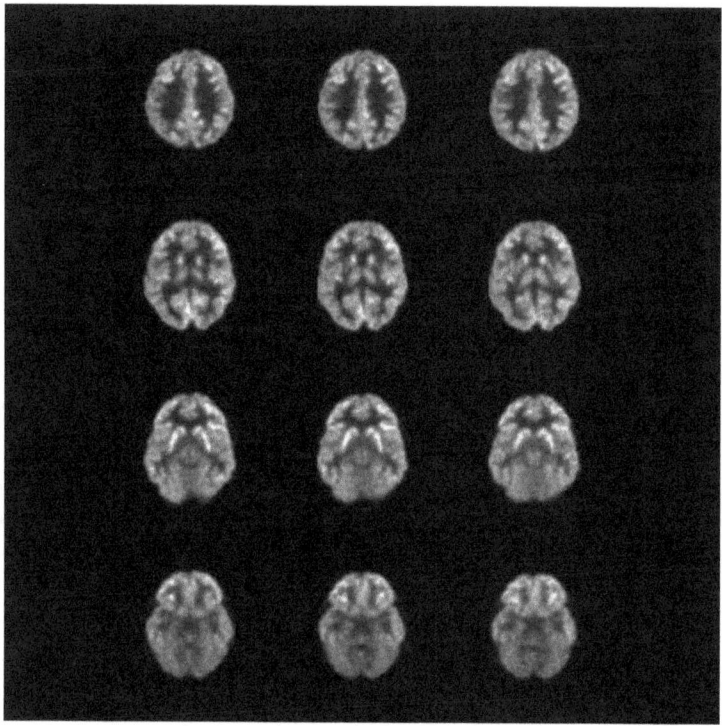

FIGURE 14.1. Normal FDG PET scan from a healthy individual without any neuropsychiatric disorder. The scan demonstrates uniform metabolism throughout the cortical and subcortical structures.

fMRI is primarily able to evaluate changes in CBF during various mental states. Such states can be evaluated as either part of the normal function of the brain or as part of the pathophysiological process of a particular disorder. The primary strength of fMRI is its ability to obtain multiple images of many different brain states in a single imaging session and compare them to each other. The most common MRI methods include blood oxygen labeled dependent (BOLD) imaging and arterial spin labeling. Both approaches can measure CBF but use slightly different approaches. BOLD imaging is the most widely used sequence in activation studies in which the person being evaluated performs one or more tasks that activate cognitive, emotional, or sensory processes in the brain. BOLD imaging can also be performed while the individual is at rest in order to determine functional connectivity. Functional connectivity is determined by observing how CBF in brain structures changes in an associated manner. Thus, in a simplistic way, if the frontal lobe activity increases and decreases in the same way as does the thalamus, they are thought to be functionally connected. A different sequence called diffusion tensor imaging observes how water diffuses along various fiber tracts, thus evaluating how those tracts are connected—structural connectivity. This chapter reviews some of the major applications and findings of functional brain imaging in the evaluation of psychiatric disorders, particularly from the perspective of integrative psychiatry.

Neuroimaging in Depression

Functional neuroimaging has been widely used to study patients with depression. Initial studies explored the pathophysiological mechanisms involved with depression, but more recent studies have started to focus on how neuroimaging might be useful in assessing individual types, determining prognosis, and developing a treatment plan. Of importance is the issue that depression, as well as many other psychiatric conditions, are heterogeneous in nature. Thus patients with depression may have abnormal function in different brain areas that relate to the interindividual differences in how depression manifests and responds to treatment. Neurotransmitter studies can also be used to determine if some patients have greater abnormalities in their serotonin system versus their dopamine system. It might be appropriate then to manage patients with approaches that focus on one system or the other. Thus, depending on the pathophysiology, different treatment strategies might be considered including antidepressant medications, dietary interventions, meditation, supplements, or other nonpharmacological approaches.

Overall, the most common finding on SPECT and PET imaging in depressed patients (see Figure 14.2) is a global decrease in CBF and cerebral metabolism. Early FDG PET studies showed that patients with late-age onset

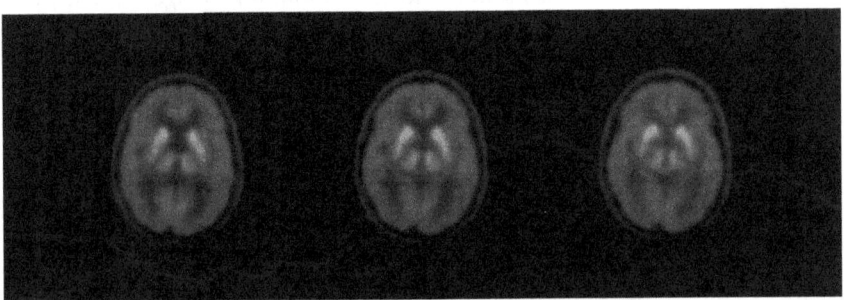

FIGURE 14.2. An FDG PET scan of a patient with major depression shows a global cortical decrease in metabolism relative to the subcortical structures.

depression have decreased metabolism throughout the cortex and even in many subcortical structures but with relative preservation of the basal ganglia. A larger meta-analysis study revealed that patients with major depression had decreased metabolism in the bilateral insula, left putamen, right caudate, and cingulate gyrus and had increased metabolism in the right thalamus and vermis (Su et al., 2014). Metabolic findings also correlate with depression ratings based on self-report versus clinician determined (Milak et al., 2010). Depressed patients with concomitant anxiety symptoms have demonstrated increased metabolism in the right parahippocampal and left anterior cingulate regions and decreased metabolism in the cerebellum, left fusiform gyrus, left superior temporal, left angular gyrus, and left insula (Reiman et al., 1989). Specific symptoms also correlate with functional changes in the brain. One study showed that depression correlated positively with metabolism in the cingulate gyrus, thalamus, and basal ganglia, but sleep problems positively correlated with limbic and basal ganglia metabolism (Milak et al., 2005). In addition, loss of motivation was negatively correlated with parietal and superior frontal lobe metabolism.

Dr. Daniel Amen and his centers have collected the largest database of SPECT scans in psychiatric patients with over 100,000 scans. His group has published an increasing number of studies on this database that includes patients with depression, anxiety, head injury, and other problems. The results from studies based on the Amen database as well as those from other researchers has suggested exciting potential for SPECT scanning in psychiatry. He has noted several different patterns including a hypofrontal pattern, a hypotemporal pattern, and a global hypoperfusion pattern (Amen, Krishnamani, Meysami, Newberg, & Raji, 2017). His clinical and research work has also utilized this type of functional neuroimaging for developing a management plan since different imaging findings can help predict response to specific types of treatment. Such a paradigm of observing initial metabolic or CBF changes might be highly useful in integrative medicine as a way of helping individualize therapy. Thus some patients might benefit from one type of antidepressant medication or another while others would benefit more from meditation or other nonpharmacological approaches. Future studies will have to determine whether similar imaging characteristics help predict response to acupuncture, meditation, or other integrative therapies. Imaging can also help assess how patients respond to various treatment approaches.

FDG PET studies have explored treatment-related effects in patients with depression. In the most general way, brain function tends toward a normalization with successful treatment. For example, several studies showed that successful treatment with paroxetine was associated with an increase toward normal metabolism in the inferior frontal gyrus and prefrontal cortex (Brody et al., 1999) and a decrease toward normal metabolism in the insula and limbic regions (Kennedy et al., 2001).

Still other studies have explored how imaging might help predict response to therapy. For example, one study showed that in depressed patients, venlafaxine and bupropion responders had decreased medial prefrontal and temporal lobe metabolism in their pretreatment scans whereas nonresponders did not have these findings (Little et al., 1996, 2005). Another small study showed that response to both paroxetine or cognitive behavioral therapy was associated with decreased metabolism in the orbitofrontal cortex and left medial prefrontal cortex, in addition to increased metabolism in the right occipital-temporal cortex (Kennedy et al., 2007). Response to cognitive-behavior therapy (CBT) and venlafaxine was differentiated on the basis of metabolism with decreased metabolism in the thalamus found in CBT responders and decreased metabolism in the right nucleus accumbens and subgenual cingulate found in venlafaxine responders.

On pretreatment scans, lower metabolism in the left ventral anterior cingulate gyrus, ventrolateral prefrontal cortex, and orbitofrontal cortex has been associated with a better treatment response to paroxetine (Brody et al., 1999). Furthermore, decreased activity in limbic and striatal regions along with increased activity in the prefrontal cortex, parietal lobe, and cingulate cortex has been associated with improvements in clinical symptoms (Mayberg et al., 2000). In a study of sleep deprivation, high pretreatment metabolic rates and posttreatment decreases in the medial prefrontal cortex and anterior cingulate metabolism were associated with a better response to sleep deprivation therapy (Smith et al., 1999; Wu et al., 1999).

More recent studies have shown that hypometabolism in the insula is associated with a good response to CBT, and a poor response to escitalopram and hypermetabolism in the insula is associated with a good response to escitalopram and poor response to CBT (McGrath et al., 2013). In a similar study, cingulate gyrus and superior temporal sulcus hypermetabolism was associated with nonresponders to both escitalopram and CBT (McGrath et al., 2014).

Related studies utilizing fMRI have shown specific brain activity patterns associated with response to treatment. For example, one study of 21 patients with major depression showed that patients responding better to pharmacological treatment had greater activation in the dorsomedial prefrontal cortex, posterior cingulate cortex, caudate nucleus, insula, and superior frontal gyrus when viewing pictures with negative emotional content (Samson et al., 2011). The ability to activate these regions pretherapy may demonstrate their role as a neurophysiological marker for treatment response and predictor for success of future therapy.

MRI scans have also been utilized to determine treatment response. Several fMRI studies indicated that response to CBT is associated with activation in the anterior cingulate cortex in response to emotional processing (Costafreda, Khanna, Mourao-Miranda, & Fu, 2009; Ritchey, Dolcos, Eddington, Strauman, & Cabeza, 2011; Siegle, Carter, & Thase, 2006). However, another study showed that dorsal anterior cingulate cortex (ACC) response during the emotion processing of sad faces showed an inverse relationship with clinical response (Fu et al., 2008). An fMRI study of elderly depressed patients showed that during an executive function test, those patients with decreased activation in the left inferior frontal and right superior frontal gyrus, as well as increased activation in the right middle frontal gyrus and left superior frontal gyrus, was associated with a positive response to CBT (Thompson et al., 2015). Another study showed that higher brain volume in the anterior cingulate correlated with response to CBT (Fujino et al., 2015). Also, early response to therapy helps predict longer term response. A study of 35 patients with major depression underwent fMRI to evaluate their response to fearful and happy emotional facial expressions before and after seven days of treatment with escitalopram (Godlewska, Browning, Norbury, Cowen, & Harmer, 2016). Depressed patients who demonstrated an early response to the selective serotonin reuptake inhibitor (SSRI) with a greater reduction in neural activity to fearful versus happy facial expressions in the anterior cingulate, insula, amygdala, and thalamus were better responders after six weeks of treatment.

With regard to transcranial magnetic stimulation (TMS) treatment several early studies showed that metabolic patterns predict response to TMS. For example, a PET study (Kimbrell et al., 1999) showed that hypermetabolism in the left dorsolateral prefrontal cortex predicted antidepressant effect of 1-Hz repetitive transcranial magnetic stimulation (rTMS) while hypometabolism predicted the positive effects of 20 Hz stimulation. An early fMRI study of 12 patients showed that an absence of a response to a mental work task at the site of TMS stimulation predicted the clinical response to active rTMS (Eschweiler et al., 2000). A SPECT study of 24 patients with major depression showed that heightened pretreatment anterior cingulate CBF was a positive predictor for successful response to rTMS (Langguth et al., 2007). A study of 26 depressed patients showed that patients with initially lower CBF in the ventromedial prefrontal cortex had a significantly better response to high-frequency regional TMS therapy (Kito, Hasegawa, & Koga, 2012a). Conversely, increased CBF in the ventromedial prefrontal cortex may show a better response to low-frequency rTMS (Kito, Hasegawa, & Koga, 2012b).

The serotonin system has been particularly explored in patients with mood disorders because of the effectiveness of SSRIs, which are believed to aid depression by affecting the serotonergic system. PET and SPECT can be performed using tracers that bind to either the postsynaptic serotonin receptors or the serotonin transporters. The serotonin type 2A postsynaptic receptor does not appear to be affected in patients with late life onset depression, although there is decreased binding in patients with Alzheimer's disease (Meltzer et al., 1999). A review of imaging studies of depression found a decrease in serotonin-2A binding in depressed patients who recently used antidepressants but no change in those without recent antidepressant use (Meyer, 2007). The clinical improvement in depressed patients treated with paroxetine has also been correlated with an increased density of serotonin type 2A receptors in the frontal cortex (Meyer et al., 2001; Zanardi et al., 2001). However, the reduction in the serotonin type 1A receptor binding in depressed patients was not changed by SSRI treatment (Sargent et al., 2000) or by electroconvulsive therapy (Saijo et al., 2010). Serotonin transporter binding in patients with major depression, measured with ^{11}C DASB PET, was found to be decreased in the brain stem, thalamus, caudate, putamen, anterior cingulate cortex, and frontal cortex (Selvaraj et al., 2011). This finding is consistent with other imaging studies of the serotonin transporter in patients with depression.

As with cerebral metabolic and blood flow studies, neuroimaging of the serotonergic system might help predict response to therapy. For example, a SPECT study of 23 patients with major depression showed that higher pretreatment diencephalic central serotonin transporter availability significantly predicted better response to treatment after four weeks (Kugaya et al., 2004). A study of 22 patients with major depression using DASB PET showed that pretherapy higher binding in the habenulae (epithalamus), amygdala-hippocampus complex, anterior insula, anterior cingulate cortex, striatum, midbrain, and cerebellar vermis was correlated with SSRI treatment response (Lanzenberger et al., 2012).

Other receptors have been studied in patients with mood disorders. One study suggested that there is decreased D2 receptor binding in depression patients after successful response to electroconvulsive therapy (Saijo et al., 2009). Finally, there appears to be decreased gamma-aminobutyric acid A (GABA-A) binding in the parahippocampus and superior temporal lobe in patients with depression, which correlates with hyperactivity in the hypothalamic-pituitary axis (Klumpers et al., 2010).

More specifically with regard to integrative therapies in depression, several neuroimaging studies have observed significant physiological effects. A study of 29 drug-naïve patients with major depressive disorder (MDD) revealed that MDD patients had initially abnormal function in their default mode network. However, electroacupuncture at the GV20 point induced increased functional connectivity between the posterior cingulate cortex and anterior cingulate cortex and decreased functional connectivity between the posterior cingulate cortex and left middle prefrontal cortex, left angular gyrus, and bilateral hippocampus/parahippocampus (Deng et al., 2016). A similar study explored the effect of laser acupuncture on the default mode network in patients with depression also showing alterations in the activity of the inferior parietal cortex and the cerebellum (Quah-Smith, Suo, Williams, & Sachdev, 2013). Meditation has been shown to have significant effects on brain function in patients with major depression. One study of 21 patients with MDD found increased functional connectivity between the right dorsal medial prefrontal cortex and both the left dorsal lateral prefrontal cortex and the left lateral orbitofrontal cortex (Chen et al., 2015). The implications of these findings suggest that acupuncture and meditation can induce specific physiological changes in the brain of patients with depression; however, these studies did not report whether there were associated improvements in depressive symptoms. Thus a more elaborate understanding of the mechanism by which such integrative therapies work will require additional studies.

Overall, one can see the potential value in functional neuroimaging in patients with depression. In addition to diagnosing and characterizing the specific physiological subtypes of the disease, it can also be useful for directing therapy and determining response to therapy. Importantly, neuroimaging can be used in patients with depression to observe how various integrative therapies, including those related to diet, nutrition, meditation, acupuncture, and others, affect the neurophysiology of depression.

Neuroimaging in Bipolar Disorder

PET has been used to study cerebral glucose metabolism in bipolar patients. Bipolar patients who are actively depressed have decreased global metabolism (Baxter et al., 1985). As their depression improves, they have increases in their cerebral metabolism. In contrast, unipolar patients are found to have normal global metabolic rates that did not correlate with clinical symptoms (Schwartz, 1987). Studies have further demonstrated that bipolar depressed patients have decreased metabolism in the frontal gyri, right cingulate gyrus, and bilateral inferior parietal lobules (Hosokawa, Momose, & Kasai, 2009). PET studies report similar decreases in global metabolism in bipolar patients in the depressive phase, while unipolar patients have global metabolism within normal limits (Phelps, Mazziotta, Baxter, & Gerner, 1984). Further, bipolar patients in the hypomanic phase have normal glucose metabolism. Studies have demonstrated that bipolar depression is associated with a pattern of prefrontal hypometabolism, while a cerebello-posterior cortical hypermetabolism may be observed in bipolar patients (Ketter et al., 2001). An FDG PET study also differentiated BD-I patients from BD-II patients with the former having significantly lower glucose metabolism in the anterior cingulate, insula, striatum, and parts of the prefrontal cortex and higher glucose metabolism in the left parahippocampus (Li et al., 2012). This study also reported correlations between executive function and abnormal glucose uptake in BD-I patients, particularly in the parahippocampus.

BD is characterized by affective alternations between elevated moods and depression. The onset of the illness is typically during early adulthood; however, early symptoms may be mild and undetectable. In MRI studies, there have been a number of findings in BD patients. For example, one volumetric study demonstrated increases in the right caudate volume in BD patients (Kozicky et al., 2013). Among 18 BD fMRI studies reviewed by Heng, Song, and Sim (2010), the most common finding was a decrease in fractional anisotropy in the frontal regions. This is consistent with other BD studies that found a decrease in white matter density in prefrontal regions (Adler et al., 2004, Bruno, Cercignani, & Ron, 2008; van der Schot et al., 2010). Additionally, several studies have reported decreased fractional anisotropy values in the white matter tracts of the corpus callosum using both region of interest (ROI) analyses and voxel based analysis (VBA; Bellani et al., 2009). Among adolescents experiencing the early stages of BD, decreased fractional anisotropy values were observed in the left superior frontal region and the right orbital frontal region (Adler et al., 2006; Kafantaris et al., 2009).

Neuroimaging may help better differentiate BD from unipolar depression as well as have the potential direct therapy and measure response to various integrative approaches. For example, an fMRI study showed that following mindfulness-based cognitive therapy bipolar patients experienced significant improvements in anxiety and emotion regulation as well as tests of working memory, spatial memory, and verbal fluency (Ives-Deliperi, Howells, Stein, Meintjes, & Horn, 2013). These clinical improvements, as well as measures of mindfulness, were associated with BOLD signal increases in the medial prefrontal cortex and posterior parietal lobe.

Neuroimaging in Anxiety

Brain regions involved in anxiety symptoms and anxiety disorders typically differ from those associated with depression. PET has been utilized to gain a better understanding of the neurophysiologic mechanisms underlying stress and anxiety. In general, the hippocampus, the amygdala, and the prefrontal cortex as part of the limbic system are believed to play prominent roles in the regulation of the hypothalamic-pituitary-adrenal axis, which leads to the regulation of the stress response. Early studies of patients with anxiety disorders using H$_2$O PET found that these patients have increased rCBF in the right parahippocampal gyrus in a resting, non-panic state, compared to controls (Reiman, Butler, Raichle, Robins, & Herscovitch, 1984, Reiman et al., 1989). During a lactate-induced panic attack, such patients have increased rCBF bilaterally in the temporal poles, the claustrum, and the lateral putamen.

In patients with generalized anxiety disorder, there are lower metabolic rates in the basal ganglia and white matter and relatively increased metabolism in the left inferior occipital lobe, right posterior temporal lobe, and right precentral frontal gyrus (Wu et al., 1991). In one study, benzodiazepine therapy resulted in reduced metabolism in cortical areas, the limbic system, and the basal ganglia. Another study showed benzodiazepines resulted in relative decreases in metabolism in the visual cortex and increases in the basal ganglia and thalamus (Buchsbaum et al., 1987). An FDG PET study found that the prefrontal cortex is activated as the result of psychosocial stress with distinct prefrontal metabolic glucose patterns linked to endocrine stress measures such as cortisol levels (Kern et al., 2008).

Several studies have explored the predictive value of neuroimaging studies in anxiety disorders. For example, one study showed that when viewing fearful facial expressions the increase in anterior cingulate cortex activity was directly correlated with response to venlafaxine treatment while decreased activity in the left amygdala was correlated with a positive response (Whalen et al., 2008). Similarly, a study showed that anterior cingulate response in anticipation of seeing negative emotional images also correlated with venlafaxine treatment response (Nitschke et al., 2009). Several neuroimaging studies have explored how anxiety might be attenuated by integrative medicine approaches. A set of studies in patients with social anxiety showed that the Mindful-Based Stress Reduction (MBSR) program resulted in increases in dorsomedial prefrontal cortex (DMPFC) activity during a negative self-view task as well as changes in the timing of neural responses in the DMPFC and posterior cingulate cortex during the negative self-view task (Goldin, Ziv, Jazaieri, & Gross, 2012; Goldin, Ziv, Jazaieri, Hahn, & Gross, 2013). Interestingly, when MBSR was compared to an aerobic exercise program, both groups had significantly reduced anxiety and there were no statistical differences between the two treatments. The MBSR and exercise groups had different brain-related changes posttherapy, which raises important future questions regarding how various integrative approaches might help patients with anxiety.

In terms of neurotransmitter systems, PET studies have demonstrated decreased serotonin type 1A receptor binding in patients with panic disorder and social anxiety disorder but not in PTSD (Akimova, Lanzenberger, & Kasper, 2009). Stressors have also been shown to be associated with a release

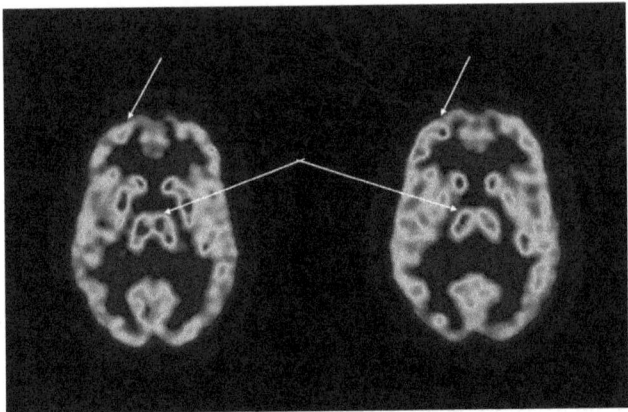

FIGURE 14.3. FDG PET scans of a subject at rest and while performing a meditation task. During meditation, there is increased metabolism in the frontal lobes (thin arrow) and decreased metabolism in the thalami (thick arrow). These structures are involved in stress and anxiety pathways, and the observed effects in these scans may provide physiological support for the antianxiety effects of such practices.

of dopamine using PET imaging (Pruessner et al., 2010). A PET study utilizing ^{11}C-Raclopride, which binds to the postsynaptic D2 receptor, demonstrated a significant increase in dopamine levels during Yoga Nidra meditation practice (Kjaer et al., 2002). This finding may help explain how such practices reduce anxiety symptoms since the dopamine release may result in an overall decrease in readiness for action and reactivity that is associated with this particular type of meditation and ultimately. In addition, FDG PET scans have shown specific changes in the frontal lobes and thalami during meditation that might contribute to its anti-anxiety effects (Figure 14.3). Future studies will be necessary to elaborate on the physiological processes associated with stress and anxiety. Finally, research has suggested that yoga may increase GABA in the brain; GABA is the primary molecule related to benzodiazepine receptor medications (Streeter et al., 2007).

Neuroimaging in Schizophrenia

PET studies of abnormal glucose metabolism in schizophrenia (see Figure 14.4) have contributed to our overall understanding of the pathophysiological basis of the disorder. However, less effort has been made in distinguishing hyper- and hypometabolic areas of activity as they correlate with various positive and negative symptoms in schizophrenia (Buchsbaum & Hazlett, 1998,

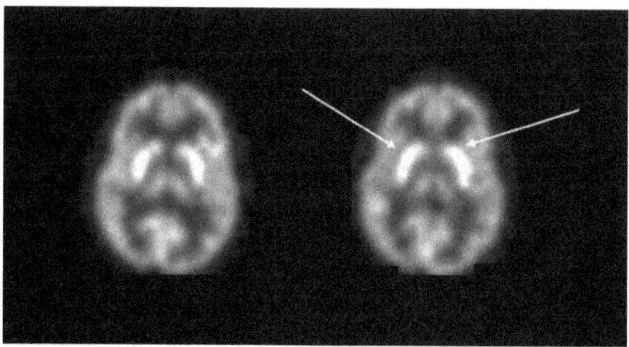

FIGURE 14.4. FDG PET scan of patient with schizophrenia showing a mild global decrease, particularly in the frontal regions (arrows) consistent with some of the reported findings in the literature of hypofrontality.

but also see Hill et al., 2004). More current, as well as older, studies of resting state FDG PET in schizophrenia provide a complex picture of the profile of regional metabolic abnormalities associated with the disorder and treatment responses, which highlight the heterogeneity in study methodologies as well as in schizophrenia itself. For example, an FDG PET study reported hypometabolism in the basal ganglia, thalamus, amygdala, and brainstem of chronic patients (under neuroleptic treatment) compared with controls, with additional reductions in parts of the cerebellum, left and right cingulate gyrus, and parietal and frontal lobes noted in a subgroup of patients exhibiting low positive symptoms (Ben-Shachar et al., 2007). A comparison of severe schizophrenics (under neuroleptic treatment) versus controls revealed a marked decrease in the frontal cortex, primary sensory regions, and anterior cingulate cortex, as well as increased levels of glucose metabolism in the basal ganglia, precentral, paracentral, precuneus, angular, temporal, occipital and cerebellar regions in both hemispheres, and most notably in the middle temporal region in the left temporal lobe (Fujimoto et al., 2007). Furthermore, a study of schizophrenic patients (either un- or never medicated; Soyka, Koch, Möller, Rüther, & Tatsch, 2005) found increased frontal lobe metabolism accompanied by mild increases in metabolic activity in the thalamus, striatum, and temporal lobes. Such findings partially contrast with results of another study reporting reduced bilateral thalamic metabolism in never-medicated patients (Clark, Kopala, Li, & Hurwitz, 2001). A study of long-term and recent-onset schizophrenic patients found hypometabolism in the visual and insular cortices, along with hypermetabolism in the motor and inferior temporal regions, in both subgroups of patients relative to controls. A study of the default mode network structures in medicated patients showed resting metabolism to be decreased in the dosromedial prefrontal cortex, and increased in the lentiform nucleus and cerebellum, in patients relative to controls (Park et al., 2009). A more recent study showed that schizophrenic patients had decreased metabolic activity in the center of large fronto-temporal and cerebellar white matter tracts compared to patients with BD (Altamura et al., 2013).

The dopamine hypothesis of schizophrenia suggests that the cardinal symptoms of the disorder can be attributed to abnormal dopaminergic function. A number of PET scan studies have supported this contention, showing increased uptake in the striatum. However, as with the variability in schizophrenic symptoms, studies have similarly reported a complex pattern of dopamine activity. For example, one study (Okubo et al., 1997) found that while there were no differences observed in binding of the D2 receptors in the striatum, binding of the D1 receptors was reduced in the prefrontal cortex of schizophrenic patients (neuroleptic naive and neuroleptic free), relative to controls. A subsequent ^{11}C-labeled L-DOPA PET study of schizophrenic patients (Lindstrom et al. 1999) showed higher dopamine synthesis in the striatum and medial prefrontal cortex in patients relative to controls. Increased presynaptic dopamine metabolism in the striatum in schizophrenic patients has been reported using ^{18}F-FDOPA (Hietala et al., 1995; Reith et al.,1994). More recently, a study reported increased striatal ^{18}F-FDOPA uptake in patients with prodromal symptoms of schizophrenia, although not to the same degree as patients with clearly diagnosed schizophrenia (Howes et al., 2009). These results have been contrasted by other studies that have either reported reduced striatal ^{18}F-FDOPA uptake in neuroleptic-free schizophrenics (Elkashef et al., 2000) or no group differences (Dao-Castellana et al., 1997). Furthermore, other studies reported significantly reduced extrastriatal D2/D3 receptor binding in the thalamus as well as the amygdala, cingulate gyrus, and temporal cortex, in neuroleptic-naive schizophrenics (Buchsbaum et al., 2006; Suhara et al., 2002; Talvik, Nordström, Olsson, Halldin, & Farde, 2003; Yasuno et al., 2004).

Schizophrenia is described by an abnormal integration of cognitive and emotional processes, and the etiology of this mental disorder still remains unknown. In individuals with chronic schizophrenia, over 50 different brain regions have been reported to be involved in the illness based on a meta-analysis of voxel based morphometry (VBM) studies looking at gray matter volume in these subjects (Honea, Crow, Passingham, & Mackay, 2005). The regions in particular that have consistently been reported across studies are the left medial temporal lobe, the left superior temporal lobe, the prefrontal cortices, and the anterior cingulate (Haznedar et al., 2004; Kakeda & Korogi, 2010; Shenton, Whitford, & Kubicki, 2010).

Recent studies measuring white matter in individuals with chronic schizophrenia have shed some light on the pathophysiology of the illness. A recent meta-analysis of 36 VBA studies looking at chronic schizophrenia identified reduced fractional anisotropy (FA) as compared to controls in several key regions including the cingulum bundle, the corpus callosum, the arcuate and uncinate fasciculi, and the frontal longitudinal fasciculi (White, Nelson, & Lim, 2008). Additional reviews looking at VBM studies are consistent with these findings as well as several other regions including the internal capsule and fornix (Kubicki et al., 2007; Kubiki, McCarley, & Shenton, 2005; Kyriakopoulos, Vyas, Barker, Chitnis, & Frangou, 2008; Williams, 2008). At this point, there appears to be concordance between white matter and gray matter deficits in schizophrenics, which may ultimately lead to a cohesive neuropathological theory to explain the disorder. In particular, reduced gray matter in temporal and frontal cortices, especially those that correspond to Wernicke's and Broca's areas, may be further explained in schizophrenics due to the reduced FA observed in the arcuate fasciculus, which connects these two structures. This anatomical deficit should have a significant effect on speech in general, a point that may help explain some of the common symptoms of schizophrenia including auditory hallucinations, delusions, and deficits in verbal memory. Additionally, the decreased FA in the cingulum bundle corresponds to the decreased gray matter observed in the anterior cingulate, which is involved in memory, emotion, and attention due to its multifarious connections. This may help explain the anatomically diffuse nature of the illness as reported by the plethora of studies looking at anatomical differences of schizophrenics compared to controls.

Recently, there has been a rise in the number of diffusion tensor imaging (DTI) studies looking at the early stages of schizophrenia referred to as first-episode schizophrenia. The hope is that the study of the illness during its early stages will allow for even earlier detection and possible intervention by better understanding the interaction of various brain structures as the illness progresses. Recent tractography studies (Price et al., 2007, 2008) identified subtle differences in the left uncinate fasciculus and the corpus callosum. The left uncinate fasciculus is of particular interest as it connects the inferior frontal gyrus with the anterior temporal lobe and is believed to be involved in memory and emotion and exhibits the longest period of development across all white matter regions, developing beyond the age of 30. Other studies found decreases in FA values in the cingulum bundle, the frontal lobe, and the perihippocampal gyrus (Hao et al., 2006; Kumra et al., 2004; Szeszko et al., 2008). One recent study (Cheung et al., 2008) looking at first-episode schizophrenia in never-medicated patients ($n = 25$) found decreases in FA values in the left fronto-occipital fasciculus, the left inferior longitudinal fasciculus, the splenium of the corpus callosum, and the right parietal white matter. Additional studies need to be conducted using medication-naïve patients to properly determine the effect of medication during the early stages of the illness.

There are a few studies related to integrative therapies in schizophrenia (Bosch et al., 2015; Deng & Adams, 2017; Langer, Cangas, Salcedo., & Fuentes, 2012), but due to the severity of the illness, integrative approaches might be less useful. In addition, there are no imaging studies of integrative approaches in schizophrenic patients, but perhaps future studies might help indicate ways in which meditation, acupuncture, or diet and nutrition might be useful as adjunct therapies in these complicated patients.

Neuroimaging in Obsessive Compulsive Disorder

Several studies have used PET and SPECT imaging to investigate patients with obsessive-compulsive disorder (OCD). The cortico-striata-thalamic circuit involving the orbiotofrontal cortex (OFC) has been implicated in the neuropathology of OCD. Studies have generally shown that OCD patients have increased cerebral metabolism in the orbitofrontal cortex and specifically the caudate nuclei (Figure 14.5; Baxter et al., 1988; Insel & Winslow, 1992; Sawle, Hymas, Lees, & Frackowiak, 1991). Another study found hypermetabolism in the cingulate gyrus of OCD patients compared to controls (Swedo et al., 1989). Several PET studies have also shown hypometabolism within the bilateral parietal lobes in OCD. Some studies show a negative correlation with between obsessive-compulsive symptoms and right parietal rCBF. It has been hypothesized that parietal lobe dysfunction, particularly within the angular and supramarginal gyri, could contribute to the cognitive deficits evident in OCD.

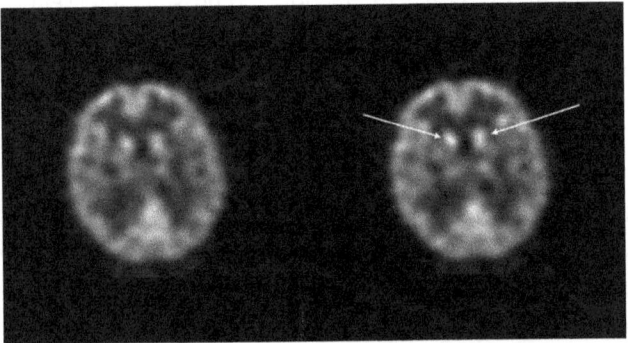

FIGURE 14.5. FDG PET of a patient with OCD showing increased glucose metabolism in the caudate nuclei bilaterally (arrow).

PET has been utilized to explore the effects of different types of therapy in OCD. One study demonstrated that higher glucose metabolism in the orbitofrontal cortex was associated with greater improvement with behavioral therapy and a worse outcome with fluoxetine treatment (Brody et al., 1998). Behavior therapy responders also had significant bilateral decreases in caudate metabolism posttreatment (Schwartz, Stoessel, Baxter, Martin, & Phelps, 1996). There is some suggestion that different patterns of metabolic activity in OCD patients predict response to behavioral therapy versus medication. In one study, behavioral therapy responders had significant bilateral decreases in caudate metabolism compared to poor responders. Further, lower pretreatment metabolism in both the left and right OFC in OCD patients predicted greater improvement with paroxetine treatment (Saxena et al., 1999).

Neurotransmitter studies have also revealed important findings in OCD patients. One PET study found a significant decrease in serotonin-2A receptor availability in the frontal, dorsolateral, and medial frontal cortex, as well as in the temporo-parietal association cortex in OCD patients (Perani et al., 2008). There was also a significant correlation between serotonin-2A receptor availability in the orbitofrontal and dorsolateral frontal cortex and the severity of clinical OCD symptoms. In addition, this same study utilized ^{11}C Raclopride PET and found a significant reduction of D2 receptor binding in the whole striatum, possibly reflecting endogenous dopaminergic hyperactivity. Furthermore, the reduction in binding was improved by treatment with fluvoxamine with a concomitant improvement in symptoms (Moresco et al., 2007). Another PET study showed that OCD patients had decreased serotonin transporter binding in the insular cortex as suggesting a potential role for the serotonergic system in the pathophysiology of OCD (Matsumoto et al., 2010).

Specific gray and white matter regions have been implicated in OCD. For example, a large study of 412 OCD patients showed these patients had significantly smaller volumes of gray and white matter in the dorsomedial prefrontal cortex, anterior cingulate cortex, and inferior frontal gyrus extending to the insula (de Wit et al., 2014). OCD patients also were found to have greater cerebellar gray matter volumes. One of the first studies to look at the diffusion of white matter tracts in patients with OCD was by Szeszko and colleagues (2005), who identified reduced FA using ROI analysis in several regions including the bilateral anterior cingulate, bilateral supramarginal, right posterior cingulated, and left lingual gyrus. Several studies have identified decreased FA in patients with OCD in the cingulate cortex (anterior body, body, and rostrum), bilateral cingulum bundle, bilateral inferior fronto-occipital fasciculus, and right inferior parietal white matter (Bora et al., 2011; Garibotto et al., 2010; Menzies et al., 2008; Nakamae et al., 2008; Saito et al., 2008). Another study using ROI analysis identified left greater than right asymmetries in the cingulum bundle in patients with OCD as well as greater FA values in patients with OCD as compared to controls in the left cingulum bundle and left anterior limb of the internal capsule (Cannistraro et al., 2007). As with schizophrenia, there are no imaging studies in OCD patients with respect to integrative approaches to treatment. There are several studies that have explored the use of neuroimaging in predicting treatment response with antidepressant or CBT. Hoexter et al. (2013) showed that OCD symptom improvement with fluoxetine treatment was significantly correlated with smaller pretreatment gray matter volume in the right middle lateral OFC, while improvement with CBT treatment was correlated with larger pretreatment gray matter volume within the right medial prefrontal cortex. Given the growing number of clinical trials exploring acupuncture, meditation, and other integrative approaches in these patients (Shannahoff-Khalsa et al., 1999; Zhang, Wang, Tan, Jin, & Yao, 2009), neuroimaging would be an important next step for assessing mechanistic effects.

Neuroimaging in Posttraumatic Stress Disorder

PTSD is an anxiety disorder associated with changes in neural circuitry typically involving the frontal lobe and limbic structures. Altered metabolism in these brain structures after a traumatic event is associated with the development of PTSD. A case report of a subject exposed to war-related sounds before and after treatment with an SSRI showed that, before treatment, trauma reminders resulted in decreased rCBF in the insula, prefrontal, and inferior frontal cortices and increased CBF in the cerebellum, precuneus, and supplementary motor cortex. These findings normalized after SSRI administration suggesting that the therapeutic effect of such medications in PTSD patients could be related to prefrontal and paralimbic areas that are involved in memory and emotional control. An FDG PET study of 15 patients showed that PTSD was associated with a specific pattern of decreased activity in the cingulate gyri, precuneus, insula, hippocampus prefrontal cortex, occipital lobe, and verbal areas (Molina, Isoardi, Prado, & Bentolila, 2010). This same study showed relatively increased activity in the fusiform gyrus, superior temporal lobe, and cerebellum in PTSD patients.

A different study reported rCBF changes associated with the recollection of traumatic events in trauma-exposed individuals with and without PTSD. This study showed that the exposure to the traumatic condition was associated with increases in the orbitofrontal cortex and anterior temporal poles in PTSD patients (Shin et al., 1999). Additionally, PTSD patients had CBF decreases in the anterior frontal regions and the left inferior frontal region. A follow-up study by the same group (Shin et al., 2004) showed that PTSD patients had CBF decreases in the medial frontal gyrus when recalling their traumatic memories. PTSD symptom severity was also positively correlated with CBF in the right amygdala and negatively correlated with CBF in medial frontal gyrus.

In terms of therapy, a recent fMRI study from our group showed that the NeuroEmotional Technique was able to significantly reduce symptoms in cancer patients with traumatic memories and that this clinical response was associated with reduced reactivity in the parahippocampus and brain stem regions (Monti et al., 2017). An fMRI study of CBT showed that greater activity in left dorsal striatum and frontal networks during an inhibitory control task was associated with improved PTSD symptom after therapy (Falconer, Allen, Felmingham, Williams, & Bryant, 2013). Another fMRI study of mindfulness-based exposure therapy (MBET) in PTSD patients showed increased default mode network functional connectivity between the posterior cingulate dorsolateral dorsolateral prefrontal cortex regions and dorsal ACC regions after MBET (King et al., 2016). These changes in connectivity were correlated with improvements in avoidant and hyperarousal symptoms in these patients.

Neuroimaging in Alcoholism

Studies of chronic alcoholic patients with PET have generally found decreased whole brain metabolism by up to 20% to 30% that includes both cortical and subcortical structures (Sachs, Russell, Christman, & Cook, 1987; Samson, Baron, Feline, Bories, & Crouzel, 1986; Wik et al., 1988). While this hypometabolism is usually distributed throughout the cortex, the parietal areas have been found to be particularly affected. Other studies have reported frontal lobe hypometabolism in patients with alcoholism. Also, studies have reported metabolic deficits in the left hemisphere more often than in the right (Volkow & Fowler, 1992).

Studies have also explored the effects of alcohol on various neurotransmitter systems within the brain. GABA receptor function is altered in alcoholics as demonstrated by a decreased impact of lorazepam on functional changes in the thalamus, basal ganglia, and cerebellum. This decreased response may be associated with the decreased sensitivity to the effects of alcohol and benzodiazepines in these patients (Volkow et al., 1995; Volkow et al., 1993). One study reported reduced binding in the striatal monoaminergic presynaptic terminals in severe chronic alcoholic patients suggesting that the damaging effects of severe chronic alcoholism on the central nervous system are more extensive than previously considered (Gilman et al., 1998). A comparison of alcoholics to controls showed that a serotoninergic challenge resulted in a blunted response in alcoholics in the basal ganglia and prefrontal areas (Hommer et al., 1997).

Another PET study using statistical parametric mapping comparing alcoholics and controls significant differences in the rate of serotonin synthesis between groups. Serotonin synthesis was significantly reduced in the medial prefrontal cortex in alcoholics, suggesting the possibility of impaired planning, self-control, and moderation of social behaviors. In addition, there were correlations between regional serotonin synthesis and the quantity-frequency measure of alcohol consumption.

Studies exploring alcohol cue reactivity have suggested that the fronto-limbic dopaminergic neuroadaptations underlie this reactivity. Alcohol ingestion has been shown to release dopamine in the ventral tegmental area, which projects to the nucleus accumbens, amygdala, and frontal areas (Heinz, Beck, Grusser, Grace, & Wrase, 2009). This dopamine release may play an important role in the motivational aspect of drug-cue learning, which is supported by studies showing activation in reinforcement-related limbic areas evoked by alcohol cues (Grüsser et al., 2004). In addition, reactivity in these areas has been correlated with craving (Myrick et al., 2004) and alcohol consumption after relapse (Beck et al., 2012).

With regard to therapeutic studies, a study of 64 recently detoxified alcoholics showed that pretreatment activation in the ventral striatum induced by alcohol images predicted response to naltrexone treatment on relapse behavior (Mann et al., 2014). One study of 38 alcohol dependent patients found that TMS to the dorsolateral prefrontal cortex resulted in an increase in fronto-parietal connectivity, suggesting that this intervention might support cognitive control in such patients (Jansen, van Wingen, van den Brink, & Goudriaan, 2015). An fMRI study of 32 abstinent alcoholics undergoing bias modification training showed reduced activation in the bilateral amygdala during alcohol cue presentation (Wiers et al., 2015). Since initial activation in the amygdala correlated with craving and arousal ratings of alcohol stimuli, the decreased response in amygdala activity correlated with decreases in craving posttreatment. No studies have specifically explored the impact of integrative approaches to the management of alcoholism, but future studies could be performed analogous to the aforementioned reports.

Neuroimaging in Chronic Concussion

Concussion is generally considered more of a neurological disorder but often results in a number of psychiatric symptoms such as depression, anxiety, fatigue, and cognitive deficits. More than 1.5 million Americans suffer traumatic brain injuries (TBIs) annually with 80,000 to 90,000 individuals with long-term disability. While neuroimaging in the acute head injury is helpful to exclude fractures and intracranial hemorrhages, patients with chronic symptoms might also benefit from neuroimaging. The goals of neuroimaging in patients with chronic concussion symptoms is to determine specific areas of abnormal brain function and to help determine potential therapeutic options. A particularly important result from imaging can be the observation of specific physiological deficits, which can be helpful for the patient to understand that his or her symptoms have a biological basis. Many patients with persistent symptoms can be labeled as malingering, so demonstrating clear physiological problems can be a great relief psychologically to chronic concussion patients. For patients with persistent postconcussive symptoms, there exists an urgent need to provide quantitative biomarkers to measure the extent of injury and clarify prognosis: Given that structural imaging techniques often deliver "normal" results in these patients, functional and metabolic imaging approaches offer a potential solution for clinical care today.

Lesions such as cortical contusions, intracranial hematomas, and resultant encephalomalacia have metabolic abnormalities on PET imaging that are confined primarily to the site of injury. Subdural and epidural hematomas can cause more widespread hypometabolism, which can also affect the contralateral hemisphere (George et al., 1989). Diffuse axonal injury has been found to cause diffuse cortical hypometabolism with a predilection for the parieto-occipital cortices, likely related to the disruption of callosal input into the visual cortex (Alavi, 1989).

There are several important challenges in evaluating FDG/PET scans in patients with chronic TBI. First, few radiologists have sufficient expertise in the interpretation of FDG PET brain scans. TBI results in many subtle findings that could be directly related to a patient's symptoms and if these metabolic findings were are missed, the clinical approach might proceed in the wrong direction. It is also important to recognize that since TBI is such a heterogeneous disorder, there may be no single pattern observed. This is particularly the case in patients with multiple head injuries, which can result in an array of findings. Focal PET findings often correspond to neuropsychological deficits and symptoms. In many circumstances, there can also be a more global cortical decrease in metabolism (see Figure 14.6). There is evidence that FDG PET imaging is superior to neuropsychological assessment in predicting cognitive decline in patients with TBI (Chetelat et al., 2005). This finding is important, especially in older patients who might experience cognitive decline related to such other etiologies such as Alzheimer's disease, stroke, Parkinson's disease, or other conditions.

CBF imaging with SPECT is a commonly available functional neuroimaging modality and can be particularly useful in patients with chronic TBI symptoms. Unfortunately, few clinicians take advantage of the widespread

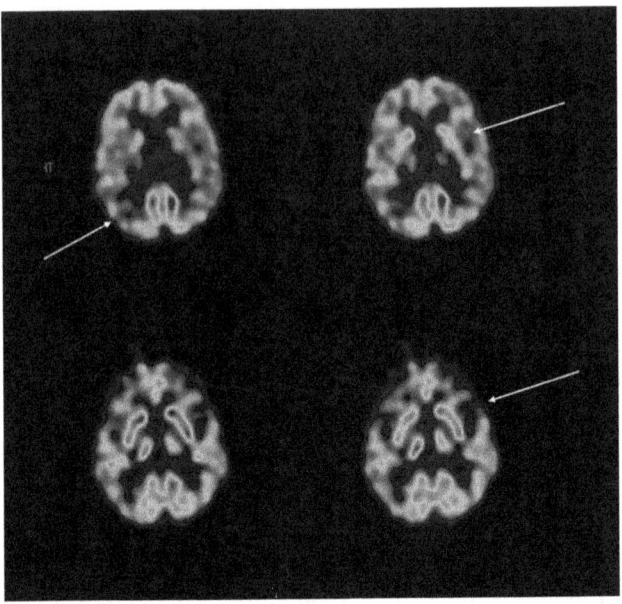

FIGURE 14.6. FDG PET of a patient with prior head injury and persistent symptoms showing areas of both increased and decreased glucose metabolism (arrow).

availability of SPECT brain imaging. However, SPECT scans often detect abnormalities that are not observed on computed tomography (CT) or MRI. Specifically, investigators have found a greater number of abnormalities in patients with TBI that were detected earlier with HMPAO SPECT scans compared to CT (Newton et al., 1992). An early study reported that 80% of brain injury patients had CBF deficits on SPECT, while only 55% were found to have abnormalities on CT scans (Gray, Ichise, Chung, Kirsh, & Franks, 1992). The lesions found on SPECT are generally larger in size than those detected with anatomical imaging.

It should be noted that future clinical applications of both PET and SPECT imaging may rely on the development of novel tracers that evaluate other aspects of brain physiology that might pertain to the specific pathophysiology of TBI, such as the elaboration of inflammatory markers, amyloid protein, or tau protein. For example, current studies have shown that TBI patients have higher tau protein binding. Tracers that observe specific neurotransmitter changes associated with TBI effects might also be helpful in ascertaining physiological effects of TBI. Neurotransmitters such as dopamine, serotonin, norepinephrine, GABA, and others might may play an important role in the persistent symptoms associated with TBI (Hayes & Dixon, 1994).

Functional MRI has been used in a variety of research studies to help document disruptions in function related to particular tasks, cognitive and affective. DTI can help evaluate the disruption in various neuronal tracts in the brain (Shenton et al., 2012). Resting BOLD imaging can evaluate functional connectivity within the brain, which could help to further demonstrate how neuronal connections are disrupted by TBI (Stevens et al., 2012). Magnetic resonance spectroscopy may help to demonstrate the concentration of different neurotransmitters or metabolites that could be altered by TBI (Gardner, Iverson, & Stanwell, 2014).

In the end, functional neuroimaging in patients with chronic concussion symptoms might be an important diagnostic tool that could also aid integrative medicine. By understanding the complex pathophysiology of a patient, therapies targeting specific brain regions might be useful. For example, meditation practices might be useful for augmenting frontal lobe function. Neurofeedback similarly might be useful in chronic concussion patients.

Conclusion

Overall, functional brain imaging has been highly valuable in providing important and useful information regarding disorders of affect and cognition. This field has greatly expanded in the past 20 years and contributed to our overall understanding of these disorders. Moving forward, there are great opportunities to utilize functional neuroimaging with PET, SPECT, and fMRI as tools for evaluating the impact of integrative therapies on these disorders. Such studies will help delineate the mechanism of action of these integrative therapies and also provide needed data to support their expanded in use in these populations. Importantly, this research can help demonstrate the most appropriate interventions for each disorder and also indicate the benefits and potential risks associated with these integrative interventions.

REFERENCES

Adler, C. M., Adams, J., DelBello, M. P., Holland, S. K., Schmithorst, V., Levine, A., et al. (2006). Evidence of white matter pathology in bipolar disorder adolescents experiencing their first episode of mania: A diffusion tensor imaging study. *The American Journal of Psychiatry, 163*(2), 322–324.

Adler, C. M., Holland, S. K., Schmithort, V., Wilke, M., Weiss, K. L., Pan, H., & Strakowski, S. M. (2004). Abnormal frontal white matter tracts in bipolar disorder: A diffusion tensor imaging study. *Bipolar Disorders, 6*, 197–203.

Akimova, E., Lanzenberger, R., & Kasper, S. (2009). The serotonin-1A receptor in anxiety disorders. *Biological Psychiatry, 66*(7), 627–635.

Alavi, A. (1989). Functional and anatomical studies of head injury. *The Journal of Neuropsychiatry and Clinical Neurosciences, 1*, S45–S50.

Altamura, A. C., Bertoldo, A., Marotta, G., Paoli, R. A., Caletti, E., Dragogna, F., et al. (2013). White matter metabolism differentiates schizophrenia and bipolar disorder: A preliminary PET study. *Psychiatry Research, 214*(3), 410–414.

Amen, D. G., Krishnamani, P., Meysami, S., Newberg, A., & Raji, C. A. (2017). Classification of depression, cognitive disorders, and co-morbid depression and cognitive disorders with perfusion SPECT neuroimaging. *Journal of Alzheimer's Disease, 57*(1), 253–266.

Baxter, L. R., Schwartz, J. M., Mazziotta, J. C., Phelps, M. E., Pahl, J. J., Guze, B. H., & Fairbanks, L. (1988). Cerebral glucose metabolic rates in nondepressed patients with obsessive-compulsive disorder. *The American Journal of Psychiatry, 145*(12), 1560–1563.

Baxter, L. R. J., Phelps, M. E., Mazziotta, J. C., Schwartz, J. M., Gerner, R. H., Selin, C. E., & Sumida, R. M. (1985). Cerebral metabolic rates for glucose in mood disorders: Studies with positron emission tomography and fluorodeoxyglucose F 18. *Archives of General Psychiatry, 42*(5), 441–447.

Beck, A., Wüstenberg, T., Genauck, A., Wrase, J., Schlagenhauf, F., Smolka, M. N., et al. (2012). Effect of brain structure, brain function, and brain connectivity on relapse in alcohol-dependent patients. *Archives of General Psychiatry, 69*(8), 842–852.

Bellani, M., Yeh, P., Tansella, M., Balestrieri, M., Soares, J. C., & Brambilla, P. (2009). DTI studies of corpus callosum in bipolar disorder. *Biochemical Society Transactions, 37*(Part 5), 1096–1098.

Ben-Shachar, D., Bonne, O., Chisin, R., Klein, E., Lester, H., Aharon-Peretz, J., et al. (2007). Cerebral glucose utilization and platelet mitochondrial complex I activity in schizophrenia: A FDG-PET study. *Progress in Neuropsychopharmacology and Biological Psychiatry, 31*, 807–813.

Bora, E., Harrison B. J., Fornito, A., Cocchi, L., Pujol, J., Fontenelle, L. F., et al. (2011). White matter microstructure in patients with obsessive-compulsive disorder. *Journal of Psychiatry and Neuroscience, 36*, 42–46.

Bosch, P., van den Noort, M., Yeo, S., Lim, S., Coenen, A., & van Luijtelaar, G. (2015). The effect of acupuncture on mood and working memory in patients with depression and schizophrenia. *Journal of Integrative Medicine, 13*(6), 380–390.

Brody, A. L., Saxena, S., Schwartz, J. M., Stoessel, P. W., Maidment, K., Phelps, M. E., & Baxter, L. R. (1998). FDG-PET predictors of response to behavioral therapy and pharmacotherapy in obsessive compulsive disorder. *Psychiatry Research: Neuroimaging, 84*(1), 1–6.

Brody, A. L., Saxena, S., Silverman, D. H. S., Fairbanks, L. A., Phelps, M. E., Huang, S., et al. (1999). Brain metabolic changes in major depressive disorder from pre- to post-treatment with paroxetine. *Psychiatry Research: Neuroimaging, 91*(3), 127–139.

Bruno, S., Cercignani, M., & Ron, M. A. (2008). White matter abnormalities in bipolar disorder: A voxel-based diffusion tensor imaging study. *Bipolar Disorders, 10*(4), 460–468.

Buchsbaum, M. S., Christian, B. T., Lehrer, D. S., Narayanan, T. K., Shi, B., Mantil, J., et al. (2006). D2/D3 dopamine receptor binding with [F-18]fallypride in thalamus and cortex of patients with schizophrenia. *Schizophrenia Research, 85*(1), 232–244.

Buchsbaum, M. S., & Hazlett, E. A. (1998). Positron emission tomography studies of abnormal glucose metabolism in schizophrenia. *Schizophrenia Bulletin, 24*(3), 343–364.

Buchsbaum, M. S., Wu, J., Haier, R., Hazlett, E., Ball, R., Katz, M., et al. (1987). Positron emission tomography assessment of effects of benzodiazepines on regional glucose metabolic rate in patients with anxiety disorder. *Life Sciences, 40*(25), 2393–2400.

Cannistraro, P. A., Makris, N., Howard, J. D., Wedig, M. M., Hodge, S. M., Wilhelm, S., & Fukui, K. (2007). A diffusion tensor imaging study of white matter in obsessive-compulsive disorder. *Depression and Anxiety, 24*(6), 440–446.

Chen, F., Lv, X., Fang, J., Yu, S., Sui, J., Fan, L., et al. (2015). The effect of body-mind relaxation meditation induction on major depressive disorder: A resting-state fMRI study. *Journal of Affective Disorders, 183*, 75–82.

Chételat, G., Eustache, F., Viader, F., De La Sayette, V., Pélerin, A., Mézenge, F., et al. (2005). FDG-PET measurement is more accurate than neuropsychological assessments to predict global cognitive deterioration in patients with mild cognitive impairment. *Neurocase, 11*(1), 14.

Cheung, V., Cheung, C., McAlonan, G., Deng, Y., Wong, J., Yip, L., et al. (2008). A diffusion tensor imaging study of structural dysconnectivity in never-medicated, first-episode schizophrenia. *Psychological Medicine, 38*(6), 877–885.

Clark, C., Kopala, L., Li, D. K., & Hurwitz, T. (2001). Regional cerebral glucose metabolism in never-medicated patients with schizophrenia. *Canadian Journal of Psychiatry. Revue Canadienne De Psychiatrie, 46*(4), 340–346.

Costafreda, S. G., Khanna, A., Mourao-Miranda, J., & Fu, C. H. Y. (2009). Neural correlates of sad faces predict clinical remission to cognitive behavioural therapy in depression. *NeuroReport, 20*(7), 637–641.

Dao-Castellana, M., Paillère-Martinot, M., Hantraye, P., Attar-Lévy, D., Rémy, P., Crouzel, C., et al. (1997). Presynaptic dopaminergic function in the striatum of schizophrenic patients. *Schizophrenia Research, 23*(2), 167–174.

de Wit, S. J., Alonso, P., Schweren, L., Mataix-Cols, D., Lochner, C., Menchón, J. M., et al. (2014). Multicenter voxel-based morphometry mega-analysis of structural brain scans in obsessive-compulsive disorder. *BMC Psychiatry, 171*(3), 340–349.

Deng, D., Liao, H., Duan, G., Liu, Y., He, Q., Liu, H., et al. (2016). Modulation of the default mode network in first-episode, drug-naïve major depressive disorder via acupuncture at Baihui (GV20) acupoint. *Frontiers in Human Neuroscience, 10*, 230.

Deng, H., & Adams, C. E. (2017). Traditional Chinese medicine for schizophrenia: A survey of randomized trials. *Asia-Pacific Psychiatry, 9*.

Elkashef, A. M., Doudet, D., Bryant, T., Cohen, R. M., Li, S. H., & Wyatt, R. J. (2000). 6-(18)F-DOPA PET study in patients with schizophrenia: Positron emission tomography. *Psychiatry Research*, *100*(1), 1–11.

Eschweiler, G. W., Wegerer, C., Schlotter, W., Spandl, C., Stevens, A., Bartels, M., & Buchkremer, G. (2000). Left prefrontal activation predicts therapeutic effects of repetitive transcranial magnetic stimulation (rTMS) in major depression. *Psychiatry Research: Neuroimaging*, *99*(3), 161–172.

Falconer, E., Allen, A., Felmingham, K. L., Williams, L. M., & Bryant, R. A. (2013). Inhibitory neural activity predicts response to cognitive-behavioral therapy for posttraumatic stress disorder. *The Journal of Clinical Psychiatry*, *74*(9), 895–901.

Fu, C. H. Y., Williams, S. C. R., Cleare, A. J., Scott, J., Mitterschiffthaler, M. T., Walsh, N. D., et al. (2008). Neural responses to sad facial expressions in major depression following cognitive behavioral therapy. *Biological Psychiatry*, *64*(6), 505–512.

Fujimoto, T., Takeuch, K., Matsumoto, T., Kamimura, K., Hamada, R., Nakamura, K., & Kato, N. (2007). Abnormal glucose metabolism in the anterior cingulate cortex in patients with schizophrenia. *Psychiatry Research: Neuroimaging*, *154*(1), 49–58.

Fujino, J., Yamasaki, N., Miyata, J., Sasaki, H., Matsukawa, N., Takemura, A., et al. (2015). Anterior cingulate volume predicts response to cognitive behavioral therapy in major depressive disorder. *Journal of Affective Disorders*, *174*, 397–399.

Gardner, A., Iverson, G. L., & Stanwell, P. (2014). A systematic review of proton magnetic resonance spectroscopy findings in sport-related concussion. *Journal of Neurotrauma*, *31*(1), 1–18.

Garibotto, V., Scifo, P., Gorini, A., Alonso, C. R., Brambati, S., Bellodi, L., & Perani, D. (2010). Disorganization of anatomical connectivity in obsessive compulsive disorder: A multi-parameter diffusion tensor imaging study in a subpopulation of patients. *Neurobiology of Disease*, *37*(2), 468–476.

George, J. K., Alavi, A., Zimmerman, R. A. (1989). Metabolic (PET) correlates of anatomic lesions (CT/MRI) produced by head trauma [Abstract]. *The Journal of Nuclear Medicine*, *30*, 802.

Gilman, S., Koeppe, R. A., Adams, K. M., Junck, L., Kluin, K. J., Johnson-Greene, D., et al. (1998). Decreased striatal monoaminergic terminals in severe chronic alcoholism demonstrated with (+)[11C]dihydrotetrabenazine and positron emission tomography. *Annals of Neurology*, *44*(3), 326–333.

Godlewska, B. R., Browning, M., Norbury, R., Cowen, P. J., & Harmer, C. J. (2016). Early changes in emotional processing as a marker of clinical response to SSRI treatment in depression. *Translational Psychiatry*, *6*(11), e957.

Goldin, P., Ziv, M., Jazaieri, H., & Gross, J. J. (2012). Randomized controlled trial of mindfulness-based stress reduction versus aerobic exercise: Effects on the self-referential brain network in social anxiety disorder. *Frontiers in Human Neuroscience*, *6*, 295.

Goldin, P., Ziv, M., Jazaieri, H., Hahn, K., & Gross, J. J. (2013). MBSR vs aerobic exercise in social anxiety: fMRI of emotion regulation of negative self-beliefs. *Social Cognitive and Affective Neuroscience*, *8*(1), 65–72.

Gray, B. G., Ichise, M., Chung, D., Kirsh, J. C., & Franks, W. (1992). Technetium-99m-HMPAO SPECT in the evaluation of patients with a remote history of traumatic brain injury: A comparison with X-ray computed tomography. *The Journal of Nuclear Medicine, 33*(1), 52–58.

Grüsser, S. M., Wrase, J., Klein, S., Hermann, D., Smolka, M. N., Ruf, M., et al. (2004). Cue-induced activation of the striatum and medial prefrontal cortex is associated with subsequent relapse in abstinent alcoholics. *Psychopharmacology, 175*(3), 296–302.

Hao, Y., Liu, Z., Jiang, T., Gong, G., Liu, H., Tan, L., et al. (2006). White matter integrity of the whole brain is disrupted in first-episode schizophrenia. *Neuroreport, 17*(1), 23–26.

Hayes, R., & Dixon, C. (1994). Neurochemical changes in mild head injury. *Seminars in Neurology, 14*(1), 25–31.

Haznedar, M. M., Buchsbaum, M. S., Hazlett, E. A., Shihabuddin, L., New, A., & Siever, L. J. (2004). Cingulate gyrus volume and metabolism in the schizophrenia spectrum. *Schizophrenia Research, 71*(2), 249–262.

Heinz, A., Beck, A., Grusser, S. M., Grace, A. A., & Wrase, J. (2009). Identifying the neural circuitry of alcohol craving and relapse vulnerability. *Addiction Biology, 14*(1), 108–118.

Heng, S., Song, A. W., & Sim, K. (2010). White matter abnormalities in bipolar disorder: Insights from diffusion tensor imaging studies. *Journal of Neural Transmission, 117*(5), 639–654.

Hietala, J., Syvälahti, E., Vuorio, K., Räkköläinen, V., Bergman, J., Haaparanta, M., Solin, O., Kuoppamäki, M., Kirvelä, O., Ruotsalainen, U., et al. (1995). Presynaptic dopamine function in striatum of neuroleptic-naive schizophrenic patients. *Lancet, 346*(8983), 1130–1131.

Hill, K., Mann, L., Laws, K. R., C. M. E. Stephenson, Nimmo-Smith, I., & McKenna, P. J. (2004). Hypofrontality in schizophrenia: A meta-analysis of functional imaging studies. *Acta Psychiatrica Scandinavica, 110*(4), 243–256.

Hoexter, M. Q., Dougherty, D. D., Shavitt, R. G., D'Alcante, C. C., Duran, F. L. S., Lopes, A. C., et al. (2013). Differential prefrontal gray matter correlates of treatment response to fluoxetine or cognitive-behavioral therapy in obsessive-compulsive disorder. *European Neuropsychopharmacology, 23*(7), 569–580.

Hommer, D., Andreasen, P., Rio, D., Williams, W., Ruttimann, U., Momenan, R., et al. (1997). Effects of m-chlorophenylpiperazine on regional brain glucose utilization: A positron emission tomographic comparison of alcoholic and control subjects. *Journal of Neuroscience, 17*(8), 2796–2806.

Honea, R., Crow, T. J., Passingham, D., & Mackay, C. E. (2005). Regional deficits in brain volume in schizophrenia: A meta-analysis of voxel-based morphometry studies. *The American Journal of Psychiatry, 162*(12), 2233–2245.

Hosokawa, T., Momose, T., & Kasai, K. (2009). Brain glucose metabolism difference between bipolar and unipolar mood disorders in depressed and euthymic states. *Progress in Neuropsychopharmacology & Biological Psychiatry, 33*(2), 243–250.

Howes, O. D., Montgomery, A. J., Asselin, M., Murray, R. M., Valli, I., Tabraham, P., et al. (2009). Elevated striatal dopamine function linked to prodromal signs of schizophrenia. *Archives of General Psychiatry, 66*(1), 13–20.

Insel, T. R., & Winslow, J. T. (1992). Neurobiology of obsessive compulsive disorder. *The Psychiatric Clinics of North America, 15*(4), 813–824.

Ives-Deliperi, V. L., Howells, F., Stein, D. J., Meintjes, E. M., & Horn, N. (2013). The effects of mindfulness-based cognitive therapy in patients with bipolar disorder: A controlled functional MRI investigation. *Journal of Affective Disorders, 150*(3), 1152–1157.

Jansen, J. M., van Wingen, G., van den Brink, W., & Goudriaan, A. E. (2015). Resting state connectivity in alcohol dependent patients and the effect of repetitive transcranial magnetic stimulation. *European Neuropsychopharmacology, 25*(12), 2230–2239.

Kafantaris, V., Kingsley, P., Ardekani, B., Saito, E., Lencz, T., Limk K., & Szeszko, P. (2009). Lower orbital frontal white matter integrity in adolescents with bipolar disorder. *Journal of American Academy of Child and Adolescent Psychiatry, 48,* 79–86.

Kakeda, S., & Korogi, Y. (2010). The efficacy of a voxel-based morphometry on the analysis of imaging in schizophrenia, temporal lobe epilepsy, and Alzheimer's disease/mild cognitive impairment: A review. *Neuroradiology, 52*(8), 711–721.

Kennedy, S. H., Evans, K. R., Krüger, S., Mayberg, H. S., Meyer, J. H., McCann, S., et al. (2001). Changes in regional brain glucose metabolism measured with positron emission tomography after paroxetine treatment of major depression. *The American Journal of Psychiatry, 158*(6), 899–905.

Kennedy, S. H., Konarski, J. Z., Segal, Z. V., Lau, M. A., Bieling, P. J., McIntyre, R. S., & Mayberg, H. S. (2007). Differences in brain glucose metabolism between responders to CBT and venlafaxine in a 16-week randomized controlled trial. *The American Journal of Psychiatry, 164*(5), 778–788.

Kern, S., Oakes, T. R., Stone, C. K., McAuliff, E. M., Kirschbaum, C., & Davidson, R. J. (2008). Glucose metabolic changes in the prefrontal cortex are associated with HPA axis response to a psychosocial stressor. *Psychoneuroendocrinology, 33*(4), 517–529.

Ketter, T. A., Kimbrell, T. A., George, M. S., Dunn, R. T., Speer, A. M., Benson, B. E., et al. (2001). Effects of mood and subtype on cerebral glucose metabolism in treatment-resistant bipolar disorder. *Biological Psychiatry, 49*(2), 97–109.

Kimbrell, T. A., Little, J. T., Dunn, R. T., Frye, M. A., Greenberg, B. D., Wassermann, E. M., et al. (1999). Frequency dependence of antidepressant response to left prefrontal repetitive transcranial magnetic stimulation (rTMS) as a function of baseline cerebral glucose metabolism. *Biological Psychiatry, 46*(12), 1603–1613.

King, A. P., Block, S. R., Sripada, R. K., Rauch, S., Giardino, N., Favorite, T., et al. (2016). Altered default mode network (DMN) resting state functional connectivity following a mindfulness-based exposure therapy for posttraumatic stress disorder (PTSD) in combat veterans of Afghanistan and Iraq. *Depression and Anxiety, 33*(4), 289–299.

Kito, S., Hasegawa, T., & Koga, Y. (2012a). Cerebral blood flow in the ventromedial prefrontal cortex correlates with treatment response to low-frequency right prefrontal repetitive transcranial magnetic stimulation in the treatment of depression. *Psychiatry and Clinical Neurosciences, 66*(2), 138–145.

Kito, S., Hasegawa, T., & Koga, Y. (2012b). Cerebral blood flow ratio of the dorsolateral prefrontal cortex to the ventromedial prefrontal cortex as a potential predictor of treatment response to transcranial magnetic stimulation in depression. *Brain Stimulation*, 5(4), 547–553.

Kjaer, T. W., Bertelsen, C., Piccini, P., Brooks, D., Alving, J., & Lou, H. C. (2002). Increased dopamine tone during meditation-induced change of consciousness. *Cognitive Brain Research*, 13(2), 255–259.

Klumpers, U. M. H., Veltman, D. J., Drent, M. L., Boellaard, R., Comans, E. F. I., Meynen, G., et al. (2010). Reduced parahippocampal and lateral temporal GABAA-[11C]flumazenil binding in major depression: Preliminary results. *European Journal of Nuclear Medicine and Molecular Imaging*, 37(3), 565–574.

Kozicky, J., Ha, T. H., Torres, I. J., Bond, D. J., Honer, W. G., Lam, R. W., & Yatham, L. N. (2013). Relationship between frontostriatal morphology and executive function deficits in bipolar I disorder following a first manic episode: Data from the systematic treatment optimization program for early mania (STOP-EM). *Bipolar Disorders*, 15(6), 657–668.

Kubicki, M., McCarley, R., Westin, C., Park, H., Maier, S., Kikinis, R., et al. (2007). A review of diffusion tensor imaging studies in schizophrenia. *Journal of Psychiatric Research*, 41(1), 15–30.

Kubicki, M., McCarley, R. W., & Shenton, M. E. (2005). Evidence for white matter abnormalities in schizophrenia. *Current Opinion in Psychiatry*, 18(2), 121–134.

Kugaya, A., Sanacora, G., Staley, J. K., Malison, R. T., Bozkurt, A., Khan, S., et al. (2004). Brain serotonin transporter availability predicts treatment response to selective serotonin reuptake inhibitors. *Biological Psychiatry*, 56(7), 497–502.

Kumra, S., Ashtari, M., McMeniman, M., Vogel, J., Augustin, R., Becker, D. E., et al. (2004). Reduced frontal white matter integrity in early-onset schizophrenia: A preliminary study. *Biological Psychiatry*, 55(12), 1138–1145.

Kyriakopoulos, M., Vyas, N. S., Barker, G. J., Chitnis, X. A., & Frangou, S. (2008). A diffusion tensor imaging study of white matter in early-onset schizophrenia. *Biological Psychiatry*, 63(5), 519–523.

Langer, Á. I., Cangas, A. J., Salcedo, E., & Fuentes, B. (2012). Applying mindfulness therapy in a group of psychotic individuals: A controlled study. *Behavioural and Cognitive Psychotherapy*, 40(1), 105–109.

Langguth, B., Wiegand, R., Kharraz, A., Landgrebe, M., Marienhagen, J., Frick, U., et al. (2007). Pre-treatment anterior cingulate activity as a predictor of antidepressant response to repetitive transcranial magnetic stimulation (rTMS). *Neuro Endocrinology Letters*, 28(5), 633–638.

Lanzenberger, R., Kranz, G. S., Haeusler, D., Akimova, E., Savli, M., Hahn, A., et al. (2012). Prediction of SSRI treatment response in major depression based on serotonin transporter interplay between median raphe nucleus and projection areas. *NeuroImage*, 63(2), 874–881.

Li, C., Hsieh, J., Wang, S., Yang, B., Bai, Y., Lin, W., et al. (2012). Differential relations between fronto-limbic metabolism and executive function in patients with remitted bipolar I and bipolar II disorder. *Bipolar Disorders*, 14(8), 831–842.

Lindström, L. H., Gefvert, O., Hagberg, G., Lundberg, T., Bergström, M., Hartvig, P., & Långström, B. (1999). Increased dopamine synthesis rate in medial prefrontal cortex and striatum in schizophrenia indicated by L-(β- 11C) DOPA and PET. *Biological Psychiatry, 46*(5), 681–688.

Little, J. T., Ketter, T. A., Kimbrell, T. A., Danielson, A., Benson, B., Willis, M. W., & Post, R. M. (1996). Venlafaxine or bupropion responders but not nonresponders show baseline prefrontal and paralimbic hypometabolism compared with controls. *Psychopharmacology Bulletin, 32*(4), 629–635.

Little, J. T., Ketter, T. A., Kimbrell, T. A., Dunn, R. T., Benson, B. E., Willis, M. W., Luckenbaugh, D. A., & Post, R. M. (2005). Bupropion and venlafaxine responders differ in pretreatment regional cerebral metabolism in unipolar depression. *Biological Psychiatry, 57*(3), 220–228.

Mann, K., Vollstädt-Klein, S., Reinhard, I., Leménager, T., Fauth-Bühler, M., Hermann, D., et al. (2014). Predicting naltrexone response in alcohol-dependent patients: The contribution of functional magnetic resonance imaging. *Alcoholism: Clinical and Experimental Research, 38*(11), 2754–2762.

Matsumoto, R., Ichise, M., Ito, H., Ando, T., Takahashi, H., Ikoma, Y., et al. (2010). Reduced serotonin transporter binding in the insular cortex in patients with obsessive-compulsive disorder: A [11C]DASB PET study. *Neuroimage, 49*(1), 121–126.

Mayberg, H. S., Brannan, S. K., Tekell, J. L., Silva, J. A., Mahurin, R. K., McGinnis, S., & Jerabek, P. A. (2000). Regional metabolic effects of fluoxetine in major depression: Serial changes and relationship to clinical response. *Biological Psychiatry, 48*(8), 830–843.

McGrath, C. L., Kelley, M. E., Dunlop, B. W., Holtzheimer, P. E, Craighead, W. E., & Mayberg, H. S. (2014). Pretreatment brain states identify likely nonresponse to standard treatments for depression. *Biological Psychiatry, 76*(7), 527–535.

McGrath, C. L., Kelley, M. E., Holtzheimer, P. E., Dunlop, B. W., Craighead, W. E., Franco, A. R., et al. (2013). Toward a neuroimaging treatment selection biomarker for major depressive disorder. *JAMA Psychiatry, 70*(8), 821–829.

Meltzer, C. C., Price, J. C., Mathis, C. A., Greer, P. J., Cantwell, M. N., Houck, P. R., et al. (1999). PET imaging of serotonin type 2A receptors in late-life neuropsychiatric disorders. *The American Journal of Psychiatry, 156*(12), 1871–1878.

Menzies, L., Chamberlain, S. R., Laird, A. R., Thelen, S. M., Sahakian, B. J., & Bullmore, E. T. (2008). Integrating evidence from neuroimaging and neuropsychological studies of obsessive-compulsive disorder: The orbitofronto-striatal model revisited. *Neuroscience and Biobehavioral Reviews, 32*(3), 525–549.

Meyer, J. H. (2007). Imaging the serotonin transporter during major depressive disorder and antidepressant treatment. *Journal of Psychiatry & Neuroscience, 32*(2), 86–102.

Meyer, J. H., Kapur, S., Eisfeld, B., Brown, G. M., Houle, S., DaSilva, J., et al. (2001). The effect of paroxetine on 5-HT (2A) receptors in depression: An [(18)F]setoperone PET imaging study. *The American Journal of Psychiatry, 158*(1), 78–85.

Milak, M. S., Keilp, J., Parsey, R. V., Oquendo, M. A., Malone, K. M., & Mann, J. J. (2010). Regional brain metabolic correlates of self-reported depression severity contrasted with clinician ratings. *Journal of Affective Disorders, 126*(1), 113–124.

Milak, M. S., Parsey, R. V., Keilp, J., Oquendo, M. A., Malone, K. M., & Mann, J. J. (2005). Neuroanatomic correlates of psychopathologic components of major depressive disorder. *Archives of General Psychiatry, 62*(4), 397–408.

Molina, M. E., Isoardi, R., Prado, M. N., & Bentolila, S. (2010). Basal cerebral glucose distribution in long-term post-traumatic stress disorder. *The World Journal of Biological Psychiatry, 11*(2 Part 2), 493–501.

Monti, D. A., Tobia, A., Stoner, M., Wintering, N., Matthews, M., He, X. S., et al. (2017). Neuro emotional technique effects on brain physiology in cancer patients with traumatic stress symptoms: Preliminary findings. *Journal of Cancer Survivorship, 11*(4), 438–446.

Moresco, R. M., Pietra, L., Henin, M., Panzacchi, A., Locatelli, M., Bonaldi, L., et al. (2007). Fluvoxamine treatment and D2 receptors: A PET study on OCD drug-naïve patients. *Neuropsychopharmacology, 32*(1), 197–205.

Myrick, H., Anton, R. F., Li, X., Henderson, S., Drobes, D., Voronin, K., & George, M. S. (2004). Differential brain activity in alcoholics and social drinkers to alcohol cues: Relationship to craving. *Neuropsychopharmacology, 29*(2), 393–402.

Nakamae, T., Narumoto, J., Shibata, K., Matsumoto, R., Kitabayashi, Y., Yoshida, T., et al. (2008). Alteration of fractional anisotropy and apparent diffusion coefficient in obsessive-compulsive disorder: A diffusion tensor imaging study. *Progress in Neuropsychopharmacology & Biological Psychiatry, 32*(5), 1221–1226.

Newton, M. R., Greenwood, R. J., Britton, K. E., Charlesworth, M., Nimmon, C. C., Carroll, M. J., & Dolke, G. (1992). A study comparing SPECT with CT and MRI after closed head injury. *Journal of Neurology, Neurosurgery, and Psychiatry, 55*(2), 92–94.

Nitschke, J. B., Davidson, R. J., Sarinopoulos, I., Kalin, N. H., Johnstone, T., Whalen, P. J., & Oathes, D. J. (2009). Anticipatory activation in the amygdala and anterior cingulate in generalized anxiety disorder and prediction of treatment response. *The American Journal of Psychiatry, 166*(3), 302–310.

Okubo, Y., Suhara, T., Suzuki, K., Kobayashi, K., Inoue, O., Terasaki, O., et al. (1997). Decreased prefrontal dopamine D1 receptors in schizophrenia revealed by PET. *Nature, 385*(6617), 634–636.

Park, K., Kim, J., Seok, J. H., Chun, J. W., Park, H., & Lee, J. D. (2009). Anhedonia and ambivalence in schizophrenic patients with fronto-cerebellar metabolic abnormalities: A fluoro-D-glucose positron emission tomography study. *Psychiatry Investigation, 6*(2), 72–77.

Perani, D., Garibotto, V., Gorini, A., Moresco, R. M., Henin, M., Panzacchi, A., et al. (2008). In vivo PET study of 5HT(2A) serotonin and D(2) dopamine dysfunction in drug-naive obsessive-compulsive disorder. *Neuroimage, 42*(1), 306–314.

Phelps, M. E., Mazziotta, J. C., Baxter, L., & Gerner, R. (1984). Positron emission tomographic study of affective disorders: Problems and strategies. *Annals of Neurology, 15*(Suppl.), S149–S156.

Price, G., Cercignani, M., Parker, G. J. M., Altmann, D. R., Barnes, T. R. E., Barker, G. J., et al. (2007). Abnormal brain connectivity in first-episode psychosis: A diffusion MRI tractography study of the corpus callosum. *Neuroimage, 35*(2), 458–466.

Price, G., Cercignani, M., Parker, G. J. M., Altmann, D. R., Barnes, T. R. E., Barker, G. J., et al. (2008). White matter tracts in first-episode psychosis: A DTI tractography study of the uncinate fasciculus. *Neuroimage, 39*(3), 949–955.

Pruessner, J. C., Pruessner, M., Dedovic, K., Lord, C., Buss, C., Collins, L., et al. (2010). Stress regulation in the central nervous system: Evidence from structural and functional neuroimaging studies in human populations—2008 Curt Richter award winner. *Psychoneuroendocrinology, 35*(1), 179–191.

Quah-Smith, I., Suo, C., Williams, M. A., & Sachdev, P. S. (2013). The antidepressant effect of laser acupuncture: A comparison of the resting brain's default mode network in healthy and depressed subjects during functional magnetic resonance imaging. *Medical Acupuncture, 25*(2), 124–133.

Reiman, E. M., Butler, F. K., Raichle, M. E., Robins, E., & Herscovitch, P. (1984). A focal brain abnormality in panic disorder, a severe form of anxiety. *Nature, 310*(5979), 683–685.

Reiman, E. M., Raichle, M. E., Robins, E., Mintun, M. A., Fusselman, M. J., Fox, P. T., et al. (1989). Neuroanatomical correlates of a lactate-induced anxiety attack. *Archives of General Psychiatry, 46*(6), 493–500.

Reith, J., Benkelfat, C., Sherwin, A., Yasuhara, Y., Kuwabara, H., Andermann, F., et al. (1994). Elevated dopa decarboxylase activity in living brain of patients with psychosis. *Proceedings of the National Academy of Sciences of the United States of America, 91*(24), 11651–11654.

Ritchey, M., Dolcos, F., Eddington, K. M., Strauman, T. J., & Cabeza, R. (2011). Neural correlates of emotional processing in depression: Changes with cognitive behavioral therapy and predictors of treatment response. *Journal of Psychiatric Research, 45*(5), 577–587.

Sachs, H., Russell, J. A. G., Christman, D. R., & Cook, B. (1987). Alteration of regional cerebral glucose metabolic rate in non-korsakoff chronic alcoholism. *Archives of Neurology, 44*(12), 1242–1251.

Saijo, T., Takano, A., Suhara, T., Arakawa, R., Okumura, M., Ichimiya, T., et al. (2010). Effect of electroconvulsive therapy on 5-HT1A receptor binding in patients with depression: A PET study with [11C]WAY 100635. *International Journal of Neuropsychopharmacology, 13*(6), 785–791.

Saijo, T., Takano, A., Suhara, T., Arakawa, R., Okumura, M., Ichimiya, T., Ito, H., & Okubo, Y. (2010). Electroconvulsive therapy decreases dopamine D-receptor binding in the anterior cingulate in patients with depression: a controlled study using positron emission tomography with radioligand [^{11}C]FLB 457. *Journal of Clinical Psychiatry, 71*(6), 793–799.

Saito, Y., Nobuhara, K., Okugawa, G., Takase, K., Sugimoto, T., Horiuchi, M., et al. (2008). Corpus callosum in patients with obsessive-compulsive disorder: Diffusion-tensor imaging study. *Radiology, 246*(2), 536–542.

Samson, A. C., Meisenzahl, E., Scheuerecker, J., Rose, E., Schoepf, V., Wiesmann, M., & Frodl, T. (2011). Brain activation predicts treatment improvement in patients with major depressive disorder. *Journal of Psychiatric Research, 45*(9), 1214–1222.

Samson, Y., Baron, J. C., Feline, A., Bories, J., & Crouzel, C. (1986). Local cerebral glucose utilisation in chronic alcoholics: A positron tomographic study. *Journal of Neurology, Neurosurgery, and Psychiatry, 49*(10), 1165–1170.

Sargent, P. A., Kjaer, K. H., Bench, C. J., Rabiner, E. A., Messa, C., Meyer, J., et al. (2000). Brain serotonin1a receptor binding measured by positron emission tomography with [11C]WAY-100635: Effects of depression and antidepressant treatment. *Archives of General Psychiatry, 57*(2), 174–180.

Sawle, G. V., Hymas, N. F., Lees, A. J., & Frackowiak, R. S. (1991). Obsessional slowness: Functional studies with positron emission tomography. *Brain: A Journal of Neurology, 114*(Part 5), 2191–2202.

Saxena, S., Brody, A. L., Maidment, K. M., Dunkin, J. J., Colgan, M., Alborzian, S., et al. (1999). Localized orbitofrontal and subcortical metabolic changes and predictors of response to paroxetine treatment in obsessive-compulsive disorder. *Neuropsychopharmacology, 21*(6), 683–693.

Schwartz, J. M. (1987). The differential diagnosis of depression. relevance of positron emission tomography studies of cerebral glucose metabolism to the bipolar-unipolar dichotomy. *JAMA, 258*(10), 1368–1374.

Schwartz, J. M., Stoessel, P. W., Baxter, L. R., Martin, K. M., & Phelps, M. E. (1996). Systematic changes in cerebral glucose metabolic rate after successful behavior modification treatment of obsessive-compulsive disorder. *Archives of General Psychiatry, 53*(2), 109–113.

Selvaraj, S., Murthy, N. V., Bhagwagar, Z., Bose, S. K., Hinz, R., Grasby, P. M., & Cowen, P. J. (2011). Diminished brain 5-HT transporter binding in major depression: A positron emission tomography study with [11C]DASB. *Psychopharmacology, 213*(2-3), 555–562.

Shannahoff-Khalsa, D. S., Ray, L. E., Levine, S., Gallen, C. C., Schwartz, B. J., & Sidorowich, J. J. (1999). Randomized controlled trial of yogic meditation techniques for patients with obsessive-compulsive disorder. *CNS Spectrums, 4*(12), 34–47.

Shenton, M. E., Hamoda, H. M., Schneiderman, J. S., Bouix, S., Pasternak, O., Rathi, Y., et al. (2012). A review of magnetic resonance imaging and diffusion tensor imaging findings in mild traumatic brain injury. *Brain Imaging and Behavior, 6*(2), 137–192.

Shenton, M. E., Whitford, T. J., & Kubicki, M. (2010). Structural neuroimaging in schizophrenia: From methods to insights to treatments. *Dialogues in Clinical Neuroscience, 12*(3), 317–332.

Shin, L. M., McNally, R. J., Kosslyn, S. M., Thompson, W. L., Rauch, S. L., Alpert, N. M., et al. (1999). Regional cerebral blood flow during script-driven imagery in childhood sexual abuse-related PTSD: A PET investigation. *The American Journal of Psychiatry, 156*(4), 575–584.

Shin, L. M., Orr, S. P., Carson, M. A., Rauch, S. L., Macklin, M. L., Lasko, N. B., et al. (2004). Regional cerebral blood flow in the amygdala and medial prefrontal cortex during traumatic imagery in male and female Vietnam veterans with PTSD. *Archives of General Psychiatry, 61*(2), 168–176.

Siegle, G. J., Carter, C. S., & Thase, M. E. (2006). Use of fMRI to predict recovery from unipolar depression with cognitive behavior therapy. *The American Journal of Psychiatry, 163*(4), 735–738.

Smith, G. S., Reynolds, C. F., Pollock, B., Derbyshire, S., Nofzinger, E., Dew, M. A., et al. (1999). Cerebral glucose metabolic response to combined total sleep deprivation and antidepressant treatment in geriatric depression. *The American Journal of Psychiatry, 156*(5), 683–689.

Soyka, M., Koch, W., Möller, H. J., Rüther, T., & Tatsch, K. (2005). Hypermetabolic pattern in frontal cortex and other brain regions in unmedicated schizophrenia patients: Results from a FDG-PET study. *European Archives of Psychiatry and Clinical Neuroscience, 255*(5), 308–312.

Stevens, M. C., Lovejoy, D., Kim, J., Oakes, H., Kureshi, I., & Witt, S. T. (2012). Multiple resting state network functional connectivity abnormalities in mild traumatic brain injury. *Brain Imaging and Behavior, 6*(2), 293–318.

Streeter, C. C., Jensen, J. E., Perlmutter, R. M., Cabral, H. J., Tian, H., Terhune, D. B., et al. (2007). Yoga asana sessions increase brain GABA levels: A pilot study. *Journal of Alternative and Complementary Medicine, 13*(4), 419–426.

Su, L., Cai, Y., Xu, Y., Dutt, A., Shi, S., & Bramon, E. (2014). Cerebral metabolism in major depressive disorder: A voxel-based meta-analysis of positron emission tomography studies. *BMC Psychiatry, 14*(1), 321.

Suhara, T., Okubo, Y., Yasuno, F., Sudo, Y., Inoue, M., Ichimiya, T., et al. (2002). Decreased dopamine D2 receptor binding in the anterior cingulate cortex in schizophrenia. *Archives of General Psychiatry, 59*(1), 25–30.

Swedo, S. E., Schapiro, M. B., Grady, C. L., Cheslow, D. L., Leonard, H. L., Kumar, A., et al. (1989). Cerebral glucose metabolism in childhood-onset obsessive-compulsive disorder. *Archives of General Psychiatry, 46*(6), 518–523.

Szeszko, P. R., Ardekani, B. A., Ashtari, M., Malhotra, A. K., Robinson, D. G., Bilder, R. M., & Lim, K. O. (2005). White matter abnormalities in obsessive-compulsive disorder: A diffusion tensor imaging study. *Archives of General Psychiatry, 62*(7), 782–790.

Szeszko, P. R., Hodgkinson, C. A., Robinson, D. G., DeRosse, P., Bilder, R. M., Lencz, T., et al. (2008). DISC1 is associated with prefrontal cortical gray matter and positive symptoms in schizophrenia. *Biological Psychology, 79*(1), 103–110.

Talvik, M., Nordström, A., Olsson, H., Halldin, C., & Farde, L. (2003). Decreased thalamic D2/D3 receptor binding in drug-naive patients with schizophrenia: A PET study with [11C]FLB 457. *International Journal of Neuropsychopharmacology, 6*(4), 361–370.

Thompson, D. G., Kesler, S. R., Sudheimer, K., Mehta, K. M., Thompson, L. W., Marquett, R. M., et al. (2015). FMRI activation during executive function predicts response to cognitive behavioral therapy in older, depressed adults. *The American Journal of Geriatric Psychiatry, 23*(1), 13–22.

van der Schot, Astrid C, Vonk, R., Brouwer, R. M., van Baal, C. M., Brans, R. G. H., et al. (2010). Genetic and environmental influences on focal brain density in bipolar disorder. *Brain, 133*(10), 3080–3092.

Volkow, N. D., & Fowler, J. S. (1992). Neuropsychiatric disorders: Investigation of schizophrenia and substance abuse. *Seminars in Nuclear Medicine, 22*(4), 254–267.

Volkow, N. D., Wang, G. J., Begleiter, H., Hitzemann, R., Pappas, N., Burr, G., et al. (1995). Regional brain metabolic response to lorazepam in subjects at risk for alcoholism. *Alcoholism, Clinical and Experimental Research, 19*(2), 510–516.

Volkow, N. D., Wang, G. J., Hitzemann, R., Fowler, J. S., Wolf, A. P., Pappas, N., et al. (1993). Decreased cerebral response to inhibitory neurotransmission in alcoholics. *The American Journal of Psychiatry, 150*(3), 417–422.

Whalen, P. J., Johnstone, T., Somerville, L. H., Nitschke, J. B., Polis, S., Alexander, A. L., et al. (2008). A functional magnetic resonance imaging predictor of treatment response to venlafaxine in generalized anxiety disorder. *Biological Psychiatry, 63*(9), 858–863.

White, T., Nelson, M., & Lim, K. O. (2008). Diffusion tensor imaging in psychiatric disorders. *Topics in Magnetic Resonance Imaging, 19*(2), 97–109.

Wiers, C. E., Wiers, R. W., Stelzel, C., Gladwin, T. E., Park, S. Q., Pawelczack, S., et al. (2015). Effects of cognitive bias modification training on neural alcohol cue reactivity in alcohol dependence. *The American Journal of Psychiatry, 172*(4), 335–343.

Wik, G., Borg, S., Sjögren, I., Wiesel, F. A., Blomqvist, G., Borg, J., & Stone-Elander, S. (1988). PET determination of regional cerebral glucose metabolism in alcohol-dependent men and healthy controls using 11C-glucose. *Acta Psychiatrica Scandinavica, 78*(2), 234–241.

Williams, L. M. (2008). Voxel-based morphometry in schizophrenia: Implications for neurodevelopmental connectivity models, cognition and affect. *Expert Review of Neurotherapeutics, 8*(7), 1049–1065.

Wu, J., Buchsbaum, M. S., Gillin, J. C., Tang, C., Cadwell, S., Wiegand, M., et al. (1999). Prediction of antidepressant effects of sleep deprivation by metabolic rates in the ventral anterior cingulate and medial prefrontal cortex. *The American Journal of Psychiatry, 156*(8), 1149–1158.

Wu, J. C., Buchsbaum, M. S., Hershey, T. G., Hazlett, E., Sicotte, N., & Chad Johnson, J. (1991). PET in generalized anxiety disorder. *Biological Psychiatry, 29*(12), 1181–1199.

Yasuno, F., Suhara, T., Ichimiya, T., Takano, A., Ando, T., & Okubo, Y. (2004). Decreased 5-HT1A receptor binding in amygdala of schizophrenia. *Biological Psychiatry, 55*(5), 439–444.

Zanardi, R., Artigas, F., Moresco, R., Colombo, C., Messa, C., Gobbo, C., et al. (2001). Increased 5-hydroxytryptamine-2 receptor binding in the frontal cortex of depressed patients responding to paroxetine treatment: A positron emission tomography scan study. *Journal of Clinical Psychopharmacology, 21*(1), 53–58.

Zhang, Z., Wang, X., Tan, Q., Jin, G., & Yao, S. (2009). Electroacupuncture for refractory obsessive-compulsive disorder: A pilot waitlist-controlled trial. *Journal of Nervous and Mental Disease, 197*(8), 619–622.

15

Commonly Encountered Sleep Disorders

KARL DOGHRAMJI

Key Points

- Sleep is not simply the absence of wakefulness; it is the product of active brain processes that produce changes throughout the mind and body.
- Insomnia and excessive daytime somnolence can have a number of causes that need to be identified first by using sleep logs, laboratory testing, and polysomnography.
- Although insomnia is often a product of psychiatric illness, the emergence of insomnia in otherwise healthy individuals, and its persistence, strongly predict the emergence of future psychiatric disorders, including depression, anxiety disorders, and substance use disorders.
- Integrative approaches focusing on sleep hygiene may be the most effective starting point for therapy.
- Cognitive therapy, relaxation therapy, and sleep restriction can also be effective therapeutic interventions.
- Pharmacological therapies include a variety of different types of medications that can all be potentially useful, but care must be taken regarding side effects and potential dependence.
- Sleep apnea is a common cause of sleep problems and can be managed using a variety of approaches including weight reduction and continuous positive airway pressure machines.
- Narcolepsy, restless legs syndrome, and parasomnias are other conditions that should be evaluated in patients with sleep problems.

The Clinical Approach to Sleep-Related Complaints

The two primary clinical manifestations of sleep disorders are insomnia and excessive daytime sleepiness (excessive daytime somnolence [EDS]). Sleepiness refers to the likelihood of falling asleep. This is considered a normal biological need or drive; an apt analogy is sleep is to sleepiness as food is to hunger. However, sleepiness is considered to be excessive when it is expressed at inappropriate times, such as during daytime activities, including driving and conversation. Insomnia is the inability to fall asleep, stay asleep, or the complaint of unrefreshing sleep despite adequate opportunity to do so. Unusual activity during sleep is also a common symptom of sleep disorders, and disorders featuring this symptom are collectively referred to as the parasomnias.

In the evaluation of sleep disturbances in clinical settings, the first task is to identify the underlying disorder(s). Following the identification of a primary sleep disorder, specific treatment can be instituted with confidence (Doghramji & Choufani, 2010).

The diagnostic process, summarized in Box 15.1, begins with a thorough history, with particular attention directed toward the hallmark symptoms of the major sleep disorders outlined earlier. In most cases, it is beneficial to interview the bed partner, who is more likely than the patient to be aware of

---

Box 15.1 The Clinical Evaluation of Sleep Disorders

1. Patient interview
2. Chief complaint: Insomnia, excessive daytime sleepiness, or parasomnia?
3. History of present illness
4. Sleep/wake habit history
5. Sleep hygiene history: meal and exercise times, ambient noise, light and temperature, etc.
6. Pattern of consumption of recreational substances (especially caffeine and alcohol) and medications
7. Medication history for both medical, psychiatric and sleep disorder
8. General medical, psychiatric, and surgical history
9. Sleep diary
10. Inventories for daytime sleepiness/alertness
11. Psychological inventories
12. Bedpartner interview
13. Physical and mental status examination
14. Serum laboratory tests
15. Polysomnography

Adapted from Doghramji & Choufani (2010).

unusual events during sleep. If the presenting symptom is excessive daytime sleepiness, its severity should be carefully evaluated. Patients almost invariably misjudge the extent of sleepiness. Therefore, direct questioning regarding how sleepy an individual feels often is not helpful. The propensity for falling asleep is a more accurate measure; in severe cases, individuals fall asleep while actively engaged in complex tasks such as speaking, writing, or even eating. They may also experience sleep attacks, which mandates rapid clinical intervention. Milder levels of daytime sleepiness result in falling asleep in passive situations, such as while reading or watching television. The Epworth Sleepiness Scale (Johns, 1991) is a useful office-based test for daytime sleepiness.

If the history is positive for naps, the possibility that they are related to narcolepsy should be examined by determining whether they are refreshing, brief in duration, or accompanied by dreams. The timing of naps also should be determined because this may alert the physician to the possibility of a circadian rhythm sleep disorder.

If the presenting symptom is insomnia, its duration should be determined. Disorders causing acute insomnia are usually transient in nature and more likely to resolve with conservative intervention and treatment with hypnotic agents. Chronic and unrelenting insomnia, which lasts more than a few months, usually requires a more careful investigation and complex treatment. A determination also should be made as to whether the patient's difficulty is in falling asleep or maintaining sleep. The former may be related to a circadian rhythm sleep disorder, while the latter is more consistent with gastroesophageal reflux disease, obstructive sleep apnea (OSA) or central sleep apnea (CSA) syndrome, or periodic limb movement disorder (PLMD), among others.

Sleep habits should be carefully reviewed, including the patient's usual bedtime, time spent awake in bed before and following the onset of sleep, and final morning awakening and arising times. Sleep logs completed daily over two weeks before the evaluation often are more revealing and accurate in this regard. The history also should include the pattern of drug, medication, and recreational substance use, as well as potential sleep hygiene difficulties.

A physical examination should be performed to assess signs of specific sleep disorders; for example, a neck circumference of 16 inches or greater in women and 17 inches or greater in men is associated with an increased risk for sleep-related breathing disorders (Chung et al., 2008). The examination can also reveal the potential for contributory medical and neurologic illnesses. A thorough psychiatric history and mental status examination are also important. Finally, serum laboratory tests, including thyroid function studies, should be considered if they have not been performed within six months before the evaluation.

If the this office-based process raises the possibility of an intrinsic sleep disorder, polysomnography should be considered. Circumstances when

> **Box 15.2 Circumstances When Appropriate to Refer to a Sleep Disorders Center**
>
> 1. Need for nocturnal or daytime polysomnography in the following situations:
>   a. Suspicion of a sleep-related breathing disorder
>   b. Assessment of efficacy of treatment for a sleep-related breathing disorder
>   c. Suspicion of PLMD or another sleep-related neuromuscular disorder that cannot be fully diagnosed by clinical interview
>   d. Paroxysmal arousals or other sleep-related behaviors thought related to a seizure disorder and an EEG and clinical evaluation are inconclusive
>   e. Suspicion of narcolepsy
>   f. When the diagnosis of insomnia is uncertain, if previous treatments have failed, or if that patient experiences abrupt arousals associated with violent behavior
> 2. Need for a consultation by a physician specializing in sleep medicine

polysomnography can be useful are outlined in Box 15.2 (Doghramji & Doghramji, 2007).

Selected Sleep Disorders

INSUFFICIENT SLEEP SYNDROME

Although not classified in the *Diagnostic and Statistical Manual of Mental Disorders* (fifth edition [DSM-5]), insufficient sleep syndrome is recognized in the International Classification of Sleep Disorders (ICSD; American Academy of Sleep Medicine [AASM], 2014). Insufficient sleep syndrome is often under-recognized as the most common cause of excessive daytime sleepiness worldwide. Persons affected with insufficient sleep syndrome curtail their time in bed, usually in response to social and occupational demands. Sleep deprivation may be acute, lasting a few hours or days, or chronic, lasting many days, months, or years. It may also be total, encompassing the entire night, or partial, involving a few hours per night. The most common type is chronic and partial. The National Sleep Foundation recently released normative sleep times by age (See Table 15.1), which is a helpful guideline for clinicians and patients. Sleep deprivation by as little as one hour per night, over long periods of time, can lead to debilitating EDS, which may necessitate long periods of recovery sleep. Sleep logs usually reveal curtailed bedtimes, occasionally with extended bedtime hours on weekends and holidays. Treatment with stimulant agents is rarely warranted because no degree of chronic curtailment in sleep needs can be soundly overcome by the habitual use of stimulant agents.

Table 15.1. National Sleep Foundation Expert Panel Guidelines for Sleep Duration

Age	Recommended (Hours)	May Be Appropriate (Hours)	Not Recommended (Hours)
Newborns 0–3 months	14 to 17	11 to 19	Less than 11. More than 19
Infants 4–11 months	12 to 15	10 to 18	Less than 10. More than 18
Toddlers 1–2 years	11 to 14	9 to 16	Less than 9. More than 16
Preschoolers 3–5 years	10 to 13	8 to 14	Less than 8. More than 14
School-aged children 6–13 years	9 to 11	7 to 12	Less than 7. More than 12
Teenagers 14–17 years	8 to 10	7 to 11	Less than 7. More than 11
Young adults 18–25 years	7 to 9	6 to 11	Less than 6. More than 11
Adults 26–64 years	7 to 9	6 to 10	Less than 6. More than 10
Older adults ≥65 years	7 to 8	5 to 9	Less than 5. More than 9

Note: Adapted from Hirshkowitz et al. (2015).

Instead, sufferers, usually younger adults, should be urged to extend bedtimes on a daily basis.

INADEQUATE SLEEP HYGIENE

This problem is also not classified as a disorder in DSM-5, but inadequate sleep hygiene bears mentioning especially since identifying this issue as the basis for the problem with insomnia may also facilitate developing a behavioral approach to address the problem. This category encompasses behaviors and external factors that impair sleep quality and quantity (Box 15.3). From a therapeutic standpoint, proper sleep hygiene behaviors may be utilized to improve sleep, although these techniques are quite variable in methodology and there are limited data substantiating their efficacy (Hauri, 2012; Morgenthaler et al., 2006). However, these measures can help at home when given to patients complaining of insomnia or EDS.

INSOMNIA DISORDER

Insomnia disorder represents the second most commonly expressed complaint (after pain) in clinical settings (Mahowald, Kader, & Schenck, 1997). Insomnia includes the complaint of an inability to fall asleep or stay asleep or the experience of frequent early morning awakenings without the ability

> **Box 15.3 Sleep Hygiene Measures**
>
> *Do's*
>
> - Increase exposure to bright light during the day
> - Establish a daily activity routine
> - Exercise regularly in the morning and/or afternoon
> - Set aside a worry time
> - Establish a comfortable sleep environment
> - Do something relaxing before bedtime
> - Try a warm bath
>
> *Don'ts*
>
> - Alcohol
> - Caffeine, nicotine, and other stimulants
> - Exposure to bright light during the night
> - Exercise within three hours of bedtime
> - Heavy meals or drinking within three hours of bedtime
> - Using bed for things other than sleep (or sexual activity)
> - Napping, unless a shift worker
> - Watching the clock
> - Trying to sleep
> - Noise
> - Excessive heat/cold in room

to return to sleep. Patients often report that sleep is unrefreshing. The sleep disturbance should cause significant distress or impairment in social settings, occupational settings, or other important areas of function. The sleep difficulty should occur despite adequate time for sleep. The DSM-5 no longer specifies whether this disorder is primary or secondary. However, it recommends that the insomnia be specified if it occurs with (a) non-sleep disorder mental comorbidity including substance use disorders, (b) other medical comorbidities, or (c) another sleep disorder. It should be further documented as *episodic* (lasting one to three months), *persistent* (three months or longer), or *recurrent* (two or more episodes within the space of one year). In the United States, 70 million people have one or more symptoms of insomnia (Ohayon, Lemoine, Arnaud-Briant, & Dreyfus, 2002; Ohayon & Partinen, 2002), but only 23.5 million (10% of the US population) meet diagnostic criteria for insomnia (National Institutes of Health, 2005) and about one-third of these patients use medications for insomnia. In a three-year longitudinal study, 74% of insomnia patients reported symptoms persisting for one year and 46% of patients stated that their symptoms had persisted for three years (Morin et al., 2008).

Insomnia sufferers place a significant burden on both the healthcare system and their employers, in both direct and indirect expenses, including medical expenses, ramifications of accidents, and reduced productivity due to absenteeism and decreased work efficiency (Walsh & Engelhardt, 1992). Insomnia costs the American public $92.5 billion to $107.5 billion annually, in both direct and indirect expenses (Stoller, 1994).

Although insomnia may be initiated by a wide variety of stressors and conditions, it may persist well beyond the resolution of these factors due to the emergence of perpetuating factors, such as learned mental associations ("I'll never be able to fall asleep") or somatized tension, which, in turn, cause arousal and prevent sleep. Patients then develop an excessive concern about the inability to fall asleep, mostly felt as bedtime approaches, leading to anticipatory anxiety over the prospect of another night of sleeplessness followed by another day of fatigue. A vicious cycle is set up, therefore, where excessive focus on sleep and "trying" to sleep cause greater tension and diminished sleep. Insomnia perpetuated by such processes is referred to as "psychophysiological insomnia" in the ICSD-3 (AASM, 2014). This insomnia is supported by a history of difficulty in falling asleep that is situational, usually occurring in the context of the patient's own bedroom. Sleep may be normal in other situations such as hotel rooms. Patients also report that they can fall asleep when they are not trying to, such as when they are watching TV or reading. Patients also report approaching bedtimes at home with intense anxiety and dread. Although they may have "hard-driving" personalities, psychiatric evaluation usually does not uncover diagnosable psychopathology. During the clinical examination, patients may appear tense. Although polysomnography is not usually necessary to confirm the diagnosis, it can be useful in ruling out other, concurrent sleep disorders. Cognitive-behavioral and pharmacologic treatments are well suited for this disorder.

Nonpharmacologic Treatments of Insomnia

Cognitive-behavioral therapies for insomnia are summarized in Table 15.2 (Morgenthaler et al., 2006; Morin et al., 2006). They include sleep hygiene education, described earlier, and stimulus control therapy. Patients are instructed to get out of bed following 15 to 20 minutes of sleeplessness while in bed, go to another room, and engage in relaxing activities but remain awake. They then return to bed only when sleepy. This therapy strives to reassociate the bedroom and bed with sleep and break the mental association between the bedroom and wakefulness. In addition, relaxation training strives to diminish tension and anxiety with various strategies, including progressive muscle relaxation,

Table 15.2. Psychological and Behavioral Treatments for Insomnia

Treatment	Method
Stimulus control therapy[a]	If unable to fall asleep within 20 minutes, get out of bed and repeat as necessary
Relaxation therapies[a]	Biofeedback, progressive muscle relaxation
Restriction of time in bed (sleep restriction)	Decrease time in bed to equal time actually asleep and increase as sleep efficiency improves
Cognitive therapy	Talk therapy to dispel unrealistic and exaggerated notions about sleep
Paradoxic intention	Try to stay awake
Sleep hygiene education	Promote habits that help sleep; eliminate habits that interfere with sleep
Cognitive-behavioral therapy[a]	Combines sleep restriction, stimulus control, and sleep hygiene education with cognitive therapy

Note: Adapted from Morgenthaler (2006) and Bootzin and Perlis (1992).
[a]Standard Treatment according to American Academy of Sleep Medicine.

biofeedback, guided imagery, autogenic training, abdominal breathing exercises, and meditation.

Sleep restriction therapy strives to curtail sleep and is especially useful in patients with multiple awakenings during the evening. It works by producing a state of sleep debt, which aids in consolidating subsequent sleep. Patients are instructed initially to limit the time spent in bed to the amount of actual time they habitually sleep, as determined using sleep logs. Sleep efficiency for the patient, which is the ratio of actual sleep time to time spent in bed, is calculated over a five-day period. When sleep efficiency increases to >90%, patients are allowed 15 to 20 minutes of additional time in bed by going to bed earlier. If sleep efficiency decreases below 85%, then their time in bed is further curtailed by a similar amount. Morning rising time is kept constant, and napping is disallowed. Over time, sleep becomes more consolidated and productive.

Cognitive therapy strives to identify and dispel thoughts that are tension producing and have a negative effect upon sleep. Many individuals develop misperceptions about sleep, such as unrealistic expectations ("I must get eight hours of sleep every night"), amplifications of consequences ("insomnia is incurable"), and sleep performance anxiety ("if I do not sleep well tonight, my performance tomorrow will be seriously jeopardized"). Once identified, misperceptions are consciously challenged, and positive perceptions about sleep are substituted. Paradoxical intention attempts to dissolve performance anxiety that prevents sleep by asking patients to stop trying to sleep and deliberately attempt to remain awake.

Pharmacologic Treatments for Insomnia

A wide array of compounds have been utilized for their sleep-promoting qualities over the years. Alcohol may be one of the most widely utilized "self-prescribed" agents by patients with insomnia because it enhances sleepiness and decreases sleep latency. However, it is a poor choice because it is associated with increased nocturnal awakenings and greater daytime somnolence (Roehrs & Roth, 2001). Alcohol can also result in further impairment in sleep-related respiration in patients with OSA. Antihistamines and over-the-counter products cannot be wholeheartedly recommended both because they have unpredictable effects on sleep and because they can cause adverse systemic effects due to their anticholinergic and sympathomimetic properties. Although barbiturates and barbiturate-like drugs (choral hydrate, glutethimide, and others) were utilized as hypnotics in the past, they are generally no longer recommended because they have a far greater potential for significant sedation and even death in overdoses when compared to benzodiazepine compounds.

Melatonin, a hormone released by the pineal gland whose secretion peaks during sleep, has long been suggested to be helpful for sleep. Melatonin has had significant popularity in recent years among patients with insomnia as an over-the-counter sleep aid. Unfortunately, studies have indicated that its beneficial effects on sleep latency and total sleep time are, at best, modest (Ferracioli-Oda, Qawasmi, & Bloch, 2013). Melatonin may, however, be useful in affecting positive changes in circadian rhythm sleep disorders, although more definitive studies are needed. In addition, concerns exist regarding the purity of certain melatonin preparations as over-the-counter herbal supplements are not regulated in the United States. Because of the lack of methodologically rigorous dose-response studies, the proper dosage of melatonin to be used in the treatment of insomnia is not well delineated.

More recently introduced medications for the treatment of insomnia are summarized in Table 15.3 (Morgenthaler et al., 2006) with regards to their effects on sleep latency or wake after sleep onset (WASO). Insomnia featuring difficulties in falling asleep can be managed with all medications listed with the exception of low-dose doxepin. On the other hand, maintenance insomnia is optimally managed by medications that are indicated for WASO. Some, such as suvorexant, eszopiclone, and zolpidem ER are effective for both types of insomnia. Recently, the AASM provided practice guidelines on the pharmacological management of insomnia (Sateia, Buysse, Krystal, Neubauer, & Heald, 2017). Whenever possible, pharmacologic agents should be supplemented with behavioral and cognitive therapies.

Table 15.3. Recently Introduced Medications for the Treatment of Insomnia

Medication	Sleep Latency	WASO
Zaleplon	Yes	No
Zolpidem	Yes	No
Zolpidem ER	Yes	Yes
Zolpidem, oral spray	Yes	No
Zolpidem, sublingual	Yes	No
Eszopiclone	Yes	Yes
Ramelteon	Yes	No
Low-dose doxepin	Yes	Yes
Suvorexant	Yes	Yes

Note: WASO = wake after sleep onset. Printed with permission from Doghramji and Doghramji (2007, p.256).

OBSTRUCTIVE AND CENTRAL SLEEP APNEA

There are two types of sleep apnea syndrome: OSA and CSA. The defining pathologic events in OSA are apneas, or pauses in ventilation and hypopneas (shallow breathing) during sleep that are due to a closure of the upper airway. In CSA, apneas are due to impaired inspiratory effort despite a patent upper airway. Isolated cases of pure CSA are rare but can be seen in patients with heart failure and neuromuscular disease. More commonly, CSA coexists with OSA, in which case the latter is considered the primary pathologic entity (AASM, 2014). The DSM-5 also recognizes central sleep apnea as (a) idiopathic central sleep apnea, (b) Cheyne-Stokes breathing, or (c) CSA comorbid with opioid use (American Psychiatric Association, 2013). OSA can only be diagnosed by means of polysomnogram, which determines the apnea-hypopnea index (AHI) and is typically classified as mild (AHI 5–14), moderate (AHI 15–29) or severe (AHI $\geq$ 30; Kryger, Roth, & Dement, 2011).

Upper airway closure in OSA is thought to occur because of the failure of the genioglossus and other upper airway dilator muscles, often in the context of existing structural changes in the upper airway that constrict resting airway patency. Apneas are accompanied by cyclic asphyxia (hypoxemia, hypercarbia, and acidosis), which in turn can cause cardiac arrhythmias, pulmonary and systemic hypertension, and a fall in cardiac output, which rises to normal levels following the termination of apneas. Apneas are terminated by arousals, episodes of sudden brain activation that are reflected by an increase in electroencephalogram (EEG) frequency to the alpha range during sleep; in turn, they cause sleep fragmentation and poor sleep quality, which is thought to be responsible for the EDS and emotional consequences of the disorder (Chokroverty, 2009).

Patients commonly present for clinical attention at the behest of their bed partner, who may be concerned about sleep-related gaps in breathing or loud snoring, or because sleepiness interferes with daytime function. Because patients are unaware of their own snoring, bed partners and family members must be interviewed to provide collateral information regarding the patient's symptoms related to possible OSA. Snoring can be exacerbated by weight gain, alcohol ingestion near bedtime, and lying on one's back. It is often a source of embarrassment and may place significant strain on interpersonal relationships, as spouses may resort to sleeping in separate beds or bedrooms. Bed partners also often observe whole-body movements, occasionally violent, during apneic episodes. Patients may talk and yell during sleep and assume unusual body positions as they attempt to inspire, yet sleepwalking is uncommon. Despite obvious discontinuous sleep, it is striking that most patients report sleep to be continuous, with the notable exception of the elderly, who may report insomnia. The consequences of and symptoms associated with OSA are caused by fragmented nocturnal sleep and asphyxia. Factors that predispose an individual to OSA are summarized in Box 15.4 (Nuckton, Glidden, Browner, & Claman, 2006; Young, Skatrud, & Peppard, 2004). The Mallampati score grades the amount of space available in the oropharynx and can independently predict apnea risk. It is defined as Class I: soft palate, uvula, fauces, tonsillar pillars visible; Class II: soft palate, uvula, fauces visible; Class III: soft palate, base of uvula visible; Class IV: only hard palate visible. Historical risk factors include a history of snoring, breathing pauses during sleep, and EDS. Other risk factors include smoking, chronic nocturnal nasal congestion, and a variety of conditions, such as hypertension, heart disease, and cerebrovascular disease.

Box 15.4 Predisposing Factors for Obstructive Sleep Apnea Syndrome

1. Obesity (body mass index >30)
2. Neck circumference >17 inches in men and >16 inches in women
3. Upper airway occlusion as judged by the Mallampati score
4. Adenotonsillar hypertrophy
5. Large uvula
6. Low-lying soft palate
7. Tonsilar hypertrophy
8. Narrow or obstructed nasal passages
9. Retrognathia, micrognathia, and other craniofacial abnormalities

OSA is associated with a heightened risk of depression, whose severity increases with the severity of the OSA; therefore, OSA should be considered in the differential diagnosis of major depression. Treatment of OSA in patients with comorbid depression has been shown to improve depression (Peppard, Szklo-Coxe, Hla, & Young, 2006; Schwartz & Karatinos, 2007). Many patients misuse alcohol to control anxiety and stimulants to stay awake. Cognitive changes in occupational and academic productivity is often impaired. Inhibited sexual desire, impotence, and ejaculatory impairment are reported by approximately one-third of OSA patients.

Dull, frontal morning headaches are common complaints of patients with OSA and are thought to be a result of episodic asphyxia and consequent cerebral vasodilatation. These headaches can last for one to two hours. Gastroesophageal reflux is a consequence of decreased intrathoracic pressure during apneas. Sleep-related enuresis is occasionally reported, and waking up to urinate is very common in patients with OSA. Sedating pharmacologic agents, including alcohol and benzodiazepine, and anxiolytic agents such as diazepam and alprazolam tend to increase the duration and frequency of apneas. Therefore, benzodiazepines are contraindicated for untreated patients.

TREATMENT OPTIONS FOR OSA

The first-line treatment for OSA is continuous positive airway pressure (CPAP) due to a high level of efficacy for many patients with OSA. CPAP is an ambulatory device that introduces room air at a high flow rate into the upper airway by a nasal mask and dissipates apneas by means of a "pneumatic splint" mechanism. The optimum pressure required to eliminate apneas is determined through polysomnography with a variable pressure device, following which patients utilize CPAP at a constant pressure at home while asleep. The primary complication in the use of CPAP is nonadherence; only half of patients prescribed CPAP actually use it regularly (Gay, Weaver, Loube, & Iber, 2006; Weaver & Grunstein, 2008; Weaver et al., 2007). Reasons for noncompliance with CPAP include upper airway irritation, discomfort at the mask site, and feelings of suffocation, among others. Various methods can enhance adherence, including in-line air humidification, mask shapes and sizes that are tailored to patients' preferences, bilevel positive airway pressure devices that deliver lower pressures during expiration than inspiration, and demand-pressure devices that tailor the pressure delivered to the severity of apneas on an ongoing basis. New masks, new data card recorders, and now smartphone applications are all constantly being developed to help patients become more compliant with CPAP therapy.

Medical weight reduction should always be encouraged, although its results are often unpredictable. Therefore, it should not be relied upon as the sole treatment modality for more severe cases but can be very effective for obese patients with mild disease. Oral appliances that prevent mandibular and tongue collapse during sleep have also seen a recent increase in popularity. Although the efficacy rates are lower than with CPAP, compliance rates are higher. Their side effects include excessive salivation and jaw pain. The AASM guidelines recommend that oral appliances are not as effective as CPAP but may be used in patients with mild or moderate OSA or in patients of any severity level who cannot tolerate CPAP (Ramar et al., 2015). If breathing disturbances are found to be more frequent in the supine position, positioning devices that promote sleep in the nonsupine position can be helpful in mild OSA cases (Permut et al., 2010).

Uvulopalatopharyngoplasty surgery is an intraoperative procedure performed under general anesthesia, where the uvula is partially removed along with the tonsils and part of the soft palate. It is highly effective for the elimination of snoring but suffers from lower efficacy than CPAP for more severe forms of apnea. Combining this with more invasive procedures, such as genioglossus advancement-hyoid myotomy and suspension, bimaxillary advancement, or maxillary and mandibular osteotomy, yields higher success rates. Tracheostomy has been performed in the past, prior to the advent of CPAP, but is now rarely performed. Nasal surgery can be helpful in patients with mild to moderate OSA who also have some degree of nasal airway compromise. Surgical intervention should be considered to be second-line therapy for OSA patients who cannot tolerate CPAP therapy (Aurora et al., 2010; Ishii et al., 2017). The determination of surgical success preoperatively has posed a clinical challenge for many years (Doghramji, Jabourian, Pilla, Farole, & Lindholm, 1995). Drug-induced endoscopy has been utilized more recently, which, when applied preoperatively, promises to help select patients who may be optimal candidates for specific surgical procedures, thereby increasing operative success rates (Huntley, Chou, Doghramji, & Boon, 2017).

Upper airway stimulation therapy, also referred to as hypoglossal nerve stimulation therapy, was recently introduced for treatment of OSA refractory to treatment with positive airway pressure devices. It is indicated for moderate to severe OSA. The neurostimulator, which is surgically implanted, delivers electrical stimulating pulses to the hypoglossal nerve through a lead that interfaces with the hypoglossal nerve, in synchrony with ventilatory chest activity as detected by a sensing lead placed at the fourth intercostal area. The first multicenter study demonstrated that the median AHI score at 12 months decreased 68%, from 29.3 events per hour to 9.0 events per hour (Strollo et al., 2014). Four-year-long postmarketing treatment studies indicate continued improvement in daytime functioning and alertness levels (Gillespie et al., 2017).

Daytime sleepiness remains problematic in some patients despite optimal management of the AHI with CPAP or other modalities. In such cases, pharmacologic agents such as modafinil and armodafinil, both wake-promoting agents, can be utilized. These are discussed further in the following sections (Roth et al., 2006).

NARCOLEPSY

The five major symptoms of narcolepsy are persistent daytime sleepiness, cataplexy, hypnagogic (or, less commonly, hypnopompic) hallucinations, sleep paralysis, and disturbed and restless sleep. Persistent daytime sleepiness is present in all patients with narcolepsy and usually accompanied by daytime naps that, unlike in OSA, are brief (typically 15 minutes) and refreshing. Naps are often accompanied by vivid dreams (AASM, 2014).

Cataplexy, an abrupt paralysis or paresis of skeletal muscles, usually follows emotional experiences such as anger, surprise, laughter, or physical exercise. Rarely, it can be generalized, in which case the patient may collapse, or, more commonly, isolated to an individual muscle group, resulting in a transient loss of function, such as a locked jaw, feeling weak at the knees, or legs buckling during an outburst of laughter. The episode typically lasts anywhere from a few seconds to a few minutes, during which the patient is awake. Following its termination, the patient typically regains function without any residual impairment. Although cataplexy is the pathognomic symptom of narcolepsy, it can only be elicited in about 70% of patient interviews. Cataplexy should not be confused with its near-homonym catalepsy, or waxy flexibility, an unrelated phenomenon noted in schizophrenia of the catatonic type.

Hypnagogic (or hypnopompic) hallucinations are vivid and often frightening dreams that occur shortly after falling asleep (or upon awakening). Sleep paralysis involves a transient global paralysis of voluntary muscles, which usually occurs shortly after falling asleep and lasts a few seconds or minutes. Cataplexy, hypnagogic hallucinations, and sleep paralysis are thought to be manifestations of an underlying aberration in the control of the timing of rapid eye movement (REM) sleep, which, in turn, results in "attacks" of REM sleep during wakefulness or partial wakefulness. Sleep in narcoleptics is also typically disturbed, characterized by numerous awakenings and arousals.

Narcolepsy is a lifelong condition. Its peak age of onset is during the second decade, yet diagnosis is established an average of 10 years later. People with narcolepsy develop significant psychosocial impairments as a result of EDS, such as job loss and interpersonal difficulties. They are also susceptible to auto accidents and to sustaining injuries as a result of falling asleep in inappropriate situations. Many patients with narcolepsy develop depression, anxiety, and substance-use difficulties. Twenty percent of narcoleptic patients develop social anxiety disorder, and 23% of patients also suffer from an eating disorder (Fortuyn et al., 2008; Ohayon, 2013).

Most cases of narcolepsy are idiopathic, but there are cases of secondary narcolepsy. A genetic factor is thought to be involved because 1% to 2% of first-degree relatives are affected by the disorder, a frequency that is 20 to 40 times higher than the population risk. However, most cases are sporadic, and only 17% to 36% of monozygotic twins are concordant for narcolepsy (Mignot, 1998). Therefore, its etiology cannot be explained solely on the basis of genetic factors; environmental triggers are thought to be involved, such as head trauma, viral illness, exposure to toxins, sleep deprivation, change in the sleep/wake cycle, and developmental factors such as puberty and aging.

The central pathological abnormality in narcolepsy is thought to be a deficiency of hypocretins. Hypocretin neuron cell bodies in the human brain are localized to the perifornical region of the posterior hypothalamus, extending into the lateral hypothalamus. These neurons densely innervate the hypothalamus, histaminergic tuberomammillary nucleus, noradrenergic locus coeruleus, serotonergic raphe nuclei, dopaminergic ventral tegmental area, midline thalamus, and nucleus of the diagonal band-nucleus basalis complex of the forebrain and are thought to be important in maintaining wakefulness. There is also a strong association between narcolepsy and human leukocyte antigens, raising the suspicion of an autoimmune destruction of wakefulness-controlling hypocretin cells (Klein, Burghaus, & Diederich, 2012).

The DSM-5 allows for the diagnosis of narcolepsy to be made on the basis of history of an irrepressible need to sleep plus cataplexy, although hypocretin deficiency or sleep testing can substitute for the latter. Sleep testing is comprised of nocturnal polysomnography (PSG), followed by a multiple sleep latency test. The ICSD-3 mandates testing for diagnosis (AASM, 2014; American Psychiatric Association, 2013).

Treatment of narcolepsy is directed at daytime somnolence, REM-related aberrations, and psychosocial consequences. In milder cases, excessive sleepiness can be managed with conservative measures such as spending an adequate time in bed, taking two or three short naps, and avoiding alcohol and other sedating agents. Even in more severe cases, judiciously timed naps can minimize the dosage of medication required to control symptoms. Commonly utilized medications for excessive sleepiness and cataplexy are described in Table 15.4. Tolerance may be minimized by prescribing the lowest effective dose and asking patients to take regular drug holidays on days when their need for alertness is lowest. It is important to note that the only drug Food and Drug Administration

Table 15.4. Pharmacologic Treatment of Narcolepsy

For EDS	For Cataplexy	For both EDS and Cataplexy
Methylphenidate	Protriptyline	Sodium oxybate (γ-hydroxybutyrate)[a]
Methamphetamine	Fluoxetine	
Amphetamine	Venlafaxine	
Modafinil[a]	Clomipramine	
Armodafinil[a]		

Note: EDS = excessive daytime somnolence.
[a]Food and Drug Administration approved for treating the listed symptom (Guilleminault & Cao, 2011).

(FDA) approved for treatment of cataplexy is sodium oxybate. It is also approved for the treatment of EDS in narcolepsy (Guilleminault & Cao, 2011).

Many patients with narcolepsy also require emotional support. Education plays a key role in management because peers, parents, teachers, and patients themselves may confuse the effects of drowsiness with laziness or lack of motivation.

RESTLESS LEGS SYNDROME AND PERIODIC LIMB MOVEMENT DISORDER

PLMD is characterized by the repetitive (usually every 20 to 40 seconds) twitches of the legs and, less commonly, arms during sleep. Patients usually present with the complaint of unrelenting insomnia, most often characterized by repeated awakenings following sleep onset. Some patients with PLMD complain of EDS. In either case, the patient with PLMD is usually unaware of the movements and the brief arousals that follow and has no lasting sensation in the extremities (AASM, 2014).

Also known as Willis-Ekbom's disease, the hallmark symptom in restless legs syndrome (RLS) is an irresistible urge to move the extremities, typically the legs but occasionally also the arms and other body parts. Patients with RLS often experience uncomfortable and unpleasant sensations in the extremities, which are described as creepy-crawly, painful, tugging, and tingling, among others. These symptoms begin, or are worsened, during periods of rest or inactivity, such as while attending the theater or reading quietly, and peak in the evening. As a result, patients commonly complain of difficulty in falling and staying asleep. Their symptoms are also typically partially or totally relieved by movement, such as walking or stretching, although relief is usually temporary. Many patients with RLS are depressed, irritable, and angry. Psychosocial impairments, such as job loss and relationship difficulties, are quite common. The two disorders are believed to be related. Approximately 80% of patients with RLS also have PLMD, yet only 30% of individuals who have PLMD also have RLS symptoms (Hening et al., 2004).

Both periodic leg movements during sleep and RLS are more common in middle and older age. The disorders can be primary (idiopathic), in which case the etiology is thought to be due to an abnormality of brain dopamine receptors, although the etiology of the disorder is unknown. They can also be secondary, in which case they coexist with a wide variety of conditions (e.g., pregnancy), the intake of certain drugs (e.g., caffeine and various antidepressants), drug withdrawal states, iron deficiency, uremia, leukemia, neuropathy, and rheumatoid arthritis and following gastric surgery. The symptoms are typically exacerbated by stress.

Polysomnography is not necessary to establish the diagnosis in RLS; its diagnosis is based on symptoms alone. However, polysomnography is necessary to confirm the diagnosis of PLMD. The results of PSG testing in this case reveal periodic leg muscle bursts during quiet wakefulness and sleep, the latter associated with arousals and awakenings. RLS should be distinguished from nocturnal leg cramps, which involve pain in the deep muscles of the lower extremities and are independent of sleep and usually worsen with movement, and from akathesia, a motor restlessness that occurs in the context of treatment with neuroleptics and antidepressants.

Once the diagnosis is established, the first goal is to identify the underlying cause. To this end, a thorough physical examination, chemistry panel, complete blood count, and serum ferritin should be performed and underlying abnormalities treated. If the serum ferritin is <50 μg/L, supplementation with ferrous sulfate should be instituted and follow-up testing should be performed to avoid iron overload (Sun, Chen, Ho, Earley, & Allen, 1998; Wang, O'Reilly, Venkataraman, Mysliwiec, & Mysliwiec, 2009). Sleep hygiene principles should be followed. For the primary disorder, treatment choices involve the use of dopamine agonists, including pramipexole, ropinirole, and rotigotine, which are all FDA approved for RLS. Typical side effects include augmentation (worsening of symptoms despite escalating dose), postural hypotension, somnolence, and nausea. Additionally, compulsive behavior can be seen at higher doses. Pramipexole should be avoided in patients with renal disease, as it primarily excreted in the urine. Gabapentin-enacarbil is also FDA approved for the treatment of RLS and differs from traditional gabapentin in that the enacarbil moiety is a prodrug that allows for better gastrointestinal absorption and enhanced bioavailability. Typical side effects include sedation, dizziness, fatigue, and peripheral edema. For refractory patients, benzodiazapines or opiates, such as codeine, can

Table 15.5. Features and Treatments of Common Parasomnias

Parasomnia	Clinical Features	PSG Findings	Treatment
Sleep Walking	Ambulation in sleep Age affected: prepubertal children Difficulty in arousal during episode Amnesia for the episode Episodes occur in the first third of night	Sleepwalking out of slow-wave sleep	Prevention: removal of sharp objects, use floor mattress Reassurance of parents Psychiatric evaluation for adults Benzodiazepines in refractory cases
Sleep Terrors	Sudden, intense scream during sleep with evidence of intense fear No dream recall	Sleep terror beginning during slow wave sleep	Reassurance in children Psychiatric evaluation for adults
Nightmare Disorder	Sudden awakening with intense fear Recall of frightening dream content Full alertness on awakening Usually occurs in latter half of night Frequent nightmares can be indicative of psychiatric conditions	Abrupt awakening from REM Tachycardia and tachypnea during episode	Psychotherapy Hypnosis
REM Sleep Behavior Disorder	Violent or injurious behavior during sleep Body movement associated with dreams Dream recall present Dreams are enacted while they occur Neurologic evaluations with MRI of the brain and evoked potentials rarely reveal structural lesions May be a harbinger for a synucleinopathy	Excessive EMG tone or phasic twitching in REM	Clonazepam Melatonin Protective measures Psychotherapy
Sleep Bruxism	Tooth grinding or clenching during sleep Tooth wear and jaw discomfort	Bursts of jaw EMG activity	Dental examination Mouth guards Relaxation training Psychotherapy

Note: PSG = polysomnography; REM = rapid eye movement; EMG = electromyogram; MRI = magnetic resonance imaging.

Adapted from Kryger et al. (2011).

be used for therapy, but these treatments are not FDA approved for this indication. Levodopa with carbidopa is no longer used for RLS, as it appears to have a high propensity for augmentation (Estivill, 2015; Montplaisir, Allen, Walters, & Ferini-Strambi, 2011; Oertel et al., 2009; Walters et al., 2009).

Parasomnias

Parasomnias are disturbing events that occur during sleep or are aggravated by sleep. Clinical aspects, including the description and treatment of the most common parasomnias, are summarized in Table 15.5.

Conclusion

Disturbances in sleep and wakefulness in the integrative psychiatric setting can be related to primary sleep disorders, whose identification and direct management can augment psychiatric care. It is important, therefore, for psychiatrists to develop strategies to recognize the disorders discussed in this chapter and either be comfortable treating them or recognize when to refer to a sleep disorders center and sleep specialist.

REFERENCES

American Academy of Sleep Medicine. (2014). *International classification of sleep disorders: A diagnostic and coding manual* (3rd ed.). Darien, IL: Author.

American Psychiatric Association. (2013). *Diagnostic and statistical manual of mental disorders* (5th ed.). Arlington, VA: Author.

Aurora, R. N., Casey, K. R., Kristo, D., Auerbach, S., Bista, S. R., Chowdhuri, S., et al. (2010). Practice parameters for the surgical modifications of the upper airway for obstructive sleep apnea in adults. *Sleep, 33*(10), 1408.

Chokroverty, S. (2009). *Sleep disorders medicine: Basic science, technical considerations, and clinical aspects.* Philadelphia: Saunders Elsevier.

Chung, F., Shapiro, C. M., Yegneswaran, B., Liao, P., Vairavanathan, S., Islam, S., et al. (2008). STOP questionnaire: A tool to screen patients for obstructive sleep apnea. *Anesthesiology, 108*(5), 812–821. doi:10.1097/ALN.0b013e31816d83e4

Doghramji, K., & Choufani, D. (2010). Taking a sleep history. In J. Winkelman & D. Plante (Eds.), *Foundations of psychiatric sleep medicine* (pp. 95–110). Cambridge, UK: Cambridge University Press.

Doghramji, K., & Doghramji, P. P. (2007). *Clinical management of insomnia.* West Islip, NY: Professional Communications.

Doghramji, K., Jabourian, Z. H., Pilla, M., Farole, A., & Lindholm, R. N. (1995). Predictors of outcome for uvulopalatopharyngoplasty. *Laryngoscope, 105*(3 Part 1), 311–314.

Estivill, E., & de la Fuente, V. (2015). The efficacy of ropinirole in the treatment of chronic insomnia secondary to restless legs syndrome: Polysomnography data. *Revista de neurologia, 29*(9), 805–807.

Ferracioli-Oda, E., Qawasmi, A., & Bloch, M. H. (2013). Meta-analysis: Melatonin for the treatment of primary sleep disorders. *PLoS One, 8*(5), e63773.

Fortuyn, H. A., Swinkels, S., Buitelaar, J., Renier, W. O., Furer, J. W., Rijnders, C. A., et al. (2008). High prevalence of eating disorders in narcolepsy with cataplexy: A case-control study. *Sleep, 31*(3), 335–341.

Gay, P., Weaver, T., Loube, D., & Iber, C. (2006). Evaluation of positive airway pressure treatment for sleep related breathing disorders in adults. *Sleep, 29*(3), 381–401.

Gillespie, M. B., Soose, R. J., Woodson, B. T., Strohl, K. P., Maurer, J. T., de Vries, N. et al. (2017). Upper airway stimulation for obstructive sleep apnea: Patient-reported outcomes after 48 months of follow-up. *Otolaryngology—Head and Neck Surgery, 156*(4), 765–771.

Guilleminault, C., & Cao, M. (2011). Narcolepsy: Diagnosis and management. In M. H. Kryger, T. Roth, & W. C. Dement (Eds.), *Principles and practice of sleep medicine* (5th ed., pp. 957–968). St. Louis, MO: Saunders.

Hauri, P. J. (2012). Sleep/wake lifestyle modifications: Sleep hygiene. In T. J. Barkoukis, J. K. Matheson, R. Ferber, & K. Doghramji (Eds.), *Therapy in sleep medicine* (pp. 151–160). Philadelphia: Elsevier Saunders.

Hening, W., Walters, A. S., Allen, R. P., Montplaisir, J., Myers, A., & Ferini-Strambi, L. (2004). Impact, diagnosis and treatment of restless legs syndrome (RLS) in a primary care population: The REST (RLS epidemiology, symptoms, and treatment) primary care study. *Sleep Medicine, 5*(3), 237–246. doi:10.1016/j.sleep.2004.03.006

Hirshkowitz, M., Whiton, K., Albert, S. M., Alessi, C., Bruni, O., DonCarlos, L., et al. (2015). National Sleep Foundation's sleep time duration recommendations: Methodology and results summary. *Sleep Health, 1*(1), 40–43. doi:10.1016/j.sleh.2014.12.010

Huntley, C., Chou, D., Doghramji, K., & Boon, M. (2017). Preoperative drug induced sleep endoscopy improves the surgical approach to treatment of obstructive sleep apnea. *The Annals of Otology, Rhinology, and Laryngology, 126*(6), 478–482.

Ishii, L. E., Tollefson, T. T., Basura, G. J., Rosenfeld, R. M., Abramson, P. J., Chaiet, S. R., et al. (2017). Clinical practice guideline: Improving nasal form and function after rhinoplasty. *Otolaryngology—Head and Neck Surgery, 156*(2 Suppl.), S30. doi:10.1177/0194599816683153.

Johns, M. W. (1991). A new method for measuring daytime sleepiness: The Epworth Sleepiness Scale. *Sleep, 14*(6), 540–545.

Klein, G., Burghaus, L., & Diederich, N. (2012). Pathogenesis of narcolepsy: From HLA association to hypocretin deficiency. *Fortschritte der Neurologie-Psychiatrie, 80*(11), 627–634.

Kryger, M., Roth, T., & Dement, W. C. (2011). *Principles and practice of sleep medicine* (5th ed.). Philadelphia: Elsevier Saunders.

Mahowald, M. W., Kader, G., & Schenck, C. H. (1997). Clinical categories of sleep disorders I. *Continuum, 3*(4), 35–65.

Mignot, E. (1998). Genetic and familial aspects of narcolepsy. *Neurology, 50*(2 Suppl. 1), 16.

Montplaisir, J., Allen, R. P., Walters, A., & Ferini-Strambi, L. (2011). Restless legs syndrome and periodic limb movements during sleep. In M. Kryger, T. Roth, & W. C. Dement (Eds.), *Principles and practice of sleep medicine* (5th ed.) (pp. 1026–1037). Philadelphia: Elsevier Saunders.

Morgenthaler, T., Kramer, M., Alessi, C., Friedman, L., Boehlecke, B., Brown, T., et al. (2006). Practice parameters for the psychological and behavioral treatment of insomnia: An update. An American Academy of Sleep Medicine report. *Sleep, 29*(11), 1415–1419.

Morin, C. M., Belanger, L., LeBlanc, M., Ivers, H., Savard, J., Espie, C. A., et al. (2009). The natural history of insomnia: A population-based 3-year longitudinal study. *Archives of Internal Medicine, 169*(5), 447–453. doi:10.1001/archinternmed.2008.610

Morin, C. M., Bootzin, R. R., Buysse, D. J., Edinger, J. D., Espie, C. A., & Lichstein, K. L. (2006). Psychological and behavioral treatment of insomnia: Update of the recent evidence (1998–2004). *Sleep, 29*(11), 1398–1414.

National Institutes of Health. (2005). National Institutes of Health State of the Science Conference statement on manifestations and management of chronic insomnia in adults, June 13–15, 2005. *Sleep, 28*(9), 1049–1057.

Nuckton, T. J., Glidden, D. V., Browner, W. S., Claman, D. M. (2006). Physical examination: Mallampati score as an independent predictor of obstructive sleep apnea. *Sleep, 29*(7), 903–908.

Oertel, W. H., Benes, H., Garcia-Borreguero, D., Geisler, P., Hogl, B., Saletu, B., et al. (2008). Efficacy of rotigotine transdermal system in severe restless legs syndrome: A randomized, double-blind, placebo-controlled, six-week dose-finding trial in Europe. *Sleep Medicine, 9*(3), 228–239.

Ohayon, M. M. (2013). Narcolepsy is complicated by high medical and psychiatric comorbidities: A comparison with the general population. *Sleep Medicine, 14*(6) 488–492.

Ohayon, M. M., Lemoine, P., Arnaud-Briant, V., & Dreyfus, M. (2002). Prevalence and consequences of sleep disorders in a shift worker population. *Journal of Psychosomatic Research, 53*(1), 577–583.

Ohayon, M. M., & Partinen, M. (2002). Insomnia and global sleep dissatisfaction in Finland. *Journal of Sleep Research, 11*(4), 339–346.

Peppard, P. E., Szklo-Coxe, M., Hla, K. M., & Young, T. (2006). Longitudinal association of sleep-related breathing disorder and depression. *Archives of Internal Medicine, 166*(16), 1709–1715. doi:10.1001/archinte.166.16.1709

Permut, I., Diaz-Abad, M., Chatila, W., Crocetti, J., Gaughan, J. P., D'Alonzo, G. E., et al. (2010). Comparison of positional therapy to CPAP in patients with positional obstructive sleep apnea. *Journal of Clinical Sleep Medicine, 6*(3), 238–243.

Ramar, K., Dort, L. C., Katz, S. G., Lettieri, C. J., Harrod, C. G., Thomas, S. M., & Chervin, R. D. (2015). Clinical practice guideline for the treatment of obstructive sleep apnea and snoring with oral appliance therapy: An update for 2015. *Journal of Clinical Sleep Medicine, 11*(7), 773–827. doi:10.5664/jcsm.4858

Roehrs, T., & Roth, T. (2001). Sleep, sleepiness and alcohol use. *Alcohol Research and Health, 25*(2), 101–109.

Roth, T., White, D., Schmidt-Nowara, W., Wesnes, K. A., Niebler, G., Arora, S., & Black, J. (2006). Effects of armodafinil in the treatment of residual excessive sleepiness associated with obstructive sleep apnea/hypopnea syndrome: A 12-week, multicenter, double-blind, randomized, placebo-controlled study in nCPAP-adherent adults. *Clinical Therapy, 28*(5), 689–706.

Sateia, M. J., Buysse, D. J., Krystal, A. D., Neubauer, D. N., Heald, J. L. (2017). Clinical practice guideline for the pharmacologic treatment of chronic insomnia in adults: An American Academy of Sleep Medicine clinical practice guideline. *Journal of Clinical Sleep Medicine, 13*(2), 307–349.

Schwartz, D. J., & Karatinos, G. (2007). For individuals with obstructive sleep apnea, institution of CPAP therapy is associated with an amelioration of symptoms of depression which is sustained long term. *Journal of Clinical Sleep Medicine, 3*(6), 631.

Stoller, M. K. (1994). Economic effects of insomnia. *Clinical Therapy, 16*(5), 97; discussion 854.

Strollo, P. J. Jr., Soose, R. J., Maurer, J. T., Maurer, M. D., de Vries, N., Cornelius, J., et al. (2014). Upper-airway stimulation for obstructive sleep apnea. *New England Journal of Medicine, 370*(2), 139–149. doi:10.1056/NEJMoa1308659

Sun, E. R., Chen, C. A., Ho, G., Earley, C. J., & Allen, R. P. (1998). Iron and the restless legs syndrome. *Sleep, 21*(4), 371–377.

Walsh, J. K., & Engelhardt, C. L. (1999). The direct economic costs of insomnia in the United States for 1995. *Sleep, 22*(Suppl. 2), 386.

Walters, A. S., Ondo, W. G., Kushida, C. A., Becker, P. M., Ellenbogen, A. L., Canafax, D. M., et al. (2009). Gabapentin enacarbil in restless legs syndrome: A phase 2b, 2-week, randomized, double-blind, placebo-controlled trial. *Clinical Neuropharmacology, 32*(6), 311.

Wang, J., O'Reilly, B., Venkataraman, R., Mysliwiec, V., & Mysliwiec, A. (2009). Efficacy of oral iron in patients with restless legs syndrome and a low-normal ferritin: A randomized, double-blind, placebo-controlled study. *Sleep Medicine, 10*(9), 973.

Weaver, T. E., & Grunstein, R. R. (2008). Adherence to continuous positive airway pressure therapy: The challenge to effective treatment. *Proceedings of the American Thoracic Society, 5*(2), 173–178. doi:10.1513/pats.200708-119MG; 10.1513/pats.200708-119MG

Weaver, T. E., Maislin, G., Dinges, D. F., Bloxham, T., George, C. F. P., Greenberg, H., et al. (2007). Relationship between hours of CPAP use and achieving normal levels of sleepiness and daily functioning. *Sleep, 30*(6), 711–719.

Young, T., Skatrud, J., & Peppard, P. E. (2004). Risk factors for obstructive sleep apnea in adults. *JAMA, 291*(16), 2013–2016.

16

Cognitive Interventions: Brain Training and Rehabilitation

THOMAS SWIRSKY-SACCHETTI AND ROBERT L. RIDER

> **Key Points**
>
> - Cognitive or brain training takes advantage of neuroplasticity, cognitive reserve, and cognitive resilience.
> - Education can protect people initially but can be associated with faster decline once disease becomes symptomatic.
> - Computerized brain training via the brain training industry is controversial with more studies required to better determine its effectiveness.
> - Studies have shown that specific brain training can help with particular domains of cognitive function.
> - Incorporating integrative elements such as dietary counseling and exercise also can benefit cognitive function.

Introduction

Cognitive intervention is any activity or technique used to maintain or improve cognitive functioning. Converging lines of research indicate that cognitive intervention has the benefit of improving brain functioning in healthy older adults as well as to slow decline in individuals with disease-related cognitive impairments (Gates & Valenzuela, 2010). There is inconsistency in the field regarding the terminology used for activities to improve cognitive functioning: cognitive remediation, cognitive rehabilitation, neurorehabilitation, cognitive enhancement therapy, cognitive training, brain training, and brain fitness are some of the terms commonly used. A major distinguishing feature lies in who is receiving the intervention: cognitive remediation and rehabilitation, for instance, employ techniques designed for individuals with known or suspected brain damage. Historically, these interventions have focused on individuals with acquired deficits (e.g., traumatic brain injury, stroke) or on those with longstanding dysfunction (e.g., schizophrenia). Although the distinction is often blurred, cognitive *rehabilitation* uses techniques that target everyday functioning (e.g., balancing a checkbook), whereas cognitive *remediation* has a narrower focus on specific cognitive functions to be remediated (i.e. memory, attention, or problem-solving) that underlie tasks of everyday functioning. By strengthening underlying brain processes, improvements made through cognitive remediation can theoretically generalize to many different tasks.

The explosion of interest in enhancing brain capabilities of individuals with normal cognitive functioning has arisen from the theoretical underpinnings of cognitive remediation. Whether techniques used to restore cognitive abilities can also be used to bolster healthy cognitive functions is a critical question facing the brain training industry. There is now tremendous interest in applying principles of neuropsychological functioning and practices of cognitive training in order to minimize or offset the loss of certain cognitive abilities due to natural decline or "normal aging." Yet, even the distinction between normal versus pathological aging is not hard and fast. When does an aging brain begin to show evidence of decline? What are the differences between normal aging, mild cognitive impairment, or early dementia? What changes in brain functioning should be expected? What, if anything, can be done to slow or even stop these changes? These questions are at the core of this chapter.

The same underlying principles of brain functioning also often unify our efforts at both restoration of lost function and enhancement of normal functioning and prevention of decline, which further obscures the aforementioned distinctions. However, in this chapter, we nonetheless provide a critical review of brain training programs and then remedial or restorative interventions with the implicit understanding that the underlying principles of neuropsychological functioning are the same. Given the recent proliferation of web-based brain fitness activities, our intent is to further clarify the extent to which cognitive interventions are evidence-based and how effective these commercially successful programs are.

Factors Impacting Cognitive Skill Acquisition

Before the further review of interventions, it is important to highlight a few important concepts that underlie any effort to change brain functioning. These concepts pertain to the "receiver characteristics" of the brain: neuroplasticity and cognitive reserve or resilience. It is also necessary to address issues of "transfer of learning" and "generalization," which reflect the extent to which something learned in one setting "transfers" to other settings.

NEUROPLASTICITY, COGNITIVE RESERVE, AND COGNITIVE RESILIENCE

Neuroplasticity refers to the brain's ability to reorganize itself by forming new neural connections in order to compensate for an injury, to adjust to new situations, or to otherwise adapt to changes in an organism's environment. Every time someone learns something new, there are corresponding changes in the brain. The adult brain, once believed to consist of a static organization of mechanistic functional areas, is capable of learning and of reorganizing through Hebbian principles of synaptic plasticity. That is, those neurons that are activated in close temporal proximity tend to make synaptic connections while those that fire out of sync with one another fail to connect and may even diverge even if once connected (i.e., neurons that fire together, wire together). Research into the nature of neuroplasticity has demonstrated a robust capacity for neuronal networks to change their structure in response to injury and, in certain cases, in response to training (Rakic, 2002). This property of neural systems is, in part, what allows for functional recovery through rehabilitation and what cognitive training companies claim underlies their purported effects on performance. As described in this chapter, however, the preponderance of empirical evidence has indicated brain training software does not produce changes in function that generalize beyond the task upon which one is trained.

While the terms *neuroplasticity, brain plasticity,* and *neural plasticity* have been used liberally in the brain training industry, the concepts of cognitive reserve and resilience are curiously absent from the brain training industry's lexicon. What makes this omission unusual is the fact that cognitive reserve and resilience are potentially more amenable to intentional manipulation and have more support for potentially protecting against cognitive decline than brain training. In fact, a number of cognitive and psychological factors have been associated with a lower incidence of dementia. These factors, it has been suggested, increase cognitive resilience. For instance, having a higher

IQ, higher level of education, a higher level of occupational attainment, and more frequent participation in stimulating leisure activities have been shown to predict lower rates of cognitive decline in older adults and in those with Alzheimer's disease pathology (Tucker & Stern, 2011). Premorbid IQ and socioeconomic status have also been associated with cognitive resilience in the presence of demonstrated hippocampal atrophy (Topiwala, 2015).

Individuals with higher educational levels can also demonstrate a more rapid decline in functioning once the disease becomes symptomatic (Scarmeas, Albert, Manly, & Stern, 2006). This is thought to be a reflection of how cognitive reserve can be neuroprotective, allowing people to maintain higher levels of functioning until the underlying neuropathology reaches a critical threshold, after which more rapid and arguably more noticeable decline occurs. One implication this has for treating cognitive decline is the possibility that individuals with factors associated with greater cognitive reserve may be more likely to benefit from techniques that engage higher level semantic or executive functions (Hampstead, Mosti, & Swirsky-Sacchetti, 2014).

It is also important to note that the impact of these "resiliency factors" is likely to be mediated by a number of other variables including sociocultural factors, the presence and severity of any underlying medical or psychiatric conditions, and the presence or absence of other genetic predisposing factors. For instance, one group of researchers found that among white ApoE4 carriers, the strongest predictors of cognitive resilience (i.e., lower rates of conversion to Alzheimer's) were an absence of recent negative life events, a higher literacy level, more advanced age, a higher educational level, and more time spent reading. By contrast, among black ApoE4 carriers, the strongest predictors of cognitive resilience were a higher literacy level, a higher educational level, female sex, and the absence of diabetes mellitus (Kaup, Nettiksimmons, LeBlanc, & Yaffe, 2015).

TRANSFER OF LEARNING AND GENERALIZATION

Transfer of learning, sometimes referred to as generalization, refers to the extent to which a learned behavior or cognitive skill set will transfer or carry over to a new or similar context. Transferability is a crucial concept in both brain training and rehabilitation because the import of a trained function is dependent upon the extent to which it transfers to real-life personally relevant situations. Parenté and Hermann (2003) present various theories of transferability of learning. The most positive transfer will occur when the content of the learned skill *and* the context in which it will be applied are identical or very similar; for example, a person learning how to drive in on-the-road driving instruction will have better transfer of learning to real-life driving than a person who learns in a driving simulator or a person who learns the rules of driving in a driver's manual. In most cases, there is a difference between a training situation (computerized training or therapy session) and real life, in which case the goal is to facilitate transferability by making both the skill set and the context as similar as possible in both the initial learning and the later application. Parenté and Hermann also emphasize, in working mainly with those suffering from traumatic brain injury, the impaired person may need to be made aware of the similarities. This necessary step has been addressed in some but not all cognitive enhancement programs for the elderly (see the Advanced Cognitive Training for Independent and Vital Elderly [ACTIVE] study described later in which those receiving memory enhancement training were specifically trained in how the memory strategies could be applied to everyday life). Transferability will also be facilitated when the skill set is maintained across different task demands. As an example, we consider the PEG method of memory rehabilitation later; this organizational structure can be used to memorize shopping lists, tomorrow's appointments, or things on a "to-do" list. The concept of negative transfer is also important to consider. In its most simplistic form, negative transfer refers to the extent to which learning one thing inhibits learning of a new thing. Negative transfer is most likely to occur when both the required skill set and the context are different.

Computerized Cognitive Training

The early 2000s saw an explosion of research devoted to the study neuroplasticity. This surge in interest was accompanied by, and likely spurred by, the emergence and now proliferation of commercially available computerized cognitive training (CCT) programs. Prior to 2000, products like Fast ForWord® reading assistant (Scientific Learning Corporation, n.d.) were available for specific segments of the population with known problems such as auditory processing deficits or delayed reading. However, the mass marketing of computerized "brain games" for the general public began in earnest at the turn of the millennium and has continued to grow. The impelling forces fueling this growth most certainly include the growing public health concern posed by Alzheimer's disease and other forms of dementia as well as the aging of a generation of baby boomers, whose longevity poses challenging questions regarding the inevitability of age-related cognitive decline. Foremost among these questions is whether normal age-related cognitive decline can be slowed, stopped, or even reversed with the right combination of interventions.

Unfortunately, there have been problems with the research literature investigating CCT that have cast some doubt on the potential for brain training to mitigate cognitive decline. Multiple reviews have highlighted the issue of heterogeneity of research designs in CCT studies, calling for a more systematic approach. Papp, Walsh, and Snyder's (2009) meta-analysis of randomized controlled trials of CCT in older adults is one example of such a review. Their analysis showed there was no evidence of any significant cognitive benefit from CCT programs across 10 studies. In a more recent and comprehensive review of the CCT literature, Simons and colleagues (2016) similarly found little evidence to support the claim that CCT can prevent or slow cognitive decline in humans.

Notably, while these reviews and many other studies have helped to identify some of the specific research challenges in assessing CCT programs, the brain training industry continues to grow at a rapid pace, and it has become clear that the science will need to keep pace. According to a study by SharpBrains, the brain training industry saw approximately $600 million in annual revenues in 2009, approximately $1 billion by 2012, and is projected by the authors of the study to reach $4 billion to $10 billion by 2020 (Selk, 2013). As the brain training industry grows in size and influence, the need for increasing scientific evaluation will only increase.

In the following sections, we offer a sampling of the products and companies comprising this industry and give a broad overview of the research studies that have attempted to evaluate their effectiveness. Due to the heterogeneity of brain training products and the speed with which this industry is growing, our overview is necessarily more a snapshot than an in-depth critique. For a more thorough review of the CCT industry, see the excellent reviews referenced earlier by Papp et al. (2009) and Simons et al. (2016).

LUMOSITY®

LumosLabs, founded in 2005 by Kunal Sarkar, Michael Scanlon, and David Drescher, launched its online subscription-based service Lumosity® in 2015. Since its launch, Lumosity has rapidly become one of the most recognizable names in the brain training industry, offering online games designed to train cognition in several domains including verbal reasoning, memory, and spatial awareness. As one of the most prominent computerized programs, Lumosity has also drawn a lot of attention from researchers in the field of cognitive neuroscience, particularly due to some of the company's early claims that users may be able to stave off cognitive decline and even dementia.

A study by Ballesteros and colleagues (2015) compared the effects of exercises from Lumosity to a control condition on memory performances in older adults. Participants underwent 20 one-hour training sessions with Lumosity. Those completing the training showed significantly faster choice reaction time, reduced distraction, increased alertness, and better immediate and delayed visual recognition memory as well as a trend toward higher self-ratings of assertivity and affection. No significant changes in visuospatial working memory or executive control were observed following training. At a three-month follow-up study, the trained group continued to report significantly higher levels of subjective well-being including higher ratings on scales assessing assertivity and affection, but the differences between trained and untrained groups was no longer significant for any of the cognitive outcome measures (Ballesteros et al., 2015).

Toril, Reales, Mayas, and Ballesteros (2016) conducted a longitudinal study of 40 older adults randomized to either a control group or a seven- to eight-week computerized training condition that employed several of Lumosity's games aimed at improving visuospatial skills. Specifically, the authors chose the Speed Match, Memory Matrix, Rotation Matrix, Face Memory, Money Comb, and Lost in Migration exercises. Each participant in the training group received 15 one-hour training sessions over the course of the study with each game being played twice. Control participants engaged in their usual activities during the study. Outcome measures included tasks designed to assess visuospatial working memory, auditory working memory, immediate and delayed facial memory, and immediate and delayed memory for visual scenes. Results showed improvement on the trained Lumosity tasks over the course of the study. More importantly, after completing the 15 sessions, trained participants performed better than those in the control group on multiple outcome measures including tests of visual working memory, auditory attention, and facial memory. This difference was maintained after a three-month, no-contact period with regard to one of the two visuospatial working memory measures as well as the tests of facial memory and auditory attention. The researchers concluded that training on these Lumosity exercises was associated with significant improvement in working memory performance. However, they cite the study's limitations, which included the absence of an active control condition, a relatively small sample size, and the absence of any measure of skill transfer or generalization.

Wentink and colleagues (2016) investigated the effects of training on several Lumosity games on cognitive performance in patients who had suffered a stroke. Patients were required to play at least 15 to 20 minutes per day, five days per week. Games were targeted to attention, speed, memory, flexibility, and problem-solving. Control group participants received information about brain function, stress, and stroke. Cognitive outcome measures included commonly used measures of attention, processing speed, visual and auditory working memory, mental flexibility, and fluid intelligence. The investigators also assessed participants' subjective self-perceived cognitive functioning, self-efficacy, and quality of life. The study found no effects of Lumosity training on cognitive functioning, quality of life, or self-efficacy after eight weeks of training.

BrainTrain®

BrainTrain® publishes the Captain's Log program, which also has some empirical support (BrainTrain 2017). Rabiner, Murray, Skinner, and Malone (2010) carried out a randomized trial assessing the effectiveness of Captain's Log in remediating attentional difficulties. Students in the Captain's Log group scored significantly higher than controls and when compared to another computerized program designed for reading problems. Lampit Ebster, and Valenzuela (2014) found that individuals who used the Captain's Log MIndPower Builder also showed faster and more accurate mental processing on bookkeeping and accounting math than controls, suggesting possible generalization of CCT-trained skills or "far transfer" of cognitive training to relevant real-world job performance.

Ecroth-Bucher and Siberski (2009) used the Captain's Log and another computerized training (SoundSmart) as part of an Integrated Cognitive Stimulation and Training Program. The program consisted of two 45-minute sessions weekly for older adults with and without cognitive compromise over a six-week period. The intervention consisted of the computerized training as well as paper and pencil based simulation and training activities targeting multiple aspects of cognition. Participants were rated based on pretraining cognitive testing as nonimpaired, mildly impaired, and moderately impaired and randomly divided into treatment and waiting list control groups. Data was collected pretraining, at the conclusion of training (six weeks), and again at follow-up eight weeks after the conclusion of training. An "integration session" was designed to blend mental stimulation into ecologically plausible activities (i.e., writing checks to pay bills). Outcome measures included the Dementia Rating Scale, immediate and delayed recall of two short stories, and a working memory task involving repetition of letter and numbers presented aurally. The results reflected significant changes in Dementia Rating Scale scores, and both short and delayed memory of stories and changes were maintained over the eight-week follow-up. Significant improvements were noted in the mild and moderately impaired groups but not in the unimpaired group.

One limitation of the study was its small sample size ($n = 15$) and the lack of an adequate placebo-control group especially in light of known placebo effects in this age group. Generalizability of findings is also limited because nearly all participants were Caucasian and women. The authors also noted a decreasing trend in mean scores after eight weeks, leaving one to question at what point the treatment effect might dissipate.

POSIT SCIENCE/BRAIN HQ

BrainHQ is a prominent online, computerized brain training program created by Posit Science. Its website features 29 exercises including tasks tapping attention, memory, and processing speed. The BrainHQ site also reports that its exercises are aimed at exercising "intelligence, navigation, and people skills" (Posit Science, n.d.). In one study, with individuals trained using BrainHQ's training program as associated with significantly higher ratings of everyday cognition, the effect was modest (Smith et al., 2009), and, in a separate study of the same intervention, the benefits that were seen in both formal cognitive testing and self-report measures also waned after three months (Zelinski et al., 2011).

Compared with Lumosity, the research into the effectiveness of BrainHQ's CCT program is less extensive. However, BrainHQ's double-decision task, which was used in association with the multisite ACTIVE study (described later), has shown some early promising results. The double-decision task requires users to view a target visual stimulus (a cartoon vehicle), which is promptly removed and replaced with the target and a distractor. During the initial presentation of the target vehicle, the user must also note the position on the screen of a second visual stimulus (e.g., a road sign) somewhere in the periphery. Within seconds, a new screen is presented with both the target vehicle and a distractor vehicle. The user must identify which of the vehicles matches the target vehicle and also click the place on the screen where the second visual stimulus appeared on the initial presentation. However, the impact of the task alone was not evaluated in the ACTIVE study, which, as described later, also involved instruction in strategies for boosting performance on the tasks, increasing self-efficacy, and applying skills to everyday tasks.

Combined Programs

A number of large-scale, multicenter studies have reported beneficial effects of programs combining CCT with other interventions such as physical exercise, nutrition, and social engagement. These studies have the benefit of a larger sample sizes with greater generalizability but the downside of being unable to determine the benefits of cognitive interventions in isolation. The use of multiple interventions also reflects common sense; that is, a healthy brain is unlikely to be maintained without a multisystem approach. These programs are covered elsewhere in this book, so the following brief descriptions focus on their cognitive intervention components.

THE ACTIVE STUDY

In 1998, a group of researchers across six sites began enrolling a large group of adults over the age of 65 in the ACTIVE trial (Jobe et al., 2001). The ACTIVE trial represents one of the most ambitious cognitive training studies to date, following over 2,800 participants in a longitudinal study to assess the effects of perceptual and cognitive interventions on cognitively demanding tasks of daily living such as everyday problem-solving, activities of daily living and instrumental activities of daily living functioning, everyday speed of processing, driving, and medication use. Secondary outcomes included health-related quality of life, mobility, and health services utilization.

The ACTIVE trial involved three groups randomized to one of three cognitive training interventions—reasoning training, memory training, and speed-of-processing training—or a no-contact control group. Interventions were administered in small groups of three to five participants during 10 one-hour sessions spread across six weeks, though some completed a two-week compressed version of the training. In the memory intervention, participants were instructed on how to use meaning, organization, visualization, and association to support memory. They practiced these strategies on tasks involving learning and recall of word lists, item sequences, text, and details and gists of stories. In the reasoning training, participants were instructed on strategies to solve problems requiring linear thinking, such as determining the next item in a sequence, medication dosing patterns, and filling a pill-reminder case. In the computerized speed of processing intervention, trainers instructed participants on a computer task aimed at improving the speed of visual search and the ability to quickly perform one or more attentional tasks. Four exercises were used for training. In the first, participants were asked to simply identify a given object at increasingly brief exposures. In the second task, participants needed to divide their attention between identifying a centrally located item and one in the periphery (see previous description of the double-decision task). Distracters were added in the third task. In the fourth task, an auditory attention demand was added.

All participants were instructed on the intervention-specific strategies and how to complete the exercises and then practiced the tasks. They were also given strategies for boosting performance on the tasks, increasing self-efficacy, and applying the skills they were learning in the training to everyday tasks. Booster sessions, occurring approximately 11 months after the end of primary training and consisting of four 75-minute sessions over a two- to three-week period, were offered to a portion of those who had completed the initial training. The researchers assessed three levels of outcome variables: (a) proximal outcomes, or performance on measures of cognitive abilities; (b) primary outcomes, or measures of daily function; and (c) secondary outcomes, or measures of health-related quality of life, everyday mobility, and health service utilization. With regard to proximal outcomes, multiple measures of memory were administered including measures of word-list learning and memory, reasoning, speed of processing, and vocabulary (which was described as a nonspecific proximal outcome).

Among the primary outcome measures were an instrument based on the Minimum Data Set for Home Care (Morris et al., 1997), which assesses tasks such as meal preparation, housework, finances, healthcare, telephone use, shopping, independence in travel, and need for support in basic activities such as dressing, personal hygiene, and bathing. The measure includes subscales to assess the degree of independence in the completion of tasks and the perceived degree of difficulty in completing tasks. Measures of everyday problem-solving, actual observed performance of tasks of daily living, a complex reaction time test, and a timed task assessing instrumental activities of daily living were used to assess the performance of everyday functions. Secondary outcomes were also included such as health-related quality of life, everyday mobility, health service utilization, self-reported falls, and motor vehicle crashes.

Immediate improvements in the proximal outcome (i.e., cognitive ability trained) was demonstrated (Ball et al., 2002) and found to persist through five years of follow-up (Willis et al., 2006). The effects were ability-specific such that those in the reasoning training did not show significant improvement in memory or speed of processing. The largest and most notable improvements were seen in the speed of processing intervention. Reasoning and Memory each showed lesser improvements, respectively. The impact of training on performance was greatest immediately after the intervention, showing some reduction over time. Nonetheless, the improvements in performance remained statistically significant at the five-year follow-up. The booster training for reasoning and speed training also produced significant added benefits to performance. All three intervention groups were found to have fewer problems with instrumental activities of daily living relative to controls at the five-year follow-up. Transfer of training effects to Everyday Problem Solving and

Everyday Speed was seen at five years for participants who had received the added "booster" sessions (Willis et al., 2006).

The ACTIVE trial was funded by the National Institute on Aging and the National Institute for Nursing Research, which addresses one of the main concerns raised by the Institute of Medicine group regarding inherent bias in studies of brain training. While a no-contact control does not meet the Institute of Medicine recommendations for the use of an active control group, the comparison across training conditions represents a form of "active control." The reasoning intervention was not uniform due to large differences in baseline reasoning measures. Participants in this group were therefore divided into two levels, varying the difficulty of the tasks presented in the early training phase, pacing and amount of time spent on training, and the relative emphasis of the trainer on modeling of strategies. The selection process for the subset of participants receiving booster sessions is unclear. Because there was no measure of participants' compliance with the interventions in daily life, it is difficult to distinguish the effects of the intervention from frequency of use, and dose-response relationships are unclear. For example, did subjects receiving computer training continue to use it, or a similar program, throughout follow-up? How does this compare to subjects who received memory or reasoning training? Because memory strategies are internal processes, measurement of how often participants used the strategies in daily life are inherently more difficult to assess than measuring time spent on a computerized brain training game. Yet this distinction is crucial if benefits noted on follow-up were truly due to the cognitive intervention (i.e., computerized brain training vs. memory) and not simply the amount of time spent on the intervention.

Neurogrow Brain Fitness

Fotuhi and colleagues (2016) have developed a multimodal program for individuals with mild cognitive impairment (MCI). The program components involve cognitive stimulation, neurofeedback training, counseling for eating a Mediterranean diet, omega-3 supplements, fitness activities, and mindfulness meditation. Cognitive stimulation was provided with The Captain's Log computerized brain training to improve working memory, attention, and processing speed. Patients also received "Brain Coaching/Counseling," which consisted of meditation training and behavior therapy as well as education regarding diet, exercise, sleep hygiene, and stress reduction. It appears that training was performed by "trained psychometricians." The remaining intervention consisted of neurofeedback, aimed to train individuals through auditory and visual feedback how to normalize brain wave activity. In addition to baseline neuropsychological testing, patients were also given a baseline quantitative EEG with noted abnormalities to be used as targets for the neurofeedback training. The authors reported on 127 patients with an average age of 70.69 and a diagnosis of MCI. Upon completing the program, patients on average improved in 4.68 of the 10 cognitive domains, with younger and higher functioning patients understandably witnessing greater gains. Furthermore, a random subset of 17 patients had a brain magnetic resonance imaging (MRI) scan at the conclusion of the program and of these, 9 showed actual growth in the size of the hippocampus. (It is unclear how these 17 patients were selected for follow-up MRI.)

One limitation of the study is not unique to the combined-program approach (i.e., one cannot determine which of the interventions was most effective in facilitating change). This study also lacked a control group, a serious omission given the power of the placebo response, especially in elderly individuals with MCI who are anxious about losing cognitive function. As described earlier, the placebo response may be especially potent if the participants' perception is that the brain training should improve performance. In light of the limited data/scores provided, it is also difficult to judge the magnitude of the effect. The study also failed to monitor compliance with the various interventions and used performance on neuropsychological testing as an outcome measure which would have been nicely supplemented by real-life measures of cognitive functioning such as those used in the ACTIVE study.

THE FINGER STUDY

The Finnish Geriatric Intervention Study to Prevent Cognitive Impairment and Disability (FINGER) represents another large, multi-center, randomized controlled trial which began in 2009 (Kivipelto et al., 2013). Unlike the ACTIVE study, which has investigated only cognitive training, the aim of FINGER was to investigate whether a "multidomain intervention" including diet, exercise, cognitive training, and vascular risk monitoring could prevent or delay cognitive impairment in older adults who were identified as at increased risk for cognitive decline but without substantial impairment. According to the study authors, this broader scope of intervention was borne out of the general failure of prior studies, investigating only one type of intervention such as cognitive activity, to show prevention benefits. In addition, participants in the FINGER study were recruited from the FINRISK database, which allowed for more detailed baseline data to be used for assessing the treatment effects. A total of 1,260 individuals were enrolled in the study ($n = 631$ in the intervention group, $n = 629$ in the control group).

As the focus of our chapter is on methods of cognitive training, we don't review the nutritional or physical exercise interventions in detail. It is important to note, however, that the intervention group received both the physical exercise training and nutritional programs alongside the cognitive training sessions. Like the ACTIVE study, the FINGER cognitive training component included group and individual sessions. Twenty group sessions allowed for 10 sessions of training by psychologists, six sessions of education on age-related cognitive changes as well as methods for applying memory and reasoning strategies to everyday activities, and four sessions for assessing participants' progress. Individual training took place over two periods of six months, with each period including 72 computer-based training sessions administered three times per week in 10- to 15-minute sessions. Sessions included tasks aimed at training (a) executive functions—updating spatial, updating letter, updating number, and mental set shifting tasks; (b) working memory functions—a mental maintenance task; (c) episodic memory functions—relational and spatial tasks; and (d) mental speed—a shape match task.

Cognitive assessment was completed at baseline and at the one- and two-year postrandomization points using an extended version of the neuropsychological test battery (NTB; Harrison et al., 2007), and cognitive outcomes were assessed in specific domains as well as in a generalized fashion (Ngandu et al., 2015). Within specific cognitive domains, executive functioning was assessed using a category fluency test, digit span, condition C of the concept shifting test, the trail making test, and a shortened version of the Stroop test. Processing speed was assessed via the letter-digit substitution test, condition A of the concept shifting test (condition A), and condition two of the Stroop test. Memory performances were assessed on a visual paired associates test, immediate and delayed recall trials, logical memory immediate and delayed recall, and word list learning and delayed recall. Ngandu and colleagues (2015) reported significant increases in the intervention group versus the control group for the measure of general cognitive functioning as well as in the specific domains of executive functioning and processing speed (Ngandu et al., 2015). Participants in the intervention group scored 25% higher than the control group at their two-year follow-up evaluation in the composite measure of cognition. Improvements at the two-year follow-up were also noted in executive functioning and processing speed, which were 83% and 150% higher, respectively, in the intervention group versus the control group. No significant difference was found between the intervention and control groups on the primary memory outcome measure.

While the combined intervention in the FINGER study was found to have significant benefits to general cognition, executive functioning, and processing speed, the study authors do not report the specific impact of the cognitive training program. Additionally, given the inclusion of individuals with known risk factors for cardiovascular and cerebrovascular disease, the inclusion of a no-treatment control group was considered ethically untenable. Thus the control group was given the same health advice typically given in primary care settings with regard to their overall health, specific risk factors, nutrition, and physical activity. Perhaps as a result of the regular contact with their healthcare providers, those in both the intervention and control groups appear to have shown improvements relative to baseline in general cognitive functioning, executive functions, processing speed, and memory. A small effect was reported for the mean change of in both groups on total NTB scores with slightly more improvement from baseline to one year than from one year to two years. Unfortunately, the authors do not report whether the performances in either group at one- and two-year follow-up were significantly different from baseline. The authors utilized z-scores, standardized to the baseline mean. Inspection of their results suggests the largest change occurred in the memory from baseline to 24 months with a z-score difference of approximately +.35. The authors do not mention the use of any alternate forms, suggesting the possibility that their results were contaminated by practice effects. The use of reliable change indices would have also been helpful to clarify whether the differences seen were clinically significant. Also, the sole outcome measure was neuropsychological testing, and an additional dimension of everyday functioning, as used in the ACTIVE study, would have been beneficial. Nonetheless, despite these limitations, the results of the FINGER study are encouraging insofar as they demonstrate some benefit to cognition from a multifactorial approach that includes diet, exercise, and cognitive training.

The SMART Trial

The Study of Mental Activity and Resistance Training (SMART) trial investigated whether, and to what degree, physical and cognitive exercise could delay cognitive decline in old age. The trial looked specifically at individuals over the age of 55 to determine whether CCT using the COGPACK program, physical resistance exercise, or a combination of the two could prevent or slow cognitive and functional decline. What sets the SMART trial apart from many other studies of this sort is the use of neuroimaging to assess for both structural and functional changes associated with the study interventions. Specifically, the investigators focused on structural and functional features of the hippocampus—a region long known to be involved in episodic memory, and the posterior cingulate region—which is functionally associated with the default mode network. The authors found that physical resistance training but not CCT was associated with significantly improved global cognition and expanded gray matter in the posterior cingulate. Those who completed the physical resistance training also showed reversed progression of white matter hyperintensities in multiple brain areas. Conversely, cognitive training was associated with slowed decline in overall memory performance, which was mediated by enhanced functional connectivity between the hippocampus and superior frontal cortex (Suo et al., 2016).

Certainly, more studies investigating the neural correlates of interventions designed for slowing cognitive decline are needed as they are particularly suited to answering questions about how these interventions might exert their effects or why some programs are more successful than others in enhancing specific cognitive functions.

THE SCIENTIFIC CONSENSUS ON THE BRAIN TRAINING INDUSTRY

On October 20, 2014, a group of 75 researchers from around the globe signed on to show their support for a letter published by the Max Planck Institute for Human Development and the Stanford Center for Longevity and (2017). The letter levels criticisms at the brain training industry, focusing on their lack of empirical support and overreaching claims regarding potential benefits to brain health and everyday cognitive performance. The authors of the letter note that assessing the effects of cognitive training is an immensely complex problem and aptly describe it as "a devil with many details" (Max Planck Institute for Human Development and Stanford Center on Longevity, n.d.). One primary issue the authors raise involves the peer-reviewed research backing many brain training companies cite as supporting their products' effectiveness. These cited studies are often only tangentially related to the brain training games in question. Moreover, while the studies cited on many brain training companies' websites may indeed show improved performance following training, the authors of the letter offer plausible, and perhaps more parsimonious, explanations for the improvements in performance such as the acquisition of strategies and the impact of motivation. While strategies that work on computerized tasks may be applicable to study outcome measures, this does not at all guarantee they will transfer to real-world tasks. And, with all else being equal, an individual who is highly motivated to improve his or her cognitive functioning will likely be more engaged in training and perhaps even perform better on outcome measures than an individual who is less motivated, simply by virtue of his or hermotivation.

As the scientific community has called for the use of more rigorous experimental controls in order to adequately assess the impact of brain training programs, the brain training industry has made efforts to respond. To this end, many studies have included active control groups as a means to address the "placebo effect" in brain training research. In a reply to the scientific community's consensus letter, the brain training industry released its own letter, in which members argued that the brain training literature not only showed the transfer of training effects but that the studies they cite often employed "control strategies to account for 'placebo' effects" (Cognitive Training Data, n.d.). However, one of the most frequently used "control strategies" may not be sufficient for fully capturing the impact of placebo effects. Despite what appears to be a widespread assumption that placebo effects are comparable across the active control and intervention conditions, none of the studies cited on the Cognitive Training Data website attempt to assess the validity of this assumption (Boot, Blakely, & Simons, 2011). In other words, if a brain training study includes an active control group (e.g., trained on a memory task) for comparison with an intervention group (e.g., trained on a reasoning task), the assumptions made by participants regarding whether and to what degree their training will impact their performance on the study's outcome measure may differ, particularly if the outcome measure appears to tap something different than the task on which the participant was trained. Thus while it is uncommon for studies to actually measure participants' perceptions of the relatedness between the training tasks to outcome measures (Boot et al., 2011), in the absence of this measurement, it cannot be said that placebo effects have been fully accounted for.

Perhaps more importantly, while motivation and expectation should not be underestimated as a potential source of contamination in studies of brain training, the authors of the consensus letter point to an even more glaring issue involving patient motivation—opportunity costs. There is a cost in time, money, and effort associated with engaging in online brain training that could be spent on some other activity. It is reasonable to assume an individual who is motivated to improve his or her cognitive performance may also pursue other means of improving brain health. However, the time and money spent using brain training sites and products could be spent instead on any number of other activities, including some which been shown to have real and reliable benefits for brain health such as physical exercise, meditation, and social engagement. These activities not only have a more well-established research base but carry with them other benefits as well that go beyond the potential boost to cognitive functioning and, in many cases, come at a much lower financial cost. The majority of research cited by brain training companies appears to rest on the statistically significant effects of training that can be demonstrated on similar laboratory-based tasks. Even meta-analytic studies, which can give some estimate of the size of the effects conferred by brain training, do not fully mitigate problems with the individual studies they include in their analyses. Also, while meta-analyses may be useful in summarizing the existing, published research, such approaches cannot fully account for null findings that are never published (i.e., the file drawer problem). The authors of the letter do, however, express enthusiasm for studies showing, for example, improvement in driving performance in older adults after computerized reasoning and speed of processing training. They also point to such studies as the exceptions, as many published investigations fail to include indices of real-world functioning as outcome measures. To date, there is little evidence that brain training games' effects go beyond the trained skills or that, as is often advertised, they promote "brain health" in any general sense.

The extent to which individuals develop strategies for completing tasks of attention and memory is, to a certain extent, a generalizable commodity, though the extent to which these constitute "enhancement" of the underlying cognitive abilities is questionable. Furthermore, the authors point to a dearth of research demonstrating the persistence of skills over an extended period of time (i.e., longer than the study period). One study is cited as showing an association between extensive computerized brain training and improved reasoning and episodic memory maintained over two years, but this study only investigated a group of younger adults and again suffers from the same questions regarding strategy acquisition and motivation.

The authors encourage further research into the potential benefit of computerized brain training games but emphasize the importance of holding companies that publish such games to the same standards for demonstrating reliability and validity to which the publishers of psychometric tests are held. They offer the following five recommendations for individuals considering using brain training programs: (a) consider the opportunity costs; (b) consider the fact that physical exercise has empirical support as an activity that clearly benefits cognitive functioning; (c) studies carried out by researchers with financial conflicts of interest are not sufficient for demonstrating effectiveness and need replication; their effects should also be clinically significant, not just statistically significant; (d) there is no evidence that any brain game can cure or prevent Alzheimer's disease or any other form of dementia; and (e) any gains made by challenging oneself once or even for a concentrated period with brain training games is likely to be short-lived and does not work like an inoculation against cognitive decline. The brain training industry remains controversial, with more studies required to better determine the long-term effectiveness of computerized cognitive exercise. Nonetheless, the industry and the field have shown a clear interest in promoting brain science as a whole and more specifically in attempting to advance our ability to maintain healthy cognitive function into late life.

Cognitive Remediation and Rehabilitation

Cognitive remediation focuses on the strengthening of specific cognitive processes such as memory or executive functioning that subserve behavior. The goal of remediation is to invoke a change that is both long-lasting and generalized to more than one behavior. Cognitive rehabilitation has a broader focus of everyday behavioral functions, such as remembering appointments or cooking a meal. Cognitive rehabilitation can, in part, rely on changes in the environment so as to minimize the underlying neural requirement. External compensatory techniques can be conceptualized as changing or rearranging the environment so that the task (e.g., remembering an appointment) is accomplished by relying upon a memory notebook or a smartphone reminder. In this scenario, the emphasis is not on changing the way the brain processes the information; rather, the task demands are altered (and often lessened) based on "crutches" or external changes in the environment. In this example, nothing is changed about the way the brain processes the information; the behavior (remembering an appointment) is completed through a change in the environment (smartphone reminder). Although the focus of this chapter is not on external compensatory techniques, these can be quite useful and sometimes most helpful in cases of more severe brain dysfunction when the ability to learn new strategies is significantly compromised. The Academy of Neurologic Communication Disorders and Sciences conducted a systematic review and meta-analysis of studies reporting the use of external memory aids, including memory notebooks and electronic aides (Sohlberg et al., 2007). It concluded that assistive devices should be included in practice guidelines to improve the functional ability of patients suffering from traumatic brain injuries. There are hundreds of effective strategies for simplification or rearranging of the environment to facilitate everyday functioning in the elderly as well as in those suffering from neurological impairment (Gitlin & Burgh, 1995). Greenway, Duncan, and Smith (2013) provide a comprehensive training in a memory notebook system designed for patients with MCI and early dementia. In this program, which requires the attendance of a caregiver who assists in homework and integration, each day is broken down into things needing to be done and things that are time-specific, with additional space allocated for important things to remember that arise in the completion of a day's activities.

The primary focus here, however, is to describe evidence-based techniques that in some way change or strengthen the underlying physiological/neural substrates in the brain to strengthen memory and other brain functions. The American Congress of Rehabilitation Medicine (ACRM) has developed a cognitive rehabilitation manual based on empirically supported techniques in the area of attention, memory, visuospatial skills, social skills, and executive functions (Haskins, Cicerone, & Trexler, 2012). This manual is designed for work with patients suffering from traumatic brain injury or stroke; further research is needed to determine the effectiveness of these techniques to other populations (e.g., normal aging and early dementia).

The cognitive rehabilitation of memory has received the most attention in clinical and research endeavors, undoubtedly due to the ubiquitous nature of memory and the natural changes in memory function in the process of aging. In the area of memory, intervention can be rehearsal based or compensatory (Hampstead et al., 2008). Rehearsal-based interventions are based upon repetition of information over time and strengthen existing neural pathways. There are variations in the way the information is presented for encoding (e.g., errorful vs. errorless learning), as well as variations in how the information is retrieved (e.g., vanishing cues). The ACRM manual provides an exhaustive review of the various approaches to memory and learning.

A common critique of early computer-based programs for cognitive remediation (and, indeed, for brain training programs) is the lack of carry-over into everyday life. Even though a patient may show improved performance on the specific computerized program, the programs lack "ecological validity"; that is, the improvement has no effect on everyday performance. Stringer (2011) has developed a manualized program, Ecologically Oriented Neurorehabilitation of Memory, in response to these limitations. One common complaint among brain-damaged individuals as well as those with normal aging is remembering names. Stringer has developed an associative technique designed to improve face-name associations entitled "Feature, Reason, and Image" (Hampstead et al., 2008). This is a three step process. In the first step, a salient feature is identified (Feature) and patients are encouraged to pick an unusual or prominent feature (e.g., Paul is "tall"). The second step (Reason) involves a verbally based reason for selecting the feature (e.g., Paul is very tall so "Paul-tall"). Last, patients are encouraged to imagine and integrate the previous steps using mental imagery (Image). This mnemonic strategy improves learning and memory in both healthy older adults and patients with MCI (Hampstead, Sathian, et al., 2012). Hampstead and colleagues (2011) also demonstrated that individuals with MCI show improvement in recalling names, which was also demonstrated in functional MRI changes before and after training. Individuals in the training group had greater activation of brain regions in the lateral frontoparietal working memory networks and the hippocampus (Hampstead, Stringer, Stilla, Giddens, & Sathian, 2012).

The American Congress of Rehabilitation Medicine's Cognitive Rehabilitation Manual contains specific evidence-based procedures for rehabilitation of attention, memory, executive functions, hemispatial neglect, and social communication (Haskins et al., 2012). One technique that has met with wide utilization is the memory peg technique described by Wilson (2009). In the visual peg method, the target items to be remembered are linked with a standard set of peg words that are already learned and memorized in a fixed order. The classic example (outlined in Haskins et al., 2012) of this mnemonic strategy is based upon learning these easy associations: one-bun, two-shoe, three-tree, four-door, five-hive, and so on. These rhyming words are committed to memory to serve as "pegs" for new learnings to be "hung on." If one wanted to remember a shopping list of five items, one would form an association by virtue of a series of visual images utilizing the peg words; the more unusual or outlandish the visual image, the better. Assume the five items to be purchased are milk, lettuce, cheese, laundry detergent, and a newspaper. Visual peg images, therefore, might be as follows:

- One-bun: imagine a quart of milk in a hot-dog bun
- Two-shoe: imagine a shoe brimming over with lettuce leaves
- Three-tree: imagine a tree with pieces of cheese replacing the leaves
- Four-door: imagine a door with a container of laundry detergent hanging from the door handle
- Five-hive: imagine a beehive covered with newspaper pages

Thus the peg system could be utilized to remember appointments, a list of things to do, the largest capital cities, or any other material that can be visualized. Also, instead of using an auditory verbal rehearsal strategy that would utilize a left hemisphere frontal/temporoparietal network (i.e., repeating the shopping list to oneself), using the visual peg system utilizes visual processing areas in the right hemisphere of the brain thereby changing the internal neural processing. An individual could certainly create his or her own peg system. Another natural sequential and automatized order is the alphabet: for example, "A" could represent an army of ants; "B" could be linked to a bumble bee. To use the aforementioned example of shopping items, one might visualize an army of ants carrying a quart of milk and a bumble bee with lettuce for wings.

Many individuals who are cognitively compromised have difficulty with the planning and organization requirements underlying many executive functions in daily life. Stringer (2011) has devised the Write-Organize-Picture-Rehearse (W-O-P-R) strategy to minimize memory and/or executive dysfunction. For example, both memory and executive functions are required in remembering the day's activities or appointments. Using the W-O-P-R method, a combination of both external (writing it down) and internal (organizing and picturing and rehearsing) processes are used. Once a patient writes down a list of appointments/activities, the next step is to organize them in a way that makes sense. Given the location of appointments, does is make sense for one to logically follow another? Are some appointments time sensitive? Can activities be chunked together? The aforementioned peg system can then be used to picture the items written down. In the rehearsal stage, the patient is encouraged to say the activities in sequential order and to use the visual peg association, as necessary, to recall all activities. If the visual peg fails, the patient can consult the written list, and so on until the day's activities are recalled without the need for the written reminders.

In general, remediation of executive function deficits as proposed by the American Congress of Rehabilitation Medicine (Haskins et al., 2012) addresses the major components of executive functioning, that is, developing an awareness of a need, formulation of a plan toward a desired outcome, enactment of a response or a series of responses toward that desired outcome, and evaluation of how well the desired outcome was achieved with any necessary modifications to follow. One such intervention often used is metacognitive strategy training. Metacognition, or thinking about thinking, involves both metacognitive knowledge (i.e., a person's ongoing moment by moment awareness of his or her thinking and more stable beliefs about one's thinking), as well as metacognitive control (i.e., self-monitoring of thoughts and the ability to adapt to changes in task demands; Kennedy et al., 2008). Individuals who are more compromised may benefit from learning a Goal-Plan-Do-Review (G-P-D-R) approach, which eventually becomes internalized with practice. Luria (1973) was among the first to advocate "self-talk" as a remedial technique with frontally damaged patients and theorized different "functional loops" or physiological activations that occur with tasks that are being conducted with the aid of self-talk. Cicerone and Giacino (1992) also describe "self-talk" procedures (i.e., the patient is taught to talk him or herself through procedures). As simple as this sounds, becoming accustomed to initially talking out loud and graduating to inner talk serves additional goals of preventing unwanted behaviors while facilitating planning and focus.

Deficits in attention are extremely common and can significantly interfere with a wide range of daily activities that require attention as a fundamental skill. One cannot remember or solve a problem if one cannot attend. There are many models of attention. Sohlberg and Mateer (1987) divide attention into five components: focused attention, sustained attention, selective attention, alternating attention, and divided attention. These are hierarchically organized, with focused attention being the most basic and referring to the ability to recognize and acknowledge sensory input. Sustained attention is the ability to maintain attention over time, and selective attention involves responding to targeted information while ignoring or inhibiting non-target (distracting) information. Alternating attention involves shifting from one focus to another, and divided attention refers to the ability to respond to two or more stimuli at the same time.

In Attention Process Training, Sohlberg and Mateer (2001) emphasize that attention training should include tasks aimed at generalization with the goal being improvements in everyday life. They provide different levels of training depending upon the level of impairment severity, and the program consists of different tracks corresponding to the components of attention noted earlier, and specific guidelines are presented for generalization activities. For example, Sohlberg, Johnson, Paule, Raskin, and Mateer (1993) suggest cooking and paying bills/balancing a checkbook as residential activities for sustained attention, while typing or answering phone calls might be vocational generalizing activities. Cooking with potentially distracting background noise represents a selective attention task, and cooking a meal with two items that require simultaneous monitoring would represent a divided attention task.

Conclusion

This chapter has described two primary types of cognitive intervention, brain training and cognitive remediation/rehabilitation. The goal of both is to improve functioning, whether that functioning is impaired due to acquired illness, subject to the effects of normal aging, or simply the focus of someone who wants to sharpen cognitive functioning. Although the research is not uniform in its support for various cognitive interventions, there is mounting support for cognitive interventions to both improve normal functioning and ameliorate cognitive dysfunction. Whereas the brain was once viewed as a fixed unmalleable system in adulthood, recent research on neuroplasticity suggests we have a robust capacity for neuronal networks to change their structure in response to both injury and learning, even into old age. Cognitive reserve or resilience further suggests that all brains are not alike in their adaptability; factors such as IQ, education and occupational attainment, stimulation with leisure activities, and even stress can affect the brain's resilience in the face of acquired injury or normal aging.

In general, research in both brain training and cognitive remediation needs adequate placebo controls that account for differential placebo effects across training conditions and outcome measures (Boot et al., 2011), larger sample sizes, long-term follow-up, outcome measures that are clinically meaningful, and careful monitoring of dose-response relationships. In particular, although the ACTIVE study accounted for many of these issues, there was no clarification as to how often the individuals continued to use their training intervention over follow-up, with obviously greater difficulty monitoring the frequency of reliance on (or practice with) internal memory strategies versus time spent on computerized brain training. Although larger samples with multicenter trials have obvious benefits, these studies tend to have programs using numerous interventions in addition to cognitive (e.g., physical exercise, nutrition), which limit conclusions about which intervention produces which effect. The preponderance of research supports the notion that brain training will result in improved performance on identical or similar games, but this improvement will not necessarily transfer or generalize to real-life situations or prevent disease. There is a need for the brain training industry and cognitive rehabilitation, based upon research on the transfer of learning and generalizability, to create games and challenges/exercises that more closely mimic real-life activities if the goal is to create real-life improvement.

REFERENCES

Ball, K., Berch, D. B., Helmers, K. F., Jobe, J. B., Leveck, M. D., Marsiske, M., et al. (2002). Effects of cognitive training interventions with older adults: A randomized controlled trial. *JAMA, 288*(18), 2271–2281.

Ballesteros, S., Mayas, J., Prieto, A., Toril, P., Pita, C., Pde, L., et al. (2015). A randomized controlled trial of brain training with non-action video games in older adults: Results of the 3-month follow-up. *Frontiers in Aging Neuroscience, 7*, 45.

Ballesteros S, Prieto A, Mayas J, Toril, P., Pita, C., de León, P., et al. (2014). Brain training with non-action video games enhances aspects of cognition in older adults: A randomized controlled trial. *Frontiers in Aging Neuroscience, 6*, 277.

Boot, W. R., Blakely, D. P., & Simons, D. J. (2011). Do action video games improve perception and cognition? *Frontiers in Psychology, 2*, 226.

BrainTrain. (n.d.). Retrieved from http://www.braintrain.com/.

Cicerone, K., & Giacino, J. (1992). Remediation of executive function deficits after traumatic brain injury. *NeuroRehabilitation, 2*, 12–22.

Cognitive Training Data. (n.d.). Cognitive training data response letter. Retrieved from http://www.cognitivetrainingdata.org/the-controversy-does-brain-training-work/response-letter/

Eckroth-Bucher, M., & Siberski, J. (2009). Preserving cognition through an integrated cognitive stimulation and training program. *American Journal of Alzheimer's Disease and Other Dementia, 24*(3), 234–245.

Fotuhi, M., Lubinski, B., Trullinger, M., Riloff, T., Hadadi, M., & Raji, C. (2016). A personalized 12-week "brain fitness program" for improving cognitive function and increasing the volume of hippocampus in elderly with mild cognitive impairment. *Journal of Prevention of Alzheimer's Disease, 3*(3), 133–137.

Gates, N., & Valenzuela, M. (2010). Cognitive exercise and its role in cognitive function in older adults. *Current Psychiatry Report, 12*, 20–27.

Gitlin, L. N., & Burgh, D. (1995). Issuing assistive devices to older patients in rehabilitation: An exploratory study. *American Journal of Occupational Therapy, 49*(10), 994–1000.

Greenaway, M. C., Duncan, N. L., & Smith, G. E. (2013). The memory support system for mild cognitive impairment: Randomized trial of a cognitive rehabilitation intervention. *International Journal of Geriatric Psychiatry, 28*(4), 402–409.

Hampstead, B. M., Mosti, C. B., & Swirsky-Sacchetti, T. (2014). Cognitively based methods of enhancing and maintaining functioning in those at risk of Alzheimer's disease. *Journal of Alzheimer's Disease, 42*(Suppl. 4), S483–S493.

Hampstead, B. M., Sathian, K., Moore, A. B., Nalisnick, C., & Stringer, A. Y. Explicit memory training leads to improved memory for face-name pairs in patients with mild cognitive impairment: Results of a pilot investigation. *Journal of International Neuropsychological Science, 14*(5), 883–889.

Hampstead, B. M., Sathian, K., Phillips, P. A., Amaraneni, A., Delaune, W. R., & Stringer, A. Y. (2012). Mnemonic strategy training improves memory for object location associations in both healthy elderly and patients with amnestic mild cognitive impairment: A randomized, single-blind study. *Neuropsychology, 26*(3), 385–399.

Hampstead, B. M., Stringer, A. Y., Stilla, R. F., Deshpande, G., Hu, X., Moore, A. B., & Sathian, K. (2011). Activation and effective connectivity changes following explicit-memory training for face-name pairs in patients with mild cognitive impairment: A pilot study. *Neurorehabilitation and Neural Repair, 25*(3), 210–222.

Hampstead, B. M., Stringer, A. Y., Stilla, R. F., Giddens, M., & Sathian, K. (2012). Mnemonic strategy training partially restores hippocampal activity in patients with mild cognitive impairment. *Hippocampus, 22*(8), 1652–1658.

Harrison, J., Minassian, S. L., Jenkins, L., Black, R. S., Koller, M., & Grundman, M. (2007). A neuropsychological test battery for use in Alzheimer disease clinical trials. *Archives of Neurology, 64*(9), 1323–1329.

Haskins, E. C., Cicerone, K. D., & Trexler, L. E. (2012). *Cognitive rehabilitation manual: Translating evidence-based recommendations into practice.* Reston, VA: ACRM Publishing.

Jobe, J. B., Smith, D. M., Ball, K., Tennstedt, S. L., Marsiske, M., Willis, S. L., et al. (2001). ACTIVE: A cognitive intervention trial to promote independence in older adults. *Controlled Clinical Trials, 22*(4), 453–479.

Kaup, A. R., Nettiksimmons, J., LeBlanc, E. S., & Yaffe, K. (2015). Memory complaints and risk of cognitive impairment after nearly 2 decades among older women. *Neurology, 85*(21), 1852–1858.

Kennedy, M. R., Coelho, C., Turkstra, L., Coelho, C., Turkstra, L., Ylvisaker, M., et al. (2008). Intervention for executive functions after traumatic brain injury: A systematic review, meta-analysis and clinical recommendations. *Neuropsychological Rehabilitation, 18*(3), 257–299.

Kivipelto, M., Solomon, A., Ahtiluoto, S., Ngandu, T., Lehtisalo, J., Antikainen, R., et al. (2013). The Finnish Geriatric Intervention Study to Prevent Cognitive Impairment and Disability (FINGER): Study design and progress. *Alzheimer's & Dementia, 9*(6), 657–665.

Lampit, A., Ebster, C., & Valenzuela, M. (2014). Multi-domain computerized cognitive training program improves performance of bookkeeping tasks: A matched-sampling active-controlled trial. *Frontiers in Psychology*, 5, 794.

Luria, A. R. (1973). *The working brain: An introduction to neuropsychology.* New York: Basic Books.

Max Planck Institute for Human Development and Stanford Center on Longevity. (n.d.). A consensus on the brain training industry from the scientific community. Retrieved from http://longevity3.stanford.edu/blog/2014/10/15/the-consensus-on-the- brain-training-industry-from-the-scientific-community/

Morris, J. N., Fries, B. E., Steel, K., Ikegami, N., Bernabei, R., Carpenter, G. I., et al. (1997). Comprehensive clinical assessment in community setting: Applicability of the MDS-HC. *Journal of the American Geriatric Society*, 45(8), 1017–1024.

Ngandu, T., Lehtisalo, J., Levalahti, E., Ahtiluoto, S., Jula, A., Laatikainen, T., et al. (2015). A 2 year multidomain intervention of diet, exercise, cognitive training, and vascular risk monitoring versus control to prevent cognitive decline in at-risk elderly people (FINGER): A randomised controlled trial. *The Lancet*, 385(9984), 2255–2263.

Papp, K. V., Walsh, S. J., & Snyder, P. J. (2009). Immediate and delayed effects of cognitive interventions in healthy elderly: A review of current literature and future directions. *Alzheimer's & Dementia*, 5(1), 50–60.

Parente, R., & Hermann, D. (2003). *Retraining cognition: Techniques and applications* (2nd ed.). Austin, TX: PRO-ED.

Posit Science. (n.d.). Brain HQ. Retrieved from http://www.brainhq.com/

Rabiner, D. L., Murray, D. W., Skinner, A. T., & Malone, P. S. (2010). A randomized trial of two promising computer-based interventions for students with attention difficulties. *Journal of Abnormal Child Psychology*, 38(1), 131–142.

Rakic P. (2002). Neurogenesis in adult primate neocortex: An evaluation of the evidence. *Nature Reviews Neuroscience*, 3(1), 65–71.

Scarmeas, N., Albert, S. M., Manly, J. J., & Stern, Y. (2006). Education and rates of cognitive decline in incident Alzheimer's disease. *Journal of Neurology, Neurosurgery & Psychiatry*, 77(3), 308–316.

Scientific Learning Corporation. (n.d.). Fast ForWord Reading Assistant. Retrieved from http://www.scilearn.com/products/fast-forword/reading-series

Selk, J. (2013). Amidst billion-dollar brain fitness industry, a free way to train your brain. *Forbes*. Retrieved from https://www.forbes.com/sites/jasonselk/2013/08/13/amidst-billion-dollar-brain-fitness-industry-a-free-way-to-train-your-brain/#63fa5f732b0d

Simons, D. J., Boot, W. R., Charness, N., Gathercole, S. E., Chabris, C. F., Hambrick, D. Z., et al. (2016). Do "brain-training" programs work? *Psychological Science in the Public Interest*, 17(3), 103–186.

Smith, G. E., Housen, P., Yaffe, K., Ruff, R., Kennison, R. F., Mahncke, H. W., & Zelinski, E. M. (2009). A cognitive training program based on principles of brain plasticity: Results from the Improvement in Memory with Plasticity-based Adaptive Cognitive Training (IMPACT) study. *Journal of the American Geriatric Society*, 57(4), 594–603.

Sohlberg, M., Johnson, L., Paule, L., Raskin, S., & Mateer, C. (1993). *Attention Process Training–II: A program to address attentional deficits for persons with mild cognitive impairment.* Puyallup, WA: Association for Neuropsychological Research and Development.

Sohlberg, M., Kennedy, M., Avery, J., Coelho, C. A., Turkstra, L., Ylvisaker, M., & Yorkston, K. (2007). Evidence based practice for the use of external aids as a memory rehabilitation technique. *Journal of Medical Speech Pathology, 15*(1), xv–li.

Sohlberg, M. M., & Mateer, C. A. (1987). Effectiveness of an attention-training program. *Journal of Clinical and Experimental Neuropsychology, 9*(2), 117–130.

Sohlberg, M. M., & Mateer, C. A. (2001). *Cognitive rehabilitation: An integrative neuropsychological approach.* New York: Guilford Press.

Stringer, A. Y. (2011). Ecologically oriented neurorehabilitation of memory: Robustness of outcome across diagnosis and severity. *Brain Injury, 25*(2), 169–178.

Suo, C., Singh, M. F., Gates, N., Leung, I., Valenzuela, M. J., Suo, C., et al. (2016). Therapeutically relevant structural and functional mechanisms triggered by physical and cognitive exercise. *Molecular Psychiatry, 21*(11), 1633–1642.

Topiwala, A., Allan, C. L., Valkanova, V., Zsoldos, E., Filippini, N., Sexton, C. E., et al. (2015). Resilience and MRI correlates of cognitive impairment in community-dwelling elders. *British Journal of Psychiatry, 207*(5), 435–439.

Toril, P., Reales, J. M., Mayas, J., & Ballesteros, S. (2016). Video game training enhances visuospatial working memory and episodic memory in older adults. *Frontiers in Human Neuroscience, 10.*

Wentink, M., Berger, M., de Kloet, A., Meesters, J., Band, G. P. H., Wolterbeek, R., et al. (2016). The effects of an 8-week computer-based brain training programme on cognitive functioning, QoL and self-efficacy after stroke. *Neuropsychological Rehabilitation, 26*(5–6), 847–865.

Willis, S. L., Tennstedt, S. L., Marsiske, M., Ball, K., Elias, J., Koepke, K. M., et al. (2006). Long-term effects of cognitive training on everyday functional outcomes in older adults. *JAMA, 296*(23), 2805–2814.

Wilson, B. A. (2009). *Memory rehabilitation: Integrating theory and practice.* New York: Guilford Press.

Zelinski, E. M., Spina, L. M., Yaffe, K., Ruff, R., Kennison, R. F., Mahncke, H. W., & Smith, G. E. (2011). Improvement in memory with plasticity-based adaptive cognitive training: Results of the 3-month follow-up. *Journal of the American Geriatric Society, 59*(2), 258–265.

17

Integrative Approaches to Cognitive Decline

THOMAS J. KELLY IV AND MIJAIL SERRUYA

Key Points

- Cognitive decline is a highly prevalent medical problem as people age.
- There are no known treatments that halt neurodegenerative processes such as Alzheimer's or Parkinson's disease.
- Physical exercise is essential to good brain health.
- Social engagement supports positive emotions and overall brain health.
- Cognitive engagement and exercises can improve specific cognitive domains.
- Eating a good, healthful diet is essential for maintaining a healthy brain and preventing cognitive decline.
- Diets such as the Mediterranean diet that are high in plant-based foods, healthy fats, and antioxidants help to maintain good brain health.
- Good sleep helps support brain health.
- Nutritional supplements such as N-acetyl-cysteine, omega-3 fatty acids, vitamin D, and antioxidants can be part of a program to maintain good brain health.
- Meditative, biofeedback, and other modulatory practices may promote healthy brain function.
- Combining these approaches together appears to have a synergistic "more than the sum of their parts" benefit on protecting and enhancing brain health.

Introduction

Prevalence studies indicate that there are over 4.5 million adults with Alzheimer's disease (AD) in the United States (Hebert, Weuve, Scherr, & Evans, 2013). Approximately 3 million people have Parkinson's disease. Approximately 800,000 patients a year suffer a stroke, and another 1 million have other types of neurodegenerative disorders. The percentage of adults with dementia rises dramatically with age: at least 5% of those aged 65 have dementia, and this rises to more than 45% for those reaching age 85. As the overall population ages, neurodegenerative diseases will become more common. In fact, the number of AD patients is likely to rise to 13.2 million by 2050. The estimated costs associated with dementia are expected to surpass $10 billion annually. The best strategy to reduce this personal and public health catastrophe is the development of disease-halting therapy combined with methods to identify the pathology at the earliest stage possible. However, a recent article in the *Journal of the American Medical Association* stated that while "no medications have proven effective for [neurodegenerative disorders]; treatments and interventions should be aimed at reducing cardiovascular risk factors and prevention of stroke. Aerobic exercise, mental activity, and social engagement may help decrease risk of further cognitive decline" (Langa & Levine, 2014).

The physiology of the neurodegenerative process includes degeneration of cholinergic neurons in the basal forebrain, which is thought to cause the loss of episodic memory in people with AD and dementia with Lewy bodies (Francis, Palmer, Snape, & Wilcock, 1999). Accordingly, acetycholinesterase inhibitors (including donepezil, galantamine, and rivastigmine) are approved to delay cognitive decline in these patients. Memantine, a metabolite of amantadine, blocks N-methyl-D-aspartate receptors, appears to block excitotoxicity in metabolically vulnerable neurons, and is approved for patients with suspected moderate to severe AD (Carter, Banister, & Blaber, 2003). Unfortunately, the benefits of these approved agents are marginal, and they do not delay the underlying disease progression (Lleó, Greenberg, & Growdon, 2006).

Development of therapeutic agents that target the underlying pathogenesis of neurodegenerative diseases is currently being investigated. The inflammatory neurodegenerative process involves hormones, calcium dysregulation, axoplasmic transport, prion proteins and protein misfolding, oxidative stress, and a variety of neurotransmitters and their receptors (Sohal, Mockett, & Orr, 2002). While single-pathway therapeutics may yet see an effective intervention become available, this is not mutually exclusive to a combination approach that could target several of these pathways simultaneously and yield a synergistic, preventative benefit. Given the efficacy of therapy that combines multiple medications and nonpharmacologic interventions for chronic illnesses including cancer, cardiovascular disease, and HIV infection, there is growing interest on the application of combination therapies for neurodegenerative conditions (Bredesen, 2014). In addition to combining medications (such as donepezil and memantine), combination therapy can include nonpharmacologic approaches including dietary modification, aerobic exercise, and meditative practice. While other chapters in this volume address some of these alternate approaches in greater detail, here we review a more targeted summary with respect to neurodegenerative disorders and cognitive decline.

The Pillars of Brain Health

We propose that normal function of the human brain relies on five pillars: (a) regular aerobic exercise, (b) regular social engagement, (c) regular cognitive engagement, (d) consistently healthy nutrition, (e) and healthy sleep. Although engaging in these activities can be considered common sense, there is a growing body of data indicating they may induce compelling changes in brain structure and function, and hence providers would be justified in counseling their patients that their pursuit is not merely about a lifestyle choice and is instead a medicine.

Sedentary habits are a risk factor for cognitive decline, and *physical activity* has protective effects. Numerous trials have demonstrated the benefits of regular exercise (Aguiar, Monteiro, Feres, Gomes, & Melo, 2014; Alghadir, Gabr, & Al-Eisa, 2016; Bonura & Tenenbaum, 2014; Bossers et al., 2015; Bruin, Zwan, & Bogels, 2016; Carter, Banister, & Blaber, 2003; Chapman et al., 2013; Colcombe et al., 2006; Douris et al., 2003; Hardy et al., 2015; Hars, Herrmann, Gold, Rizzoli, & Trombetti, 2014; Hogan et al., 2013; Ide & Secher, 2000; Iyalomhe et al., 2015; Köbe et al., 2016; Küster et al., 2016; Leavitt et al., 2014; Liu-Ambrose et al., 2016; Masley, Roetzheim, & Gualtieri, 2009; Ngandu, Lehtisalo, & Solomon, 2015; Patterson et al. 2008; Predovan, Fraser, Renaud, & Bherer, 2012; Rush University Medical Center, 2015; Särkämö et al., 2014; Smith et al., 2014; ten Brinke et al., 2015; Van den Heuvel et al., 2009; van der Zwan et al., 2015; van Praag, Fleshner, Schwartz, & Mattson, 2014; Yu et al., 2013), with the greatest benefits seen in aerobic exercise. Stretching, resistance training, and weight training each also bring benefits and appear to be most helpful when combined with aerobic exercise. Exercise is associated with increased volume in several brain areas, including the hippocampus (Chapman et al., 2013; Colcombe et al., 2006; Leavitt et al., 2014; Smith et al., 2014; ten Brinke et al., 2015). Additionally, exercise improves brain metabolism (Ide & Secher, 2000; van Praag, Fleshner, Schwartz, & Mattson, 2014). For patients with mobility constraints, aquatherapy, the use of a reclined bicycle or a rowing machine, provide opportunities for exercise, and for those who cannot tolerate those approaches, chair-based exercises (e.g., chair yoga) have been shown to have benefits (Bonura & Tenenbaum, 2014; Carter et al., 2003; Douris et al., 2003; Köbe et al., 2016; Leavitt et al., 2014; Rush University Medical Center, 2015). Physical activity, and aerobic exercise in particular, has been found to improve memory, executive functioning, visuospatial skills, and information processing speeds found in aging adults. Aerobic exercise, reinforced by a monthly one-hour training session, was enough to bring significant changes to a cohort of sedentary results: a post hoc analysis showed that the participants had an elevated resting cerebral blood flow within the anterior cingulate and hippocampal regions and improved memory (Chapman et al., 2013).

Aside from a few exceptions (Madden, Blumenthal, Allen, & Emery, 1989; Young, Angevaren, Rusted, & Tabet, 2015), physical activity, more specifically aerobic exercise, is a well-researched treatment for cognitive issues involving attention (Hogan et al., 2013), executive functioning (Predovan et al., 2012), cognitive flexibility (Masley et al., 2009), neuroplasticity (Chapman et al., 2013), and mood (Yu et al., 2013) in aging adults. Exercise increases total antioxidant capacity and lowers serum levels malondialdehyde and 8-hydroxyguanine oxidants (Alghadir et al., 2016). Exercisers experience increases in overall brain volume (Colcombe et al., 2006), hippocampal volume (Leavitt et al., 2014; ten Brinke et al., 2015), and hippocampal blood flow (Chapman et al., 2013). There are increases in maximal oxygen uptake, downregulations in inflammation promoting genes, and upregulation in anti-inflammatory genes that promote immunity, neuron survival, and axon growth (Iyalomhe et al., 2015). Although aerobic cardiovascular exercise is the most studied, less strenuous strength and resistance training also confer a benefit in and of themselves and may augment the effects of aerobic exercise (Bossers et al., 2015).

If a patient encounters difficulty in creating an exercise plan due to a medical constraint (e.g., neuropathy or imbalance), a reclined bicycle, a rowing machine, supervised aquatherapy, or hiring a physical therapist or personal trainer are viable alternatives. It has been shown that lower-body exercise can retrain balance, and both aqua and land training are equally effective mediums for doing so (Douris et al., 2003). Hiring a personal trainer and making a financial commitment to exercising may improve compliance with the exercise regimen. Delegating a workout partner is a useful way to stay in line with exercise and is essential in adults with depression or neurodegenerative conditions that cause apathy and lack of insight.

Social engagement has been shown to protect the brain from degeneration and appears to protect cognition from the changes associated with normal aging and neurodegenerative disease (Kuiper et al., 2015; Küster et al., 2016). Patients should be advised to get out of the house more than once per week, engage with other people beyond their immediate families, attend religious services or cultural events, visit a petting zoo or engage with animals, have a poker night, go bowling, play a sport with others, attend a musical concert, or visit museums and art galleries. The premise is to place the mind in a socially and ideally intellectually stimulating environment, where new circumstances can be introduced to the brain.

Engaging daily in cognitively challenging tasks may boost cognitive reserve and overall brain health. If a professional athlete were to stop training for a month, his or her skills and endurance would decline. Likewise, people should be mentally challenging themselves every day in order to maintain a level of "mental fitness." Crossword puzzles, sudoku (Nozawa et al., 2015), listening to music (Chu et al., 2013; Guétin et al. 2009; Hars et al., 2014; Innes, Selfe, Brown, Rose, & Thompson-Heisterman, 2012; Svansdottir & Snaedal, 2006; Thompson, Moulin, Hayre, & Jones, 2006), playing an instrument (Bugos, Perlstein, McCrae, Brophy, & Bedenbaugh, 2007), singing (Särkämö et al., 2014), art work (Bolwerk, Mack-Andrick, Lang, Dörfler, & Maihöfner, 2014), attending lectures, taking classes, and reading books (Bostrom & Sandberg, 2009) have all been shown to improve cognition and quality of life. Passive mental activity, such as watching television or passively browsing the Internet, should be limited to, on average, no more than one hour per day (Johnson, Cohen, Kasen, & Brook, 2007; Lin, Cherng, Chen, Chen, & Yang, 2015; Takeuchi et al., 2013).

Cognitive training software has become quite popular in the marketplace in recent years, and the games are designed to benefit everyday living. However, only a minority of those playing brain training games experience a generalized improvement in their memory and attention in daily life (Hardy et al., 2015; Kwok, Bai, Li, Ho, & Lee, 2013; Mayas, Parmentier, Andrés, & Ballesteros, 2014; Toril, Reales, Mayas, & Ballesteros, 2016). Most adults engaged in these games only improve at playing the games themselves (van Heugten, Ponds, & Kessels, 2016; Wentink et al., 2016; Zickefoose, Hux, Brown, & Wulf, 2013). Computerized training studies have been hampered by methodological flaws (Cavallo, Signorino, & Perucchini, 2016; Moreau, Kirk, & Waldie, 2016) and remarkable placebo effects (Foroughi, Monfort, Paczynski, McKnight, & Greenwood, 2016). These games appear to be more effective if they are customized and integrated into one's daily routine (e.g., bank account management, using technological devices; Chan, Haber, Drew, & Park, 2014; Dewar, Kapur, & Kopelman, 2016). For adults interested in computerized training to enhance cognition, the most prudent advice may be to pursue training within a clinical trial, or to work with a neuropsychologist, occupational therapist, or speech therapist who can help them select an optimal product and develop a customized regimen.

Diet is a necessary facet to be addressed in lowering the risk of developing cognitive decline (Marcason, 2015). The MIND diet combines the Mediterranean diet; with the Dietary Approaches to Stop Hypertension (DASH) diets (Rush University Medical Center, 2015; thus it is called MIND for Mediterranean-DASH Intervention for Neurodegenerative Delay). Brain healthy foods in the MIND diet include vegetables with an emphasis on green leafy vegetables ("the darker the better"), nuts, berries, beans, whole grains, fish, poultry, olive oil, and modest amounts of wine. Fiber, healthy fats, and antioxidants are important. Brain unhealthy foods include red meat, butter/stick margarine, cheese, pastries and sweets, and fried or fast foods. General guidelines involve eating at least three servings of whole grains, a salad, one vegetable, and an optional single glass of wine per day. One or two servings of nuts are encouraged daily, and beans should be frequently included in the diet as they are low glycemic, high fiber, high protein sources. Poultry and berries are recommended at least once weekly. Butter should be eaten in quantities less than one tablespoon/day while cheese and fried or fast foods should be eaten less than once a week (Marcason, 2015; Rush University Medical Center, 2015). The MIND diet was found to lower the risk of developing AD by as much as 53% in participants who strictly adhered to it and approximately 35% in those who moderately followed it. This diet reduces cardiovascular risk for hypertension, heart attack, and stroke. A benefit to the MIND diet is that it is easier to follow than the Mediterranean diet. Those who follow these general dietary guide lines for a longer period of time experience more protection than others who start later (Rush University Medical Center, 2015).

Getting regular *sufficient and healthy sleep* appears neuroprotective, and irregular sleep risks cognitive impairment and dementia (Chen et al., 2015; Peter-Derex, Yammine, Bastuji, & Croisile, 2015). Correcting breathing difficulties should be prioritized as they can greatly impair overall sleep quality and can have deleterious or contributory effects on the cognition of a person. For sleep apnea, an eight-year study found that the implementation of continuous positive airway pressure therapy slowed decline in Mini-Mental Status Examination (MMSE) scores (Troussière et al., 2014). Too much exposure to artificial light (e.g., mobile phone) can disrupt sleep (Cho, Joo, Koo, & Hong, 2013; Higuchi, Motohashi, Liu, & Maeda, 2005) and may negatively affect cognition (Cajochen et al., 2011). For those with insomnia, or who simply do not wake up feeling rested enough, reinforcement of melatonin's circadian rhythm with supplementation may help (Wade et al., 2014; Xu et al., 2015). Normally, sunlight suppresses melatonin secretion and darkness enhances secretion: to reinforce this cycle, a small amount of melatonin may be taken soon after sunset and a second, larger amount 14 hours after waking up or 1 hour prior to bedtime.

Behavioral symptoms of neurodegenerative diseases may include disturbed sleep-wake patterns, sleepwalking, and agitation. Typically, in mild and severe cases, a patient may sleep during the day and be awake for as much as 40% of the night (Bonanni et al., 2005). Both light therapy and melatonin (e.g., 3 mg in the afternoon, plus additional doses closer to bedtime) have been shown to be efficacious in promoting a proper sleep schedule and are additive in their effects as a combination therapy (Paul et al., 2011). Furthermore, 30 minutes of 10,000 lux treatment (using the same "light box" deployed for adults with seasonal affective disorder) in the morning has also been shown to reduce aggression in those impaired with AD-related cognitive decline (Thorpe, Middleton, Russell, & Stewart, 2000). Once-daily light treatment for 30 minutes should be encouraged, as it is risk-free and may be very effective in correcting sleep problems in both normal and psychiatrically disturbed dementia patients, who may or may not experience agitation or other sleep and mood-related symptoms (Burns, Allen, Tomenson, Duignan, & Byrne, 2009; Chong, Tan, Tay, & Wong, 2013; Forbes, Blake, Thiessen, Peacock, & Hawranik, 2014; van Maanen, Meijer, van der Heijden, & Oort, 2016).

Reducing Risk Factors

Hypertension, the metabolic syndrome or diabetes mellitus, hyperlipidemia, low vitamin D, low vitamin B12, depression, polypharmacy, untreated obstructive sleep apnea, obesity, physical inactivity, and smoking are each modifiable risk factors for cognitive decline and have clear, evidence-based treatments.

Three of the key goals of primary care medicine are maintenance of healthy blood pressure, blood sugar, and lipid levels. Careful management of these *vascular risk factors* is associated with healthy aging with intact cognition (Mcmaster, Kristinsson, Turesson, Bjorkholm, & Landgren, 2010; Patterson et al. 2008; Shinohara et al., 2014; Van den Heuvel et al., 2009), while uncontrolled blood control may be related to white matter lesions and medial temporal lobe atrophy in AD (Korf, Scheltens, Barkhof, & Leeuw, 2005). In adults who have had a stroke, or have evidence of significant vascular disease on brain imaging, an antiplatelet agent such as aspirin may also be indicated. Cholesterol-lowering and blood pressure lowering medications may also have neuroprotective benefits beyond their known vascular benefits. Atorvastatin has been shown to increase cerebral blood flow in adults at risk for AD (Carlsson et al., 2012) and appears to have neuroprotective effects via modulation of the heme oxygenase/biliverdin reductase system in the brain (Barone, Di Domenico, & Butterfield, 2014). Diuretics and centrally acting angiotensin enzyme inhibitors appear to reduce lifetime risk of cognitive impairment and dementia, respectively (O'Caoimh et al., 2014; Yasar et al., 2013; Ye et al., 2015).

Vitamin B12 levels positively correlate with memory, concentration, and hippocampal structure, and low vitamin B12 levels are associated with cognitive decline (Horvat et al., 2016). Methyl-cobalamin, a vitamin-B isomer, when taken with methyl-folate and N-acetyl-cysteine, appears to slow cognitive decline. While most laboratories offer a cutoff of 290 pg/mL as "normal," this threshold appears historical rather than evidence-based: given that vitamin B12, in particular as methyl-cobalamin, is a benign, water-soluble vitamin, it may be reasonable to advise supplementation in those with objective evidence of cognitive impairment and either a B12 level of less than 500 pg/mL or indirect evidence suggestive of B12 insufficiency, such as macrocytic anemia (or even erythrocytes with a mean corpuscular volume on the higher end of the normal range and hemoglobin on the lower end of the normal range) or methyl malonic acidemia.

Even without B12 or folate insufficiency, hyperhomocysteinemia by itself appears to be a modifiable risk factor for cognitive decline, as higher levels of homocysteine are associated with cognitive impairments (Hooshmand et al., 2010). A high homocysteine may be lowered with folic acid (.8mg/d) vitamin B6 (.5mg/d), and vitamin B12 (20ug/d); using this protocol, participants with a homocysteine of >13umol/L had a reduced rate in brain atrophy by 53% and exhibited improved cognitive testing scores (Smith et al., 2010).

Vitamin D3 is a secosteroid hormone that shares a synthetic pathway with cholesterol (Dursun et al., 2016). Vitamin D3 helps in regulating calcium homeostasis, has anti-inflammatory and anti-oxidant effects, and appears neuroprotective as it aids in the clearance phagocytosis and degradation of Aβ peptides (Keeney & Butterfield, 2015; Miller, Whisner, & Johnston, 2016). Age-related vitamin D3 insufficiency and cognitive decline has been reported by numerous cross-sectional and long-term studies that report associations between lower vitamin D3 concentrations, brain changes, and cognition related to executive dysfunction (Annweiler, 2016; Balion et al., 2012; Kuźma et al., 2016; Llewellyn et al., 2010; Mohajeri, Troesch, & Weber, 2015; Shen & Ji, 2015; van der Schaft et al., 2013). The treating physician should be aware that vitamin D2 does not have any effect in reducing Alzheimer's disease and related dementia (ADRD; Przybelski et al., 2008; Stein, Scherer, Ladd, & Harrison, 2011). In the Framingham Heart Study, low vitamin D3 was associated with reduced cognition and lower hippocampal volume (Karakis et al., 2016). The consensus for an "at-risk" person would be a vitamin D3 concentration of <50nmol/L whereas one with >50nmol/L would be expected to perform better on cognitive tasks and have larger volumetric measures of particular brain structures that would be indicated in AD (Annweiler, 2016; Balion et al., 2012; Hooshmand et al., 2014; Littlejohns et al., 2014; Llewellyn et al., 2010; Morley, 2014; Przybelski & Binkley, 2007; Przybelski et al., 2008). While there is inadequate data to defend supplementation in cognitively normal people with normal levels of vitamin D as a neuroprotectant (Yeshokumar, Saylor, Kornberg, & Mowry, 2015), there is data to advocate for repletion in those with insufficiency and supplementation in those with cognitive impairment on the low end of the normal range (Gangwar et al., 2015). Interestingly, memantine combined with vitamin D3 may afford synergistic properties in reducing Aβ-induced axonal degeneration (Annweiler, Brugg, Peyrin, Bartha, & Beauchet, 2014; Annweiler et al., 2011).

Rosacea is a chronic inflammatory skin disorder that involves upregulation of matrix metalloproteinases and antimicrobial peptides (Egeberg, Hansen, Gislason, & Thyssen, 2016). A longitudinal study following 5.5 million Danish individuals found that those with rosacea were at a 25% increased risk for developing ADRD when compared to those who did not have it. Women had a 28% increased risk, whereas men had a 16% increased risk (Egeberg et al., 2016). Given these epidemiological findings, and the putative pathophysiological roles of peptides (Soscia et al., 2010) and metalloproteinases (Rosenberg, 2009) in neurodegeneration, treatment of rosacea as a risk factor could play a role in slowing cognitive decline. Testosterone replacement, as compared to placebo, in men improves mood and quality of life (Snyder et al., 2016). While most men do not experience improvements in cognition with testosterone (Lu et al., 2006; Seidl & Massman, 2015), a subset may find spatial memory enhanced (Cherrier et al., 2001; Holland, Bandelow, & Hogervorst, 2011; Janowsky, Oviatt, & Orwoll, 1994).

Medications typically come with their own unique sets of side effects and should be continually reviewed to ensure that their usage is justified and discontinued otherwise. Many medications can impair memory, attention, and mood. Reflux medication proton-pump inhibitors might disrupt stomach absorption of iron and B vitamins and increase the risk of dementia in certain individuals (Akter et al., 2015; Gomm et al., 2016).

Clinical depression can cause significant declines in cognitive function at any age and in the elderly may even manifest as a "psuedodementia." Proper screening and prompt treatment are crucial, and a wide array of evidence-based interventions, including psychotherapy and certain medications, are available.

Supplements for Cognitive Decline

Over-the-counter supplements are not subject to the safety and efficacy scrutiny the Food and Drug Administration gives to prescription medications, and hence providers and consumers should exercise caution prior to adding any such supplements to a daily regimen. Likewise, unless the supplements were taken in the exact formulation, brand, and dosages used in a particular study, there is no guarantee that a particular supplement will have the same safety and efficacy. It is important to ensure that the prescribing provider is aware of over-the-counter supplements and to ask a pharmacist to run an interaction check of the supplements with prescription medications. All other things being equal, it is likely best for the brain for particular vitamins and supplements to be incorporated into the diet in the food in which they naturally occur (e.g., omega-3-fatty acids from seafood, polyphenols from pomegranate). When such dietary changes are not feasible, over-the-counter formulations may be considered. A recent meta-analysis found no benefits of omega-3, B vitamins, and vitamin E supplements on cognition in nondemented adults (Forbes et al., 2014), hence a skeptical eye is encouraged in considering the putative benefits of any supplement.

MEDIUM CHAIN TRIGLYCERIDES

AD is accompanied by a 20% to 40% decrease in the brain's ability to utilize glucose (Hoyer, 1992). Decreased glucose metabolism in the bilateral parietal lobes, and to a secondary degree in the temporal lobes, is a hallmark of AD, and disturbed glucose metabolism is seen in all neurodegenerative diseases and correlates to histopathological changes (e.g., plaque density in AD; McCall, 1992). Ketone bodies such as acetoacetate, β-hydroxybuterate (BHB), and acetone can be used as non-glucose energy sources in the brain and are made in large quantities by fat metabolism when the body cannot access glucose; this effect can be witnessed in prolonged fasting, untreated diabetes mellitus, or with a low-carbohydrate, high-protein, and high-fat diet (Henderson, 2008; VanItallie & Nufert 2003). Glycolysis flows into the citric acid cycle: in the absence of glycolysis, ketone bodies can enter the citric acid cycle directly as BHB. BHB has a variety of neuroprotective effects and appears to counter the effects of cytotoxic agents, hypoxia, traumatic brain injury, and glutamate toxicity (Henderson et al., 2009; Izumi, Ishii, Katsuki, Benz, & Zorumski, 1998; Kashiwaya et al., 2013; Yin et al., 2016). Ketone bodies also appear to increase mitochondrial efficiency and functioning in the absence of glucose (Sato et al., 1995). While a strict ketogenic diet may be appropriate for certain children with medically refractory epilepsy, it might not be feasible in an adult with AD (Keene & Hope, 1997; Mungas et al., 1990). Medium chain triglycerides (MCTs, fatty acids derived from coconut oil, palm oil and dairy fat), which are metabolized into BHB, may improve cognitive function in ADRD cases for patients who are not carriers for the APOE4 genotype but are ineffective in those who are positive for the allele (Henderson et al., 2009; Reger et al., 2004; Sharma, Bemis, & Desilets, 2014). Without offering instructions to abstain from glucose, administration of an oral ketogenic compound Axona (AC-1202) can significantly elevate average serum BHB levels, especially when given chronically over several weeks. Higher serum ketone levels have been correlated with higher scores on standardized cognitive testing (Henderson et al., 2009). Except for those with brittle diabetes, MCTs may be considered.

OMEGA-3-FATTY ACIDS

Fishery products are highly recommended as dietary sources of omega-3 for the MIND diet (Rush University Medical Center, 2015), and their intake is associated with lower risk of cognitive impairment (Cansev, Wurtman, Sakamoto, & Ulus, 2008; Köbe et al., 2016; Konagai et al., 2013; Strike, Carlisle, Gibson, & Dyall, 2016; Vakhapova, Richter, Cohen, Herzog, & Korczyn, 2011; van der Wurff et al., 2016). Marine-derived docosahexaenoic acid (DHA) was associated with lower risk of ADRD (Zhang et al., 2016). Omega-3 supplementation has been shown to enhance cognition in randomized, controlled trials for cohorts ranging from adolescents to the elderly (Strike et al., 2016; van der Wurff et al., 2016). When taken at the same time as engaged in an aerobic exercise routine, omega-3-fatty acid supplementation appears to lower homocysteine and increase gray matter volume throughout the brain (Köbe et al., 2016). Omega-3-supplements derived from lower-in-the-food-chain organisms appears to have less mercury contamination (Foran, Flood, & Lewandrowski, 2003); krill oil has been shown to be higher in polyunsaturated fatty acids and with more dose effectiveness in treating cognition than sardine-derived oil (Konagai et al., 2013; Ulven et al., 2011).

Phosphatidyl serine (PS) is a phospholipid found in the inner, hydrophobic portion of mammalian plasma membranes. When PS is placed in a preparation with marine sourced −3 long-chain polyunsaturated fatty acids attached to its backbone (in particular to DHA, i.e., PS-DHA), PS-DHA can bypass the blood–brain barrier and appears to benefit cognition. PS-DHA is a functional form of brain PS and may be utilized without further biosynthesis by the body (Mozzi, Buratta, & Goracci, 2003). Commercially available as Vayacog, this unique proprietary combination links PS and omega-3 fatty acids, though a similar benefit might be achieved by taking separate PS and omega-3 supplements simultaneously once per day. After 15 weeks of supplementation in nondemented elderly, Vayacog was shown to significantly improve memory and learning ability in those with higher baseline cognition (Vakhapova, Cohen, Richter, Herzog, & Korczyn, 2010). PS-DHA may cause slight weight gain and reduced resting diastolic blood pressure in certain individuals and overall appears to be well-tolerated (Vakhapova et al., 2011).

Upon oral administration of *N-acetyl-cysteine* (NAC), L-cysteine is quickly metabolized to cystine within the brain. Cystine is a rate-limiting constituent of glutathione, a key endogenous antioxidant that modulates glutamatergic, neurotropic, and inflammatory pathways (Lushchak & Lushchak, 2012). Cystine is the antiport substrate for the cystine-glutamate antiporter and as a result improves extra- and intracellular glutamate regulation, reducing overall intracellular glutamate (Kau et al., 2008). In a small, controlled trial of adults with AD, those given NAC 50mg/kg/day for six months had improved cognitive performance in a subset of tasks (Adair, Knoefel, & Morgan, 2001). NAC may also boost cognition in adults following traumatic brain injury (Hoffer, Balaban, Slade, Tsao, & Hoffer, 2013) and may also work to protect dopaminergic neurons in Parkinson's disease (Monti et al., 2016).

ADAPTOGENS

Adapt-232 is a standardized combination of extracts of *Rhodiola rosea L., Schisandra chinensis (turcz.),* and *Eleutherococcus senticosus (Eleuthero)* (Panossian, 2004). These supplements appear to increase resistance to mental exhaustion and can increase attention in cases of fatigue and weakness while also having no negative side effects or a "come down" like other stimulants (Aslanyan et al., 2010). Eleuthero can increase the concentration of digoxin when they are taken concurrently and requires monitoring in that case (Gardiner, Phillips, & Shaughnessy, 2008). Adaptogens interact with the hypothalamic-pituitary-adrenal axis, a part of the stress system that primarily functions to respond to chronic stress and adaptation (Aslanyan et al., 2010; Panossian & Wikman, 2009). In a cohort of adult women reporting fatigue, a 270 mg dose of Adapt-232, attention, speed, and accuracy during a stressful cognitive task improved significantly with lower percentages of errors, indicating a more efficient quality of work (Aslanyan et al., 2010).

Polyphenols and pomegranate juice can be used for oxidative stress. As the normal aging process continues, intracellular macromolecules may accumulate and, if targeted by oxidative stress, exacerbate neurodegeneration (Bokov, Chaudhuri, & Richardson, 2004; Sohal et al., 2002; Swomley et al., 2014). In a diet that lacks antioxidants, or AD pathology that could cause a decrease in plasma antioxidants, tau phosphorylation may occur as a compensatory response to oxidative stress (Koudinov, Kezlya, Koudinova, & Berezov, 2009; Rinaldi et al., 2003). A variety of fruits are abundant in numerous antioxidants such as ascorbic acid, carotenoids, and phenols. Each fruit has a varying antioxidant profile and differences in its potency as an antioxidant. Typically, whole foods are high in antioxidant phenolic substances. There is evidence that polyphenols interact synergistically, and taking multiple polyphenols as part of a rounded diet is more effective than a treatment regimen composed of isolated polyphenols (Seeram et al., 2005). Pomegranates in particular have a high concentration of polyphenols (Kelawala & Ananthanarayan, 2004). Mice given pomegranate juice from age 6 to 12½ months cognitively outperformed those given sugar water. In addition, the pomegranate-treated mice had 53% less thioflavine-S (a dye used to test for protein aggregation) positive fibrillar amyloid deposition and 51% less hippocampal soluble amyloid deposition (Kelawala & Ananthanarayan, 2004). In humans, older subjects with age-related memory complaints who drank 8 oz daily for 28 days experienced an increase in their memory, plasma trolox-equivalent antioxidant capacity values, and urolithin A-glucuronide values. On functional magnetic resonance imaging, there was increased bilateral activity in the basal ganglia, thalamus, left inferior frontal gyrus, and left middle frontal gyrus that was related to spatial and memory tasks, resulting in an increase in performance (Bookheimer et al., 2013). A study on older patients undergoing cardiac surgery found that daily supplementation of pomegranate had a significant protective effect on their postoperative memory retention (Mandal, Williams, & Mandal, 2007; Ropacki, Patel, & Hartman, 2013).

Probiotics can represent another line of defense. The gut and brain communicate through numerous pathways, and the gut plays a primary environmental influence on brain function and behavior (Cryan & Dinan, 2012; Moloney, Desbonnet, Clarke, Dinan, & Cryan, 2014). Gut microbiota and well-being have recently been linked to a series of conditions such as major depression, Parkinson's, autism, obesity, and other related disorders (Cryan & Dinan, 2012; Mu, Yang, & Zhu, 2016). The research shows that aging individuals with poor health are more likely to show weaning microbial population diversity (Moloney et al., 2014). In relation to psychological health, probiotic bacteria and antibiotic supplements have been proven effective in the treatment of anxiety, mood, cognition, and pain Cryan & Dinan, 2012). Polyphenols help regulate the microbiome as microorganisms convert polyphenols into bioavailable metabolites that stimulate growth of beneficial bacteria (ex: *Lactobacilli*, bifidobacteria) and inhibit production of pathogenic bacterium (Cardona, Andrés-Lacueva, Tulipani, Tinahones, & Queipo-Ortuño, 2013; Dueñas et al., 2015). Microbiome integrity is best formed by habituation, as long-term and consistent dietary choices will shape the characteristics of the population. High consumption of Mediterranean diet–related foods is positively associated with beneficial microbiome profiles (De Filippis et al., 2016). The gut responds quickly to its inputs, as measurable microbiome composition can change within 24 hours of a change in diet.

Resveratrol is an antioxidant (de la Lastra & Villegas, 2007), occurring naturally in certain fruits and berries, that appears to targets multiple pathways (López-Otín, Blasco, Partridge, Serrano, & Kroemer, 2013) involved in neurodegenerative cognitive decline including misfolding of the amyloid-beta

(Porat, Abramowitz, & Gazit, 2006; Turner et al., 2015) and tau proteins (Min et al., 2010), cellular metabolic state (Gomes et al., 2013), inflammation (Chen et al., 2013; Rahman, Biswas, & Kirkham, 2006), mitochondrial dysfunction (Leonard et al., 2003), apoptotic reactive oxygen species (Desquiret-Dumas et al., 2013), and telomere shortening (Jayasena et al., 2013; Uchiumi et al., 2011). Research exploring regimens of resveratrol from 500 mg once daily to 1000 mg twice daily indicate that this supplement may increase hippocampal functional connectivity, memory retention, and glucose metabolism in healthy older adults (Turner, et al., 2015a, 2015b; Wightman et al., 2015; Witte, Kerti, Margulies, & Flöel, 2014). While generally benign, some participants develop side effects such as fatigue, increased diastolic blood pressure, gastrointestinal symptoms, diarrhea, or weight loss (Wightman et al., 2015). Although serum antibody concentrations positively correlate with neuropsychological impairment (Luis et al., 2009), resveratrol does not prevent the formation of antibody oligomers and rather appears to inhibit their cytotoxicity (Feng et al., 2009).

Vitamin E (d-alpha-tocopherol) is a term used to collectively describe eight lipid soluble antioxidant compounds: the tocopherols (α-, β-, γ-, and δ-) and the tocotrienols (α-, β-, γ-, and δ-). α-tocopherol is the most common form in human tissues and is well studied on its antioxidant properties, treatment effects on cognitive impairment, and inhibition of androgen-binding protein induced cell death (Behl, Davis, Cole, & Schubert, 1992; Grimm, Mett, & Hartmann, 2016). In addition to functioning as antioxidants, vitamin E species may also be neuroprotective, anti-inflammatory, and hypocholesterolemic (Brigelius-Flohe & Traber, 1999; Jiang, 2014; Reiter, Jiang, & Christen, 2007). Plasma vitamin E levels in patients suffering from ADRD are typically lower than average (Lopes da Silva et al., 2014; Mangialasche et al., 2012) and are higher in those with reduced risk (Li & Shen, 2012; Mangialasche et al., 2010; Morris et al., 2005). However, other literature suggests vitamin E is ineffective (Petersen et al., 2005) in preventing or treating cognitive impairment (Blacker, 2005). A recent meta-analysis of several clinical trials showed that the smaller trials have inconsistent results with an overall effect near zero, with a significant increase in all-cause mortality observed in vitamin E doses greater than 400 IU/day (Miller et al., 2005). Some of the confounds against vitamin E's efficacy may be explained by a lack of bioavailability of γ-tocopherol. In postmortem analyses, higher levels of γ-tocopherol were associated with reduced AD pathology. In contrast, higher concentrations of α-tocopherol were linked to an increased Aβ load in the absence of sufficient γ-tocopherol levels (Morris et al., 2015). γ-tocopherol is a more effective scavenger of free radicals and inflammation causing species, and the intake of α-tocopherol supplements causes a reduction in γ-tocopherol (Usoro & Mousa, 2010). Since vitamin E is an antioxidant, it is expected to receive an unpaired electron ("free radical") from an oxidized conjugated lipid. If the oxidized vitamin E is not removed from the environment, it will continue to accumulate or pass the radical electron to another lipid, further damaging the membrane. An oxidized vitamin E molecule can be removed by donating the extra electron to a water-soluble electron-accepting molecule like ascorbate (vitamin C), urea, pyruvate, nicotinamide adenine dinucleotide hydride, cysteine, or glutathione. Animal studies have shown that brain glutathione (a potent antioxidant) levels do not rise in mice fed dietary vitamin E (Gaedicke et al., 2009) and do increase significantly in those fed a combination of vitamins E and C, with 13 additional bioflavonoids, polyphenols, and carotenoids (Rebrin et al., 2005). Vitamin E can interact with warfarin, further preventing coagulation (Gardiner et al., 2008).

Huperzine A is an extract from club moss (*Huperzia serrata*) that is an alkaloid with reversible acetylcholinesterase-inhibiting ability. For centuries, the Chinese have used the moss as a treatment for swelling, fever, and blood disorders, and it appears to have memory-enhancing and neuroprotective effects in certain animal and human studies (Zangara, 2003). Huperzine A can lessen iron concentration in the brain, which would buffer against the course of neurodegenerative disorders (Qian & Ke, 2014), likewise, it may protect against amyloid-beta oxidation and mitochondrial dysfunction and increase the regulation of nerve growth factor while also working as an antagonist on N-methyl-D-aspartate receptors (Qian & Ke, 2014; Xu et al., 2012; Yang, Wang, Tian, & Liu, 2013). While a large randomized, controlled trial in adults with AD did not show any benefit of 200 μg daily of huperzine A, a smaller study in adults with mild to moderate vascular dementia did suggest a benefit, with an increase in MMSE scores by 1 to 5 points (Rafii et al., 2011). The dose-response data suggests that while 100 μg was effective in those with vascular dementia, doses of 400 μg appear needed to manifest effects in adults with AD (Desilets, Gickas, & Dunican, 2009; Rafii et al., 2011; Xu et al., 2012).

Ginkgo biloba is an extract from leaves of the maidenhair tree that has been used for centuries in China to improve memory, concentration, confusion, mood, anxiety, dizziness, tinnitus, and headache. Ginkgo's effects are thought to occur by dilating blood vessels, thinning blood, reducing free radicals, and having effect on neurotransmitter systems (Birks, Grimley, & Van Dongen, 2002). Clinical trials of a standardized extract of ginkgo (EGb 761) suggest a benefit in those diagnosed with AD, vascular, and mixed dementia (Wang et al., 2010; Weinmann, Roll, Schwarzbach, Vauth, & Willich, 2010). Gingko extracts increase the risk of bleeding, including for intracranial hemorrhage, in those already taking a non-steroid anti-inflammatory drug or anticoagulation such as warfarin and hence should be avoided in patients taking those agents (Abebe, 2002; Bebbington, Kulkarni, & Roberts, 2005; Bent, Goldberg, Padula, & Avins, 2005; Gardiner et al., 2008). While two studies (including one powered with over 1,000 participants) found improvements on the Alzheimer's Disease Assessment Scale for adults with AD taking up to 240 mg daily of ginkgo extract (Oken, Storzbach, & Kaye, 1998; Wang et al., 2010), a subsequent meta-analysis performed found no convincing evidence that ginkgo was effective in treating dementia and cognitive impairment (Birks et al., 2009). Trials may be flawed with small cohorts and publication bias (incorrectly implying a benefit when there were none) or may use samples with poor quality control and insufficient concentration (absence of proof is not proof of absence; Birks et al., 2002; Fransen, Pelgrom, Stewart-Knox, De Kaste, & Verhagen, 2010).

Other supplements that have been shown to have a cognitive benefit in double-blind placebo-controlled, randomized trials include standardized extracts from *Bacopa monnieri* (Dave et al., 2014; Morgan & Stevens, 2010), *Rhodiola rosea* (Darbinyan et al., 2000), Pycnogenol from *Pinus pinaster* (Bayeta & Lau, 2000; D'Andrea, 2010; Trebatická et al., 2006), Enzogenol from *Pinus radiata*, theacrine from kucha tea *Camellia assamica* (Ziegenfuss et al., 2016), choline (as choline alphoscerate, CDP-choline, citicholine; Amenta et al., 2012; Arenth, Russell, Ricker, & Zafonte, 2011; Fioravanti & Yanagi, 2005; Knott et al., 2015), and zinc (Brewer & Kaur, 2013). Case series showing an improvement in cognition with pyrroloquinoline (Itoh et al., 2016) and ganglioside (Jeon et al., 2016) suggest these may be worth further investigation. Cell culture and animal studies suggest that extracts from *Curcuma longa* (e.g., curcumin in turmeric; Begum et al., 2008), acetyl-L-carnitine (Taglialatela et al., 1994), and *Withania somnifera* (Sehgal et al., 2012) could have neuroprotective effects and likewise merit further exploration.

In addition to evaluating the effects of individual nutrients, several studies have investigated the effects of multivitamin combinations to prevent cognitive decline, both in those with suspected AD and in normal, nondemented adults. Sometimes termed "nutrient pharmaceuticals" or "nutraceuticals," several of these combination formulations have demonstrated cognitive benefits in randomized, controlled trials (summarized in Box 17.1). All of these combination therapies included vitamin E, and most include omega-3 fatty acids, vitamin B12, and folate. Other components tested include phosphatidylserine, *Ginkgo biloba*, selenium, choline, S-adenosyl-L-methionine, N-acetylcysteine, acetyl-L-carnitine, *Bacopa monierri*, and astaxanthin.

Neuromodulatory Approaches

Yoga appears to improve function in older adults who are experiencing cognitive decline. Adults engaged in regular yoga may experience improved verbal memory and increased connectivity in numerous neural regions/networks

> **Box 17.1 Supplements That Have Been Studied as Combination Formulations in Clinical Trials**
>
> *Combination Supplement Ingredients*
>
> 1g Docosahexaenoic (DHA), 160mg eicosapentaenoic acid, (EPA) 240mg *Ginkgo biloba*, 60mg phospatidylserine, 20mg d-α tocoopherol, 1mg folic acid, 20µg B12 ("Elaflex Active") (Strike et al., 2016)
>
> Eicospentaenoic acid, 300 mg, Docosahexaenoic acid, 1200 mg, Phospholipids 106 mg, Choline, 400 mg, Uridine monophosphate, 625 mg, Vitamin E (alpha-tocopherol equivalents) 40 mg, Selenium, 60 µg, Vitamin B12, 3 µg, Vitamin B6, 1 mg, Folic acid, 400 µg, Vitamin C, 80mg ("Souvenaid") (De Waal et al., 2014; Pardini et al., 2015; Shah et al., 2013)
>
> Folate, alpha-tocopherol, B12, S-adenosyl methioinine, N-acetyl cysteine, acetyl-L-carnitine (Strike et al., 2016)
>
> Curcumin, piperine, epigallocatechin gallate, α-lipoic acid, N-acetylcysteine, B vitamins, vitamin C, folate (Parachikova, Green, Hendrix, & Laferla, 2010)
>
> *Bacopa monnieri*, astaxanthin, phosphatidylserine, and vitamin E (Zanotta, Puricelli, & Bonoldi, 2014)

related to verbal memory, language processing, and visuospatial memory (Eyre et al., 2016). Yoga also improves psychological health, showing improvement in anger, depression, anxiety, well-being, general self-efficacy, morale, self-control, cortisol levels, and self-reported pain (Bonura & Tenenbaum, 2014; Curtis, Osadchuk, & Katz, 2011). Unreliable gait is a hazard for progressing patients; those with moderate to severe AD who participated in an eight-week chair yoga program had improved physical function, walking, and balance (McCaffrey et al., 2014).

Regular meditation (e.g., 12 minutes a day for eight weeks) has been associated positive changes in mood, anxiety, and other neuropsychological parameters, which correlated with increased cerebral blood flow (Moss et al., 2012). Practicing mindfulness meditation may also enhance parasympathetic influence on heart rate and work to increase heart rate variability (HRV) measures in higher anxiety individuals (Mankus, Aldao, Kerns, Mayville, & Mennin, 2013). Mindfulness practice also encourages people to report more acceptance and psychological flexibility, as they show increased awareness, self-compassion, and less judgment (Moss et al., 2014).

HRV is defined as the standard deviation of the interbeat ("R-R") interval on the electrocardiogram. HRV reflects "vagal tone:" the ability of the autonomic nervous system to respond dynamically to second-to-second changes in cardiovascular demands. HRV normally declines in healthy aging (Jandackova, Scholes, Britton, & Steptoe, 2016). Having a lower than average HRV is significantly related to lower cognitive performance, memory recall, and language (Frewen et al., 2013). HRV measures can be increased as a compensatory mechanism when the body is becoming more accustomed to cardiovascular endurance training (Carter et al., 2003). For those with generalized anxiety, HRV can be improved through practicing mindfulness (Mankus, Aldao, Kerns, Mayville, & Mennin, 2013). Biofeedback options may improve HRV by strengthening baroreceptor homeostasis and vagal afferent frontal cortical representation (Lehrer & Gevirtz, 2014). HRV biofeedback appears effective in inoculating against posttraumatic stress disorder (Hourani et al., 2016; Lewis et al., 2015). Practicing HRV biofeedback also appears to enhance self-control and improve the ability to navigate stress and cognitive tasks (Dziembowska et al., 2016; Pusenjak, Grad, Tusak, Leskovsek, & Schwarzlin, 2015).

Noninvasive electromagnetic stimulation may be another mechanism to modulate brain activity and sustain cognition across the lifetime. Repetitive transcranial magnetic stimulation (rTMS), when used in conjunction with cognitive training, may improve cognitive performance in those with AD (Rabey et al., 2012). Patients in mild stage AD had significant improvement in memory and language scores after undergoing a 10 Hz rTMS protocol configured for six cortical areas (both dorsolateral prefrontal and parietal somatosensory associated cortices and Broca's and Wernicke's areas), five days a week for six weeks (Lee, Choi, Oh, Sohn, & Lee, 2016). Transcranial direct current stimulation is different from rTMS in that it delivers a low current to points of interest on the brain via electrodes placed on the scalp. Originally developed for those with brain injury or psychiatric conditions such as major depressive disorder, it also shows some promise in treating AD. Those who underwent ten 20-minute treatments at 2 mA, with the anode over the left dorsolateral prefrontal cortex, who then performed computerized tasks targeting their most deficient cognitive processed showed stabilization in global cognitive function over those who did not receive stimulation; the stabilization effect lasted for approximately three months (Penolazzi et al., 2015). In healthy older adults, 2 mA 15-minute treatments improved their scored in trained cognitive tasks over the sham group (Stephens & Berryhill, 2016).

Integrating Approaches

Integrating multiple treatment approaches together may yield a synergistic benefit. The long-term FINGER study—a randomized controlled trial in a cohort of several thousand of at-risk elderly adults—deployed an intervention in its active arm that comprised regular group meetings with nutritionists, personally tailored physical exercise including resistance and aerobic exercise, and group and individualized cognitive training sessions (Solomon et al., 2014). After a two-year duration, participants in the active arm experienced significant improvements in executive functioning, processing speed, and reduced body mass index; improved dietary habits; and increased physical activity. The "NeuroGrow BrainFitness" program is another combined-treatment approach that incorporates cognitive skills training, counseling, meditation training, treatment for medical conditions including depression and sleep apnea, weekly neurofeedback, weekly cognitive stimulation, coaching and counseling for stress reduction, diet coaching (Mediterranean diet with omega 3 supplementation), exercise, and goal-oriented behavioral modifications. An evaluation of the effects of a this program over a 12-week period found improvements in cognitive function and a subset of patients that experienced stability (absence of atrophy) or actual growth in the hippocampus on structural imaging (Fotuhi, Lubinski, Riloff, Hadadi, & Raji, 2016). Several other combination-therapy trials have also demonstrated significant cognitive benefits by building on a core intervention of aerobic exercise training and combining this with a Mediterranean diet (Hardman, Kennedy, Macpherson, Scholey, & Pipingas, 2015), coordination and balance exercises (Tarazona-Santabalbina et al., 2016), yoga (Lin et al., 2015) and omega-3-fatty acids and cognitive stimulation (Köbe et al., 2016). A key role for the healthcare provider is to identify a set of approaches, such as those used in these combination-therapy trials, and "integrate" them into a coherent treatment plan customized to each patient.

Conclusion

Benefitting from the miracles of modern medicine and infrastructure, human beings can live well into their eighth and ninth decades. Although some degree of change in cognitive function—such as slowed reaction time and processing speed—is inevitable even in healthy aging, healthy adults can reach the century mark and beyond with their intelligence, memory, and attention intact. By implementing techniques reviewed briefly here, and in more detail in other chapters, patients and providers can be reassured they were doing everything humanly possible to keep their cognition as sharp as it possibly can be.

With overall life expectancy higher than ever, AD and stroke have risen to epidemic proportions. Finding cures for neurodegenerative conditions such as AD, dementia with Lewy bodies, and frontotemporal dementia remain areas of active research, and numerous evidence-based approaches are available to prevent stroke, enhance recovery, and reduce the risk of recurrence. As we wait for the arrival of definitive treatments to prevent or reverse the effects of these diseases, the approaches outlined this chapter offer approaches that may delay or slow illness in some and enhance quality of life in most. The techniques discussed, in particular nonpharmacologic approaches, offer little to no risk, have a foundational evidence basis, and can be adapted to each person's unique situation. It bears repeating that interventions such as aerobic exercise, mindfulness practice, and healthy nutrition are not mere lifestyle choices and instead constitute a medical intervention that can fundamentally and positively alter the structure and function of the brain.

REFERENCES

Abebe W. (2002). Herbal medication: Potential for adverse interactions with analgesic drugs. *Journal of Clinical Pharmacy and Therapeutics, 27*(6), 391–401. doi:10.1046/j.1365-2710.2002.00444.x.

Adair, J. C., Knoefel, J. E., & Morgan, N. (2001). Controlled trial of N-acetylcysteine for patients with probable Alzheimer's disease. *Neurology, 57*(8), 1515–1517. doi:10.1212/WNL.57.8.1515

Aguiar, P., Monteiro, L., Feres, A., Gomes, I., & Melo, A. (2014). Rivastigmine transdermal patch and physical exercises for Alzheimer's disease: A randomized clinical trial. *Current Alzheimer's Research, 11*(6), 532–537. doi:10.2174/1567205011666140618102224

Akter, S., Hassan, M. R., Shahriar, M., Akter, N., Abbas, M. G., & Bhuiyan, M. A. (2015). Cognitive impact after short-term exposure to different proton pump inhibitors: Assessment using CANTAB software. *Alzheimer's Research & Therapy, 7*(1), 79. doi:10.1186/s13195-015-0164-8.

Alghadir, A. H., Gabr, S. A., & Al-Eisa, E. S. (2016). Effects of moderate aerobic exercise on cognitive abilities and redox state biomarkers in older adults. *Oxidative Medicine and Cellular Longevity, 5*, 1–8. doi:10.1155/2016/2545168

Amenta, F., Fasanaro, A. M., Rea, R., & Traini, E. (2012). The ASCOMALVA trial: Association between the cholinesterase inhibitor donepezil and the cholinergic precursor choline alphoscerate in Alzheimer's disease with cerebrovascular injury: Interim results. *Journal of Neurological Science, 322*(1–2), 96–101. doi:10.1016/j.jns.2012.07.003

Annweiler, C. (2016). Vitamin D in dementia prevention. *Annals of the New York Academy of Science, 1367*(1), 57–63. doi:10.1111/nyas.13058

Annweiler, C., Brugg, B., Peyrin, J. M., Bartha, R., & Beauchet, O. (2014). Combination of memantine and vitamin D prevents axon degeneration induced by amyloid-beta and glutamate. *Neurobiology of Aging, 35*(2), 331–335. doi:10.1016/j.neurobiolaging.2013.07.029

Annweiler, C., Fantino, B., Parot-Schinkel, E., Thiery, S., Gautier, J., & Beauchet, O. (2011). Alzheimer's disease—input of vitamin D with mEmantine assay (AD-IDEA trial): Study protocol for a randomized controlled trial. *Trials, 12*(1), 230. doi:10.1186/1745-6215-12-230

Arenth, P. M., Russell, K. C., Ricker, J. H., & Zafonte, R. D. (2011). CDP-choline as a biological supplement during neurorecovery: A focused review. *PM and R, 3*(6 Suppl. 1), S123–S131. doi:10.1016/j.pmrj.2011.03.012

Aslanyan, G., Amroyan, E., Gabrielyan, E., Nylander, M., Wikman, G., & Panossian, A. (2010). Double-blind, placebo-controlled, randomised study of single dose effects of ADAPT-232 on cognitive functions. *Phytomedicine, 17*(7), 494–499. doi:10.1016/j.phymed.2010.02.005

Balion, C., Griffith, L. E., Strifler, L., Henderson, M., Patterson, C., Heckman, G., et al. (2012). Vitamin D, cognition, and dementia: A systematic review and meta-analysis. *Neurology, 79*(13), 1397–1405. doi:10.1212/WNL.0b013e31826c197f

Barone, E., Di Domenico, F., & Butterfield, D. A. (2014). Statins more than cholesterol lowering agents in Alzheimer disease: Their pleiotropic functions as potential therapeutic targets. *Biochemical Pharmacology, 88*(4), 605–616. doi:10.1016/j.bcp.2013.10.030

Bayeta, E., & Lau, B. H. S. (2000). Pycnogenol inhibits generation of inflammatory mediators in macrophages. *Nutrition Research, 20*(2), 249–259. doi:10.1016/S0271-5317(99)00157-8

Bebbington, A., Kulkarni, R., & Roberts, P. (2005). Ginkgo biloba: Persistent bleeding after total hip arthroplasty caused by herbal self-medication. *Journal of Arthroplasty, 20*(1), 125–126. doi:10.1016/j.arth.2004.02.031

Begum, A. N., Jones, M. R., Lim, G. P., Morihara, T., Kim, P., Heath, D. D., et al. (2008). Curcumin structure-function, bioavailability, and efficacy in models of neuroinflammation and Alzheimer's disease. *Journal of Pharmacology and Experimental Therapeutics, 326*(1), 196–208. doi:10.1124/jpet.108.137455

Behl, C., Davis, J., Cole, G. M., & Schubert, D. (1992). Vitamin E protects nerve cells from amyloid β-protein toxicity. *Biochemical and Biophysical Research Communications, 186*(2), 944–950. doi:10.1016/0006-291X(92)90837-B

Bent, S., Goldberg, H., Padula, A., & Avins, A. L. (2005). Spontaneous bleeding associated with Ginkgo biloba: A case report and systematic review of the literature. *Journal of General Internal Medicine, 20*(7), 657–661. doi:10.1111/j.1525-1497.2005.0121.x

Birks, J., Grimley, E. V., & Van Dongen, M. (2002). Ginkgo biloba for cognitive impairment and dementia. *Cochrane Database of Systematic Reviews, 4*, CD003120. doi:10.1002/14651858.CD003120

Blacker, D. (2005). Mild cognitive impairment—no benefit from vitamin E, little from donepezil. *New England Journal of Medicine, 352*(23), 2439–2441. doi:10.1056/NEJMe058086

Bokov, A., Chaudhuri, A., & Richardson, A. (2004). The role of oxidative damage and stress in aging. *Mechanisms of Ageing and Development, 125*(10–11), 811–826. doi:10.1016/j.mad.2004.07.009

Bolwerk, A., Mack-Andrick, J., Lang, F. R., Dörfler, A., & Maihöfner, C. (2014). How art changes your brain: Differential effects of visual art production and cognitive art evaluation on functional brain connectivity. *PLoS One, 9*(7). doi:10.1371/journal.pone.0101035

Bonanni, E., Maestri, M., Tognoni, G., Fabbrini, M., Nucciarone, B., Manca, M. L., et al. (2005). Daytime sleepiness in mild and moderate Alzheimer's disease and its relationship with cognitive impairment. *Journal of Sleep Research, 14*(3), 311–317. doi:10.1111/j.1365-2869.2005.00462.x

Bonura, K. B., & Tenenbaum, G. (2014). Effects of yoga on psychological health in older adults. *Journal of Physical Activity & Health, 11*(7), 1334–1341. doi:10.1123/jpah.2012-0365

Bookheimer SY, Renner BA, Ekstrom A, Li, Z., Henningm S. M., Brown, J. A., et al. (2013). Pomegranate juice augments memory and fMRI activity in middle-aged and older adults with mild memory complaints. *Evidence-Based Complementary and Alternative Medicine, 2013*. doi:10.1155/2013/946298.

Bossers, W. J. R., van der Woude, L. H. V., Boersma, F., Hortobágyi, T., Scherder, E. J. A., & van Heuvelen, M. J. G. (2015). A 9-week aerobic and strength training program improves cognitive and motor function in patients with dementia : A randomized, controlled trial. *American Journal of Geriatric Psychiatry, 23*(11), 1–11. doi:10.1016/j.jagp.2014.12.191

Bostrom, N., & Sandberg, A. (2009). Cognitive enhancement: Methods, ethics, regulatory challenges. *Science and Engineering Ethics, 15*(3), 311–341. doi:10.1007/s11948-009-9142-5

Bredesen, D. E. (2014). Reversal of cognitive decline: A novel therapeutic program. *Aging, 6*(9), 707–717. doi:10.3410/f.725000619.793501159

Brewer, G. J., & Kaur, S. (2013). Zinc deficiency and zinc therapy efficacy with reduction of serum free copper in Alzheimer's disease. *International Journal of Alzheimer's Disease, 2013*. doi:10.1155/2013/586365

Brigelius-Flohe, R., & Traber, M. G. (1999). Vitamin E: Function and metabolism. *FASEB Journal, 13*(10), 1145–1155.

Bruin, E. I., Zwan, J. E., & Bogels, S. M. (2016). A RCT comparing daily mindfulness meditations, biofeedback exercises, and daily physical exercise on attention control, executive functioning, mindful awareness, self-compassion, and worrying in stressed young adults. *Mindfulness.* doi:10.1007/s12671-016-0561-5

Bugos, J. A., Perlstein, W. M., McCrae, C. S., Brophy, T. S., & Bedenbaugh, P. H. (2007). Individualized piano instruction enhances executive functioning and working memory in older adults. *Aging and Mental Health, 11*(4), 464–471. doi:10.1080/13607860601086504

Burns, A., Allen, H., Tomenson, B., Duignan, D., & Byrne, J. (2009). Bright light therapy for agitation in dementia: A randomized controlled trial. *International Psychogeriatrics, 21*(4), 711–721. doi:10.1017/S1041610209008886

Cajochen, C., Frey, S., Anders, D., Späti, J., Bues, M., Pross, A., et al. (2011). Evening exposure to a light-emitting diodes (LED)-backlit computer screen affects circadian physiology and cognitive performance. *Journal of Applied Physiology, 110*(5), 1432–1438. doi:10.1152/japplphysiol.00165.2011

Cansev, M., Wurtman, R. J., Sakamoto, T., & Ulus, I. H. (2008). Oral administration of circulating precursors for membrane phosphatides can promote the synthesis of new brain synapses. *Alzheimer's & Dementia, 4*(1 Suppl. 1). doi:10.1016/j.jalz.2007.10.005

Cardona, F., Andrés-Lacueva, C., Tulipani, S., Tinahones, F. J., & Queipo-Ortuño, M. I. (2013). Benefits of polyphenols on gut microbiota and implications in human health. *Journal of Nutritional Biochemistry, 24*(8), 1415–1422. doi:10.1016/j.jnutbio.2013.05.001.

Carlsson, C. M., Xu, G., Wen, Z., Barnet, J. H., Blazel, H. M., Chappell, R. J., et al. (2012). Effects of atorvastatin on cerebral blood flow in middle-aged adults at risk for Alzheimer's disease: A pilot study. *Current Alzheimer's Research, 9*(8), 990–997. doi:10.2174/1567205128032510*75

Carter, J. B., Banister, E. W., & Blaber, A. P. (2003). The effect of age and gender on heart rate variability after endurance training. *Medicine & Science in Sports & Exercise, 35*(8), 1333–1340. doi:10.1249/01.MSS.0000079046.01763.8F

Cavallo, M., Signorino, A., & Perucchini, M. L. (2016). Benefits of cognitive treatments administered to patients affected by mild cognitive impairment/mild neurocognitive disorder. *Drug Development Research*. doi:10.1002/ddr.21339

Chan, M. Y., Haber, S., Drew, L. M., & Park, D. C. (2014). Training older adults to use tablet computers: Does it enhance cognitive function? *Gerontologist*. doi:10.1093/geront/gnu057

Chapman, S. B., Aslan, S., Spence, J. S., Defina, L. F., Keebler, M. W., Didehbani, N., & Lu, H. (2013). Shorter term aerobic exercise improves brain, cognition, and cardiovascular fitness in aging. *Frontiers in Aging Neuroscience, 5*, 1–9. doi:10.3389/fnagi.2013.00075

Chen, J.-C., Espeland, M. A., Brunner, R. L., Lovato, L. C., Wallace, R. B., Leng, X., et al. (2015). Sleep duration, cognitive decline, and dementia risk in older women. *Alzheimer's & Dementia, 12*(1), 1–13. doi:10.1016/j.jalz.2015.03.004

Chen, M. L., Yi, L., Jin, X., Liang, X.-Y., Zhou, Y., Zhang, T., et al. (2013). Resveratrol attenuates vascular endothelial inflammation by inducing autophagy through the cAMP signaling pathway. *Autophagy, 9*(12), 2033–2045. doi:10.4161/auto.26336

Cherrier, M. M., Asthana, S., Plymate, S., Baker, L., Matsumoto, A. M., Peskind, E., et al. (2001). Testosterone supplementation improves spatial and verbal memory in healthy older men. *Neurology, 57*(1), 80–88. doi:10.1212/WNL.57.1.80

Cho, J. R., Joo, E. Y., Koo, D. L., & Hong, S. B. (2013). Let there be no light: The effect of bedside light on sleep quality and background electroencephalographic rhythms. *Sleep Medicine, 14*(12), 1422–1425. doi:10.1016/j.sleep.2013.09.007

Chong, M. S., Tan, K. T., Tay, L., Wong, Y. M., & Ancoli-Israel, S. (2013). Bright light therapy as part of a multicomponent management program improves sleep and functional outcomes in delirious older hospitalized adults. *Clinical Interventions in Aging, 8*, 565–572. doi:10.2147/CIA.S44926

Chu, H., Yang, C.-Y., Lin, Y., Ou, K.-L., Lee, T.-Y., O'Brien, A. P., & Chou, K.-R. (2013). The impact of group music therapy on depression and cognition in elderly persons with dementia: A randomized controlled study. *Biological Research for Nursing*, 16(2), 209–217. doi:10.1177/1099800413485410

Colcombe, S. J., Erickson, K. I., Scalf, P. E., Kim, J. S., Prakash, R., McAuley, E., et al. (2006). Aerobic exercise training increases brain volume in aging humans. *Journal of Gerontology*, 61A(11), 5. doi:10.1093/gerona/61.11.1166

Cryan, J. F., & Dinan, T. G. (2012). Mind-altering microorganisms: The impact of the gut microbiota on brain and behaviour. *Nature Reviews Neuroscience*, 13(10), 701–712. doi:10.1038/nrn3346

Curtis, K., Osadchuk, A., & Katz, J. (2011). An eight-week yoga intervention is associated with improvements in pain, psychological functioning and mindfulness, and changes in cortisol levels in women with fibromyalgia. *Journal of Pain Research*, 4, 189–201. doi:10.2147/JPR.S22761

D'Andrea, G. (2010). Pycnogenol: A blend of procyanidins with multifaceted therapeutic applications? *Fitoterapia*, 81(7), 724–736. doi:10.1016/j.fitote.2010.06.011

Darbinyan, V., Kteyan, A., Panossian, A., Gabrielian, E., Wikman, G., & Wagner, H. (2000). Rhodiola rosea in stress induced fatigue—a double blind cross-over study of a standardized extract SHR-5 with a repeated low-dose regimen on the mental performance of healthy physicians during night duty. *Phytomedicine*, 7(5), 365–371. doi:10.1016/S0944-7113(00)80055-0

Dave, U. P., Dingankar, S. R., Saxena, V. S., Joseph, J. A., Bethapudi, B., Agarwal, A., & Kudiganti, V. (2014). An open-label study to elucidate the effects of standardized bacopa monnieri extract in the management of symptoms of attention-deficit hyperactivity disorder in children. *Advances in Mind-Body Medicine*, 28(2), 10–15.

De Filippis, F., Pellegrini, N., Vannini, L., Jeffery, I. B., La Storia, A., Laghi, L., et al. (2016). High-level adherence to a Mediterranean diet beneficially impacts the gut microbiota and associated metabolome. *Gut*, 65(11), 1812–1821. doi:10.1136/gutjnl-2015-309957

de la Lastra, C. A., & Villegas, I. (2007). Resveratrol as an antioxidant and pro-oxiant agent: Mechanisms and clinical implications. *Biochemical Society Transactions*, 35(Part 5), 1156–1160. doi:10.1042/BST0351156

De Waal, H., Stam, C. J., Lansbergen, M. M., Wieggers, R. L., Kamphuis, P. J., Scheltens, P., et al. (2014). The effect of souvenaid on functional brain network organisation in patients with mild Alzheimer's disease: A randomised controlled study. *PLoS One*, 9(1), 1–11. doi:10.1371/journal.pone.0086558

Desilets, A. R., Gickas, J. J., & Dunican, K. C. (2009). Role of huperzine A in the treatment of Alzheimer's disease. *Annals of Pharmacotherapy*, 43(3), 514–518. doi:10.1345/aph.1L402

Desquiret-Dumas, V., Gueguen, N., Leman, G., Baron, S., Nivet-Antoine, V., Chupin, S., et al. (2013). Resveratrol induces a mitochondrial complex I-dependent increase in NADH oxidation responsible for sirtuin activation in liver cells. *Journal of Biological Chemistry*, 288(51), 36662–36675. doi:10.1074/jbc.M113.466490

Dewar, B.-K., Kapur, N., & Kopelman, M. (2016). Do memory aids help everyday memory? A controlled trial of a Memory Aids Service. *Neuropsychological Rehabilitation*, 1–19. doi:10.1080/09602011.2016.1189342.

Douris, P., Southard, V., Varga, C., Schauss, W., Gennaro, C., & Reiss, A. (2003). The effect of land and aquatic exercise on balance scores in older adults. *Journal of Geriatric Physical Therapy*, 26(1), 3–6. doi:10.1519/00139143-200304000-00001

Dueñas. M., Muñoz-González, I., Cueva, C., Jiménez-Girón, A., Sánchez-Patán, F., Santos-Buelga, C., et al. (2015). A survey of modulation of gut microbiota by dietary polyphenols. *BioMed Research International*. doi:10.1155/2015/850902

Dursun, E., Alayhoğlu, M., Bilgiç, B., Hanağası, H., Lohmann, E., Atasoy, I. L., et al. (2016). Vitamin D deficiency might pose a greater risk for ApoEε4 non-carrier Alzheimer's disease patients. *Neurological Sciences*, 37(10), 1633–1643.

Dziembowska, I., Izdebski, P., Rasmus, A., Brudny, J., Grzelczak, M., & Cysewski, P. (2016). Effects of heart rate variability biofeedback on EEG alpha asymmetry and anxiety symptoms in male athletes: A pilot study. *Applied Psychophysiology and Biofeedback*, 41(2), 141–150. doi:10.1007/s10484-015-9319-4

Egeberg, A., Hansen, P. R., Gislason, G. H., & Thyssen, J. P. (2016). Patients with rosacea have increased risk of dementia. *Annals of Neurology*, 79(6), 921–928. doi:10.1002/ana.24645

Eyre, H. A., Acevedo, B., Yang, H., Siddarth, P., Van Dyk, K., Ercoli, L., et al. (2016). Changes in neural connectivity and memory following a yoga intervention for older adults: A pilot study. *Journal of Alzheimer's Disease,* 52(2), 673–684. doi:10.3233/JAD-150653

Feng, Y., Wang, X.-P., Yang, S.-G., Wang, Y.-J., Zhang, X., Du, X.-T., et al. (2009). Resveratrol inhibits beta-amyloid oligomeric cytotoxicity but does not prevent oligomer formation. *Neurotoxicology,* 30(6), 986–995. doi:10.1016/j.neuro.2009.08.013

Fioravanti, M., & Yanagi, M. (2005). Cytidinediphosphocholine (CDP-choline) for cognitive and behavioural disturbances associated with chronic cerebral disorders in the elderly. *Cochrane Database of Systematic Reviews*, 2, CD000269. doi:10.1002/14651858.CD000269.pub3

Foran, S. E., Flood, J. G., & Lewandrowski, K. B. (2003). Measurement of mercury levels in concentrated over-the-counter fish oil preparations: Is fish oil healthier than fish? *Archives of Pathology & Laboratory Medicine*, 127(12), 1603–1605. doi:10.1043/1543-2165(2003)127<1603:MOMLIC>2.0.CO;2

Forbes, D., Blake, C. M., Thiessen, E. J., Peacock, S., & Hawranik, P. (2014). Light therapy for improving cognition, activities of daily living, sleep, challenging behaviour, and psychiatric disturbances in dementia. *Cochrane Database of Systematic Reviews*, 2(2), Cd003946. doi:10.1002/14651858.CD003946.pub4

Foroughi, C. K., Monfort, S. S., Paczynski, M., McKnight, P. E., & Greenwood, P. M. (2016). Placebo effects in cognitive training. *Proceedings of the National Academy of Sciences of the United States of America*, 113(27), 7470–7474. doi:10.1073/pnas.1601243113

Fotuhi, M., Lubinski, B., Riloff, T., Hadadi, M., & Raji, C. A. (2016). A personalized 12-week "brain fitness program" for improving cognitive function and increasing the volume of hippocampus in elderly with mild cognitive impairment. *Journal of the Prevention of Alzheimer's Disease*, 2(3), 1–5.

Francis, P. T., Palmer, A. M., Snape, M., & Wilcock, G. K. (1999). The cholinergic hypothesis of Alzheimer's disease: A review of progress. *Journal of Neurology, Neurosurgery, and Psychiatry*, 66, 137–147.

Fransen, H. P., Pelgrom, S. M. G. J., Stewart-Knox, B., De Kaste, D., & Verhagen, H. (2010). Assessment of health claims, content, and safety of herbal supplements containing Ginkgo biloba. *Food and Nutrition Research*, 54. doi:10.3402/fnr.v54i0.5221

Frewen, J., Finucane, C., Savva, G. M., Boyle, G., Coen, R. F., & Kenny, R. A. (2013). Cognitive function is associated with impaired heart rate variability in ageing adults: The Irish Longitudinal Study on Ageing wave one results. *Clinical Autonomic Research*, 23(6), 313–323. doi:10.1007/s10286-013-0214-x

Gaedicke, S., Zhang, X., Huebbe, P., Boesch-Saadatmandi, C., Lou, Y., Wiswedel, I., et al. (2009). Dietary vitamin E, brain redox status and expression of Alzheimer's disease-relevant genes in rats. *British Journal of Nutrition*, 102(3), 398–406. doi:10.1017/S000711450819122X

Gangwar, A. K., Rawat, A., Tiwari, S. S. C., Tiwari, S. S. C., Narayan, J., & Tiwari, S. S. C. (2015). Role of vitamin-D in the prevention and treatment of Alzheimer's disease. *Indian Journal of Physiology and Pharmacology*, 59(1), 94–99.

Gardiner, P., Phillips, R., & Shaughnessy, A. F. (2008). Herbal and dietary supplement-drug interactions in patients with chronic illnesses. *American Family Physician*, 77(1), 73–80.

Geldenhuys, W. J., & Darvesh, A. S. (2015). Pharmacotherapy of Alzheimer's disease: Current and future trends. *Expert Review of Neurotherapeutics*, 15(1), 3–5. doi:10.1586/14737175.2015.990884

Gomes, A. P., Price, N. L., Ling, A. J. Y., Rajman, L., Hubbard, B. P., Sinclair, D. A., et al. (2015). Declining NAD+ induces a pseudohypoxic state disrupting nuclear-mitochondrial communication during aging. *Cell*, 155(7), 1624–1638. doi:10.1016/j.cell.2013.11.037

Gomm, W., von Holt, K., Thomé, F., Broich, K., Maier, W., Fink, A., et al. (2016). Association of proton pump inhibitors with risk of dementia. *JAMA Neurology*, 73(4), 410–416. doi:10.1001/jamaneurol.2015.4791

Grimm, M., Mett, J., & Hartmann, T. (2016). The impact of vitamin E and other fat-soluble vitamins on Alzheimer's disease. *International Journal of Molecular Science*, 17(11), 1785. doi:10.3390/ijms17111785

Guétin, S., Portet, F., Picot, M. C., Pommie, C., Messaoudi, M., Djabelkir, L., et al. (2009). Effect of music therapy on anxiety and depression in patients with Alzheimer's type dementia: Randomised, controlled study. *Dementia and Geriatric Cognitive Disorders*, 28(1), 36–46. doi:10.1159/000229024

Hardman, R. J., Kennedy, G., Macpherson, H., Scholey, A. B., & Pipingas, A. (2015). A randomised controlled trial investigating the effects of Mediterranean diet and aerobic exercise on cognition in cognitively healthy older people living independently within aged care facilities: The Lifestyle Intervention in Independent Living Aged Car. *Nutrition Journal*, 14(1), 1–10. doi:10.1186/s12937-015-0042-z

Hardy, J. L., Nelson, R. A., Thomason, M. E., Farzin, F., Scanlon, M., Nelson, R. A., et al. (2015). Enhancing cognitive abilities with comprehensive training: A large, online, randomized, active-controlled trial. *PLoS One, 10*(9). doi:10.1371/journal.pone.0134467

Hars, M., Herrmann, F. R., Gold, G., Rizzoli, R., & Trombetti, A. (2014). Effect of music-based multitask training on cognition and mood in older adults. *Age and Ageing, 43*(2), 196–200. doi:10.1093/ageing/aft163

Henderson, S. T., Vogel, J. L., Barr, L. J., Garvin, F., Jones, J. J., & Costantini, L.C. (2009). Study of the ketogenic agent AC-1202 in mild to moderate Alzheimer's disease: A randomized, double-blind, placebo-controlled, multicenter trial. *Nutrition & Metabolism, 6*, 31. doi:10.1186/1743-7075-6-31

Henderson, S. T. (2008). Ketone bodies as a therapeutic for Alzheimer's disease. *Neurotherapeutics, 5*(3), 470–480. doi:10.1016/j.nurt.2008.05.004

Hebert, L. E., Weuve, J., Scherr, P. A., & Evans, D. A. (2013). Alzheimer disease in the United States (2010–2050) estimated using the 2010 census. *Neurology, 80*(19), 1778–1783.

Higuchi, S., Motohashi, Y., Liu, Y., & Maeda, A. (2005). Effects of playing a computer game using a bright display on presleep physiological variables, sleep latency, slow wave sleep and REM sleep. *Journal of Sleep Research, 14*(3), 267–273. doi:10.1111/j.1365-2869.2005.00463.x

Hoffer, M. E., Balaban, C., Slade, M. D., Tsao, J. W., & Hoffer, B. (2013). Amelioration of acute sequelae of blast induced mild traumatic brain injury by N-acetyl cysteine: A double-blind, placebo controlled study. *PLoS One, 8*(1). doi:10.1371/journal.pone.0054163

Hogan, M., Kiefer, M., Kubesch, S., Collins, P., Kilmartin, L., & Brosnan, M. (2013). The interactive effects of physical fitness and acute aerobic exercise on electrophysiological coherence and cognitive performance in adolescents. *Experimental Brain Research, 229*(1), 85–96. doi:10.1007/s00221-013-3595-0

Holland, J., Bandelow, S., & Hogervorst, E. (2011). Testosterone levels and cognition in elderly men: A review. *Maturitas, 69*(4), 322–327. doi:10.1016/j.maturitas.2011.05.012

Hooshmand, B., Lökk, J., Solomon, A., Mangialasche, F., Miralbell, J., Spulber, G., et al. (2014). Vitamin D in relation to cognitive impairment, cerebrospinal fluid biomarkers, and brain volumes. *Journals of Gerontology Series A: Biomedical Sciences and Medical Sciences, 69*(9), 1132–1138. doi:10.1093/gerona/glu022

Hooshmand, B., Solomon, A., Kareholt, I., Leiviska, J., Rusanen, M., Ahtiluoto, S., et al. (2010). Homocysteine and holotranscobalamin and the risk of Alzheimer disease: A longitudinal study. *Neurology, 75*(16), 1408–1414. doi:10.1212/WNL.0b013e3181f88162

Horvat, P., Gardiner, J., Kubinova, R., Bobak, M., Gardiner, J., Kubinova, R., et al. (2016). Serum folate, vitamin B-12 and cognitive function in middle and older age: The HAPIEE study. *Experimental Gerontology, 76*, 33–38. doi:10.1016/j.exger.2016.01.011

Hourani, L., Tueller, S., Kizakevich, P., Lewis, G., Strange, L., Weimer, B., et al. (2016). Toward preventing post-traumatic stress disorder: Development and testing of a pilot predeployment stress inoculation training program. *Military Medicine, 181*(9), 1151–1160. doi:10.7205/MILMED-D-15-00192

Hoyer, S. (1992). Oxidative energy metabolism in Alzheimer brain—studies in early-onset and late-onset cases. *Molecular and Chemical Neuropathology, 16*(3), 207–224. doi:10.1007/BF03159971

Ide, K., & Secher, N. H. (2000). Cerebral blood flow and metabolism during exercise. *Progress in Neurobiology, 61*(4), 397–414. doi:10.1152/japplphysiol.00853.2007

Innes, K., Selfe, T., Brown, C., Rose, K., & Thompson-Heisterman, A. (2012). Effects of meditation on perceived stress, mood, sleep, memory and blood pressure in cognitively impaired adults and their caregivers: A pilot trial. *BMC Complementary and Alternative Medicine, 12*(Suppl. 1), 1. doi:10.1186/1472-6882-12-S1-P187

Itoh Y, Hine K, Miura H, Uetake, T., Nakano, M., Takemura, N., & Sakatani, K. (2016). Effect of the antioxidant supplement pyrroloquinoline quinone disodium salt (BioPQQ™) on cognitive functions. *Advances in Experimental Medicine and Biology, 876*, 319–325. doi:10.1007/978-1-4939-3023-4_40

Iyalomhe, O., Chen, Y., Allard, J., Ntekim, O., Johnson, S., Bond, V., et al. (2015). A standardized randomized 6-month aerobic exercise-training down-regulated pro-inflammatory genes, but up-regulated anti-inflammatory, neuron survival and axon growth-related genes. *Experimental Gerontology, 69*, 159–169. doi:10.1016/j.exger.2015.05.005

Izumi, Y., Ishii, K., Katsuki, H., Benz, A. M., & Zorumski, C. F. (1998). Beta-hydroxybutyrate fuels synaptic function during development: Histological and physiological evidence in rat hippocampal slices. *Journal of Clinical Investigation 101*(5), 1121–1132. doi:10.1172/JCI1009

Jandackova, V. K., Scholes, S., Britton, A., & Steptoe, A. (2016). Are changes in heart rate variability in middle-aged and older people normative or caused by pathological conditions? Findings from a large population-based longitudinal cohort study. *Journal of the American Heart Association, 5*(2). doi:10.1161/JAHA.115.002365

Janowsky, J. S., Oviatt, S. K., & Orwoll, E. S. (1994). Testosterone influences spatial cognition in older men. *Behavioral Neuroscience, 108*(2), 325–332. doi:10.1037//0735-7044.108.2.325

Jayasena, T., Poljak, A., Smythe, G., Braidy, N., Münch, G., & Sachdev, P. (2013). The role of polyphenols in the modulation of sirtuins and other pathways involved in Alzheimer's disease. *Ageing Research Reviews, 12*(4), 867–883. doi:10.1016/j.arr.2013.06.003.

Jeon, Y., Kim, B., Kim, J. E., Kim, B. R., Ban, S., Jeong, J. H., et al. (2016). Effects of ganglioside on working memory and the default mode network in individuals with subjective cognitive impairment: A randomized controlled trial. *American Journal of Chinese Medicine, 44*(3), 489–514. doi:10.1142/S0192415X16500270

Jiang, Q. (2014). Natural forms of vitamin E: Metabolism, antioxidant, and anti-inflammatory activities and their role in disease prevention and therapy. *Free Radical Biology and Medicine, 72*(765), 76–90. doi:10.1016/j.freeradbiomed.2014.03.035

Johnson, J. G., Cohen, P., Kasen, S., & Brook, J. S. (2007). Extensive television viewing and the development of attention and learning difficulties during adolescence. *Archives of Pediatric and Adolescent Medicine, 161*(5), 480–486. doi:10.1001/archpedi.161.5.480

Karakis, I., Pase, M. P., Beiser, A., Booth, S. L., Jacques, P. F., Rogers, G., et al. (2016). Association of serum vitamin D with the risk of incident dementia and subclinical indices of brain aging: The Framingham Heart Study. *Journal of Alzheimer's Disease, 51*, 1–11. doi:10.3233/JAD-150991

Kashiwaya, Y., Bergman, C., Lee, J. H., Wan, R., King, M. T., Mughal, M. R., et al. (2012). A ketone ester diet exhibits anxiolytic and cognition-sparing properties, and lessens amyloid and tau pathologies in a mouse model of Alzheimer's disease. *Neurobiology of Aging, 34*(6), 1530–1539. doi:10.1016/j.neurobiolaging.2012.11.023.

Kau, K. S., Madayag, A., Mantsch, J. R., Grier, M. D., Abdulhameed, O., & Baker, D. A. (2008). Blunted cystine-glutamate antiporter function in the nucleus accumbens promotes cocaine-induced drug seeking. *Neuroscience, 155*(2), 530–537. doi:10.1016/j.neuroscience.2008.06.010.

Keene, J. M., & Hope, T. (1997). Hyperphagia in dementia: 2. Food choices and their macronutrient contents in hyperphagia, dementia and ageing. *Appetite, 28*(2), 167–175. doi:10.1006/appe.1996.0068

Keeney, J. T., & Butterfield, D. A. (2015). Vitamin D deficiency and Alzheimer disease: Common links. *Neurobiology of Disease, 84*, 84–98. doi:10.1016/j.nbd.2015.06.020.

Kelawala, N. S., & Ananthanarayan, L. (2004). Antioxidant activity of selected foodstuffs. *International Journal of Food Science Nutrition, 55*(6), 511–516. doi:10.1080/09637480400015794

Knott, V., De La Salle, S., Choueiry, J., Impey, D., Smith, D., Smith, M., et al. (2015). Neurocognitive effects of acute choline supplementation in low, medium and high performer healthy volunteers. *Pharmacology, Biochemistry, and Behavior, 131*, 119–129. doi:10.1016/j.pbb.2015.02.004

Köbe, T., Witte, A. V., Schnelle, A., Lesemann, A., Fabian, S., Tesky, V. A., et al. (2016). Combined omega-3 fatty acids, aerobic exercise and cognitive stimulation prevents decline in gray matter volume of the frontal, parietal and cingulate cortex in patients with mild cognitive impairment. *Neuroimage, 131*, 226–238. doi:10.1016/j.neuroimage.2015.09.050

Konagai, C., Yanagimoto, K., Hayamizu, K., Li, H., Tsuji, T., & Koga, Y. (2013). Effects of krill oil containing n-3 polyunsaturated fatty acids in phospholipid form on human brain function: A randomized controlled trial in healthy elderly volunteers. *Clinical Inverventions in Aging, 8*, 1247–1257. doi:10.2147/CIA.S50349

Korf, E. S. C., Scheltens, P., Barkhof, F., & Leeuw, F.-E. (2005). Blood pressure, white matter lesions and medial temporal lobe atrophy: Closing the gap between vascular pathology and Alzheimer's disease? *Dementia and Geriatric Cognitive Disorders, 20*, 331–337.

Koudinov, A., Kezlya, E., Koudinova, N., & Berezov, T. (2009). Amyloid-β, tau protein, and oxidative changes as a physiological compensatory mechanism to maintain CNS plasticity under Alzheimer's disease and other neurodegenerative conditions. *Journal of Alzheimer's Disease, 18*(2), 381–400. doi:10.3233/JAD-2009-1202

Kuiper, J. S., Zuidersma, M., Oude Voshaar, R. C., Zuidema, S., van den Heuvel, E. R., Stolk, R. P., & Smidt, N. (2015). Social relationships and risk of dementia: A systematic review and meta-analysis of longitudinal cohort studies. *Ageing Research Review, 22*, 39–57. doi:10.1016/j.arr.2015.04.006

Küster, O. C., Fissler, P., Laptinskaya, D., Kolassa, I.-T., Thurm, F., Scharpf, A., et al. (2016). Cognitive change is more positively associated with an active lifestyle than with training interventions in older adults at risk of dementia: A controlled interventional clinical trial. *BMC Psychiatry, 16*(1). doi:10.1186/s12888-016-1018-z

Kuźma, E., Soni, M., Littlejohns, T. J., Ranson, J. M., van Schoor, N. M., Deeg, D. J., et al. (2016). Vitamin D and memory decline: Two population-based prospective studies. *Journal of Alzheimer's Disease, 50*(4), 1099–1108. doi:10.3233/JAD-150811

Kwok, T. C. Y., Bai, X., Li, J. C. Y., Ho, F. K. Y., & Lee, T. M. C. (2013). Effectiveness of cognitive training in Chinese older people with subjective cognitive complaints: A randomized placebo-controlled trial. *International Journal of Geriatric Psychiatry, 28*(2), 208–215. doi:10.1002/gps.3812

Langa, K. M., & Levine, D. A. (2014). The diagnosis and management of mild cognitive impairment: A clinical review. *JAMA, 312*(23), 2551–2561.

Leavitt, V. M., Cirnigliaro, C., Cohen, A., Farag, A., Brooks, M., Wecht, J. M., et al. (2014). Aerobic exercise increases hippocampal volume and improves memory in multiple sclerosis: Preliminary findings. *Neurocase, 20*(6), 695–697. doi:10.1080/13554794.2013.841951

Lee, J., Choi, B. H., Oh, E., Sohn, E. H., & Lee, A. Y. (2016). Treatment of Alzheimer's disease with repetitive transcranial magnetic stimulation combined with cognitive training: A prospective, randomized, double-blind, placebo-controlled study. *Journal of Clinical Neurology, 12*(1), 57–64. doi:10.3988/jcn.2016.12.1.57

Lehrer, P. M., & Gevirtz, R. (2014). Heart rate variability biofeedback: How and why does it work? *Frontiers in Psychology, 5*. doi:10.3389/fpsyg.2014.00756

Leonard, S. S., Xia, C., Jiang, B. H., Stinefelt, B., Klandorf, H., Harris, G. K., & Shi, X. (2003). Resveratrol scavenges reactive oxygen species and effects radical-induced cellular responses. *Biochemical and Biophysical Research Communications, 309*(4), 1017–1026. doi:10.1016/j.bbrc.2003.08.105

Lewis, G. F., Hourani, L., Tueller, S., Kizakevich, P., Bryant, S., Weimer, B., & Strange, L. (2015). Relaxation training assisted by heart rate variability biofeedback: Implication for a military predeployment stress inoculation protocol. *Psychophysiology, 52*(9), 1167–1174. doi:10.1111/psyp.12455

Li, F.-J., & Shen, L. (2013). Dietary intakes of vitamin E, vitamin C, and β-carotene and risk of Alzheimer's disease: A meta-analysis. *Journal of Alzheimer's Disease, 31*(2), 253–258. doi:10.3233/JAD-2012-120349

Lin, J., Chan, S. K. W., Lee, E. H. M., Chang, W. C., Tse, M., Su, W. W., et al. (2015). Aerobic exercise and yoga improve neurocognitive function in women with early psychosis. *NPJ Schizophrenia, 1*. doi:10.1038/npjschz.2015.47

Lin, L. Y., Cherng, R. J., Chen, Y. J., Chen, Y. J., & Yang, H. M. (2015). Effects of television exposure on developmental skills among young children. *Infant Behavior and Development, 38*, 20–26. doi:10.1016/j.infbeh.2014.12.005

Littlejohns, T. J., Henley, W. E., Lang, I. A., Annweiler, C., Beauchet, O., Chaves, P., et al. (2014). Vitamin D and the risk of dementia and Alzheimer disease. *Neurology, 83*(10), 920–928. doi:10.1212/WNL.0000000000000755

Liu-Ambrose, T., Best, J. R., Davis, J. C., Eng, J. J., Lee, P. E., Jacova, C., et al. (2016). Aerobic exercise and vascular cognitive impairment: A randomized controlled trial. *Neurology, 87*(20), 2082–2090. doi:10.1212/WNL.0000000000003332

Lleó, A., Greenberg, S. M., & Growdon, J. H. (2006). Current pharmacotherapy for Alzheimer's disease. *Annual Review of Medicine, 57*(1), 513–533. doi:10.1146/annurev.med.57.121304.131442

Llewellyn, D. J., Lang, I. A., Langa, K. M., Muniz-Terrera, G., Phillips, C. L., Cherubini, A., et al. (2010). Vitamin D and risk of cognitive decline in elderly persons. *Archives of Internal Medicine, 170*(13), 1135. doi:10.1001/archinternmed.2010.173

Lopes da Silva, S., Vellas, B., Elemans, S., Luchsinger, J., Kamphuis, P., Yaffe, K., et al. (2014). Plasma nutrient status of patients with Alzheimer's disease: Systematic review and meta-analysis. *Alzheimer's & Dementia, 10*, 485–502. doi:10.1016/j.jalz.2013.05.1771

López-Otín, C., Blasco, M. A., Partridge, L., Serrano, M., & Kroemer, G. (2013). The hallmarks of aging. *Cell, 153*(6). doi:10.1016/j.cell.2013.05.039

Lu, P. H., Masterman, D. A., Mulnard, R., Cotman, C., Miller, B., Yaffe, K., et al. (2006). Effects of testosterone on cognition and mood in male patients with mild Alzheimer disease and healthy elderly men. *Archives of Neurology, 63*(2), 177–185. doi:63.2.nct50002 [pii]\r10.1001/archneur.63.2.nct50002

Luis, C., Abdullah, L., Paris, D., Quadros, A., Mullan, M., Mouzon, B., et al. (2009). Serum beta-amyloid correlates with neuropsychological impairment. *Neuropsychology, Development, and Cognition. Section B, Aging, Neuropsychology and Cognition, 16*(2), 203–218. doi:10.1080/13825580802411766

Lushchak, V. I., & Lushchak, V. I. (2012). Glutathione homeostasis and functions: Potential targets for medical interventions. *Journal of Amino Acids, 2012*, 1–26. doi:10.1155/2012/736837

Madden, D. J., Blumenthal, J., Allen, P., & Emery, C. F. (1989). Improving aerobic capacity in healthy older adults does not necessarily lead to improved cognitive performance. *Psychology and Aging, 4*(3), 307–320. doi:10.1037/0882-7974.4.3.307

Mandal, P. K., Williams, J. P., & Mandal, R. (2007). Molecular understanding of Aβ peptide interaction with isoflurane, propofol, and thiopental: NMR spectroscopic study. *Biochemistry, 46*(3), 762–771. doi:10.1021/bi0621841

Mangialasche, F., Kivipelto, M., Mecocci, P., Rizzuto, D., Palmer, K., Winblad, B., & Fratiglioni, L. (2010). High plasma levels of vitamin E forms and reduced Alzheimer's disease risk in advanced age. *Journal of Alzheimer's Disease, 20*(4), 1029–1037. doi:10.3233/JAD-2010-091450

Mangialasche, F., Xu, W., Kivipelto, M., Costanzi, E., Ercolani, S., Pigliautile, M., et al. (2012). Tocopherols and tocotrienols plasma levels are associated with cognitive impairment. *Neurobiology of Aging, 33*(10), 2282–2290. doi:10.1016/j.neurobiolaging.2011.11.019

Mankus, A. M., Aldao, A., Kerns, C., Mayville, E. W., & Mennin, D. S. (2013). Mindfulness and heart rate variability in individuals with high and low generalized anxiety symptoms. *Behaviour Research and Therapy, 51*(7), 386–391. doi:10.1016/j.brat.2013.03.005

Marcason, W. (2015). What are the components to the MIND diet? *Journal of the Academy of Nutrition and Dietetics, 115*(10), 1744. doi:10.1016/j.jand.2015.08.002

Masley, S., Roetzheim, R., & Gualtieri, T. (2009). Aerobic exercise enhances cognitive flexibility. *Journal of Clinical Psychology in Medical Settings, 16*(2), 186–193. doi:10.1007/s10880-009-9159-6

Mayas, J., Parmentier, F. B. R., Andrés, P., & Ballesteros, S. (2014). Plasticity of attentional functions in older adults after non-action video game training: A randomized controlled trial. *PLoS One, 9*(3). doi:10.1371/journal.pone.0092269

McCaffrey, R., Park, J., Newman, D., & Hagen, D. (2014). The effect of chair yoga in older adults with moderate and severe Alzheimer's disease. *Research in Gerontology Nursing, 7*(4), 171–177. doi:10.3928/19404921-20140218-01

McCall, A. L. (1992). The impact of diabetes on the CNS. *Diabetes, 41*(5), 557–570. doi:10.2337/diab.41.5.557

Mcmaster, M. L., Kristinsson, S. Y., Turesson, I., Bjorkholm, M., & Landgren, O. (2010). Association of the Northern Manhattan Study Global Vascular Risk Score and successful aging. *Clinical Lymphoma, 9*(1), 19–22. doi:10.3816/CLM.2009.n.003.Novel

Miller, B. J., Whisner, C. M., & Johnston. C. S. (2016). Vitamin D supplementation appears to increase plasma Aβ40 in vitamin D insufficient older adults: A pilot randomized controlled trial. *Journal of Alzheimer's Disease, 52*(3), 843–847. doi:10.3233/JAD-150901

Miller, E. R., Pastor-Barriuso, R., Dalal, D., Riemersma, R. A., Appel, L. J., & Guallar, E. (2005). Meta-analysis: High-dosage vitamin E supplementation may increase all-cause mortality. *Annals of Internal Medicine, 142*(1). doi:10.7326/0003-4819-142-1-200501040-00110

Min, S. W., Cho, S. H., Zhou, Y., Schroeder, S., Haroutunian, V., Seeley, W. W., et al. (2010). Acetylation of tau inhibits its degradation and contributes to tauopathy. *Neuron, 67*(6), 953–966. doi:10.1016/j.neuron.2010.08.044

Mohajeri, M. H., Troesch, B., & Weber, P. (2015). Inadequate supply of vitamins and DHA in the elderly: Implications for brain aging and Alzheimer-type dementia. *Nutrition, 31*(2), 261–275. doi:10.1016/j.nut.2014.06.016

Moloney, R. D., Desbonnet, L., Clarke, G., Dinan, T. G., & Cryan, J. F. (2014). The microbiome: Stress, health and disease. *Mammalian Genome, 25*(1–2), 49–74. doi:10.1007/s00335-013-9488-5

Monti, D. A., Zabrecky, G., Kremens, D., Bazzan, A. J., Zhong, L., Bowen, B., et al. (2016). N-acetyl cysteine may support dopamine neurons in Parkinson's disease: Preliminary clinical and cell line data. *PLoS One, 11*(6), e0157602. doi:10.1371/journal.pone.0157602

Moreau, D., Kirk, I. J., & Waldie, K. E. (2016). Seven pervasive statistical flaws in cognitive training interventions. *Frontiers in Human Neuroscience, 10*(153), 1–17. doi:10.3389/fnhum.2016.00153

Morgan, A., & Stevens, J. (2010). Does Bacopa monnieri improve memory performance in older persons? Results of a randomized, placebo-controlled, double-blind trial. *Journal of Alternative and Complementary Medicine, 16*(7), 753–759. doi:10.1089/acm.2009.0342

Morley, J. E. (2014). Dementia: Does vitamin D modulate cognition? *Nature Reviews Neurology, 10*(11), 613–614. doi:10.1038/nrneurol.2014.193

Morris, M. C., Evans, D. A., Tangney, C. C., Bienias, J. L., Wilson, R. S., Aggarwal, N. T., & Scherr, P. A. (2005). Relation of the tocopherol forms to incident Alzheimer disease and to cognitive change. *American Journal of Clinical Nutrition, 81*(2), 508–514. doi:81/2/508 [pii]

Morris, M. C., Schneider, J. A., Li, H., Tangney, C. C., Nag, S., & Bennett, D. A. (2015). Brain tocopherols related to Alzheimer's disease neuropathology in humans. *Alzheimer's & Dementia, 11*(1), 32–39. doi:10.1016/j.jalz.2013.12.015

Moss, A. S., Reibel, D. K., Greeson. J. M., Newberg, A. B., Greeson, J. M., Thapar, A., & Bubb, R. (2014). An adapted mindfulness-based stress reduction program for elders in a continuing care retirement community: Quantitative and qualitative results from a pilot randomized controlled trial. *Journal in Applied Gerontology, 2014*, 733464814559411. doi:10.1177/0733464814559411

Moss, S., Wintering, N., Roggenkamp, H., Khalsa, D. S., Waldman, M. R., Monti, D., & Newberg, A. B. (2012). Effects of an 8-week meditation program on mood and anxiety in patients with memory loss. *Journal of Alternative and Complementary Medicine, 18*(1), 48–53. doi:10.1089/acm.2011.0051

Mozzi, R., Buratta, S., & Goracci, G. (2003). Metabolism and functions of phosphatidylserine in mammalian brain. *Neurochemical Research, 28*(2), 195–214. doi:10.1023/A:1022412831330

Mu, C., Yang, Y., & Zhu, W. (2016). Gut microbiota: The brain peacekeeper. *Frontiers in Microbiology, 7*. doi:10.3389/fmicb.2016.00345

Mungas, D., Cooper, J. K., Weiler, P. G., Gietzen, D., Franzi, C., & Bernick, C. (1990). Dietary preference for sweet foods in patients with dementia. *Journal of American Geratric Society, 38*(9), 999–1007.

Ngandu, T., Lehtisalo, J., Solomon, A., Levälahti, E., Ahtiluoto, S., Antikainen, R., et al. (2015). A 2 year multidomain intervention of diet, exercise, cognitive training, and vascular risk monitoring versus control to prevent cognitive decline in at-risk elderly people (FINGER): A randomised controlled trial. *The Lancet, 385*(9984), 2255–2263. doi:10.1016/S0140-6736(15)60461-5

Nozawa, T., Taki, Y., Kanno, A., Nouchi, R., Kawashima, R., Taki, Y., et al. (2015). Effects of different types of cognitive training on cognitive function, brain structure, and driving safety in senior daily drivers: A pilot study. *Behavioural Neurology*. doi:10.1155/2015/525901

O'Caoimh, R., Healy, L., Gao, Y., Svendrovski, A., Kerins, D. M., Eustace, J., et al. (2014). Effects of centrally acting angiotensin converting enzyme inhibitors on functional decline in patients with Alzheimer's disease. *Journal of Alzheimer's Disease, 40*(3), 595–603. doi:10.3233/JAD-131694

Oken, B. S., Storzbach, D. M., & Kaye, J. A. (1998). The efficacy of Ginkgo biloba on cognitive function in Alzheimer disease. *Archiches of Neurology, 55*(11), 1409–1415. doi:10.1001/archneur.55.11.1409

Panossian, A. G. (2004). Adaptogens: Tonic herbs for fatigue and stress. *Alternative & Complementary Therapies, 9*(6), 327–331.

Panossian, A., & Wikman, G. (2009). Evidence-based efficacy of adaptogens in fatigue, and molecular mechanisms related to their stress-protective activity. *Current Clinical Pharmacology, 4*(3), 198–219. doi:10.2174/157488409789375311

Parachikova, A., Green, K. N., Hendrix, C., & Laferla, F. M. (2010). Formulation of a medical food cocktail for Alzheimer's disease: Beneficial effects on cognition and neuropathology in a mouse model of the disease. *PLoS One, 5*(11). doi:10.1371/journal.pone.0014015

Pardini, M., Serrati, C., Guida, S., Mattei, C., Abate, L., Massucco, D., et al. (2015). Souvenaid reduces behavioral deficits and improves social cognition skills in frontotemporal dementia: A proof-of-concept study. *Neurodegenerative Diseases, 15*(1), 58–62. doi:10.1159/000369811

Patterson, C., Feightner, J. W., Garcia, A., Hsiung, G.-Y. R., MacKnight, C., & Sadovnick, A. D. (2008). Diagnosis and treatment of dementia: 1. Risk assessment and primary prevention of Alzheimer disease. *CMAJ: Canadian Medical Association Journal, 178*(5), 548–556. doi:10.1503/cmaj.070796

Paul, M. A., Gray, G. W., Lieberman, H. R., Love, R. J., Miller, J. C., Trouborst, M., & Arendt, J. (2011). Phase advance with separate and combined melatonin and light treatment. *Psychopharmacology, 214*(2), 515–523. doi:10.1007/s00213-010-2059-5

Penolazzi, B., Bergamaschi, S., Pastore, M., Villani, D., Sartori, G., & Mondini, S. (2015). Transcranial direct current stimulation and cognitive training in the rehabilitation of Alzheimer disease: A case study. *Neuropsychological Rehabilitation, 25*(6), 799–817. doi:10.1080/09602011.2014.977301

Peter-Derex, L., Yammine, P., Bastuji, H., & Croisile, B. (2015). Sleep and Alzheimer's disease. *Sleep Medicine Review, 19*, 29–38. doi:10.1016/j.smrv.2014.03.007

Petersen, R. C., Thomas, R. G., Grundman, M., Bennett, D., Doody, R., Ferris, S., et al. (2005). Vitamin E and donepezil for the treatment of mild cognitive impairment. *New England Journal of Medicine, 352*(23), 2379–2388. doi:10.1056/NEJMoa050151

Porat, Y., Abramowitz, A., & Gazit, E. (2006). Inhibition of amyloid fibril formation by polyphenols: Structural similarity and aromatic interactions as a common inhibition mechanism. *Chemical Biology & Drug Design, 67*(1), 27–37. doi:10.1111/j.1747-0285.2005.00318.x

Predovan, D., Fraser, S. A., Renaud, M., & Bherer, L. (2012). The effect of three months of aerobic training on stroop performance in older adults. *Journal of Aging Research, 2012*, e269815. doi:10.1155/2012/269815, 10.1155/2012/269815

Przybelski, R., Agrawal, S., Krueger, D., Engelke, J. A., Walbrun, F., & Binkley, N. (2008). Rapid correction of low vitamin D status in nursing home residents. *Osteoporosis International, 19*(11), 1621–1628. doi:10.1007/s00198-008-0619-x

Przybelski, R. J., & Binkley, N. C. (2007). Is vitamin D important for preserving cognition? A positive correlation of serum 25-hydroxyvitamin D concentration with cognitive function. *Archives of Biochemistry and Biophysics, 460*(2), 202–205. doi:10.1016/j.abb.2006.12.018

Pusenjak, N., Grad, A., Tusak, M., Leskovsek, M., & Schwarzlin, R. (2015). Can biofeedback training of psychophysiological responses enhance athletes' sport performance? A practitioner's perspective. *The Physician and Sportsmedicine, 43*(3), 287–299. doi:10.1080/00913847.2015.1069169

Qian, Z. M., & Ke, Y. (2014). Huperzine A: Is it an effective disease-modifying drug for Alzheimer's disease? *Frontiers in Aging Neuroscience, 6*. doi:10.3389/fnagi.2014.00216

Rabey, J. M., Dobronevsky, E., Aichenbaum, S., Gonen, O., Marton, R. G., & Khaigrekht, M. (2012). Repetitive transcranial magnetic stimulation combined with cognitive training is a safe and effective modality for the treatment of Alzheimer's disease: A randomized, double-blind study. *Journal of Neural Trasmission, 120*(5), 813–819. doi:10.1007/s00702-012-0902-z

Rafii, M., Walsh, S., Little, J., Behan, K., Reynolds, B., Ward, C., et al. (2011). A phase II trial of huperzine A in mild to moderate Alzheimer disease. *Neurology, 76*(17), 1389–1394

Rahman, I., Biswas, S. K., & Kirkham, P. A. (2006). Regulation of inflammation and redox signaling by dietary polyphenols. *Biochemical Pharmacology, 72*(11), 1439–1452. doi:10.1016/j.bcp.2006.07.004

Rebrin, I., Zicker, S., Wedekind, K. J., Paetau-Robinson, I., Packer, L., & Sohal, R. S. (2005). Effect of antioxidant-enriched diets on glutathione redox status in tissue homogenates and mitochondria of the senescence-accelerated mouse. *Free Radical Biology and Medicine, 39*(4), 549–557. doi:10.1016/j.freeradbiomed.2005.04.008

Reger, M. A., Henderson, S. T., Hale, C., Cholerton, B., Baker, L. D., Watson, G. S., et al. (2004). Effects of β-hydroxybutyrate on cognition in memory-impaired adults. *Neurobiology of Aging, 25*(3), 311–314. doi:10.1016/S0197-4580(03)00087-3

Reiter, E., Jiang, Q., & Christen, S. (2007). Anti-inflammatory properties of a- and γ-tocopherol. *Molecular Aspects of Medicine, 28*(5–6), 668–691. doi:10.1016/j.mam.2007.01.003

Richard, E., Van den Heuvel, E., Moll van Charante, E. P., Achthoven, L., Vermeulen, M., Bindels, P. J., & Van Gool, W. A. (2009). Prevention of dementia by intensive vascular care (PreDIVA): A cluster-randomized trial in progress. *Alzheimer Disease and Associated Disorders, 23*(3), 198–204. doi:10.1097/WAD.0b013e31819783a4

Rinaldi, P., Polidori, M. C., Metastasio, A., Mariani, E., Mattioli, P., Cherubini, A., et al. (2003). Plasma antioxidants are similarly depleted in mild cognitive impairment and in Alzheimer's disease. *Neurobiology of Aging, 24*(7), 915–919. doi:10.1016/S0197-4580(03)00031-9

Ropacki, S., Patel, S. M., & Hartman, R. E. (2013). Pomegranate supplementation protects against memory dysfunction after heart surgery: A pilot study. *Evidence-Based Complementary and Alternative Medicine, 2013*, 932401. doi:10.1155/2013/932401

Rosenberg, G. (2009). Matrix metalloproteinases and their multiple roles in neurodegenerative diseases. *Lancet Neurology, 8*(2), 205–216. doi:10.1016/S1474-4422(09)70016-X

Rush University Medical Center. (2015). *MIND diet may help prevent Alzheimer's*. Chicago: Author.

Särkämö, T., Tervaniemi, M., Laitinen, S., Numminen, A., Kurki, M., Johnson, J. K., & Rantanen, P. (2014). Cognitive, emotional, and social benefits of regular musical activities in early dementia: Randomized controlled study. *Gerontologist, 54*(4), 634–650. doi:10.1093/geront/gnt100

Sato, K., Kashiwaya, Y., Keon, C., Tsuchiya, N., King, M. T., Radda, G. K., et al. (1995). Insulin, ketone bodies, and mitochondrial energy transduction. *FASEB Journal, 9*, 651–658.

Seeram, N. P., Adams, L. S., Henning, S. M., Niu, Y., Zhang, Y., Nair, M. G., & Heber, D. (2005). In vitro antiproliferative, apoptotic and antioxidant activities of punicalagin, ellagic acid and a total pomegranate tannin extract are enhanced in combination with other polyphenols as found in pomegranate juice. *Journal of Nutritional Biochemistry, 16*(6), 360–367. doi:10.1007/3-540-35375-5

Sehgal, N., Gupta, A., Valli, R. K., Joshi, S. D., Mills, J. T., Hamel, E., et al. (2012). Withania somnifera reverses Alzheimer's disease pathology by enhancing low-density lipoprotein receptor-related protein in liver. *Proceedings of the National Academy of Sciences of the United States of America, 109*(9), 3510–3515. doi:10.1073/pnas.1112209109

Seidl, J. N. T., & Massman, P. J. (2015). Relationships between testosterone levels and cognition in patients with Alzheimer disease and nondemented elderly men. *Journal of Geratric Psychiatry and Neurology, 28*(1), 27–39.

Shah, R. C., Kamphuis, P. J., Leurgans, S., Swinkels, S. H., Sadowsky, C. H., Bongers, A., et al. (2013). The S-Connect study: Results from a randomized, controlled trial of Souvenaid in mild-to-moderate Alzheimer's disease. *Alzheimer's Research & Therapy, 5*(6), 59. doi:10.1186/alzrt224

Sharma, A., Bemis, M., & Desilets, A. R. (2014). Role of medium chain triglycerides (Axona) in the treatment of mild to moderate Alzheimer's disease. *American Journal of Alzheimer's Disease and Other Dementias, 29*(5), 409–414. doi.org/10.1177/1533317513518650

Shen, L., & Ji, H.-F. (2015). Vitamin D deficiency is associated with increased risk of Alzheimer's disease and dementia: Evidence from meta-analysis. *Nutrition Journal, 14*(1), 76. doi:10.1186/s12937-015-0063-7

Shinohara, M., Sato, N., Shimamura, M., Kurinami, H., Hamasaki, T., Chatterjee, A., et al. (2014). Possible modification of Alzheimer's disease by statins in midlife: Interactions with genetic and non-genetic risk factors. *Frontiers in Aging and Neuroscience, 6*, 1–12. doi:10.3389/fnagi.2014.00071

Smith, A. D., Smith, S. M., de Jager, C. A., Johnston, C., Agacinski, G., Oulhaj, A., et al. (2010). Homocysteine-lowering by B vitamins slows the rate of accelerated brain atrophy in mild cognitive impairment: A randomized controlled trial. *PLoS One, 5*(9), 1–10. doi:10.1371/journal.pone.0012244

Smith, J. C., Nielson, K. A., Woodard, J. L., Figueroa, C. M., Nielson, K. A., Durgerian, S., et al. (2014). Physical activity reduces hippocampal atrophy in elders at genetic risk for Alzheimer's disease. *Frontiers in Aging and Neuroscience, 6*. doi:10.3389/fnagi.2014.00061

Snyder, P. J., Bhasin, S., Cunningham, G. R., Matsumoto, A. M., Stephens-Shields, A. J., Cauley, J. A., et al. (2016). Effects of testosterone treatment in older men. *New England Journal of Medicine, 374*(7), 611–624. doi:10.1056/NEJMoa1506119

Sohal, R. S., Mockett, R. J., & Orr, W. C. (2002). Mechanisms of aging: An appraisal of the oxidative stress hypothesis. *Free Radical Biology and Medicine, 33*(5), 575–586. doi:10.1016/S0891-5849(02)00886-9

Solomon, A., Levälahti, E., Soininen, H., Tuomilehto, J., Lindström, J., Lehtisalo, J., et al. (2014). A multidomain, two-year, randomized controlled trial to prevent cognitive impairment: The Finger study. *Alzheimer's & Dementia, 10*(4), P137–P138. doi:10.1016/j.jalz.2014.04.083

Soscia, S. J., Kirby, J. E., Washicosky, K. J., Hyman, B., Tanzi, R. E., Moir, R. D., et al. (2010). The Alzheimer's disease-associated amyloid β-protein is an antimicrobial peptide. *PLoS One, 5*(3), 1–10. doi:10.1371/journal.pone.0009505

Stein, M. S., Scherer, S. C., Ladd, K. S., & Harrison, L. C. (2011). A randomized controlled trial of high-dose vitamin D2 followed by intranasal insulin in Alzheimer's disease. *Journal of Alzheimer's Disease, 26*(3), 477–484. doi:10.3233/JAD-2011-110149

Stephens, J. A., & Berryhill, M. E. (2016). Older adults improve on everyday tasks after working memory training and neurostimulation. *Brain Stimulation, 9*(4), 553–559. doi:10.1016/j.brs.2016.04.001

Strike, S. C., Carlisle, A., Gibson, E. L., & Dyall, S. C. (2016). A high omega-3 fatty acid multinutrient supplement benefits cognition and mobility in older women: A randomized, double-blind, placebo-controlled pilot study. *Journals of Gerontology Series A: Biological Sciences and Medical Sciences, 71*(2), 236–242. doi:10.1093/gerona/glv109

Svansdottir, H. B., & Snaedal, J. (2006). Music therapy in moderate and severe dementia of Alzheimer's type: A case-control study. *International Psychogeriatrics, 18*(4), 613–621. doi:10.1017/S1041610206003206

Swomley, A. M., Förster, S., Keeney, J. T., Zhang, Z., Sultana, R., Butterfield, D. A., et al. (2014). Abeta, oxidative stress in Alzheimer disease: Evidence based on proteomics studies. *Biochimica et Biophysica Acta, 1842*(8), 1248–1257. doi:10.1016/j.bbadis.2013.09.015

Taglialatela, G., Navarra, D., Cruciani, R., Ramacci, M. T., Alema, G. S., & Angelucci, L. (1994). Cetyl-L-carnitine treatment increases nerve growth factor levels and choline acetyltransferase activity in the central nervous system of aged rats. *Experimental Gerontology, 29*(1), 55–66.

Takeuchi, H., Taki, Y., Hashizume, H., Asano, K., Asano, M., Sassa, Y., et al. (2013). The impact of television viewing on brain structures: Cross-sectional and longitudinal analyses. *Cerebral Cortex*. doi:10.1093/cercor/bht315

Tan, C. C., Yu, J. T., Wang, H. F., Tan, M. S., Meng, X. F., Wang, C., et al. (2014). Efficacy and safety of donepezil, galantamine, rivastigmine, and memantine for the treatment of Alzheimer's disease: A systematic review and meta-analysis. *Journal of Alzheimer's Disease, 41*(2), 615–631.

Tarazona-Santabalbina, F. J., Gómez-Cabrera, M. C., Pérez-Ros, P., Martínez-Arnau, F. M., Cabo, H., Tsaparas, K., et al. (2016). A multicomponent exercise intervention that reverses frailty and improves cognition, emotion, and social networking in the community-dwelling frail elderly: A randomized clinical trial. *Journal of the American Medical Directors Association, 17*(5), 426-433. doi:10.1016/j.jamda.2016.01.019

ten Brinke, L. F., Bolandzadeh, N., Nagamatsu, L. S., Hsu, C. L., Davis, J. C., Miran-Khan, K., & Liu-Ambrose, T. (2015). Aerobic exercise increases hippocampal volume in older women with probable mild cognitive impairment: A 6-month randomised controlled trial. *British Journal of Sports Medicine, 49*(4), 248–254. doi:10.1136/bjsports-2013-093184

Thompson, R. G., Moulin, C. J., Hayre, S., & Jones, R. W. (2006). Music enhances category fluency in healthy older adults and Alzheimer's disease patients. *Experiential Aging Research, 31*, 91–99. doi:10.1080/03610730590882819

Thorpe, L., Middleton, J., Russell, G., & Stewart, N. (2000). Bright light therapy for demented nursing home patients with behavioral disturbance. *American Journal of Alzheimer's Disease and Other Dementias, 15*(1), 18–26. doi:10.1177/153331750001500109

Toril, P., Reales, J. M., Mayas, J., & Ballesteros, S. (2016). Video game training enhances visuospatial working memory and episodic memory in older adults. *Frontiers in Human Neuroscience, 10*, 206. doi:10.3389/fnhum.2016.00206

Trebatická, J., Kopasová, S., Hradecná, Z., Cinovský, K., Skodácek, I., Suba, J., et al. (2006). Treatment of ADHD with French maritime pine bark extract, Pycnogenol. *European Child & Adolescent Psychiatry, 15*(6), 329–335. doi:10.1007/s00787-006-0538-3

Troussière, A.-C., Monaca Charley, C., Salleron, J., Richard, F., Delbeuck, X., Derambure, P., et al. (2014). Treatment of sleep apnoea syndrome decreases cognitive decline in patients with Alzheimer's disease. *Journal of Neurology, Neurosurgery, and Psychiatry, 85*, 1405–1408. doi:10.1136/jnnp-2013-307544

Turner, R. S., Thomas, R. G., Craft, S., van Dyck, C. H., Mintzer, J., Reynolds, B. A., et al. (2015a). A randomized, double-blind, placebo-controlled trial of resveratrol for Alzheimer disease. *Neurology, 85*(16), 1383–1391. doi:10.1212/WNL.0000000000002035

Turner, R., Thomas, R., Craft, S., van Dyck, C. H., Mintzer, J., Reynolds, B., et al. (2015b). Resveratrol is safe and well-tolerated in individuals with mild-moderate dementia due to Alzheimer's disease. *Neurology, 84*. doi:84:S33-009

Uchiumi, F., Watanabe, T., Hasegawa, S., Hoshi, T., Higami, Y., & Tanuma, S. (2011). The effect of resveratrol on the Werner syndrome RecQ helicase gene and telomerase activity. *Current Aging Science, 4*(1), 1–7. doi:10.2174/1874609811104010001

Ulven, S. M., Kirkhus, B., Lamglait, A., Lamglait, A., Basu, S., Haider, T., et al. (2011). Metabolic effects of krill oil are essentially similar to those of fish oil but at lower dose of EPA and DHA, in healthy volunteers. *Lipids, 46*(1), 37–46. doi:10.1007/s11745-010-3490-4

Usoro, O. B., & Mousa, S. A. (2010). Vitamin E forms in Alzheimer's disease: A review of controversial and clinical experiences. *Critical Reviews in Food Science and Nutrition, 50*(5), 414–419. doi:10.1080/10408390802304222

Vakhapova, V., Cohen, T., Richter, Y., Herzog, Y., & Korczyn, A. D. (2010). Phosphatidylserine containing ω-3 fatty acids may improve memory abilities in non-demented elderly with memory complaints: A double-blind placebo-controlled trial. *Dementia and Geriatric Cognitive Disorders, 29*(5), 467–474. doi:10.1159/000310330

Vakhapova, V., Richter, Y., Cohen, T., Herzog, Y., & Korczyn, A. D. (2011). Safety of phosphatidylserine containing omega-3 fatty acids in non-demented elderly: A double-blind placebo-controlled trial followed by an open-label extension. *BMC Neurology, 11*, 79. doi:10.1186/1471-2377-11-79

van der Schaft, J., Koek, H. L., Dijkstra, E., Verhaar, H. J. J., van der Schouw, Y. T., & Emmelot-Vonk, M. H. (2013). The association between vitamin D and cognition: A systematic review. *Ageing Research Reviews, 12*(4), 1013–1023. doi:10.1016/j.arr.2013.05.004.

van der Wurff, I. S. M., von Schacky, C., Berge, K., Zeegers, M. P., Kirschner, P. A., & de Groot, R. H. M. (2016). Association between blood omega-3 index and cognition in typically developing Dutch adolescents. *Nutrients, 8*(1). doi:10.3390/nu8010013

van der Zwan, J. E., de Vente, W., Huizink, A.C., Bögels, S. M., & de Bruin, E. I. (2015). Physical activity, mindfulness meditation, or heart rate variability biofeedback for stress reduction: A randomized controlled trial. *Applied Psychophysiological Biofeedback, 40*(4), 257–268. doi:10.1007/s10484-015-9293-x

van Heugten, C. M., Ponds, R. W., & Kessels, R. P. (2016). Brain training: Hype or hope? *Neuropsychological Rehabilitation, 26*(5–6), 639–644. doi.org/10.1080/09602011.2016.1186101

van Maanen, A., Meijerm A, M., van der Heijden, K. B., & Oort, F. J. (2016). The effects of light therapy on sleep problems: A systematic review and meta-analysis. *Sleep Medicine Reviews, 29*, 52–62. doi:10.1016/j.smrv.2015.08.009

van Praag, H., Fleshner, M., Schwartz, M. W., & Mattson, M. P. (2014). Exercise, energy intake, glucose homeostasis, and the brain. *Journal of Neuroscience, 34*(46), 15139–15149. doi:10.1523/JNEUROSCI.2814-14.2014

VanItallie, T. B., & Nufert, T. H. (2003). Ketones: Metabolism's ugly duckling. *Nutrition Review, 61*(10), 327–341. doi:10.131/nr.2003.oct.327

Wade, A. G., Farmer, M., Harari, G., Fund, N., Laudon, M., Nir, T., et al. (2014). Add-on prolonged-release melatonin for cognitive function and sleep in mild to moderate Alzheimer's disease: A 6-month, randomized, placebo-controlled, multicenter trial. *Clinical Interventions in Aging, 9*, 947–961. doi:10.2147/CIA.S65625

Wang, B. S., Wang, H., Song, Y. Y., Qi, H., Rong, Z.-X., Wang, B.-S., et al. (2010). Effectiveness of standardized ginkgo biloba extract on cognitive symptoms of dementia with a six-month treatment: A bivariate random effect meta-analysis. *Pharmacopsychiatry, 43*(3), 86–91. doi:10.1055/s-0029-1242817

Weinmann, S., Roll, S., Schwarzbach, C., Vauth, C., & Willich, S. N. (2010). Effects of Ginkgo biloba in dementia: Systematic review and meta-analysis. *BMC Geriatrics, 10*, 14. doi:10.1186/1471-2318-10-14

Wentink, M. M., Berger, M. A. M., de Kloet, A. J., Meesters, J., Band, G. P. H., Wolterbeek, R., et al. (2016). The effects of an 8-week computer-based brain training programme on cognitive functioning, QoL and self-efficacy after stroke. *Neuropsychological Rehabilitation, 26*, 847–865. doi:10.1080/09602011.2016.1162175

Wightman, E. L., Haskell-Ramsay, C. F., Reay, J. L., Williamson, G., Dew, T., Zhang, W., & Kennedy, D. O. (2015). The effects of chronic trans-resveratrol supplementation on aspects of cognitive function, mood, sleep, health and cerebral blood flow in healthy, young humans. *British Journal of Nutrition, 114*, 1427–1437. doi:10.1017/S0007114515003037

Witte, A. V., Kerti, L., Margulies, D. S., & Flöel, A. (2014). Effects of resveratrol on memory performance, hippocampal functional connectivity, and glucose metabolism in healthy older adults. *Journal of Neuroscience, 34*(23), 7862–7870. doi:10.1523/JNEUROSCI.0385-14.2014

Xu, J., Wang, L.-L., Dammer, E. B., Li, C.-B., Xu, G., Chen, S.-D., & Wang, G. (2015). Melatonin for sleep disorders and cognition in dementia: A meta-analysis of randomized controlled trials. *American Journal of Alzheimer's Disease and Other Dementias, 30*(5), 439–447. doi:10.1177/1533317514568005

Xu, Z. Q., Liang, X. M., Wu, J., Zhang, Y. F., Zhu, C. X., & Jiang, X. J. (2012). Treatment with huperzine A improves cognition in vascular dementia patients. *Cell Biochemistry and Biophysics, 62*(1), 55–58. doi:10.1007/s12013-011-9258-5

Yang, G., Wang, Y., Tian, J., & Liu, J.-P. (2013). Huperzine A for Alzheimer's disease: A systematic review and meta-analysis of randomized clinical trials. *PLoS One, 8*(9), e74916. doi:10.1371/journal.pone.0074916

Yasar, S., Xia, J., Yao, W., Xue, Q.-L., Carlson, M. C., Furberg, C. D., et al. (2013). Antihypertensive drugs decrease risk of Alzheimer disease: Ginkgo Evaluation of Memory Study. *Neurology, 81*(10), 896–903. doi:10.1212/WNL.0b013e3182a35228

Ye, R., Hu, Y., Yao, A., Yang, Y., Shi, Y., Jiang, Y., & Zhang, J. (2015). Impact of renin-angiotensin system-targeting antihypertensive drugs on treatment of Alzheimer's disease: A meta-analysis. *International Journal of Clinical Practice*. doi:10.1111/ijcp.12626

Yeshokumar, A. K., Saylor, D., Kornberg, M. D., & Mowry, E. M. (2015). Evidence for the importance of vitamin D status in neurologic conditions. *Current Treatment Options in Neurology, 17*(12), 1–13. doi:10.1007/s11940-015-0380-3

Yin, J. X., Maalouf, M., Han, P., Zhao, M., Gao, M., Dharshaun, T., et al. (2015). Ketones block amyloid entry and improve cognition in an Alzheimer's model. *Neurobiology of Aging, 39*, 25–37. doi:10.1016/j.neurobiolaging.2015.11.018

Young, J., Angevaren, M., Rusted, J., & Tabet, N. (2015). Aerobic exercise to improve cognitive function in older people without known cognitive impairment. *Cochrane Database of Systematic Reviews, 4*, CD005381. doi:10.1002/14651858.CD005381.pub4

Yu, F., Nelson, N. W., Savik, K., Wyman, J. F., Dysken, M., & Bronas, U. G. (2013). Affecting cognition and quality of life via aerobic exercise in Alzheimer's disease. *Western Journal of Nursing Research, 35*(1), 24–38. doi:10.1177/0193945911420174

Zangara, A. (2003). The psychopharmacology of huperzine A: An alkaloid with cognitive enhancing and neuroprotective properties of interest in the treatment of Alzheimer's disease. *Pharmacology, Biochemistry, and Behavior, 75*(3), 675–686. doi:10.1016/S0091-3057(03)00111-4

Zanotta, D., Puricelli, S., & Bonoldi, G. (2014). Cognitive effects of a dietary supplement made from extract of Bacopa monnieri, astaxanthin, phosphatidylserine, and vitamin E in subjects with mild cognitive impairment: A noncomparative, exploratory clinical study. *Neuropsychiatric Disease and Treatment, 10*, 225–230. doi:10.2147/NDT.S51092

Zhang, Y., Chen, J., Qiu, J., Li, Y., Wang, J., & Jiao, J. (2016). Intakes of fish and polyunsaturated fatty acids and mild-to-severe cognitive impairment risks: A dose-response meta-analysis of 21 cohort studies. *American Journal of Clinical Nutrition, 103*(8), 330–340. doi:10.3945/ajcn.115.124081

Zickefoose, S., Hux, K., Brown, J., & Wulf, K. (2013). Let the games begin: A preliminary study using Attention Process Training-3 and Lumosity™ brain games to remediate attention deficits following traumatic brain injury. *Brain Injury, 27*(6), 707–716. doi:10.3109/02699052.2013.775484

Ziegenfuss, T. N., Habowski, S. M., Sandrock, J. E., Kedia, A. W., Kerksick, C. M., & Lopez, H. L. (2016). A two-part approach to examine the effects of theacrine (TeaCrine®) supplementation on oxygen consumption, hemodynamic responses, and subjective measures of cognitive and psychometric parameters. *Journal of Dietary Supplements, 211*, 1–15. doi:10.1080/19390211.2016.1178678

18

Integrative Approaches to Depression

NANCY WINTERING AND ANDREW B. NEWBERG

> **Key Points**
>
> - Integrative medicine therapies are commonly used by patients for the management of mood disorders such as depression.
> - A variety of natural products and botanicals have been shown to be useful in the management of mood disorders.
> - Meditation-based practices such as mindfulness can help to improve levels of stress, depression, and anxiety.
> - Maintaining proper diet and nutrition is an important aspect of managing mood disorders.
> - It is important to recognize potential adverse effects of integrative medicine therapies used for mood disorders.

Introduction

Mood disorders, also referred to as affective disorders, are a group of diagnoses that include major depression, seasonal affective disorder, dysthymia, cyclothymia, and bipolar disorder. Mood disorders have a significant impact upon public health due to their prevalence (Kessler et al., 1994), associated healthcare costs, and high rate of morbidity and mortality (Greenberg, Stiglin, Finkelstein, & Berndt, 1993; Rice & Miller, 1998; Simon, Ormel, Vonkorff, & Barlow, 1995). According to a National Institutes of Mental Health 2015 report, approximately 16 million or 6.7% of American adults experienced at least one depressive episode during the previous year. Major depression as a single or recurring episode is the most common disorder. In a World Health Organization 2010 report, major depression accounted for the equivalent of 3.7% of all disability adjusted life years and 8.3% of all years lived with disability in the United States. A 2015 National Report on Drug Use and Health provided 12-month prevalence data for major depressive episode; the highest rates of depression (10.3%) are among 18- to 25-year-old adults. For the general population, prevalence among females of all ages (8.5%) was greater than males (4.7%). The economic burden of depression of $210.5 billion in 2010 continues to rise. The direct cost for treatment of depression was 45.5%; suicide-related costs were 5%, and 50% of costs were related to workplace costs. These estimates do not include the direct costs associated with self-payment for integrative medicine and complementary and alternative medicine (CAM) practitioners for services that are not billable to insurance. The costs for comorbid physical and psychiatric medical conditions associated with treatment of depression and other disorders are on the rise (Greenberg, Fournier, Sisitsky, Pike, & Kessler, 2015).

An integrated psychiatry approach that includes CAM in the treatment of mood disorders has the capacity to treat the whole person. Many persons with mood disorders do not seek treatment or may receive treatment that is not effective (Alegría, Bijl, Lin, Walters, & Kessler, 2000; Bijl et al., 2003). Despite the availability of a variety of pharmacological and psychotherapeutic treatment options, epidemiological data indicates that many persons with depressive symptoms do not seek traditional mental health treatments (Wang, Berglund, & Kessler, 2000). Barriers to treatment appear to be greater among underserved groups of society, including persons in late-life, racial-ethnic minorities, persons with lower socioeconomic status, persons without insurance, and persons who live in rural areas (Katz, Kessler, Frank, Leaf, & Lin, 1997; Kessler et al., 2005; Keyes et al., 2008; Wang et al., 2005).

Many persons with depression seek interventions that fall within the realm of integrative medicine or CAM (Mao, Farrar, Xie, Bowman, & Armstrong, 2007). Many persons prefer a holistic approach that is patient centered and adapts treatment to their specific circumstances and values (Luberto, White, Sears, & Cotton, 2013).

The 2007 National Health Interview Survey (NHIS) reported 4 out of 10 American adults and 1 in 9 children used CAM (Barnes, Bloom, & Nahin, 2008). The NHIS report indicated approximately 96,200 adults and 11,000 children used integrative approaches for the treatment of depression. The prevalence of CAM use is greater among women and persons with higher education and persons managing a health condition. Native American and Alaskan Natives received 50.3% of CAM; Caucasians received 43.1% of services and treatments. Americans with depression reported that they are more likely to use integrative remedies than conventional antidepressants or psychotherapy

(Kessler et al., 2001). Depression, insomnia and anxiety symptoms, allergies, and chronic pain are among the most frequently cited reasons for the use of integrative medicine therapeutic approaches (Kessler et al., 2001). Persons who seek integrative medicine interventions are often from vulnerable populations such as the uninsured or racial and ethnic minorities (Givens, Houston, Van Voorhees, Ford, & Cooper, 2007; Givens, Katz, Bellamy, & Holmes, 2007; Pagan & Pauly, 2005).

Typically, integrative medicine approaches combine traditional medical therapy with appropriate evidence-based CAM therapies. Unfortunately, sometimes CAM therapies are provided outside the dominant or conventional medical and psychological approach or are provided by practitioners who may not be licensed in a medical profession. When a patient uses CAM techniques, it is always ideal for that patient to also receive care from a trained physician. The National Center for Complementary and Integrative Health, formerly known as the National Center for Complementary and Alternative Medicine (2008), classified CAM modalities/practices into broad categories:

- Mind–body interventions that include meditation, prayer, spiritual practices, mental healing and art, music and dance therapy;
- Biologically based therapies that include herbs, foods, vitamins, and supplements including natural products and dietary interventions;
- Manipulative and body-based methods including chiropractic, osteopathic manipulation, and massage; and
- Energy therapies that include Qi gong, Reiki, therapeutic touch, and acupuncture.

A treatment modality can belong to more than one category. In this chapter we focus on the mind–body, biologically based, and energy practices that have been evaluated for their effectiveness for the treatment of persons with mood disorders.

Depression

Results from an extensive 1990–1997 national survey on utilization of CAM services and treatments found that CAM treatment for chronic conditions including depression and anxiety was more prevalent than CAM use for other medical conditions (Eisenberg et al., 1998). Many patients with mood disorders who receive conventional treatment with antidepressants augment their treatment with CAM. The estimated expenditure for alternative medicine professional services increased 45.2%, from 1990 to 1997, and $14.8 billion paid out-of-pocket on CAM has been shown in a recent survey (Eisenberg et al., 1998; Purohit et al., 2015).CAM is often believed to be more effective that conventional treatment for symptom relief. In many cases patients believe that natural products are safer than conventional medicine (Badger & Nolan, 2007). Some of the reasons for preferring CAM include fewer side effects or adverse event than from pharmaceutical antidepressants, an incomplete treatment response, or a desire for more personal autonomy in healthcare decisions. The prevalence of CAM use by persons with depression is 10% to 30% and 20% to 50% among persons with bipolar disorder (Brown & Gerbarg, 2001; Solomon & Adams, 2015; Stratton & McGivern-Snofsky, 2008; Wu et al. 2007). In a survey of CAM use from 1997 to 2002, the herbal remedies for depression rose from 12.1% to 18.6% (Tindle, Davis, Phillips, & Eisenberg, 2005). In a survey of over 2,000 American adults, 53.6% of respondents with depressive symptoms reported using CAM therapy and often used botanicals in the previous 12 months (Kessler et al., 2001).

Despite their widespread use, randomized clinical trials (RCTs) in specific CAM interventions have significant methodological issues due to small sample size, duration of the intervention, open label studies, or no control groups (van der Watt, Laugharne, & Janca, 2008). A literature review of CAM studies of late-life mood and anxiety disorders identified 885 trials; only 33 trials met the minimal design criteria of ≥ 30 subjects treated for ≥ 2 weeks (Meeks, Wetherell, Irwin, Redwine, & Jeste, 2007). Despite the absence of rigorous RCTs, many CAM research studies report positive benefits in treating depressive symptoms.

Hypericum perforatum (St. John's Wort)

St. John's wort (SJW), known as hypericum perforatum, is a medical herb with antidepressant activity (Freeman et al., 2010). Several constituents of hypericum, hypericin and hyperforin, exert an antidepressant action; however, a combination of several of the plant's naturally occurring compounds may account for its activity (Greeson, Sanford, & Monti, 2001). The herb SJW has been shown to inhibit monoamine reuptake and downregulate monoamine receptors in the brain (Field, Monti, Greeson, & Kunkel, 2000). In a meta-analysis of 37 double-blind RCTs found that SJW was generally superior to placebo; however, it was equivalent to conventional antidepressant therapy for mild depression and less effective for severe depression (Linde & Knüppel, 2005). A six-week, placebo-controlled study of SJW versus citalopram, in patients with mild to moderate depression, found noninferiority of SJW versus citalopram. In this study, both SJW and citalopram were found to be superior to placebo. SJW was tolerated better with fewer side effects when compared to citalopram (Gastpar, Singer, & Zeller, 2005). A multisite RCT compared SJW to placebo for six weeks in a study that enrolled 332 persons with mild to moderate depression. The findings indicated that SJW treatment provided significant reductions in depression ratings when compared to placebo (Kasper, Anghelescu, Szegedi, Dienel, & Kieser, 2006). In another four-week, multisite RCT of SJW versus fluoxetine or placebo in 163 patients with mild to moderate depression, no superiority of either treatment versus placebo was found with the possible exception of a greater remission rate with SJW and fluoxetine when compared to placebo (Bjerkenstedt, Edman, Alken, & Mannel, 2005). Additional studies comparing SJW, fluoxetine, and placebo demonstrated conflicting results regarding efficacy (Fava et al., 2005; Moreno, Teng, Almeida, & Tavares, 2006). SJW had better tolerability and fewer adverse effects (Kasper et al., 2010).

SJW use is not without risks; in large doses photosensitivity is observed, and the herb induces cytochrome P450 enzymes. These enzymes can interfere with absorption and can increase clearance of drugs including antiretrovirals, benzodiazepines, oral contraception, digoxin, phenobarbital, and theophylline (Gurley, Swain, Williams, Barone, & Battu, 2008). Additionally, there may be an increased serious risk of toxic interactions when SJW is combined with a number of antidepressants that can result in serotonin syndrome (Boyer & Shannon, 2005).

S-ADENOSYL-METHIONINE

S-adenosyl-methionine (SAMe) is an amino acid that is distributed widely throughout the brain and is the major donor of methyl groups needed in the synthesis of monoamine neurotransmitters: dopamine, norepinephrine, and serotonin and membranes. SAMe is available as an over-the-counter supplement in the United States and is widely prescribed in Europe as an antidepressant. Preclinical studies suggest that naturally occurring SAMe levels may be reduced in patients with major depressive disorder (MDD; Bottiglieri & Hyland, 1994). The results of RCTs suggest that SAMe has been found to be generally as effective with fewer side effects as a number of standard antidepressants (Mischoulon & Fava, 2002). One review of 14 RCTs advised caution about the use of SAMe and concluded that any consideration of SAMe as a clinically significant antidepressant monotherapy therapy was premature (Echols, Naidoo, & Salzman, 2000). However, another meta-analysis that examined 28 studies concluded that SAMe was clinically and statistically superior to placebo and found no significant differences in treatment outcomes between SAMe and conventional antidepressants (Agency for Healthcare Research and Quality (AHRQ; 2002). Another review of 11 SAMe research studies concluded that SAMe produced a significant effect when compared to placebo that was supported by a reduction of depressive symptom measures (Williams, Girard, Jui, Sabina, & Katz, 2005). One study showed that SAMe enhanced the effectiveness of serotonin reuptake inhibitors in patients with depression who were originally nonresponders (Papakostas, Mischoulon, Shyu, Alpert, & Fava, 2010). SAMe has also been used clinically with children and adolescents (Schaller, Thomas, & Bazzan, 2004). However, there are no RCTs in these populations.

Some of the adverse effects of SAMe include insomnia and mild gastrointestinal problems; however, there are a few reported cases mania induced from SAMe treatment (Janicak, Lipinski, Davis, Altman, & Sharma, 1989). Some anti-parkinsonian medications may have reduced effectiveness in patients with Parkinson's disease who are also taking SAMe.

OMEGA-3 FATTY ACID

Omega-3 fatty acids are essential fatty acids (EFAs) that play a role in supporting brain structure and healthy brain function. The mechanism by which EFAs have their effect is most likely by stabilizing neuronal membranes and facilitating monoamine neurotransmission (Haag, 2003; Stahl, Begg, Weisinger, & Sinclair, 2008). The human body is unable to synthesize EFAs; therefore EFAs must be consumed through food or dietary supplements. The primary EFAs are eicosapentaenoic acid (EPA) and docosahexaenoic acid (DHA). The most common source of EPA and DHA is in fish oil. Flax and hemp are sources of alpha linolenic acid, which is a fatty acid that converts into EPA and DHA.

Reduced levels of EFAs have been associated with depression in some research studies (Dyall & Michael-Titus, 2008); EFA supplements may enhance mood (Williams et al., 2006). One study that compared a combination of EPA and DHA versus placebo in 28 patients with MDD found EPA/DHA to produce a greater reduction in symptoms ratings (Su, Huang, Chiu, & Shen, 2003). Another RCT found that 2gm of EPA daily for four weeks was an effective adjunctive therapy inpatients with MDD who had incomplete response in symptoms previously (Nemets, Stahl, & Belmaker, 2002). Many studies of omega-3 fatty acids have similar methodological issues as other integrative interventions. Nonetheless, general meta-analyses of RCTs have demonstrated benefits of omega-3 fatty acid supplementation in patients with unipolar and bipolar depression (Freeman et al., 2006; Parker et al., 2006).

Chamomile

Chamomile has been used extensively as a medical remedy in formulations such as teas, aromatic oils, and skin lotions (Rho, Han, Kim, & Lee, 2006; Wilkinson, Aldridge, Salmon, Cain, & Wilson, 1999). Several constituents of chamomile are believed to be responsible for its medicinal actions; these include terpenoids (e.g., bisabolol, chamazulene), flavonoids (e.g., apigenin, luteolin, quercitin), and coumarin (umbelliferone; Salamon, 1992). Chamomile and several of its constituent flavonoids may exert antidepressant effects via modulation of central noradrenaline, dopamine (DA), 5-hydroxytrytophan, and gamma amino butyric acid (GABA) neurotransmission and via reducing hypothalamic-pituitary-adrenal axis activity. Morita et al. (1990) found that apigenin stimulated the uptake of L-[^{14}C]-tyrosine, a DA precursor, into cultured adrenal chromaffin cells. In contrast, flavone produced an increase in [^{14}C]-catecholamine production without altering [^{14}C]-tyrosine turnover. Fifty-eight studies suggest that chamomile may exert an antidepressant and anxiolytic activity via modulation of GABA neurotransmission (Marder & Paladini, 2002). Paladini et al. (1999) found several flavonoid constituents of chamomile (e.g., chrysin, apigenin, flavone) that have antidepressant and anxiolytic activity via their effect on GABA neurotransmission (Campbell, Chebib, & Johnston, 2004).

There was only one RCT on 57 participants with anxiety and depression. The study results demonstrated a significantly greater reduction of depression symptoms and improved mood over time in the total Hamilton Depression (HAM-D) scores for chamomile versus placebo in all participants ($p < .05$). Thus chamomile may provide effective antidepressant activity in addition to anxiolytic activity in persons with depression and anxiety symptoms.

Rhodiola rosea

There are few human trials with *Rhodiola rosea* (*R. rosea*); however, animal studies suggest that *R. rosea* may have antidepressant properties. For example, Panossian et al. (2007) examined the antidepressant activity of *R. rosea* extract and several of its constituents (i.e., rhodioloside, rosavin, rosin, rosarin, tyrosol, cinnamic alcohol, cinnamaldehyde, cinnamic acid) in laboratory rats. The study showed antidepressant behavioral responses with the components, rhodioloside, and tyrosol, but rosavin, rosarin, rosin, cinnamol, cinnamaldehyde, and cinnamate were inactive. Van Diermen et al. (2009) studied the influence of *R. rosea* root extracts on monoamine oxidase (MAO)-A and MAO-B in a microtiter plate bioassay and found significant inhibition of MAO-A and

MAO-B. In a six-week RCT, *R. rosea* was studied for antidepressant efficacy in persons with mild to moderate depression using 340 mg versus 680 mg versus placebo and found a significant reduction in mean depression ratings for both *R. rosea* groups, but no change was found with the placebo group (Darbinyan et al., 2007).

TRYPTOPHAN AND HYDROXYTRYPTOPHAN

There is some evidence that supports the use of tryptophan (TRP) and 5-hydroxytryptophan (5-HTP) in patients with depression. Both supplements are amino acid precursors of the neurotransmitter serotonin that play an important role in the pathophysiology of depression. TRP and 5-HTP may exert their antidepressant effects via serotonin modulation. A literature review of 108 TRP and 5-HTP trials suggested that these agents may be effective for reducing symptoms in patients with MDD. A number of methodological limitations such as small sample size, lack of placebo control, and general study design represent a substantial problem with respect to confirming the efficacy of these supplements (Shaw, Turner, & Del Mar, 2002). Subsequently, an analysis of 27 RCTs in which 11 were placebo-controlled, 5-HTP was found to be statistically superior to placebo in five of the trials (Turner, Loftis, & Blackwell, 2006).

MINDFULNESS-BASED INTERVENTIONS

An AHRQ report conducted a review of the current state of research on a variety of meditation-based practices (Ospina et al., 2007). The AHRQ report indicated the therapeutic benefits derived from meditation-based practices for health conditions. Mindfulness meditation has incorporated two well-studied, clinically based meditation interventions for treatment of mood disorders: mindfulness-based stress reduction (MBSR) and mindfulness-based cognitive therapy (MBCT ;Bishop et al., 2004). Mindfulness approaches are not considered relaxation or mood management techniques but rather practices for cultivating greater self-awareness and acceptance.

Meta-analyses have reached conflicting conclusions regarding the efficacy of MBSR in patients with mood disorders. One review of 15 studies found no clear beneficial effects of the MBSR program on depressive symptoms in patients who had comorbid medical disorders or in patients with mood disorders alone (Toneatto & Nguyen, 2007). However, another systematic review and meta-analysis found mindfulness-based therapies to have robust within-group effect sizes in patients with anxiety and mood disorders that were maintained at follow up (Hofman, Sawyer, Witt, & Oh, 2010).

One study found a decrease in symptoms in the MBCT group in patients with chronic depression and found no significant change in the standard of care treatment group (Barnhofer et al., 2009). Another study found that patients who received MBCT training along with their usual treatment had significantly fewer episodes of relapse/recurrence when compared to those who did not receive MBCT training (Teasdale et al., 2000). It appears that MBCT programs, as an adjunct therapy may be an effective intervention in conjunction with conventional antidepressant treatment even though MBCT may not be sufficient as a stand-alone treatment for depression (Luberto, White, Sears, & Cotton, 2013).

SPIRITUALITY

Spiritual and religious practices and self-prayer are often not included in meta-analyses of CAM practices. A comprehensive review article excluded data on prayer from CAM analyses (Solomon & Adams, 2015). While prayer is not specifically an integrative intervention, spiritual and religious practices can have potent antidepressant activity. A variety of research studies have shown that persons who view themselves as more religious or spiritual have lower levels of depression. Prospective cohort studies have shown religious activity to be associated with remission of depression (Braam, Beekman, Deeg, Smit, & van Tilburg, 1997; Koenig, George, & Peterson, 1998). A strong protective effect against depression was reported in prospective studies of Christian offspring who shared the same religion as their mother (Miller, Warner, Wickramaratne, & Weissman, 1997). In elderly and oncology patients, cross-sectional studies have reported significant and nonsignificant associations between a lower prevalence of depression and indicators of religiosity (Koenig, 1998; Musick, Koenig, Hays, & Cohen, 1998). Chen, Cheal, McDonel Herr, Zubritsky, and Levkoff (2007) reported that religious participation may contribute to better treatment outcomes in patients already diagnosed with depression.

An inverse correlation between religiosity and suicide has been reported in several studies including those in older adults (Nisbet, Duberstein, Conwell, & Seiditz, 2000). Suicide may be a less acceptable option among people who hold high levels of religious devotion and orthodox religious beliefs (Neeleman, Wessely, & Lewis, 1998). However, the exact role of religion and spirutalty is unclear and to what extent religious or spiritual beliefs and practices are a deterrent to suicidal behavior. Research studies have not shown whether persons for whom suicide is a viable option are less likely to hold strong religious or spiritual beliefs or whether persons with strong beliefs are less likely to be suicidal.

Prayer can have a beneficial effect that is similar to meditation-based practices in patients with depression. One RCT demonstrated that both directed and nondirected intercessory prayer correlated favorably with measures of self-esteem, anxiety, and depression (O'Laoire, 1997).

Religion-based cognitive therapy had a favorable impact on Christian patients with clinical depression in one RCT. Due to the multiple comparison groups, it was difficult to demonstrate a strong causal relationship between the intervention and the favorable outcomes (Propst, Ostrom, Watkins, Dean, & Mashburn, 1992). A group of RCTs that used Islamic-based psychotherapy was conducted with Muslim Malays appeared to speed recovery from anxiety and depression. However, the RCT findings were not controlled for the impact of the participants' use of antidepressants and benzodiazepines (Azhar, Varma, & Dharap, 1994; Razali, Hasanah, Aminah, & Subramaniam, 1998).

YOGA

There are only a few studies that have explored the specific effect of yoga practices in patients with depression. One study of deep yoga relaxation found it reduced depression among otherwise healthy university students (Kessler et al., 2005). One pilot study of Vinyasa yoga was conducted as an adjunct intervention for persons with depression who were nonresponders to antidepressant medication. After two months, participants exhibited significant increases in mindfulness measures and in behavior activation and significant decreases in depressive symptoms (Uebelacker et al., 2010). A number of RCTs suggest that yoga can be effective in the treatment of depressive symptoms (Butler et al., 2008; Janakiramaiah et al., 2000; Woolery, Myers, Sternlieb, & Zeltzer, 2004). One study with yoga instructors found that weekly yoga sessions led to increased alpha waves and decreased cortisol (Kamei et al., 2000). Physiologically, decreased depression reported during the practice of yoga postures may related to changes in brain waves and the decreased cortisol levels. The overall findings with yoga research studies are similar to meditation in that yoga practices can be helpful as an adjunctive therapy, but there is insufficient evidence to support its use as a primary therapy in patients with depression.

ACUPUNCTURE

Acupuncture originated as an aspect of the traditional Chinese medicine (TCM) several thousand years ago. Acupuncture is based upon the notion that the energy of one's life force, called qi, runs throughout the body in a network of channels called meridians. These meridians can be accessed at specific points on the skin. In TCM, illness is understood as being caused by blockages or disruption in the flow of qi on the meridians associated with specific organ systems. One goal of acupuncture is to restore the balance of flow of qi to restore wellness. This is achieved through stimulation with acupuncture needles at specific points on meridians. When electric stimulation is applied to the acupuncture needles to act on the meridians, it is called electroacupuncture (Luo, Meng, Jia, & Zhao, 1998).

Reviews of acupuncture for depression vary in their conclusions (Ernst, Lee, & Choi, 2011). Much of the literature on acupuncture is published in the Chinese language and have not been included in English-language meta-analyses of acupuncture (Freeman et al., 2010). There are many different acupuncture techniques; however, acupuncture studies rarely distinguished the subtype of acupuncture. There is some evidence to suggest a potential role for the use of acupuncture in depression. Two RCTs were conducted to evaluate the effect of acupuncture in patients with depression (Luo, Meng, Jia, & Zhao, 1998). In the first cohort, 29 inpatients with depression were assigned randomly into three groups: electroacupuncture + placebo; amitriptyline; and electro-acupuncture + amitriptyline for six weeks. In the second cohort, a multisite study of 241 inpatients with depression were assigned to two treatment groups: electro-acupuncture + placebo and an amitriptyline group. The results from both substudies demonstrated the antidepressant effect of electroacupuncture was similar to amitriptyline; electroacupuncture showed a better therapeutic effect for anxiety somatization and cognitive process disturbance. There were fewer side effects of electro-acupuncture than amitriptyline. Findings from this research study suggest that acupuncture treatment of depression results in comparable relapse rates to antidepressant treatments (Gallagher, Allen, Hitt, Schnyer, & Manber, 2001).

A recent meta-analysis of eight RCTs that enrolled 477 participants found that acupuncture could reduce significantly the severity of depression as measured by decreased scores on the HAM-D or the Beck Depression Inventory. However, acupuncture was not found to have a significant effect on the treatment response rate or remission rate (Wang et al., 2008). A review of seven RCTs that enrolled 517 patients identified only one trial of 23 participants that compared acupuncture with sham acupuncture (Allen, Schnyer, & Hitt, 1998; Smith, Hay, & Macpherson, 2010). The analysis found a reduction in depression scores in patients who received acupuncture. The results from five trials (enrolling a total of 409 participants) that compared acupuncture with antidepressant treatment showed no difference in the reduction of depression symptoms. Another review suggested that acupuncture was as effective as antidepressants (Leo & Ligot, 2007). A report of two acupuncture RCTs, conducted in 20 patients who experienced symptoms of hypomania and a group of 26 patients who experienced symptoms of depression associated with bipolar disease, revealed that all participants experienced improvement over the course of study participation (Dennehy et al., 2009). Acupuncture treatment appeared to target the depression symptoms associated with interest and attention in both groups. Few negative side effects were reported; there was a high level of compliance with the acupuncture treatment.

DIET, NUTRITION, AND EXERCISE

Diet and nutrition are increasingly important in the context of mood disorders. Research has shown that people who are obese have approximately a 55% increased likelihood of developing depression (Luppino et al., 2010). Patients with depression are more likely to become obese due to poor food choices, increased caloric intake, and decreased physical activity. The potential pathophysiological mechanism related to inflammation appears to be associated with foods that are high in saturated fats and their various chemical constituents (Hryhorczuk, Sharma, & Fulton, 2013). The relationship between diet, health, and weight in the management of depression is unclear. Ameta-analysis of 31 studies ($n = 7,937$) evaluated the effects of programs for lifestyle modification, nondieting, dietary counseling, diet alone, exercise alone, pharmacotherapy, and placebo or control interventions (Fabricatore et al., 2011). The results showed that lifestyle modification programs were more effective at reducing depressive symptoms compared to control and nondieting interventions. Lifestyle modifications were found to be slightly better than dietary counseling and exercise-alone programs. The exercise-alone programs were found to be superior to the control intervention. No relationship was found between changes in weight and changes in depressive symptoms. The authors concluded that obese individuals in weight loss trials generally experienced reductions in symptoms of depression. Diet composition that includes essential fatty acid intake or the use of low and high-glycemic foods may alleviate depressive symptoms (Bruinsma & Taren, 2000; Cheatham et al., 2009). There is not adequate data to recommend weight loss programs and anti-inflammatory diets at this time for the treatment of depression.

Exercise has been found to be mildly useful in the management of depressive symptoms. Two RCTs found no difference between exercise, selective serotonin reuptake inhibitors, or placebo; the results suggest that patient expectancy plays a significant role (Blumenthal et al., 2007; Brenes et al., 2007). The combination of exercise programs with pharmacological interventions may improve depressive symptoms. Two RCTs and one open label trial demonstrated the superiority of combined exercise and medication over medication alone even in severe depression (Knubben et al., 2007; Mather et al., 2002; Trivedi, Greer, Grannemann, Chambliss, & Jordan, 2006).

Bipolar Disorder

Among mood disorders, bipolar disorder has been the least studied with respect to the use of integrative psychiatric interventions. Magnesium has been found to be an effective adjunctive therapy for the treatment of acute mania or rapidly cycling bipolar disorder. A small, open-label trial demonstrated that oral magnesium supplementation had comparable efficacy to lithium in patients with rapid cycling bipolar disorder (Chouinard, Beauclair, Geiser, & Etienne, 1990). A small case series showed that intravenous magnesium sulfate could be used effectively along with lithium, haloperidol, and a benzodiazepine in patients with bipolar disorder with severe treatment-resistant mania (Heiden et al., 1999). One RCT of 20 participants with prior diagnosed mania and six months on a stable mood stabilizer used 375mg of magnesium oxide versus placebo over 16 weeks demonstrated a significant reduction in mania symptoms (Giannini, Nakoneczie, Melemis, Ventresco, & Condon, 2000). In two clinical trials, Inositol was evaluated for over six weeks as an adjunct to mood stabilizers (Chengappa, Levine, & Gershon, 2000; Eden Evins et al., 2006). No statistically significant changes were observed between the inositol and placebo group; however, 12 out of 21 participants in the inositol group did demonstrate a response. More data is required to determine whether inositol might be a useful adjunct therapy in the treatment of bipolar patients.

A high prevalence of folic acid deficiency in patients with psychiatric conditions such as depression and bipolar disorder has been reported (Reynolds, 2002). There may be a potential role for folic acid supplementation in these patient populations. Behzadi et al. (2009) conducted a RCT of 88 bipolar patients who received either folic acid plus sodium valproate or just the valproate alone for three weeks. The study results revealed that patients with bipolar disorder experienced significantly greater improvement in their mania symptoms with the combined treatment after three weeks. One 52-week RCT of 102 patients with bipolar disorder stabilized on lithium who received either 200mg of folic acid or placebo showed significantly lower Beck Depression Inventory scores than the folic acid group (Coppen, Chaudhry, & Swade, 1986). Findings of a small, open-label study that used phosphatidylcholine (15 g to 30 g/day) showed decreased severity of mania symptoms and depressed mood in bipolar patients (Stoll et al., 1996).

Regarding integrative treatment approaches to the management of patients with bipolar disorder, it has been noted that in countries where there is high fish consumption there is a lower prevalence of bipolar disorder (Dyall & Michael-Titus, 2008). This observation has led to several clinical trials that used omega-3 fatty acids in the treatment of bipolar patients. Such studies have utilized fish oils and purified eicosapentaenoic acid (EPA) or docosahexaenoic acid (DHA). One RCT that enrolled 44 patients with bipolar disorder used a combination of EPA and DHA (9.6 g/day) along with conventional drug therapies. Improvements in depressed symptoms but no significant effect on mania symptoms was observed (Hamilton, 1960; Stoll et al., 1999). A small 26-week open-label study showed that 8 of 10 participants treated with one month of EPA reported substantial improvements in their depressive symptoms (Osher, Bersudsky, & Belmaker, 2005). A 12-week, three-arm controlled study involving 75 patients with bipolar disorder who received 1 g or 2 g of EPA combined with any class of psychotropic medication demonstrated a small but significant improvement in depressive symptoms in the active groups, but no change was observed in mania symptoms (Frangou, Lewis, & McCrone, 2006; Young, Biggs, Ziegler, & Meyer, 1978). Other studies, including a RCT of 121 patients, did not demonstrate significant effects on depressive or mania symptoms in bipolar patients (Hirashima et al., 2004; Keck et al., 2006). One review article stated that the evidence weakly supports the use of omega-3 in combination with conventional medications in the depressive phase of bipolar disorder; however, omega-3 fatty acids do not appear to be effective in attenuating mania symptoms (Sarris, Lake, & Hoenders, 2011).

Nutritional supplements with specific amino acids or nutrients have been used in the management of patients with bipolar disorder. Two small RCTs suggested that some branch-chained amino acids may improve acute mania by interfering with synthesis of norepinephrine and dopamine. One study treated 25 patients with bipolar disorder with an oral blend of 60 g/day branch-chained amino acids such as leucine, isoleucine, and valine or placebo. Participants in the amino acid group experienced significant reductions in the severity of mania symptoms within six hours (Scarna et al., 2003). Furthermore, the symptom reductions were sustained with repeated administration of the branch-chained amino acids. Another study used N-acetyl cysteine (NAC), an amino acid with strong antioxidant properties, at a dose of 1 g twice per day versus placebo in 75 participants on stable treatment for bipolar disorder. The findings indicated that the NAC significantly reduced bipolar depression, yet no significant effect was observed on mania symptoms (Berk et al., 2008).

A separate review of 18 RCTs reached similar conclusions regarding the use of various supplements in bipolar disorder (Sarris, Mischoulon, & Schweitzer, 2011). In bipolar depression, NAC and a chelated mineral and vitamin formula both reduced depressive symptoms. A chelated mineral formula, L-tryptophan, magnesium, folic acid, and branched-chain amino acids formulations, all appeared to reduce manic symptoms in bipolar patients. The report indicated an overall positive but mixed evidence for omega-3 fatty acids in the treatment of depressive symptoms in bipolar disorder but found no evidence for the management of mania symptoms.

A small, 12-week RCT of choline supplementation (50 mg/kg/day of choline bitartrate or placebo) in eight lithium-treated patients with patients with rapid cycling type, used magnetic resonance spectroscopy to evaluate brain purine, choline, and lithium levels before and during treatment (Lyoo, Demopulos, Hirashima, Ahn, & Renshaw, 2003). The results demonstrated a significant decrease in purine metabolite ratios from baseline in the choline supplementation group when compared to the placebo group. There were no significant differences in brain choline/creatine ratios. The study results suggest that the oral choline supplementation resulted in a significant decrease in brain purine levels, which may be related to the antimanic effects of adjuvant choline. The authors indicate that the result is "consistent with mitochondrial dysfunction in bipolar disorder inadequately meeting the demand for increased ATP production as exogenous oral choline administration increases membrane phospholipid synthesis" (Lyoo et al., 2003).

It should be mentioned that supplements with antidepressant effects such as SJW or SAMe can potentially be useful for the treatment of depressive symptoms. However, a potential concern is that such supplements can potentially induce manic symptoms in patients with bipolar disorder (Moses & Mallinger, 2000). Caution is encouraged when administering CAM interventions that have been effective specifically in patients with depression to patients with bipolar disorder.

There is limited data on the use of acupuncture in patients with bipolar disorder. One randomized study compared targeted acupuncture to "sham" acupuncture in 20 bipolar patients with symptoms of hypomania and 26 patients with symptoms of depression (Dennehy et al., 2009). The results demonstrated that both the targeted and sham acupuncture groups experienced improvement in their clinical symptoms with few side effects.

Conclusion

Many patients with depression and affective disorders may not seek conventional treatment for their symptoms. Current treatment options such as antidepressants and psychotherapeutic approaches often do not benefit many patients, although the benefit does increase with the severity of depression symptoms (Fournier et al., 2010). Questions remain regarding the adequacy of research findings on integrative treatments for mood disorders. The popularity of integrative interventions and treatments within the general population continues to grow. The data on the interventions highlighted in this chapter such as nutritional supplements, botanicals, mind-body practices, acupuncture, and spiritual practices indicates a potential for inclusion in the treatment of depressive symptoms. Further studies with a greater number of subjects, improved methodologies, better control conditions, and physiological correlates can better guide the use of integrative medicine interventions in patients with mood and affective disorders. While the use of CAM interventions as a monotherapy has not been established, the literature does affirm the adjuvant role of many of these interventions to support current medical and psychiatric approaches for an overall integrative treatment approach for mood disorders.

REFERENCES

Agency for Healthcare Research and Quality. (2002, August). S-adenosyl-l-methionine (SAMe) for depression, osteoarthritis, and liver disease (No. 02-E034). Retrieved from https://archive.ahrq.gov/clinic/tp/sametp.htm

Alegría, M., Bijl, R. V., Lin, E., Walters, E. E., & Kessler, R. C. (2000). Income differences in persons seeking outpatient treatment for mental disorders: A comparison of the US with Ontario and the Netherlands. *Archives of General Psychiatry, 57*(4), 383–391.

Allen J. J. B., Schnyer, R. N., & Hitt, S. K. (1998). The efficacy of acupuncture in the treatment of major depression in women. *Psychological Science, 9*(5), 397–401.

Azhar, M. Z., Varma, S. L., & Dharap, A. S. (1994). Religious psychotherapy in anxiety disorder patients. *Acta Psychiatrica Scandinavica, 90*(1), 1–3.

Badger, F., & Nolan, P. (2007). Use of self-chosen therapies by depressed people in primary care. *Journal of Clinical Nursing, 16*(7), 1343–1352.

Barnes, P. M., Bloom, B., & Nahin, R. L. (2008). Complementary and alternative medicine use among adults and children: United States, 2007. *National Health Statistics Reports, 12*, 1.

Barnhofer, T., Crane, C., Hargus, E., Amarasinghe, M., Winder, R., & Williams, J. M. G. (2009). Mindfulness-based cognitive therapy as a treatment for chronic depression: A preliminary study. *Behaviour Research and Therapy, 47*(5), 366–373.

Behzadi, A. H., Omrani, Z., Chalian, M., Asadi, S., & Ghadiri, M. (2009). Folic acid efficacy as an alternative drug added to sodium valproate in the treatment of acute phase of mania in bipolar disorder: A double-blind randomized controlled trial. *Acta Psychiatrica Scandinavica, 120*(6), 441–445.

Berk, M., Copolov, D. L., Dean, O., Lu, K., Jeavons, S., Schapkaitz, I., et al. (2008). N-acetyl cysteine for depressive symptoms in bipolar disorder—a double-blind randomized placebo-controlled trial. *Biological Psychiatry, 64*(6), 468–475.

Bijl, R. V., de Graaf, R., Hiripi, E., Kessler, R. C., Kohn, R., Offord, D. R., et al. (2003). The prevalence of treated and untreated mental disorders in five countries. *Health Affairs, 22*(3), 122–133.

Bishop, S. R., Lau, M., Shapiro, S., Carlson, L., Anderson, N. D., Carmody, J. et al. (2004). Mindfulness: A proposed operational definition. *Clinical Psychology: Science and Practice, 11*(3), 230–241.

Bjerkenstedt, L., Edman, G. V., Alken, R. G., & Mannel, M. (2005). Hypericum extract LI 160 and fluoxetine in mild to moderate depression: A randomized, placebo-controlled multi-center study in outpatients. *European Archives of Psychiatry and Clinical Neuroscience, 255*(1), 40–47.

Blumenthal, J. A., Babyak, M. A., Doraiswamy, P. M., Watkins, L., Hoffman, B. M., Barbour, K. A., et al. (2007). Exercise and pharmacotherapy in the treatment of major depressive disorder. *Psychosomatic Medicine, 69*(7), 587–596.

Bottiglieri, T., & Hyland, K. (1994). S-adenosylmethionine levels in psychiatric and neurological disorders: A review. *Acta Neurologica Scandinavica, Supplementum, 154*, 19.

Boyer, E. W., & Shannon, M. (2005). The serotonin syndrome. *The New England Journal of Medicine, 352*(11), 1112–1120.

Braam, A. W., Beekman, A. T., Deeg, D. J., Smit, J. H., & van Tilburg, W. (1997). Religiosity as a protective or prognostic factor of depression in later life: Results from a community survey in the Netherlands. *Acta Psychiatrica Scandinavica, 96*(3), 199–205.

Brenes, G. A., Williamson, J. D., Messier, S. P., Rejeski, W. J., Pahor, M., Ip, E., & Penninx, B. W. J. H. (2007). Treatment of minor depression in older adults: A pilot study comparing sertraline and exercise. *Aging & Mental Health, 11*(1), 61–68.

Brown, R. P., & Gerbarg, P. L. (2001). Herbs and nutrients in the treatment of depression, anxiety, insomnia, migraine, and obesity. *Journal of Psychiatric Practice, 7*(2), 75–91.

Bruinsma, K. A., & Taren, D. L. (2000). Dieting, essential fatty acid intake, and depression. *Nutrition Reviews, 58*(4), 98–108.

Butler, L. D., Waelde, L. C., Hastings, T. A., Chen, X., Symons, B., Marshall, J., et al. (2008). Meditation with yoga, group therapy with hypnosis, and psychoeducation for long-term depressed mood: A randomized pilot trial. *Journal of Clinical Psychology, 64*(7), 806–820.

Campbell, E. L., Chebib, M., & Johnston, G. A. R. (2004). The dietary flavonoids apigenin and (−)-epigallocatechin gallate enhance the positive modulation by diazepam of the activation by GABA of recombinant GABA A receptors. *Biochemical Pharmacology, 68*(8), 1631–1638.

Cheatham, R. A., Roberts, S. B., Das, S. K., Gilhooly, C. H., Golden, J. K., Hyatt, R., et al. (2009). Long-term effects of provided low and high glycemic load low energy diets on mood and cognition. *Physiology & Behavior, 98*(3), 374–379.

Chen, H., Cheal, K., McDonel Herr, E. C., Zubritsky, C., & Levkoff, S. E. (2007). Religious participation as a predictor of mental health status and treatment outcomes in older persons. *International Journal of Geriatric Psychiatry, 22*(2), 144–153.

Chengappa, K., Levine, J., & Gershon, S. (2000). Inositol as an add-on treatment for bipolar depression. *Bipolar Disorders, 2*(1), 47–55.

Chouinard, G., Beauclair, L., Geiser, R., & Etienne, P. (1990). A pilot study of magnesium aspartate hydrochloride (Magnesiocard ®) as a mood stabilizer for rapid cycling bipolar affective disorder patients. *Progress in Neuropsychopharmacology & Biological Psychiatry, 14*(2), 171–180.

Coppen, A., Chaudhry, S., & Swade, C. (1986). Folic acid enhances lithium prophylaxis. *Journal of Affective Disorders, 10*(1), 9–13.

Darbinyan, V., Aslanyan, G., Amroyan, E., Gabrielyan, E., Malmström, C., & Panossian, A. (2007). Clinical trial of Rhodiola rosea L. extract SHR-5 in the treatment of mild to moderate depression. *Nordic Journal of Psychiatry, 61*(5), 343–348.

Dennehy, E. B., Schnyer, R., Bernstein, I. H., Gonzalez, R., Shivakumar, G., Kelly, D. I., et al. (2009). The safety, acceptability, and effectiveness of acupuncture as an adjunctive treatment for acute symptoms in bipolar disorder. *The Journal of Clinical Psychiatry, 70*(6), 897–905.

Dyall, S. C., & Michael-Titus, A. T. (2008). Neurological benefits of omega-3 fatty acids. *NeuroMolecular Medicine, 10*(4), 219–235.

Echols, J. C., Naidoo, U., & Salzman, C. (2000). SAMe (S-adenosylmethionine). *Harvard Review of Psychiatry, 8*, 84–90.

Eden Evins, A., Demopulos, C., Yovel, I., Culhane, M., Ogutha, J., Grandin, L. D., et al. (2006). Inositol augmentation of lithium or valproate for bipolar depression. *Bipolar Disorders, 8*(2), 168–174.

Eisenberg, D. M., Davis, R. B., Ettner, S. L., Appel, S., Wilkey, S., Van Rompay, M., & Kessler, R. C. (1998). Trends in alternative medicine use in the United States, 1990–1997: Results of a follow-up national survey. *JAMA, 280*(18), 1569–1575.

Ernst, E., Lee, M. S., & Choi, T. (2011). Acupuncture for depression? A systematic review of systematic reviews. *Evaluation and the Health Professions, 34*(4), 403–412.

Fabricatore, A. N., Wadden, T. A., Higginbotham, A. J., Faulconbridge, L. F., Nguyen, A. M., Heymsfield, S. B., & Faith, M. S. (2011). Intentional weight loss and changes in symptoms of depression: A systematic review and meta-analysis. *International Journal of Obesity, 35*(11), 1363–1376.

Fava, M., Alpert, J., Nierenberg, A. A., Mischoulon, D., Otto, M. W., Zajecka, J., et al. (2005). A double-blind, randomized trial of St. John's wort, fluoxetine, and placebo in major depressive disorder. *Journal of Clinical Psychopharmacology, 25*(5), 441–447.

Field, H. L., Monti, D. A., Greeson, J. M., & Kunkel, E. J. S. (2000). St. John's wort. *The International Journal of Psychiatry in Medicine, 30*(3), 203–219.

Fournier, J. C., DeRubeis, R. J., Hollon, S. D., Dimidjian, S., Amsterdam, J. D., Shelton, R. C., & Fawcett, J. (2010). Antidepressant drug effects and depression severity: A patient-level meta-analysis. *JAMA, 303*(1), 47–53.

Frangou, S., Lewis, M., & McCrone, P. (2006). Efficacy of ethyl-eicosapentaenoic acid in bipolar depression: Randomised double-blind placebo-controlled study. *The British Journal of Psychiatry, 188*(1), 46–50.

Freeman, M. P., Fava, M., Lake, J., Trivedi, M. H., Wisner, K. L., & Mischoulon, D. (2010). Complementary and alternative medicine in major depressive disorder: The American Psychiatric Association Task Force report. *The Journal of Clinical Psychiatry, 71*(6), 669–681.

Freeman, M. P., Hibbeln, J. R., Wisner, K. L., Davis, J. M., Mischoulon, D., Peet, M., et al. (2006). Omega-3 fatty acids: Evidence basis for treatment and future research in psychiatry. *The Journal of Clinical Psychiatry, 67*(12), 1954–1967.

Gallagher, S. M., Allen, J. J. B., Hitt, S. K., Schnyer, R. N., & Manber, R. (2001). Six-month depression relapse rates among women treated with acupuncture. *Complementary Therapies in Medicine, 9*(4), 216–218.

Gastpar, M., Singer, A., & Zeller, K. (2005). Efficacy and tolerability of hypericum extract STW3 in long-term treatment with a once-daily dosage in comparison with sertraline. *Pharmacopsychiatry, 38*(2), 78–86.

Giannini, A. J., Nakoneczie, A. M., Melemis, S. M., Ventresco, J., & Condon, M. (2000). Magnesium oxide augmentation of verapamil maintenance therapy in mania. *Psychiatry Research, 93*(1), 83–87.

Givens, J. L., Houston, T. K., Van Voorhees, B. W., Ford, D. E., & Cooper, L. A. (2007). Ethnicity and preferences for depression treatment. *General Hospital Psychiatry, 29*(3), 182–191.

Givens, J. L., Katz, I. R., Bellamy, S., & Holmes, W. C. (2007). Stigma and the acceptability of depression treatments among African Americans and Whites. *Journal of General Internal Medicine, 22*(9), 1292–1297.

Greenberg, P. E., Fournier, A., Sisitsky, T., Pike, C. T., & Kessler, R. C. (2015). The economic burden of adults with major depressive disorder in the United States (2005 and 2010). *The Journal of Clinical Psychiatry, 76*(2), 155–162.

Greenberg, P. E., Stiglin, L. E., Finkelstein, S. N., & Berndt, E. R. (1993). The economic burden of depression in 1990. *The Journal of Clinical Psychiatry, 54*(11), 405–418.

Greeson, J. M., Sanford, B., & Monti, D. A. (2001). St. John's Wort (hypericum perforatum): A review of the current pharmacological, toxicological, and clinical literature. *Psychopharmacology, 153*(4), 402–414.

Gurley, B. J., Swain, A., Williams, D. K., Barone, G., & Battu, S. K. (2008). Gauging the clinical significance of P-glycoprotein-mediated herb-drug interactions: Comparative effects of St. John's wort, echinacea, clarithromycin, and rifampin on digoxin pharmacokinetics. *Molecular Nutrition & Food Research, 52*(7), 772–779.

Haag, M. (2003). Essential fatty acids and the brain. *Canadian Journal of Psychiatry, 48*(3), 195–203.

Hamilton, M. (1960). A rating scale for depression. *Journal of Neurology Neurosurgery Psychiatry, 23*, 56–62.

Heiden, A., Frey, R., Presslich, O., Blasbichler, T., Smetana, R., & Kasper, S. (1999). Treatment of severe mania with intravenous magnesium sulphate as a supplementary therapy. *Psychiatry Research, 89*(3), 239–246.

Hirashima, F., Parow, A. M., Stoll, A. L., Demopulos, C. M., Damico, K. E., Rohan, M. L., et al. (2004). Omega-3 fatty acid treatment and T(2) whole brain relaxation times in bipolar disorder. *The American Journal of Psychiatry, 161*(10), 1922–1924.

Hofmann, S. G., Sawyer, A. T., Witt, A. A., & Oh, D. (2010). The effect of mindfulness-based therapy on anxiety and depression: A meta-analytic review. *Journal of Consulting and Clinical Psychology, 78*(2), 169–183.

Hryhorczuk, C., Sharma, S., & Fulton, S. E. (2013). Metabolic disturbances connecting obesity and depression. *Frontiers in Neuroscience, 7*, 177.

Janakiramaiah, N., Gangadhar, B. N., Naga Venkatesha Murthy, P. J., Harish, M. G., Subbakrishna, D. K., & Vedamurthachar, A. (2000). Antidepressant efficacy of sudarshan kriya yoga (SKY) in melancholia: A randomized comparison with electroconvulsive therapy (ECT) and imipramine. *Journal of Affective Disorders, 57*(1), 255–259.

Janicak, P. G., Lipinski, J., Davis, J. M., Altman, E., & Sharma, R. P. (1989). Parenteral S-adenosyl-methionine (SAMe) in depression: Literature review and preliminary data. *Psychopharmacology Bulletin, 25*(2), 238–242.

Kamei, T., Toriumi, Y., Kimura, H., Ohno, S., Kumano, H., & Kimura, K. (2000). Decrease in serum cortisol during yoga exercise is correlated with alpha wave activation. *Perceptual and Motor Skills, 90*(3 Part 1), 1027–1032.

Kasper, S., Anghelescu, I., Szegedi, A., Dienel, A., & Kieser, M. (2006). Superior efficacy of St John's wort extract WS 5570 compared to placebo in patients with major depression: A randomized, double-blind, placebo-controlled, multi-center trial. *BMC Medicine, 4*(1), 14.

Kasper, S., Gastpar, M., Möller, H., Müller, W. E., Volz, H., Dienel, A., & Kieser, M. (2010). Better tolerability of St. John's wort extract WS 5570 compared to treatment with SSRIs: A reanalysis of data from controlled clinical trials in acute major depression. *International Clinical Psychopharmacology, 25*(4), 204–213.

Katz, S. J., Kessler, R. C., Frank, R. G., Leaf, P., & Lin, E. (1997). Mental health care use, morbidity, and socioeconomic status in the United States and Ontario. *Inquiry, 34*(1), 38–49.

Keck, P. E., Mintz, J., McElroy, S. L., Freeman, M. P., Suppes, T., Frye, M. A., et al. (2006). Double-blind, randomized, placebo-controlled trials of ethyl-eicosapentanoate in the treatment of bipolar depression and rapid cycling bipolar disorder. *Biological Psychiatry, 60*(9), 1020–1022.

Kessler, R. C., Davis, R. B., Foster, D. F., Maria I. Van Rompay, Walters, E. E., Wilkey, S. A., et al. (2001). Long-term trends in the use of complementary and alternative medical therapies in the United States. *Annals of Internal Medicine, 135*(4), 262–268.

Kessler, R. C., Demler, O., Frank, R. G., Olfson, M., Pincus, H. A., Walters, E. E., et al. (2005). Prevalence and treatment of mental disorders, 1990 to 2003. *The New England Journal of Medicine, 352*(24), 2515–2523.

Kessler, R. C., McGonagle, K. A., Zhao, S., Nelson, C. B., Hughes, M., Eshleman, et al. (1994). Lifetime and 12-month prevalence of DSM-III-R psychiatric disorders in the United States: Results from the national comorbidity survey. *Archives of General Psychiatry, 51*(1), 8–19.

Kessler, R. C., Soukup, J., Davis, R. B., Foster, D. F., Wilkey, S. A., Van Rompay, M. I., & Eisenberg, D. M. (2001). The use of complementary and alternative therapies to treat anxiety and depression in the United States. *The American Journal of Psychiatry, 158*(2), 289–294.

Keyes, K. M., Hatzenbuehler, M. L., Alberti, P., Narrow, W. E., Grant, B. F., & Hasin, D. S. (2008). Service utilization differences for axis I psychiatric and substance use disorders between White and Black adults. *Psychiatric Services, 59*(8), 893–901.

Knubben, K., Reischies, F. M., Adli, M., Schlattmann, P., Bauer, M., & Dimeo, F. (2007). A randomised, controlled study on the effects of a short-term endurance training programme in patients with major depression. *British Journal of Sports Medicine, 41*(1), 29–33.

Koenig, H. G. (1998). Religious attitudes and practices of hospitalized medically ill older adults. *International Journal of Geriatric Psychiatry, 13*(4), 213–224.

Koenig, H. G., George, L. K., & Peterson, B. L. (1998). Religiosity and remission of depression in medically ill older patients. *The American Journal of Psychiatry, 155*(4), 536–542.

Leo, R. J., & Ligot, J. S. A. (2007). A systematic review of randomized controlled trials of acupuncture in the treatment of depression. *Journal of Affective Disorders, 97*(1), 13–22.

Linde, K., & Knüppel, L. (2005). Large-scale observational studies of hypericum extracts in patients with depressive disorders—a systematic review. *Phytomedicine, 12*(1), 148–157.

Luberto, C. M., White, C., Sears, R. W., & Cotton, S. (2013). Integrative medicine for treating depression: An update on the latest evidence. *Current Psychiatry Reports, 15*(9), 391.

Luo, H., Meng, F., Jia, Y., & Zhao, X. (1998). Clinical research on the therapeutic effect of the electro-acupuncture treatment in patients with depression. *Psychiatry and Clinical Neurosciences, 52*(Suppl. 6), S338–S340.

Luppino, F. S., de Wit, L. M., Bouvy, P. F., Stijnen, T., Cuijpers, P., Penninx, Brenda W. J. H, & Zitman, F. G. (2010). Overweight, obesity, and depression: A systematic review and meta-analysis of longitudinal studies. *Archives of General Psychiatry, 67*(3), 220–229.

Lyoo, I. K., Demopulos, C. M., Hirashima, F., Ahn, K. H., Renshaw, P. F. (2003). Oral choline decreases brain purine levels in lithium-treated subjects with rapid-cycling bipolar disorder: A double-blind trial using proton and lithium magnetic resonance spectroscopy. *Bipolar Disorders, 5*(4), 300–306.

Mao, J. J., Farrar, J. T., Xie, S. X., Bowman, M. A., & Armstrong, K. (2007). Use of complementary and alternative medicine and prayer among a national sample of cancer survivors compared to other populations without cancer. *Complementary Therapies in Medicine, 15*(1), 21–29.

Marder, M., & Paladini, A. C. (2002). GABA(A)-receptor ligands of flavonoid structure. *Current Topics in Medicinal Chemistry, 2*(8), 853–867.

Mather, A. S., Rodriguez, C., Guthrie, M. F., McHarg, A. M., Reid, I. C., & McMurdo, M. E. (2002). Effects of exercise on depressive symptoms in older adults with poorly responsive depressive disorder: Randomised controlled trial. *The British Journal of Psychiatry, 180*(5), 411–415.

Meeks, T. W., Wetherell, J. L., Irwin, M. R., Redwine, L. S., & Jeste, D. V. (2007). Complementary and alternative treatments for late-life depression, anxiety, and sleep disturbance: A review of randomized controlled trials. *The Journal of Clinical Psychiatry, 68*(10), 1461–1471.

Miller, L., Warner, V., Wickramaratne, P., & Weissman, M. (1997). Religiosity and depression: Ten-year follow-up of depressed mothers and offspring. *Journal of the American Academy of Child & Adolescent Psychiatry, 36*(10), 1416–1425.

Mischoulon, D., & Fava, M. (2002). Role of S-adenosyl-L-methionine in the treatment of depression: A review of the evidence. *The American Journal of Clinical Nutrition, 76*(5), 1158S–1161S.

Moreno, R. A., Teng, C. T., Almeida, K. M., & Tavares Junior, H. (2006). Hypericum perforatum versus fluoxetine in the treatment of mild to moderate depression: A randomized double-blind trial in a Brazilian sample. *Revista Brasileira De Psiquiatria, 28*(1), 29–32.

Morita, K., Hamano, S., Oka, M., & Teraoka, K. (1990). Stimulatory actions of bioflavonoids on tyrosine uptake into cultured bovine adrenal chromaffin cells. *Biochemical and Biophysical Research Communications, 171*(3), 1199.

Moses, E. L., & Mallinger, A. G. (2000). St. John's wort: Three cases of possible mania induction. *Journal of Clinical Psychopharmacology, 20*(1), 115–117.

Musick, M. A., Koenig, H. G., Hays, J. C., & Cohen, H. J. (1998). Religious activity and depression among community-dwelling elderly persons with cancer: The moderating effect of race. *The Journals of Gerontology. Series B, Psychological Sciences and Social Sciences, 53*(4), S218.

National Center for Complementary and Alternative Medicine. (2008). *The use of complementary and alternative medicine in the united States*. Retrieved from https://nccih.nih.gov/research/statistics/2007/camsurvey_fs1.htm

National Institute of Mental Health. (2015). *Major depression among adults*. Retrieved from https://www.nimh.nih.gov/health/statistics/prevalence/major-depression-among-adults.shtml

Neeleman, J., Wessely, S., & Lewis, G. (1998). Suicide acceptability in African- and White Americans: The role of religion. *Journal of Nervous and Mental Disease, 186*(1), 12–16.

Nemets, B., Stahl, Z., & Belmaker, R. H. (2002). Addition of omega-3 fatty acid to maintenance medication treatment for recurrent unipolar depressive disorder. *The American Journal of Psychiatry, 159*(3), 477–479.

Nisbet, P. A., Duberstein, P. R., Conwell, Y., & Seiditz, L. (2000). The effect of participation in religious activities on suicide versus natural death in adults 50 and older. *The Journal of Nervous and Mental Disease, 188*(8), 543–546.

O'Laoire, S. (1997). An experimental study of the effects of distant, intercessory prayer on self-esteem, anxiety, and depression. *Alternative Therapies in Health and Medicine, 3*(6), 38–53.

Osher, Y., Bersudsky, Y., & Belmaker, R. H. (2005). Omega-3 eicosapentaenoic acid in bipolar depression: Report of a small open-label study. *The Journal of Clinical Psychiatry, 66*(6), 726–729.

Ospina, M., Bond, K., Karkhaneh, M., Tjosvold, L., Vandermeer, B., Liang, Y., et al. (2007). Meditation practices for health: State of the research. *Evidence Report/Technology Assessment, 155*, 1–263.

Pagan, J. A., & Pauly, M. V. (2005). Access to conventional medical care and the use of complementary and alternative medicine. *Health Affairs, 24*(1), 255–262.

Paladini, A. C., Marder, M., Viola, H., Wolfman, C., Wasowski, C., & Medina, J. H. (1999). Flavonoids and the central nervous system: From forgotten factors to potent anxiolytic compounds. *Journal of Pharmacy and Pharmacology, 51*(5), 519–526.

Panossian, A., Hambardzumyan, M., Hovhanissyan, A., & Wikman, G. (2007). The adaptogens rhodiola and schizandra modify the response to immobilization stress in rabbits by suppressing the increase of phosphorylated stress-activated protein kinase, nitric oxide and cortisol. *Drug Target Insights, 2*, 39–54.

Papakostas, G. I., Mischoulon, D., Shyu, I., Alpert, J. E., & Fava, M. (2010). S-adenosyl methionine (SAMe) augmentation of serotonin reuptake inhibitors for antidepressant nonresponders with major depressive disorder: A double-blind, randomized clinical trial. *The American Journal of Psychiatry, 167*(8), 942–948.

Parker, G., Gibson, N. A., Brotchie, H., Heruc, G., Rees, A., & Hadzi-Pavlovic, D. (2006). Omega-3 fatty acids and mood disorders. *The American Journal of Psychiatry, 163*(6), 969–978.

Propst, L. R., Ostrom, R., Watkins, P., Dean, T., & Mashburn, D. (1992). Comparative efficacy of religious and nonreligious cognitive-behavioral therapy for the treatment of clinical depression in religious individuals. *Journal of Consulting and Clinical Psychology, 60*(1), 94–103.

Purohit, M. P., Zafonte, R. D., Sherman, L. M., Davis, R. B., Giwerc, M. Y., Shenton, M. E., & Yeh, G. Y. (2015). Neuropsychiatric symptoms and expenditure on complementary and alternative medicine. *The Journal of Clinical Psychiatry, 76*(7), e870.

Razali, S. M., Hasanah, C. I., Aminah, K., & Subramaniam, M. (1998). Religious-sociocultural psychotherapy in patients with anxiety and depression. *Australian and New Zealand Journal of Psychiatry, 32*(6), 867–872.

Reynolds, E. H. (2002). Folic acid, ageing, depression, and dementia. *BMJ, 324*(7352), 1512–1515.

Rho, K., Han, S., Kim, K., & Lee, M. S. (2006). Effects of aromatherapy massage on anxiety and self-esteem in Korean elderly women: A pilot study. *The International Journal of Neuroscience, 116*(12), 1447–1455.

Rice, D. P., & Miller, L. S. (1998). Health economics and cost implications of anxiety and other mental disorders in the United States. *The British Journal of Psychiatry,* (34), 4.

Salamon, I. (1992). Chamomile, a medicinal plant. *Herb Spice Medicinal Plant Digest*, 10, 1–4.

Sarris, J., Lake, J., & Hoenders, R. (2011). Bipolar disorder and complementary medicine: Current evidence, safety issues, and clinical considerations. *Journal of Alternative and Complementary Medicine*, 17(10), 881–890.

Sarris, J., Mischoulon, D., & Schweitzer, I. (2011). Adjunctive nutraceuticals with standard pharmacotherapies in bipolar disorder: A systematic review of clinical trials. *Bipolar Disorders*, 13(5-6), 454–465.

Scarna, A., Gijsman, H. J., McTavish, S. F. B., Harmer, C. J., Cowen, P. J., & Goodwin, G. M. (2003). Effects of a branched-chain amino acid drink in mania. *The British Journal of Psychiatry*, 182(3), 210–213.

Schaller, J. L., Thomas, J., & Bazzan, A. J. (2004). SAMe use in children and adolescents. *European Child & Adolescent Psychiatry*, 13(5), 332–334.

Shaw, K., Turner, J., & Del Mar, C. (2002). Tryptophan and 5-hydroxytryptophan for depression. *Cochrane Database of Systematic Reviews*, 1, CD003198.

Simon, G., Ormel, J., Vonkorff, M., & Barlow, W. (1995). Health care costs associated with depressive and anxiety disorders in primary care. *The American Journal of Psychiatry*, 152(3), 352–357.

Smith, C. A., Hay, P. P., & Macpherson, H. (2010). Acupuncture for depression. *Cochrane Database of Systematic Reviews*, 1, CD004046.

Solomon, D., & Adams, J. (2015). The use of complementary and alternative medicine in adults with depressive disorders. A critical integrative review. *Journal of Affective Disorders*, 179, 101–113.

Stahl, L. A., Begg, D. P., Weisinger, R. S., & Sinclair, A. J. (2008). The role of omega-3 fatty acids in mood disorders. *Current Opinion in Investigational Drugs*, 9(1), 57–64.

Stoll, A. L., Sachs, G. S., Cohen, B. M., Lafer, B., Christensen, J. D., & Renshaw, P. F. (1996). Choline in the treatment of rapid-cycling bipolar disorder: Clinical and neurochemical findings in lithium-treated patients. *Biological Psychiatry*, 40(5), 382–388.

Stoll, A. L., Severus, W. E., Freeman, M. P., Rueter, S., Zboyan, H. A., Diamond, E., et al. (1999). Omega 3 fatty acids in bipolar disorder: A preliminary double-blind, placebo-controlled trial. *Archives of General Psychiatry*, 56(5), 407–412.

Stratton, T. D., & McGivern-Snofsky, J. L. (2008). Toward a sociological understanding of complementary and alternative medicine use. *Journal of Alternative and Complementary Medicine*, 14(6), 777–783.

Su, K., Huang, S., Chiu, C., & Shen, W. W. (2003). Omega-3 fatty acids in major depressive disorder. A preliminary double-blind, placebo-controlled trial. *European Neuropsychopharmacology*, 13(4), 267–271.

Teasdale, J. D., Segal, Z. V., Williams, J. M. G., Ridgeway, V. A., Soulsby, J. M., & Lau, M. A. (2000). Prevention of relapse/recurrence in major depression by mindfulness-based cognitive therapy. *Journal of Consulting and Clinical Psychology*, 68(4), 615–623.

Tindle, H. A., Davis, R. B., Phillips, R. S., & Eisenberg, D. M. (2005). Trends in use of complementary and alternative medicine by US adults: 1997–2002. *Alternative Therapies in Health and Medicine, 11*(1), 42–49.

Toneatto, T., & Nguyen, L. (2007). Does mindfulness meditation improve anxiety and mood symptoms? A review of the controlled research. *The Canadian Journal of Psychiatry, 52*(4), 260–266.

Trivedi, M. H., Greer, T. L., Grannemann, B. D., Chambliss, H. O., & Jordan, A. N. (2006). Exercise as an augmentation strategy for treatment of major depression. *Journal of Psychiatric Practice, 12*(4), 205–213.

Turner, E. H., Loftis, J. M., & Blackwell, A. D. (2006). Serotonin a la carte: Supplementation with the serotonin precursor 5-hydroxytryptophan. *Pharmacology and Therapeutics, 109*(3), 325–338.

Uebelacker, L. A., Tremont, G., Epstein-Lubow, G., Gaudiano, B. A., Gillette, T., Kalibatseva, Z., & Miller, I. W. (2010). Open trial of vinyasa yoga for persistently depressed individuals: Evidence of feasibility and acceptability. *Behavior Modification, 34*(3), 247–264.

van der Watt, G., Laugharne, J., & Janca, A. (2008). Complementary and alternative medicine in the treatment of anxiety and depression. *Current Opinion in Psychiatry, 21*(1), 37–42.

van Diermen, D., Marston, A., Bravo, J., Reist, M., Carrupt, P., & Hostettmann, K. (2009). Monoamine oxidase inhibition by rhodiola rosea L. roots. *Journal of Ethnopharmacology, 122*(2), 397–401.

Wang, H., Qi, H., Wang, B. S., Cui, Y. Y., Zhu, L., Rong, Z. X., & Chen, H. Z. (2008). Is acupuncture beneficial in depression? A meta-analysis of 8 randomized controlled trials. *Journal of Affective Disorders, 111*(2), 125–134.

Wang, P. S., Berglund, P., & Kessler, R. C. (2000). Recent care of common mental disorders in the United States: Prevalence and conformance with evidence-based recommendations. *Journal of General Internal Medicine, 15*(5), 284–292.

Wang, P. S., Lane, M., Olfson, M., Pincus, H. A., Wells, K. B., & Kessler, R. C. (2005). Twelve-month use of mental health services in the United States: Results from the National Comorbidity Survey replication. *Archives of General Psychiatry, 62*(6), 629–640.

World Health Organization. (2010). *World health statistics: 2010.* Geneva: World Health Organization.

Williams, A., Girard, C., Jui, D., Sabina, A., & Katz, D. L. (2005). S-adenosylmethionine (SAMe) as treatment for depression: A systematic review. *Clinical and Investigative Medicine, 28*(3), 132.

Williams, A., Katz, D., Ali, A., Girard, C., Goodman, J., & Bell, I. (2006). Do essential fatty acids have a role in the treatment of depression? *Journal of Affective Disorders, 93*(1), 117–123.

Wilkinson, S., Aldridge, J., Salmon, I., Cain, E., & Wilson, B. (1999). An evaluation of aromatherapy massage in palliative care. *Palliative Medicine, 13*(5), 409–417.

Woolery, A., Myers, H., Sternlieb, B., & Zeltzer, L. (2004). A yoga intervention for young adults with elevated symptoms of depression. *Alternative Therapies in Health and Medicine, 10*(2), 60–63.

Wu, P., Fuller, C., Liu, X., Lee, H., Fan, B., Hoven, C. W., et al. (2007). Use of complementary and alternative medicine among women with depression: Results of a national survey. *Psychiatric Services, 58*(3), 349–356.

Young, R., Biggs, J., Ziegler, V., & Meyer, D. (1978). A rating scale for mania: Reliability, validity and sensitivity. *The British Journal of Psychiatry, 133*(5), 429–435.

19

Integrative Treatment of Anxiety

BIRGIT RAKEL

Key Points

- Anxiety and anxiety disorders are among the most common complaints of people in all populations.
- Fear and anxiety are similar, but fear relates to immediate threats while anxiety refers to anticipation of future threats.
- Patients with anxiety frequently seek integrative approaches to help reduce their symptoms.
- Medications are useful in certain anxiety conditions but have a number of side effects and may be addictive.
- Dietary influences can have a significant effect of augmenting or alleviating anxiety.
- Gut microbiota may play an important role in anxiety and other emotions.
- Mind–body techniques such as meditation or mindfulness programs have been shown to significantly reduce anxiety symptoms.
- Several supplements such as kava kava, lavender, and chamomile may also have anti-anxiety effects.

Introduction

In 1948 the World Health Organization (WHO) defined health as "a state of complete physical, mental and social well-being and not merely the absence of disease." This definition is a very holistic and integrative way of looking at disease, but it does not take into account how stress and anxiety intersect with health and well-being. We are living in difficult and uncertain times, and many people in the United States live with a substantial level of stress and anxiety on a daily basis. An important question is, "When does reactionary fear, stress, and anxiety become debilitating to the extent that it becomes a disorder in which the person needs professional help?" More important for the purposes of this review are the many integrative approaches people may take to help improve stress and anxiety.

Anxiety disorders affect about 40 million American adults per year. Women have a higher risk then men for both anxiety and other mood disorders (McLean, Asnaani., Litz, & Hofmann, 2011). In a six-month observational study, 6% of men and 13% of women in the United States met the criteria for an anxiety disorder (Leon, Fulkerson, Perry, & Early-Zald, 1995). Anxiety is estimated to cause 1% of all disability adjusted life years lost worldwide in the form of posttraumatic stress disorder (PTSD), obsessive compulsive disorder (OCD), and panic attacks (WHO, 2004).

Anxiety is defined as "the apprehensive anticipation of future danger or misfortune accompanied by a feeling of dysphoria or somatic symptoms of tension. The focus of anticipated danger may be internal or external" (Jacob & Kuruvilla, 2017, p. 83). Anxiety is characterized by excessive and persistent nervousness, worrying, fear, irritability, and sleep disturbances, occurring more days then not for at least six months (Gaby, 2011). These symptoms might be accompanied by physical symptoms such as sweating, palpitations, chest pain, fatigue, headaches, difficulty concentrating, and muscle tension.

The *Diagnostic and Statistical Manual of Mental Disorders* (fifth edition [DSM-V]) describes a collection of anxiety-related conditions including generalized anxiety disorder (GAD), anxiety disorder due to a medical condition, substance-induced anxiety disorder, anxiety disorder not otherwise specified, acute stress disorder, panic attack, agoraphobia, panic disorder, specific phobia, social phobia, OCD, and PTSD.

Anxiety disorders refer to those disorders that consist of excessive fear and anxiety along with related behavioral disturbances related to those fears. *Fear* is defined as the emotional response to any real or perceived imminent threat. *Anxiety* refers to the anticipation of future threats. Fear and anxiety states overlap but are also different since fear is more often associated with acute increases in sympathetic nervous system activity necessary for the fight-or-flight response. Anxiety is more often associated with muscle tension and vigilance in preparation for future dangers. Anxiety is also associated with proactive cautious or avoidant behaviors. Currently, the criteria from the DSM-V (American Psychiatric Association, 2013) for GAD is

A. Too much anxiety or worry over more than six months. This is present most of the time in regards to many activities.
B. Inability to manage these symptoms
C. At least three of the following occur (Note: Only one item is required in children):
   1. Restlessness
   2. Tires easily
   3. Problems concentrating
   4. Irritability
   5. Muscle tension
   6. Problems with sleep
D. Symptoms result in problems with functioning
E. Symptoms are not due to medications, drugs, other physical health problems
F. Symptoms do not fit better with another psychiatric problem such as panic disorder

What virtually all patients with anxiety have in common is that they want to find ways to feel better, feel healthier, and feel more whole. Although medications for anxiety are available, they can have side effects such as drowsiness, and they can be addicting (see following discussion). Thus patients with anxiety frequently want to integrate the best of both worlds using Western and Eastern medicinal approaches. Patients want to be heard and acknowledged in their suffering and want to ease their pain.

Patients can suffer from an anxiety disorder in and of itself such as GAD, but many patients with chronic medical conditions such as cancer, diabetes, heart disease, chronic pain syndromes, or other psychiatric diseases like depression can all report significant levels of anxiety and stress in their clinical picture. Often, it is not easy to clarify whether the anxiety arose as the result of the other disease, whether the disease arose from having too much stress and anxiety, or whether the disease and anxiety co-occurred.

As clinicians, it is important to fully understand the complex relationship between anxiety and health for each individual patient. Mindful listening to patients' stories is a crucial part of the exploration as a clinician. It is important to help a patient learn to be less affected by circumstances and offer techniques or lifestyle modifications that can be incorporated into their already busy lives without imposing new stressors (i.e., the cost of therapy). In an ever-changing world in the field of medicine with computers dictating how we can practice and an ever-expanding body of evidence of physician burnout, it is important to be with our patients with an open heart, compassion, and nonjudgment to meet them as human beings we can help through our expertise. This chapter reviews the available evidence on the most effective ways of helping patients deal with stress and anxiety using an integrative approach.

Pathophysiology

Before considering therapeutic interventions for stress and anxiety, it is important to briefly review some of the underlying pathophysiology. Knowledge of the pathophysiology of stress and anxiety will inform the best therapeutic options. In humans, the stress response is most often triggered when survival of the organism is threatened and involves a cascade of different neurological, autonomic, and hormonal events. Specifically, there is activation of the sympathetic nervous system that results in increased heart rate, blood pressure, and respiratory rate. There is typically activation of alerting areas of the brain such as the hypothalamus and amygdala. The amygdala in particular becomes activated with fearful stimuli (Sander, Grafman, & Zalla, 2003); however, the network of structures involved in the fear response is much more complicated and may also incorporate the prefrontal cortex, insula, and cerebellum (Lange et al., 2015; Ohman, 2005). Cortisol, thyroid hormone, and adrenaline are the stress hormones that play a role in the stress response (Nemeroff, 1989; Ninan, 1999).

Multiple proposed (biochemical) mechanisms are at work in patients dealing with excessive stress and anxiety. Overall, the current evidence suggests that anxiety disorders are related to dysregulation of a number of neurotransmitter systems including serotonergic, noradrenergic, glutamatergic, and gamma-aminobutyric acid (GABA)-ergic transmission (Nutt, Ballenger, Sheehan, & Wittchen, 2002). GABA is the primary inhibitory central nervous system (CNS) neurotransmitter, and levels appear to be decreased in the cortex of patients with panic disorders (Goddard et al., 2001). This implies that the individual is not able to modulate the fear or stress response effectively, causing increased and sustained anxiety. Serotonin also appears to be involved in the pathogenesis of anxiety disorders as well. There is evidence that drugs that enhance serotonin neurotransmission may stimulate 5-HT_{1A} receptors in the hippocampus, which subsequently promotes neuroprotection and neurogenesis as well as reduces anxiety symptoms (Nutt, 1998).

A number of brain imaging studies implicate the amygdala hyperactivity in relation to anxiety and anxiety disorders (Brooks & Stein, 2015; Cremers & Roelofs, 2016). In addition, the amygdala is connected to other brain regions involved in emotional processing and regulation such as the hippocampus and insula (Ahmed-Leitao, Spies, van den Heuvel, & Seedat, 2016; Mochcovitch, da Rocha Freire, Garcia, & Nardi, 2014). The stress response involves activation of the hypothalamic-pituitary-adrenal axis. This axis, which is primarily related to the autonomic nervous system, is *hyperactive* in depression and in anxiety disorders.

Medical Treatment

In view of the aforementioned pathophysiological pathways, a number of drugs are considered beneficial to combat anxiety disorders including selective serotonin reuptake inhibitors (SSRIs), selective serotonin and noradrenaline reuptake inhibitors (SNRIs), and benzodiazepines (Liu et al., 2015). However, these medications are associated with a variety of side effects, and long-term use may be associated with addiction and/or tolerance.

The recommended first-line treatment strategies for most anxiety disorders include antidepressants and/or cognitive behavioral therapy (CBT; Bandelow, Seidler-Brandler, Becker, Wedekind, & Rüther, 2007). SSRIs are useful first-line agents, and there are several large reviews that have supported the use of SSRI therapies for anxiety (Gorman & Kent, 1999). Many psychiatrists also take the "start low and go slow" approach in which patients start with low (i.e., half the normal) dose used for depression and then titrate the dose up to an effective range (Bystritsky, Khalsa, Cameron, & Schiffman., 2013). Commonly used SSRIs include Celexa (citalopram), Lexapro (escitalopram), Prozac (fluoxetine), Zoloft (sertraline), and Paxil (paroxetine; Hoffman & Mathew, 2008).

Although these SSRIs can be effective, antidepressants have significant limitations including a slow onset of action and delayed time to maximal clinical effect (Hidalgo, Tupler, & Davidson, 2007). These medications also result in a number of possible side effects, including initial increase in anxiety, weight gain, and sexual side effects, which are experienced by as many as 50% of users in the long term (Schweitzer, Maguire, & Ng, 2009). Sexual dysfunction, in particular, leads many patients to discontinue their treatment (Sussman & Ginsberg, 1998). While pharmacotherapy is a common treatment strategy, 30% to 60% of patients do not achieve remission after treatment (Dugas et al., 2010; Rickels, Rynn, Iyengar, & Duff, 2006; Simon et al., 2010; Zinbarg, Eun Lee, & Lira Yoon, 2007). A recent report in *JAMA Psychiatry* found that the effectiveness of SSRIs in the treatment of anxiety has been overestimated. In fact, there is some suggestion that SSRIs may be no better than placebo under certain conditions (Roest et al., 2015).

Another class of medications in current use for anxiety is SNRIs such as venlafaxine and duloxetine. Although abnormal serotonergic neurotransmission is involved in the pathophysiology of anxiety disorders, the role of norepinephrine is less clear. However, existing evidence supports the notion that a abnormalities in norepinephrine neurotransmission is associated with anxiety symptoms as well as depression (Montoya, Bruins, Katzman, & Blier,

2016). Therefore, drugs that modulate both serotonin and norepinephrine may be useful in the treatment of anxiety disorders (Dell'Osso, Buoli, Baldwin, & Altamura, 2010; Silverstone, 2004). Several randomized trials have shown that such medications that function as dual-reuptake inhibitors may be effective in patients with anxiety disorder. One randomized controlled trial (RCT) in 251 patients with GAD showed significant improvements in anxiety symptoms at six months with venlafaxine-SR compared to placebo although the placebo group also showed substantial improvements (Gelenberg et al., 2000). However, more data is needed, especially in patients with less severe anxiety symptoms.

Benzodiazepines have long been a primary medication utilized in patients with anxiety symptoms and disorders. These medications, such as alprazolam, clonazepam, diazepam, and lorazepam, facilitate GABA neurotransmission and therefore can improve anxiety. Their key advantage over SSRIs is the rapid onset of action. Although benzodiazepines were widely used in the past for the treatment of anxiety and anxiety disorders, they are no longer considered to be first-line therapies because of the risk associated with their chronic use. The primary problem is dependence or addiction to benzodiazepines, making it difficult or impossible for patients to stop these medications (Ravindran & Stein, 2010). Other problems include substantial side effects such as somnolence and diminished cognition, which can lead to accidents/injuries, sleep disturbances, and other psychiatric issues (Murphy, Wilson, Goldner, & Fischer, 2016).

Another long-standing approach, primarily for performance anxiety, has been the use of beta blockers (Tyrer, 1988). The goal is that the beta blocker reduces heart rate and blood pressure and other autonomic symptoms associated with anxiety (Brugués, 2011). By reducing the body's anxiety response, the patient feels less anxious. However, the use of beta blockers is typically limited to specific anxiety-provoking circumstances; one particular study showed its effectiveness in helping residents perform during surgery (Elman et al., 1998). A systematic review suggested that propranolol is not significantly different compared to benzodiazepines in the management of panic disorder but concluded that routine use could not be recommended at this time (Steenen et al., 2016). In addition, beta blockers can have side effects including low blood pressure, light-headedness, and syncope.

Buspirone is a newer anxiolytic/psychotropic drug approved in the United States by the Food and Drug Administration (FDA) for short- or long-term use for GAD but is not as effective in other types of anxiety. The onset of action is about two weeks and works primarily as an agonist of the serotonin 5-HT1A receptor with high affinity (Celada, Bortolozzi, & Artigas, 2013). A large review (Chessick et al., 2006) of 36 trials on 5,908 participants generally showed that buspirone (and other azapirones) was superior to placebo in treating GAD. However, this review also noted that azapirones may be less effective than benzodiazepines. As with the other medications, there is a long list of potential side effects including the most common ones of nervousness, insomnia, depression, confusion, and gastrointestinal symptoms.

Newer pharmacological approaches for the treatment of anxiety are continually being explored. Drugs that have psychedelic effects, such as psilocybin, have even been studied. One small randomized cross-over trial in 29 patients with life-threatening cancer showed significant reductions in anxiety and depression after a single moderate dose of psilocybin combined with psychotherapy.

Integrative medicine physicians should be well aware of the pharmacological options for the management of anxiety and anxiety disorders. Many patients will present having already been on one or more of these medications. While these medications certainly can be useful, integrative psychiatry offers a number of other options that can be used either alone or in conjunction with the anti-anxiety medications.

Psychotherapeutic Interventions

As mentioned, the recommended first-line treatment strategy for most anxiety disorders include antidepressants and/or CBT (Bandelow et al., 2007). CBT is a common short-term, goal-oriented talk/psychotherapy intervention that takes a practical approach to problem-solving. Its goal is to change maladaptive patterns of thinking that underlie a patient's psychological or physical difficulties with a goal to change behavior and affect (Hassett & Gevirtz, 2009). Further, it can be used not only for basic anxiety disorders but for other disorders that incorporate anxiety as part of the constellation of symptoms such as fibromyalgia, chronic pain, or chronic fatigue.

There is a substantial body of evidence that CBT, which typically utilizes a combination of psychoeducation, relaxation training, cognitive restructuring, and behavioral aspects (Bandelow et al., 2007), is beneficial in anxiety disorders. The data show that approximately 50% to 65% of patients with anxiety disorders benefit from CBT or antidepressants (Baldwin & Polkinghorn, 2005; Nutt et al., 2002). However, even though CBT has good efficacy, it does not always work to reduce anxiety symptoms, especially when patients are not suited or motivated for face-to-face CBT. Access to effective CBT can also be an issue whether it is related to a lack of local psychologists/psychiatrists or the prohibitive costs when multiple sessions are required (Andrews & Titov, 2010). In order to respond to these limitations, a number of studies support the notion of Internet-based cognitive therapy, which has been shown to be as beneficial as face-to-face CBT (Olthuis, Watt, Bailey, Hayden, & Stewart, 2016).

More recently, mindfulness-based approaches (see later discussion) have now been combined with cognitive therapy in Mindfulness-Based Cognitive Therapy (MBCT) (Evans et al., 2008; Kim et al., 2009). Although MBCT has been effective in patients with anxiety, differentiating the impact of the cognitive therapy component from the mindfulness component has been difficult. Understanding the contribution of the different components of MBCT will be important for determining this technique's future use in patients with anxiety.

Other psychotherapeutic approaches have also been developed for anxiety disorders. Exposure therapy for anxiety is based on exposing patients in a systematic manner to stressful or anxiety-provoking situations and stimuli (Kaczkurkin & Foa, 2015). This approach is also referred to as systematic desensitization in which the patient goes step by step through a fear-related event and works toward reducing the stress response. Psychodynamic therapy is an approach that typically focuses on core conflictual relationship themes and specifically on unconscious processes that affect a person's emotions, thoughts, and behaviors. The goals of psychodynamic therapy are to create a deeper self-awareness and understanding within the patient with respect to past dysfunctional relationships. Psychodynamic therapy has been shown to be as effective as CBT with effects lasting up to at least 12 months (Salzer, Winkelbach, Leweke, Leibing, & Leichsenring, 2011).

Rational emotive behavior therapy is a therapeutic system that considers emotions, actions, and thoughts as not separate but interwoven and holds that, early in life, many people develop ineffectual or detrimental modes of managing these aspects of their lives. This therapeutic approach attempts to show patients the various ways that they needlessly upset themselves and retrain them on how to alter these negative approaches and then empower them to lead happier, more fulfilling lives (Ellis, 2003). There are some studies that have shown this therapeutic approach to be beneficial in the management of anxiety, but more studies are required to compare its effectiveness to other therapies (Warren, Smith, & Velten, 1984).

Integrative Approaches to Anxiety

We might consider a variety of integrative medicine approaches to the management of anxiety as following three tiers. The first tier brings together diet, exercise, and mind–body therapies for which there is generally strong support for such lifestyle modifications. Supplements and herbal remedies represent the second tier, and medications when necessary represent the third tier. Since we have already considered medications, we next explore the first and second tiers in more detail.

DIETARY INFLUENCES ON ANXIETY

An early study exploring the relationship between an individual's diet and anxiety and depressive illnesses was conducted in a population-based sample of Australian women (Jacka et al., 2010). The results showed that a "traditional" dietary pattern characterized by vegetables, fruit, meat, fish, and whole grains was associated with lower odds for depression and anxiety disorders. This association held even after adjusting for age, socioeconomic status, education, and health behaviors. A "Western" diet of processed and fried foods, refined grains, foods with added sugars, and beer was associated with higher anxiety scores (Jacka et al., 2010). In a follow-up study, this same group showed that the Standard American Diet, comprised of processed meats, pizza, salty snacks, chocolates, sugars and sweets, soft drinks, French fries, beer, cake, and ice cream, was also associated with a significantly higher likelihood of having anxiety symptoms (Jacka, Mykletun, Berk, Bjelland, & Tell, 2011).

When it comes to diet, it is not just what foods are eaten but sometimes how the body reacts after food is eaten. For example, an excessive fall in blood sugar leads to a compensatory response by the sympathetic nervous system, including the release of epinephrine and norepinephrine (Hoffman, 2007). While this response helps restore glucose levels to normal, it also induces a "fight-or-flight" response, which can manifest in anxiety, palpitations, and irritability. To relieve reactive hypoglycemia, the National Institutes of Health recommends avoiding or limiting glucose intake, exercising regularly since exercise increases glucose uptake and decreases insulin release, eating a variety of foods that are higher in proteins and healthy fats, and choosing high-fiber foods. Thus a high protein, low-carbohydrate diet as well as more frequent small meals is the first treatment of this condition. This diet consists of primarily vegetables, plant proteins, lean meats, and healthy oils from nuts, seeds, and olive oil. Whole grains are better than processed grains and sugars. Reducing excess sugars in foods is also very important.

Specific nutrients in the diet may have anti-anxiety effects. For example, numerous studies have identified a relationship between omega-3 and omega-6 fatty acids and anxiety symptoms. One study showed that supplemental omega-3 fatty acids reduced anxiety symptoms and levels of various inflammatory mediators in a group of medical students compared to placebo (Kiecolt, Belury, Andridge, Malarkey, & Glaser, 2011). The students who received omega-3 supplementation showed a 14% reduction in lipopolysaccharide stimulated interleukin 6 and a 20% reduction in anxiety symptoms.

In addition to the foods we eat, it has more recently been realized that the gut bacteria milieu (or microbiota) has a substantial impact on brain function and likely on anxiety. Emerging work notes that alterations in the microbiota modulate neuroplasticity-related serotonergic and GABAergic signaling systems in the CNS (Maqsood & Stone, 2016; Patterson et al., 2014). Newer studies are beginning to show that bacteria in the gastrointestinal tract, including commensal, probiotic, and pathogenic bacteria, can influence neuronal pathways and neurotransmitter systems, ultimately leading to changes in cognition and mood. As additional studies in both animal and humans clarify the relationship between the gut microbiota and the brain, novel approaches for preventing and treating mental illness, such as anxiety disorders, may be developed (Foster & Neufeld, 2013). Bidirectional communication between the brain and the gut has long been recognized and likely plays a role in various psychological disorders such as anxiety and depression.

Animal studies have shown that increased inflammation in the body may be associated with increased anxiety-like behaviors. Furthermore, these studies suggest that probiotic treatment designed to improve the gut microbiota can help reduce inflammation and associated anxiety-like behaviors (Bercik et al., 2010, 2011). Although probiotics have shown a benefit in animal studies (Ait-Belgnaoui et al., 2014), there is little data regarding the potential benefit of probiotics for reducing anxiety symptoms in humans. Although the early data suggests that probiotics might be useful for reducing anxiety in human beings, larger RCTs will be needed before establishing probiotics as a recommended therapy for patients with anxiety disorders.

There is encouraging preliminary data to suggest that avoidance of caffeine, alcohol, and smoking may reduce anxiety symptoms in the short term (Sarris et al., 2012). However, there is also evidence that the use of tobacco and/or alcohol predisposes people to the development of anxiety over time, particularly by producing chronic withdrawal symptoms, reducing health quality, and possibly precipitating somatic or emotional symptoms that maintain anxiety (McLeish et al., 2009).

Caffeine is perhaps the most commonly used psychoactive substance in the general population. Most individuals who intake caffeine through beverages or other means described increased attention, alertness, cognition, and mood. Some individuals with depressed mood may even be predisposed to using caffeine more heavily for its mood-elevating potential. The improved mood related to caffeine is likely the results of activation of noradrenergic and dopaminergic pathways (Nehlig, Daval, & Debry, 1992). If caffeine is overused, individuals may experience anxiety and insomnia, especially when the caffeine intake occurs at night (Broderick & Benjamin, 2004). There are also suggestions that caffeine can result in dependence (Meredith, Juliano, Hughes, & Griffiths, 2013). One study demonstrated that patients with anxiety disorders may be particularly sensitive to the anxiogenic effects of caffeine. The effects of oral administration of caffeine (10 mg/kg) produced significantly greater increases in anxiety, nervousness, fear, and palpitations in patients with existing anxiety disorders compared to healthy controls (Charney, Heninger, & Jatlow, 1985). Thus caffeine can cause symptoms that are difficult to distinguish from those of anxiety itself and can therefore enhance anxiety symptoms or confuse them for both patients and clinicians (Greden, 1974).

Alcohol consumption is also associated with anxiety. The "self-medication" hypothesis suggests that people use alcohol as a remedy for reducing anxiety, emotional distress, or negative mood symptoms (Kushner, Sher, & Beitman, 1990). Because of this relationship, patients with anxiety disorders should be routinely screened for alcohol misuse. In addition, almost half of people undergoing treatment for alcohol or substance abuse problems also express anxiety symptoms or even have a frank anxiety disorder (Kushner et al., 2005). In addition, alcohol withdrawal can mimic many symptoms of anxiety (Saitz, 1998). Chronic alcohol consumption also appears to be a significant stressor on the brain (Becker, 2017).

Smoking is another psychoactive habit that is common in those with anxiety disorders (Mathew, Norton, Zvolensky, Buckner, & Smits, 2011). Cigarettes, through the effect of nicotine on postsynaptic nicotinic receptors, can result in changes in mood or cognition. Nicotinic effects can downregulate dopamine D2 receptors in the nucleus accumbens, the site of the reward system (Volkow, Fowler, Wang, Baler, & Telang, 2009). Smoking can sometimes reduce anxiety in patients, but the withdraw of nicotine can subsequently increase anxiety. However, research suggests that smoking cessation does not appear to increase anxiety after quitting and may actually reduce symptoms in the long run (Bolam, West, & Gunnell, 2011).

EXERCISE

Regular physical activity has been shown to be associated with improved emotional well-being (Steptoe & Butler, 1996) and inactivity with poorer emotional well-being (Galper, Trivedi, Barlow, Dunn, & Kampert, 2006). Physical inactivity has been demonstrated to be a risk factor for the development of a variety of psychiatric illnesses, including anxiety (Bhui & Fletcher, 2000; Deslandes et al., 2009; Goodwin, 2003). North American guidelines recommend that adults participate in at least 150 minutes of moderate to vigorous physical activity every week in order to obtain clinically meaningful health benefits. However, only about one-quarter of American adults report meeting or exceeding this recommendation (Dunn, Trivedi, & O'Neal, 2001), Thus over half of all adults lead generally sedentary lifestyles, which has been associated with an increased risk for mental disorders like anxiety.

The specific therapeutic effect of physical activity or exercise in reducing anxiety is likely the result of complex interactions between physiological, neurobiological, and psychological processes (Cotman & Berchtold, 2002). Possible mechanisms by which regular activity can reduce anxiety include changes in central serotonergic systems (Chaouloff, 1997) and increases in endorphin production (Hoffman, 1997).

Current best practice guidelines for the treatment of anxiety disorders include regular physical activity such as walking for 60 minutes or running 20 to 30 minutes at least four days per week (American Psychiatric Association, 2009). The antianxiety effects of exercise generally are less than antidepressants for clinical anxiety disorders but can be beneficial as part of an integrative treatment plan (Jayakody, Gunadasa, & Hosker, 2014). Prescriptive exercise has demonstrated efficacy as a treatment strategy for anxiety symptoms since patients are more likely to engage in activity when directed by their clinician. In a recent meta-analysis, exercise as a therapeutic intervention was found to be as effective as psychotherapy, and almost as effective as medication, for the treatment of anxiety symptoms (Wipfli, Rethorst, & Landers, 2008).

MIND–BODY MODALITIES

In 1979 mindfulness meditation was introduced into medical settings by Jon Kabat Zinn at the University of Massachusetts Medical Center. He has been instrumental in promoting its use as a treatment in Western medicine, and his research has set the stage for the wider acceptance of mind–body therapies (Kabat-Zinn et al., 1992). Derived from ancient Buddhist and yoga practices, mindfulness-based therapies include the eight-week standardized Mindfulness-Based Stress Reduction Program (MBSR; e.g., Kabat-Zinn, 1982), and also MBCT (e.g., Baer, 2003; Bishop, 2002; Salmon, Lush, Jablonski, & Sephton, 2009; Segal, Williams, & Teasdale, 2002). Both approaches have been widely studied and shown to be effective in patients with various stressors and anxiety symptoms.

MBSR (Kabat-Zinn, 1990) has been one of the most studied meditation-based programs with over 300 articles and has been shown to reduce symptoms of stress, depression, and anxiety (Hofmann, Sawyer, Witt, & Oh, 2010). MBSR is an eight-week program with standardized elements so that it is relatively the same regardless of the location or teacher. The basic premise is to try to remain in the present moment using nonjudgmental awareness of thoughts and feelings. It consists of weekly group meetings, a one-day workshop, and daily individual practice at home and includes (a) training in mindfulness meditation; (b) mindful awareness, for example, during a body scan or while engaged in yoga postures; and (c) mindfulness during stressful everyday situations and social interaction. The MBSR program is associated with decreases in the habitual tendency to react to or ruminate on various thoughts, feelings, and experiences (Ramel, Goldin, Carmona, & McQuaid, 2004; Teasdale et al., 2000), stress, depression, and anxiety symptoms (Chiesa & Serretti, 2011; Evans et al., 2008; Segal et al., 2002).

Kabat-Zinn et al. (1992) first investigated the efficacy of the eight-week MBSR program on anxiety scores in 22 patients who met the DSM criteria for panic disorder or GAD, as well as 58 subjects who did not meet formal criteria for an anxiety disorder but rated in the 70th percentile or above in anxiety symptoms based upon the Symptom Check List-90–Revised. At the end of the MBSR program, as well as at three-month follow-up, there was an overall reduction in anxiety and panic symptoms.

One study of 93 patients with GAD showed a nonsignificant difference between the MBSR and Stress Management Education program on one measure of anxiety but significant improvements with the MBSR group in other measures (Hoge et al., 2013). A meta-analysis published in 2010 suggested that mindfulness-based therapy is a promising intervention for treating anxiety and mood problems in clinical populations (Hoffman et al., 2010).

A number of psychological mechanisms have been proposed by which meditation and mindfulness techniques might reduce anxiety. One hypothesis is that meditation helps view negative thoughts and stressors with a more neutral approach and as transient events. The result is a decreased propensity for developing strong secondary emotional reactions that increase subjective distress (Roemer, Orsillo, & Salters-Pedneault, 2008). It has also been suggested that meditation programs such as mindfulness function as a form of gradual exposure therapy since people are asked to allow themselves to perceive stressors while remaining calm (Treanor, 2011).

From a physiological perspective, there is data that suggests that meditation practices may alter brain function by increasing frontal lobe activity that downregulates emotional responses (Yu et al., 2011). Data also suggests that meditation programs may alter serotonin and dopamine levels, contributing to more positive emotional responses (Newberg et al., 2017; Yu et al., 2011).

An approach that is related to meditation techniques is Herbert Benson's "relaxation response," which has been shown to result in a reduction of heart rate and stress levels (Benson, 1982). The relaxation response, similarly to other meditation-based programs, has been shown in RCTs to reduce anxiety and distress significantly. A randomized study of relaxation therapy compared to alprazolam showed that both interventions significantly decreased anxiety and depression in patients. However, the effect of alprazolam was slightly quicker for anxiety and stronger for depressive symptoms (Holland et al., 1991).

One study compared self-reported speech anxiety of students who were asked to visualize themselves making an effective speech with those who were not asked to visualize themselves making an effective presentation. Students who were asked to visualize reported lower anxiety levels than those who were not asked to do so (Ayres & Hopf, 1985). It was argued that visualization can be an effective, nondisruptive method that can reduce anxiety associated with public speaking.

Movement therapy using the Alexander Technique is aimed at reeducating people to do everyday tasks with less muscular and mental tension. It has been particularly used for people who have performance anxiety (Klein, Bayard, & Wolf, 2014). For example, evidence from randomized controlled trials suggests that Alexander Technique sessions can reduce performance anxiety in musicians. Additional studies will be necessary to determine if this technique is useful for other performance activities and anxiety in general.

Yoga and tai chi are mind–body practices that both derive from more historical approaches to health and well-being. Yoga is an ancient Indian tradition and a practice that consists of three components: gentle stretching, exercises for breath control, and meditation as a mind–body intervention. More recent yoga programs have removed much of the underlying spiritual elements so that it can be performed in a secular and nondenominational manner. A systematic review of eight studies for the effect of yoga in ameliorating anxiety showed that yoga reduced anxiety in a variety of populations for durations up to three months. Patients involved in the reported studies included psychiatric outpatients, patients with OCD, and patients with phobias. While yoga appeared beneficial, the studies evaluated suffered from methodological limitations such as inadequate randomization and high dropout rates. A more recent review also showed that yoga was beneficial for reducing anxiety in children and adolescents (Weaver & Darragh, 2015). However, there are few large-scale trials to assess efficacy.

Tai chi and chi gong are two forms of movement practices that have been used in China for centuries and have been shown to help reduce stress. A randomized controlled study by Lee et al. (2001) reported that Qi Gong Therapy could significantly reduce anxiety and cortisol levels and increase natural killer cells and neutrophil levels. Tai chi is practiced in China as both a form of exercise and as a martial art. The practice generally involves moving from a standing position through a series of postures and movements much like a choreographed dance. Sequences of postures are known as "forms," which require considerable time and concentration to master (Field, 2011). A recent systemic review 68 studies suggested that tai chi is likely to benefit individuals by reducing symptoms of anxiety and depression, especially in students of higher education (Webster, Luo, Krägeloh, Moir, & Henning, 2016).

Other Integrative Therapies for Anxiety

There are a number of alternative therapeutic options for patients with anxiety. Music therapy has generally been shown to be effective at reducing anxiety. Music therapy itself is typically defined as a controlled form of listening to music with the specific goal of trying to improve a person's psychological or physical health (Mofredj, Alaya, Tassaioust, Bahloul, & Mrabet, 2016). Several studies have demonstrated that music can reduce anxiety in the medical setting, such as in surgical suites, in intensive care units, with burn patients, and with the elderly, among other groups (Daniel, 2016; Li, Zhou, & Wang, 2017; Zhang et al., 2017). Since these areas are frequently associated with high levels of stress and anxiety, music provides a way of filtering out various unpleasant and unfamiliar sounds while also reducing the need for sedation (Bradt & Dileo, 2014). The mechanism most likely relates to the slow rhythms of music, which can affect the autonomic nervous system, specifically the parasympathetic system, which results in reduced heart rate, reduced blood pressure, and better muscle tone (Peng, Koo, & Yu, 2009). The most important element of music therapy is to find music that works for each specific individual. This usually requires several sessions with a music therapist in order to determine which style of music is the most beneficial for inducing a feeling of relaxation and decreased anxiety. This can be more problematic in the intensive care setting with patients who are unresponsive. Although music therapy has not been widely studied for the treatment of GAD, it has been shown to be effective in reducing anxiety in specific patient populations such as those with anorexia, amyotrophic lateral sclerosis, and various neurodegenerative diseases (Bibb, Castle, & Newton, 2015; Peck, Girard, Russo, & Fiocco, 2016; Raglio et al., 2016).

Art therapy is a more active process that involves the person participating in the production of various works of art, such as painting or sculpture. The goal is not simply to create art but to use the creative process as a way of expressing various issues and anxieties to help the patient identify and overcome them. As with music therapy, there is little specific data on anxiety disorders. However, several studies have demonstrated reductions in anxiety and depressive symptoms in various patient populations such as those with cancer or stroke (Eum & Yim, 2015; Monti & Peterson, 2004; Monti et al., 2006).

Aromatherapy uses essential oils from plants. There are a variety of different ways in which the oils can be used. They can be absorbed by the body through topical application on the skin including through the use of massage. The oils can be directly inhaled or can be dispersed via aerial diffusion systems such as via steam baths or diffusers. Several studies have explored the use of aromatherapy approaches to reduce anxiety during various medical interventions such as colonoscopy or surgery. However, these results have generally found that aromatherapy as applied in most of these studies does not significantly reduce anxiety (Hanprasertpong et al., 2015; Hu, Peng, Lin, Chang, & Ou, 2010; Schellhammer, Ostermann, Krüger, Berger, & Heusser, 2013). A systematic review of 16 aromatherapy studies concluded that this intervention does improve anxiety symptoms, but the studies included evaluated aromatherapy on secondary anxiety in patients with a variety of other medical disorders such as cancer or dementia or who were pregnant (Lee, Tsang, Leung, & Cheung, 2011). More studies will be required to ascertain whether aromatherapy is useful in patients with primary anxiety disorders.

Finally, massage therapy has similarly been explored in specific patient populations such as those with cancer or eating disorders. Therapeutic massage is a popular way that people manage anxiety, but there are few rigorous scientific evaluations for patients diagnosed with anxiety disorders. One study showed that massage in patients with chronic neck pain also had decreased anxiety symptoms (Celenay, Kaya, & Akbayrak, 2016). Black and colleagues (2010) performed the first controlled study of chair massage that reduced anxiety in 82 inpatients withdrawing from alcohol, cocaine, and opiates.

Ancient Medical Systems

Traditional Chinese medicine (TCM) is a medical system used in China for over 2,000 years. It is based on specific principles regarding how the body and its basic energy, Qi, work. The general theory is that distortions in the natural flow and content of Qi result in disease. In addition, other factors such as the "six excesses" of wind, cold, fire, dampness, dryness, and summerheat also influence the body's processes and lead to illness. Typically, TCM utilizes a combination of acupuncture, herbal remedies, exercise and meditation, and diet as a way of managing disorders such as anxiety.

Acupuncture is a popular integrative intervention that has a more substantive body of evidence from clinical trials regarding its efficacy in the treatment of anxiety symptoms. For example, there is evidence that acupuncture is comparable with CBT, which is a common intervention in the treatment of this condition (Chae et al., 2008; Hollifield, Sinclair-Lian, Warner, & Hammerschlag, 2007). A review by Pilkington, Kirkwood, Rampes, Cummings, and Richardson (2007) identified 10 randomized and two non-randomized clinical trials of acupuncture for generalized anxiety or other anxiety disorders and generally showed positive improvements in anxiety symptoms. A study of acupuncture in women undergoing in vitro fertilization showed reductions in anxiety and actually showed improvements in clinical pregnancy rates (Qian et al., 2017). Auricular acupuncture has been shown to be beneficial in reducing anxiety symptoms in patients undergoing dental treatments in a randomized trial (Michalek-Sauberer, Gusenleitner, Gleiss, Tepper, & Deusch, 2012). Potential mechanisms of action of acupuncture that may induce anxiolysis include increased release of serotonin and norepinephrine and cortisol modulation (Cheng, 2014).

Ayurveda is an ancient medical system from India and can be traced back about 8,000 years (Feuerstein, 1998). Over many centuries different forms of yoga developed with the goal to help restore and maintain health and elevate self-awareness and consciousness (Sovik, 2000). From the Ayurvedic perspective, anxiety is a dosha imbalance where excess vata accumulates in the nervous system. Doshas are three functional energies—vata, pitta, and kapha—which, when out of balance, cause symptoms and illness. Ayurvedic approaches to treatment focus on diet, yoga, and breathing exercises. For anxiety, patients are encouraged to avoid cold food, raw food, spicy food, and caffeinated beverages. In yoga, a common approach is to focus on bringing the legs up the wall, knee to chest, and using the child's pose. A small study of 34 patients showed that 12 weeks of performing yoga three times per week was more effective at reducing anxiety symptoms compared to a similar-duration walking program (Streeter et al., 2010). Using magnetic resonance spectroscopy, subjects were also found to have a positive correlation between changes in mood scales and changes in GABA levels in the thalamus. The scientific exploration of pranayama, which is the ancient science of breath, is in its infancy but has potential to relieve anxiety and stress-related illness by reducing sympathetic and increasing parasympathetic nervous system activity.

Use of Supplements for Anxiety

A wide variety of supplements has been explored for their potential use in patients with anxiety. Since these are described in some detail elsewhere in this book, we focus here only on supplements with anxiolytic properties. In terms of anxiety, some supplements are designed to help replete nutritional deficiencies, such as with magnesium or other vitamins and minerals. Botanicals have a variety of compounds that also can have an anxiolytic effect. However, it must always be realized that the use of supplements should be regarded in a similar manner to the use of medications in terms of both effectiveness as well as potential side effects. The response, side effects, and potential drug interactions should be carefully monitored in any patient started on the supplements.

Magnesium is important in many different biochemical reactions (Wester, 1987) and involved in a wide range of physiological processes in the body including normal nerve function, neuronal activity, cardiac excitability, and electrical properties of cell membranes (Altura, 1991). Magnesium also plays a role in blood vessel dilatation, platelet aggregation, and carbohydrate and lipid metabolism and has antispasmodic effects on skeletal and smooth muscle. It is a cofactor for more than 300 different enzymes. Food sources rich in magnesium include nuts, whole grains, legumes, and green leafy vegetables. The ideal dosage of magnesium is 100 to 750 mg/day with the primary side effect being loose stools. Magnesium oxide is widely used because it has a low cost and high elemental magnesium. Magnesium citrate might be better absorbed in the gastrointestinal tract, and there is some suggestion that magnesium glycinate may be less likely to cause diarrhea (Gaby, 2011, p. 139). One large double-blind RCT showed that magnesium supplementation, when combined with an herbal formula, decreased anxiety in patients with mild to moderate anxiety over a three-month period compared to placebo (Hanus, Lafon, & Mathieu, 2004).

Several studies of multivitamins and other nutrients have also shown some benefit for anxiety symptoms. Carroll, Ring, Suter, and Willemsen (2000) reported in a double-blind RCT in 80 healthy individuals that a multivitamin containing B vitamins, vitamin C, calcium, magnesium, and zinc significantly reduced anxiety symptoms. Another study in 44 women with premenstrual syndrome showed that combining magnesium with vitamin B6 significantly reduced anxiety symptoms (De Souza, Walker, Robinson, & Bolland, 2000).

Myoinositol is a natural isomer of glucose and is also a precursor in the intracellular phosphatidyl-inositol second-messenger cycle. As a supplement, there are several studies that have demonstrated its potential benefit in patients with depression, panic disorder, and OCD (Benjamin et al., 1995; Fux, Levine, Aviv, & Belmaker, 1996; Levine et al., 1995). Another small study showed that one month of inositol up to 18 g/day was comparable to one month of fluvoxamine up to 150 mg/day in patients with panic disorder (Palatnik, Frolov, Fux, & Benjamin, 2001). However, a meta-analysis approach did not find that inositol was beneficial in anxiety disorders (Mukai, Kishi, Matsuda, & Iwata, 2014), and thus more data is needed.

Botanicals

Lavender oil (currently prepared in a capsule as Silexan) has been shown in several studies to produce a calming and soothing response. One study randomized 77 patients with GAD to receive lavender oil or a benzodiazepine and found that both groups had similar reductions in anxiety symptoms of about 45% over a six-week period (Woelk & Schläfke, 2010). A related RCT showed that in 221 patients with anxiety disorders, lavender oil given 80 mg/day for 10 weeks resulted in significant reductions in anxiety symptoms compared to placebo (Kasper et al., 2010). A recent meta-analysis of five studies (n = 1,165) with patients with a variety of anxiety-related disorders showed significant improvements in symptoms (Generoso, Soares, Taiar, Cordeiro, & Shiozawa, 2017).

Lemon balm (*Melissa officinalis*) has calming, soothing, antispasmodic, and anxiolytic effects (Shakeri, Sahebkar, & Javadi, 2016). Several small RCTs suggest that lemon balm increases feelings of calmness in healthy participants (Kennedy, Little, & Scholey, 2004; Kennedy, Scholey, Tildesley, Perry, & Wesnes, 2002). Interestingly, these studies reported significant effects on self-rated calmness even though different dosages of lemon balm were used (ranging from 300 to 1600mg). The effects of lemon balm have not yet been investigated in patients with a formal diagnosis of anxiety or depression. It should be noted that lemon balm may be a mild thyroxine inhibitor so it should be used cautiously in patients with hypothyroidism (Shakeri et al., 2016).

Passionflower is another botanical that has also been shown to reduce anxiety symptoms. Akhondzadeh et al. (2001) reported that 45 drops of passionflower extract reduced anxiety symptoms in a comparable manner compared to oxazepam in 36 patients with GAD. In this study, oxazepam had a more rapid onset of effect but also resulted in more side effects compared to passionflower. Two double-blind RCTs reported that 500mg of passionflower significantly reduced anxiety symptoms relative to placebo in patients undergoing surgical procedures (Akhondzedah et al., 2001; Aslanargun, Cuvas, Dikmen, Aslan, & Yuksel, 2012). Importantly, no negative interactions with anesthesia and surgical outcomes were observed.

Valerian (*Valeriana officinalis*) has calming, anxiolytic, antispasmodic, and sedative effects. It is typically given in doses of 300 mg three times per day. Only one study of 36 patients with GAD has been performed with valerian. That study showed that valerian was comparable to diazepam in terms of reducing anxiety, but the study size precluded any definitive evaluation of valerian for anxiety. In addition, valerian is not suitable for the acute treatment of anxiety as it may take several weeks for a beneficial effect to occur. Valerian may potentiate the effect of antidepressants.

German chamomile (*Matricaria recutita*) has been shown to have anxiolytic, sedative, and calming effects when given at doses of approximately 200 to 220mg daily. A study by Amsterdam et al. (2009) showed that eight weeks of daily capsules containing 220mg of pharmaceutical-grade extract from German chamomile, standardized to 1.2% of the constituent apigenin, significantly reduced anxiety symptoms in patients with GAD. A larger ($N = 179$ patients with GAD), long-term RCT showed that 26 weeks of chamomile 500mg given three times per day resulted in significant reductions in anxiety symptoms compared to placebo with minimal side effects (Mao et al., 2016).

Kava kava (*Piper methysticum*) has anxiolytic, hypnotic, sedative, muscle relaxant, and mild analgesic properties. It is a perennial plant native to various regions of the South Pacific (Pittler & Ernst, 2003). Traditionally, the roots of the kava plant are prepared as a water-based beverage, which is used for medicinal and psychotropic effects (Witte, Loew, & Gaus, 2005). The anti-anxiety properties of kava appear to be attributed to a group of compounds called kavalactones (Bilia, Scalise, Bergonzi, & Vincieri, 2004). Kavalactones appear to function by modulating calcium and sodium channels (Gleitz, Gottner, Ameri, & Peters, 1996), modifying binding of ligands to GABA receptors (Boonen & Häberlein, 1998), and inhibiting noradrenaline uptake (Seitz, Schüle, & Gleitz, 1997). The result of these mechanisms is to reduce neuronal firing and the stress response. Standardized preparations typically contain 100 to 200mg of kavalactones per day. In 2002 the German drug regulatory authority (Bundesinstitut fur Arzeneimittel und Medizinproducte) banned kava kava and the FDA issued an advisory notice to consumers and healthcare professionals regarding the risk of rare but severe liver injury associated with the use of kava containing dietary supplements. On June 11, 2014, 12 years after the ban of kava, the German court ruling was reversed (Am Bot Council, 2014). In 2003, a Cochrane review evaluated seven RCTs regarding the effectiveness of kava in treating anxiety (Pittler & Ernst, 2003). The meta-analysis found kava to be effective in reducing anxiety scores relative to placebo. Another pooled analysis of six studies found kava effective at reducing anxiety compared to placebo (Sarris, LaPorte, & Schweitzer, 2011).

Conclusion

There are a number of potentially effective integrative approaches for the management of anxiety disorders and anxiety symptoms. While practices like mindfulness and yoga are useful nonpharmacological interventions, various supplements along with dietary and nutritional approaches can also be useful. The mechanism of action for these different interventions is likely distinct depending on whether there are peripheral or central effects. Ultimately, much more data is required to better determine which integrative interventions are most effective for specific types of anxiety.

REFERENCES

Ahmed-Leitao, F., Spies, G., van den Heuvel, L., & Seedat, S. (2016). Hippocampal and amygdala volumes in adults with posttraumatic stress disorder secondary to childhood abuse or maltreatment: A systematic review. *Psychiatry Research: Neuroimaging, 256*, 33–43.

Ait-Belgnaoui, A., Colom, A., Braniste, V., Ramalho, L., Marrot, A., Cartier, C., et al. (2014). Probiotic gut effect prevents the chronic psychological stress-induced brain activity abnormality in mice. *Neurogastroenterology and Motility, 26*(4), 510–520.

Akhondzadeh, S., Naghavi, H. R., Vazirian, M., Shayeganpour, A., Rashidi, H., & Khani, M. (2001). Passionflower in the treatment of generalized anxiety: A pilot double-blind randomized controlled trial with oxazepam. *Journal of Clinical Pharmacy and Therapeutics, 26*(5), 363–367.

Altura, B. M. (1991). Basic biochemistry and physiology of magnesium: A brief review. *Magnesium and Trace Elements, 10*(2–4), 167–171.

American Psychiatric Association. (2009). *Practice guideline for the treatment of patients with panic disorder* (2nd ed.). Washington, DC: Author.

American Psychiatric Association. (2013). *Diagnostic and statistical manual of mental disorders* (5th ed.). Washington, DC: Author.

Amsterdam, J. D., Li, Y., Soeller, I., Rockwell, K., Mao, J. J., & Shults, J. (2009). A randomized, double-blind, placebo-controlled trial of oral Matricaria recutita (chamomile) extract therapy for generalized anxiety disorder. *Journal of Clinical Psychopharmacology, 29*(4), 378–382.

Andrews, G., & Titov, N. (2010). Is Internet treatment for depressive and anxiety disorders ready for prime time? *The Medical Journal of Australia, 192*(11 Suppl.), S45–S47.

Aslanargun, P., Cuvas, O., Dikmen, B., Aslan, E., & Yuksel, M. U. (2012). Passiflora incarnata linneaus as an anxiolytic before spinal anesthesia. *Journal of Anesthesia, 26*(1), 39–44.

Ayres, J., & Hopf, T. S. (1985). Visualization: A means of reducing speech anxiety. *Communication Education, 34*(4), 318–323.

Baer, R. A. (2003). Mindfulness training as a clinical intervention: A conceptual and empirical review. *Clinical Psychology: Science and Practice, 10*(2), 125–143.

Baldwin, D. S., & Polkinghorn, C. (2005). Evidence-based pharmacotherapy of generalized anxiety disorder. *International Journal of Neuropsychopharmacology, 8*(2), 293–302.

Bandelow, B., Seidler-Brandler, U., Becker, A., Wedekind, D., & Rüther, E. (2007). Meta-analysis of randomized controlled comparisons of psychopharmacological and psychological treatments for anxiety disorders. *The World Journal of Biological Psychiatry, 8*(3), 175–187.

Becker, H. C. (2017). Influence of stress associated with chronic alcohol exposure on drinking. *Neuropharmacology, 122*, 115–126.

Benjamin, J., Levine, J., Fux, M., Aviv, A., Levy, D., & Belmaker, R. H. (1995). Double-blind, placebo-controlled, crossover trial of inositol treatment for panic disorder. *The American Journal of Psychiatry, 152*(7), 1084–1086.

Benson, H. (1982). The relaxation response: History, physiological basis and clinical usefulness. *Acta Medica Scandinavica Supplementum, 660*, 231–237.

Bercik, P., Park, A. J., Sinclair, D., Khoshdel, A., Lu, J., Huang, X., et al. (2011). The anxiolytic effect of Bifidobacterium longum NCC3001 involves vagal pathways for gut–brain communication. *Neurogastroenterology & Motility, 23*(12), 1132–1139.

Bercik, P., Verdu, E. F., Foster, J. A., Macri, J., Potter, M., Huang, X., et al. (2010). Chronic gastrointestinal inflammation induces anxiety-like behavior and alters central nervous system biochemistry in mice. *Gastroenterology, 139*(6), 2102–2112.

Bhui, K., & Fletcher, A. (2000). Common mood and anxiety states: Gender differences in the protective effect of physical activity. *Social Psychiatry and Psychiatric Epidemiology, 35*(1), 28–35.

Bibb, J., Castle, D., & Newton, R. (2015). The role of music therapy in reducing post meal related anxiety for patients with anorexia nervosa. *Journal of Eating Disorders, 3*, 50.

Bilia, A. R., Scalise, L., Bergonzi, M. C., & Vincieri, F. F. (2004). Analysis of kavalactones from piper methysticum (kava-kava). *Journal of Chromatography B, 812*(1), 203–214.

Bishop, S. R. (2002). What do we really know about mindfulness-based stress reduction? *Psychosomatic Medicine, 64*(1), 71–83.

Black, S., Jacques, K., Webber, A., Spurr, K., Carey, E., Hebb, A., & Gilbert, R. (2010). Chair massage for treating anxiety in patients withdrawing from psychoactive drugs. *Journal of Alternative and Complementary Medicine, 16*(9), 979–987.

Bolam, B., West, R., & Gunnell, D. (2011). Does smoking cessation cause depression and anxiety? Findings from the ATTEMPT cohort. *Nicotine & Tobacco Research, 13*(3), 209–214.

Boonen, G., & Häberlein, H. (1998). Influence of genuine kavapyrone enantiomers on the GABA-A binding site. *Planta Medica, 64*(6), 504–506.

Bradt, J., & Dileo, C. (2014). Music interventions for mechanically ventilated patients. *Cochrane Database of Systematic Reviews, 12*, CD006902.

Broderick, P., & Benjamin, A. B. (2004). Caffeine and psychiatric symptoms: A review. *Journal of Oklahoma State Medical Association, 97*(12), 538–542.

Brooks, S. J., & Stein, D. J. (2015). A systematic review of the neural bases of psychotherapy for anxiety and related disorders. *Dialogues in Clinical Neuroscience, 17*(3), 261–279.

Brugués, A. O. (2011). Music performance anxiety, part 2: A review of treatment options. *Medical Problems of Performing Artists, 26*(3), 164–171.

Bystritsky, A., Khalsa, S. S., Cameron, M. E., & Schiffman, J. (2013). Current diagnosis and treatment of anxiety disorders. *Pharmacy and Therapeutics, 38*(1), 30–38, 41–44, 57.

Carroll, D., Ring, C., Suter, M., & Willemsen, G. (2000). The effects of an oral multivitamin combination with calcium, magnesium, and zinc on psychological well-being in healthy young male volunteers: A double-blind placebo-controlled trial. *Psychopharmacology, 150*(2), 220–225.

Celada, P., Bortolozzi, A., & Artigas, F. (2013). Serotonin 5-HT1A receptors as targets for agents to treat psychiatric disorders: Rationale and current status of research. *CNS Drugs, 27*(9), 703–716.

Celenay, S. T., Kaya, D. O., & Akbayrak, T. (2016). Cervical and scapulothoracic stabilization exercises with and without connective tissue massage for chronic mechanical neck pain: A prospective, randomised controlled trial. *Manual Therapy, 21*, 144–150.

Chae, Y., Yeom, M., Han, J., Park, H., Hahm, D., Shim, I., et al. (2008). Effect of acupuncture on anxiety-like behavior during nicotine withdrawal and relevant mechanisms. *Neuroscience Letters, 430*(2), 98–102.

Chaouloff, F. (1997). Effects of acute physical exercise on central serotonergic systems. *Medicine and Science in Sports and Exercise, 29*(1), 58–62.

Charney, D. S., Heninger, G. R., & Jatlow, P. I. (1985). Increased anxiogenic effects of caffeine in panic disorders. *Archives of General Psychiatry, 42*(3), 233–243.

Cheng, K. J. (2014). Neurobiological mechanisms of acupuncture for some common illnesses: A clinician's perspective. *Journal of Acupuncture and Meridian Studies, 7*(3), 105–114.

Chessick, C. A., Allen, M. H., Thase, M., Batista Miralha da Cunha, A. B., Kapczinski, F. F., de Lima, M. S., & dos Santos Souza, J. J. (2006). Azapirones for generalized anxiety disorder. *Cochrane Database of Systematic Reviews, 3*, CD006115–CD006115.

Chiesa, A., & Serretti, A. (2011). Mindfulness-based cognitive therapy for psychiatric disorders: A systematic review and meta-analysis. *Psychiatry Research, 187*(3), 441–453.

Cotman, C. W., & Berchtold, N. C. (2002). Exercise: A behavioral intervention to enhance brain health and plasticity. *Trends in Neurosciences, 25*(6), 295–301.

Cremers, H. R., & Roelofs, K. (2016). Social anxiety disorder: A critical overview of neurocognitive research. *Wiley Interdisciplinary Reviews: Cognitive Science, 7*(4), 218–232.

Daniel, E. (2016). Music used as anti-anxiety intervention for patients during outpatient procedures: A review of the literature. *Complementary Therapies in Clinical Practice, 22*, 21–23.

De Souza, M. C., Walker, A. F., Robinson, P. A., & Bolland, K. (2000). A synergistic effect of a daily supplement for 1 month of 200 mg magnesium plus 50 mg vitamin B6 for the relief of anxiety-related premenstrual symptoms: A randomized, double-blind, crossover study. *Journal of Women's Health & Gender-Based Medicine, 9*(2), 131–139.

Dell'Osso, B., Buoli, M., Baldwin, D. S., & Altamura, A. C. (2010). Serotonin norepinephrine reuptake inhibitors (SNRIs) in anxiety disorders: A comprehensive review of their clinical efficacy. *Human Psychopharmacology, 25*(1), 17–29.

Deslandes, A., Moraes, H., Ferreira, C., Veiga, H., Silveira, H., Mouta, R., et al. (2009). Exercise and mental health: Many reasons to move. *Neuropsychobiology, 59*(4), 191–198.

Dugas, M. J., Brillon, P., Savard, P., Turcotte, J., Gaudet, A., Ladouceur, R., et al. (2010). A randomized clinical trial of cognitive-behavioral therapy and applied relaxation for adults with generalized anxiety disorder. *Behavior Therapy*, *41*(1), 46–58.

Dunn, A. L., Trivedi, M. H., & O'Neal, H. A. (2001). Physical activity dose-response effects on outcomes of depression and anxiety. *Medicine and Science in Sports and Exercise*, *33*(6 Suppl.), S587–S597.

Ellis, A. (2003). Early theories and practices of rational emotive behavior therapy and how they have been augmented and revised during the last three decades. *Journal of Rational-Emotive and Cognitive-Behavior Therapy*, *21*(3), 219–243.

Elman, M. J., Sugar, J., Fiscella, R., Deutsch, T. A., Noth, J., Nyberg, M., et al. (1998). The effect of propranolol versus placebo on resident surgical performance. *Transactions of the American Ophthalmological Society*, *96*, 283–294.

Eum, Y., & Yim, J. (2015). Literature and art therapy in post-stroke psychological disorders. *The Tohoku Journal of Experimental Medicine*, *235*(1), 17–23.

Evans, S., Ferrando, S., Findler, M., Stowell, C., Smart, C., & Haglin, D. (2008). Mindfulness-based cognitive therapy for generalized anxiety disorder. *Journal of Anxiety Disorders*, *22*(4), 716–721.

Feuerstein G. (1998). *The yogic tradition: Its history, literature, philosophy and practice*. Prescott, AZ: Hohm Press.

Field, T. (2011). Tai chi research review. *Complementary Therapies in Clinical Practice*, *17*(3), 141–146.

Foster, J. A., & McVey Neufeld, K. (2013). Gut-brain axis: How the microbiome influences anxiety and depression. *Trends in Neurosciences*, *36*(5), 305–312.

Fux, M., Levine, J., Aviv, A., & Belmaker, R. H. (1996). Inositol treatment of obsessive-compulsive disorder. *The American Journal of Psychiatry*, *153*(9), 1219–1221.

Gaby, A. R. (2011). Nutritional therapy in medical practice. 1011–1015.

Galper, D. I., Trivedi, M. H., Barlow, C. E., Dunn, A. L., & Kampert, J. B. (2006). Inverse association between physical inactivity and mental health in men and women. *Medicine and Science in Sports and Exercise*, *38*(1), 173–178.

Gelenberg, A. J., Lydiard, R. B., Rudolph, R. L., Aguiar, L., Haskins, J. T., & Salinas, E. (2000). Efficacy of venlafaxine extended-release capsules in nondepressed outpatients with generalized anxiety disorder: A 6-month randomized controlled trial. *JAMA*, *283*(23), 3082–3088.

Gleitz, J., Gottner, N., Ameri, A., & Peters, T. (1996). Kavain inhibits non-stereospecifically veratridine-activated Na+ channels. *Planta Medica*, *62*(6), 580–581.

Goddard, A. W., Mason, G. F., Almai, A., Rothman, D. L., Behar, K. L., Petroff, O. A. C., et al. (2001). Reductions in occipital cortex GABA levels in panic disorder detected with 1H-magnetic resonance spectroscopy. *Archives of General Psychiatry*, *58*(6), 556–561.

Goodwin, R. D. (2003). Association between physical activity and mental disorders among adults in the United States. *Preventive Medicine*, *36*(6), 698–703.

Gorman, J. M., & Kent, J. M. (1999). SSRIs and SNRIs: Broad spectrum of efficacy beyond major depression. *The Journal of Clinical Psychiatry*, *60*(Suppl. 4), 33–38.

Greden, J. F. (1974). Anxiety or caffeinism: A diagnostic dilemma. *The American Journal of Psychiatry, 131*(10), 1089–1092.

Greenlee, H., DuPont-Reyes, M. J., Balneaves, L. G., Carlson, L. E., Cohen, M. R., Deng, G., et al. (2017). Clinical practice guidelines on the evidence-based use of integrative therapies during and after breast cancer treatment. *CA: A Cancer Journal for Clinicians, 67*(3), 194–232.

Hanprasertpong, T., Kor-anantakul, O., Leetanaporn, R., Suwanrath, C., Suntharasaj, T., Pruksanusak, N., & Pranpanus, S. (2015). Reducing pain and anxiety during second trimester genetic amniocentesis using aromatic therapy: A randomized trial. *Journal of the Medical Association of Thailand = Chotmaihet Thangphaet, 98*(8), 734–738.

Hanus, M., Lafon, J., & Mathieu, M. (2004). Double-blind, randomised, placebo-controlled study to evaluate the efficacy and safety of a fixed combination containing two plant extracts (Crataegus oxyacantha and Eschscholtzia californica) and magnesium in mild-to-moderate anxiety disorders. *Current Medical Research and Opinion, 20*(1), 63–71.

Hassett, A. L., & Gevirtz, R. N. (2009). Nonpharmacologic treatment for fibromyalgia: Patient education, cognitive-behavioral therapy, relaxation techniques, and complementary and alternative medicine. *Rheumatic Disease Clinics of North America, 35*(2), 393–407.

Hidalgo, R. B., Tupler, L. A., & Davidson, J. R. T. (2007). An effect-size analysis of pharmacologic treatments for generalized anxiety disorder. *Journal of Psychopharmacology, 21*(8), 864–872.

Holland, J. C., Morrow, G. R., Schmale, A., Derogatis, L., Stefanek, M., Berenson, S., et al. (1991). A randomized clinical trial of alprazolam versus progressive muscle relaxation in cancer patients with anxiety and depressive symptoms. *Journal of Clinical Oncology, 9*(6), 1004–1011.

Hollifield, M., Sinclair-Lian, N., Warner, T. D., & Hammerschlag, R. (2007). Acupuncture for posttraumatic stress disorder: A randomized controlled pilot trial. *The Journal of Nervous and Mental Disease, 195*(6), 504–513.

Hoffman, E. J., & Mathew, S. J. (2008). Anxiety disorders: A comprehensive review of pharmacotherapies. *The Mount Sinai Journal of Medicine, 75*(3), 248–262.

Hoffman, P. (1997). The endorphin hypothesis. In W. P. Morgan (Ed.), *Physical activity & mental health* (pp. 161-177) Washington, DC: Taylor & Francis.

Hoffman, R. P. (2007). Sympathetic mechanisms of hypoglycemic counterregulation. *Current Diabetes Reviews, 3*(3), 185–193.

Hofmann, S. G., Sawyer, A. T., Witt, A. A., & Oh, D. (2010). The effect of mindfulness-based therapy on anxiety and depression: A meta-analytic review. *Journal of Consulting and Clinical Psychology, 78*(2), 169–183.

Hoge, E. A., Bui, E., Marques, L., Metcalf, C. A., Morris, L. K., Robinaugh, D. J., et al. (2013). Randomized controlled trial of mindfulness meditation for generalized anxiety disorder: Effects on anxiety and stress reactivity. *The Journal of Clinical Psychiatry, 74*(8), 786–792.

Hu, P., Peng, Y., Lin, Y., Chang, C., & Ou, M. (2010). Aromatherapy for reducing colonoscopy related procedural anxiety and physiological parameters: A randomized controlled study. *Hepato-Gastroenterology, 57*(102–103), 1082–1086.

Jacka, F. N., Mykletun, A., Berk, M., Bjelland, I., & Tell, G. S. (2011). The association between habitual diet quality and the common mental disorders in community-dwelling adults: The Hordaland Health Study. *Psychosomatic Medicine, 73*(6), 483–490.

Jacka, F. N., Pasco, J. A., Mykletun, A., Williams, L. J., Hodge, A. M., O'Reilly, S. L., et al. (2010). Association of Western and traditional diets with depression and anxiety in women. *The American Journal of Psychiatry, 167*(3), 305–311.

Jacob, K. S., & Kuruvilla, A. (2017). *Psychiatric Presentations in General Practice*. CRC Press: Boca Raton. P 83.

Jayakody, K., Gunadasa, S., & Hosker, C. (2014). Exercise for anxiety disorders: Systematic review. *British Journal of Sports Medicine, 48*(3), 187–196.

Kabat-Zinn, J. (1982). An outpatient program in behavioral medicine for chronic pain patients based on the practice of mindfulness meditation: Theoretical considerations and preliminary results. *General Hospital Psychiatry, 4*(1), 33–47.

Kabat-Zinn, J. (1990). *Full catastrophe living*. New York: Dell.

Kabat-Zinn, J., Massion, A. O., Kristeller, J., Peterson, L. G., Fletcher, K. E., Pbert, L., et al. (1992). Effectiveness of a meditation-based stress reduction program in the treatment of anxiety disorders. *The American Journal of Psychiatry, 149*(7), 936–943.

Kaczkurkin, A. N., & Foa, E. B. (2015). Cognitive-behavioral therapy for anxiety disorders: An update on the empirical evidence. *Dialogues in Clinical Neuroscience, 17*(3), 337–346.

Kasper, S., Gastpar, M., Müller, W. E., Volz, H., Möller, H., Dienel, A., & Schläfke, S. (2010). Silexan, an orally administered Lavandula oil preparation, is effective in the treatment of "subsyndromal" anxiety disorder: A randomized, double-blind, placebo controlled trial. *International Clinical Psychopharmacology, 25*(5), 277–287.

Kennedy, D. O., Little, W., & Scholey, A. B. (2004). Attenuation of laboratory-induced stress in humans after acute administration of Melissa officinalis (lemon balm). *Psychosomatic Medicine, 66*(4), 607–613.

Kennedy, D. O., Scholey, A. B., Tildesley, N. T. J., Perry, E. K., & Wesnes, K. A. (2002). Modulation of mood and cognitive performance following acute administration of Melissa officinalis (lemon balm). *Pharmacology, Biochemistry and Behavior, 72*(4), 953–964.

Kiecolt-Glaser, J. K., Belury, M. A., Andridge, R., Malarkey, W. B., & Glaser, R. (2011). Omega-3 supplementation lowers inflammation and anxiety in medical students: A randomized controlled trial. *Brain Behavior and Immunity, 25*(8), 1725–1734.

Kim, Y. W., Lee, S., Choi, T. K., Suh, S. Y., Kim, B., Kim, C. M., et al. (2009). Effectiveness of mindfulness-based cognitive therapy as an adjuvant to pharmacotherapy in patients with panic disorder or generalized anxiety disorder. *Depression and Anxiety, 26*(7), 601–606.

Klein, S. D., Bayard, C., & Wolf, U. (2014). The Alexander technique and musicians: A systematic review of controlled trials. *BMC Complementary and Alternative Medicine, 14*(1), 414.

Kushner, M. G., Abrams, K., Thuras, P., Hanson, K. L., Brekke, M., & Sletten, S. (2005). Follow-up study of anxiety disorder and alcohol dependence in comorbid alcoholism treatment patients. *Alcoholism: Clinical and Experimental Research, 29*(8), 1432–1443.

Kushner, M. G., Sher, K. J., & Beitman, B. D. (1990). The relation between alcohol problems and the anxiety disorders. *The American Journal of Psychiatry, 147*(6), 685–695.

Lange, I., Kasanova, Z., Goossens, L., Leibold, N., De Zeeuw, C. I., van Amelsvoort, T., & Schruers, K. (2015). The anatomy of fear learning in the cerebellum: A systematic meta-analysis. *Neuroscience & Biobehavioral Reviews, 59*, 83–91.

Lee, M. S., Huh, H. J., Hong, S., Jang, H., Ryu, H., Lee, H., & Chung, H. (2001). Psychoneuroimmunological effects of Qi-therapy: Preliminary study on the changes of level of anxiety, mood, cortisol and melatonin and cellular function of neutrophil and natural killer cells. *Stress and Health, 17*(1), 17–24.

Lee, Y., Wu, Y., Tsang, H. W. H., Leung, A. Y., & Cheung, W. M. (2011). A systematic review on the anxiolytic effects of aromatherapy in people with anxiety symptoms. *Journal of Alternative and Complementary Medicine, 17*(2), 101–108.

Leon, G. R., Fulkerson, J. A., Perry, C. L., & Early-Zald, M. B. (1995). Prospective analysis of personality and behavioral vulnerabilities and gender influences in the later development of disordered eating. *Journal of Abnormal Psychology, 104*(1), 140–149.

Levine, J., Barak, Y., Gonzalves, M., Szor, H., Elizur, A., Kofman, O., & Belmaker, R. H. (1995). Double-blind, controlled trial of inositol treatment of depression. *The American Journal of Psychiatry, 152*(5), 792–794.

Li, J., Zhou, L., & Wang, Y. (2017). The effects of music intervention on burn patients during treatment procedures: A systematic review and meta-analysis of randomized controlled trials. *BMC Complementary and Alternative Medicine, 17*(1), 158.

Liu, L., Liu, C., Wang, Y., Wang, P., Li, Y., & Li, B. (2015). Herbal medicine for anxiety, depression and insomnia. *Current Neuropharmacology, 13*(4), 481–493.

Mao, J. J., Xie, S. X., Keefe, J. R., Soeller, I., Li, Q. S., & Amsterdam, J. D. (2016). Long-term chamomile (Matricaria chamomilla L.) treatment for generalized anxiety disorder: A randomized clinical trial. *Phytomedicine: International Journal of Phytotherapy & Phytopharmacology, 23*(14), 1735–1742.

Maqsood, R., & Stone, T. W. (2016). The gut-brain axis, BDNF, NMDA and CNS disorders. *Neurochemical Research, 41*(11), 2819–2835.

Mathew, A. R., Norton, P. J., Zvolensky, M. J., Buckner, J. D., & Smits, J. A. J. (2011). Smoking behavior and alcohol consumption in individuals with panic attacks. *Journal of Cognitive Psychotherapy, 25*(1), 61–70.

McLean, C. P., Asnaani, A., Litz, B. T., & Hofmann, S. G. (2011). Gender differences in anxiety disorders: Prevalence, course of illness, comorbidity and burden of illness. *Journal of Psychiatric Research; 45*(8), 1027–1035.

McLeish, A. C., Zvolensky, M. J., Del Ben, K. S., & Burke, R. S. (2009). Anxiety sensitivity as a moderator of the association between smoking rate and panic-relevant symptoms among a community sample of middle-aged adult daily smokers. *American Journal on Addictions, 18*(1), 93–99.

Meredith, S. E., Juliano, L. M., Hughes, J. R., & Griffiths, R. R. (2013). Caffeine use disorder: A comprehensive review and research agenda. *Journal of Caffeine Research, 3*(3), 114–130.

Michalek-Sauberer, A., Gusenleitner, E., Gleiss, A., Tepper, G., & Deusch, E. (2012). Auricular acupuncture effectively reduces state anxiety before dental treatment—a randomised controlled trial. *Clinical Oral Investigations, 16*(6), 1517–1522.

Mochcovitch, M. D., da Rocha Freire, R. C., Garcia, R. F., & Nardi, A. E. (2014). A systematic review of fMRI studies in generalized anxiety disorder: Evaluating its neural and cognitive basis. *Journal of Affective Disorders, 167*, 336–342.

Mofredj, A., Alaya, S., Tassaioust, K., Bahloul, H., & Mrabet, A. (2016). Music therapy, a review of the potential therapeutic benefits for the critically ill. *Journal of Critical Care, 35*, 195–199.

Monti, D., & Peterson, C. (2004). Mindfulness-based art therapy (MBAT): Results from a 2 year study. *Psychiatry Times, 21*, 63–66.

Monti, D. A., Peterson, C., Kunkel, E. J. S., Hauck, W. W., Pequignot, E., Rhodes, L., & Brainard, G. C. (2006). A randomized, controlled trial of mindfulness-based art therapy (MBAT) for women with cancer. *Psycho-Oncology, 15*(5), 363–373.

Montoya, A., Bruins, R., Katzman, M. A., & Blier, P. (2016). The noradrenergic paradox: Implications in the management of depression and anxiety. *Neuropsychiatric Disease and Treatment, 12*, 541–557.

Mukai, T., Kishi, T., Matsuda, Y., & Iwata, N. (2014). A meta-analysis of inositol for depression and anxiety disorders. *Human Psychopharmacology: Clinical and Experimental, 29*(1), 55–63.

Murphy, Y., Wilson, E., Goldner, E. M., & Fischer, B. (2016). Benzodiazepine use, misuse, and harm at the population level in Canada: A comprehensive narrative review of data and developments since 1995. *Clinical Drug Investigation, 36*(7), 519–530.

Nehlig, A., Daval, J. L., & Debry, G. (1992). Caffeine and the central nervous system: Mechanisms of action, biochemical, metabolic and psychostimulant effects. *Brain Research Reviews, 17*(2), 139–169.

Nemeroff, C. B. (1989). Clinical significance of psychoneuroendocrinology in psychiatry: Focus on the thyroid and adrenal. *The Journal of Clinical Psychiatry, 50*(Suppl.), 13–20.

Ninan, P. T. (1999). The functional anatomy, neurochemistry, and pharmacology of anxiety. *The Journal of Clinical Psychiatry, 60*(Suppl. 22), 12–17.

Nutt, D. J. (1998). Antidepressants in panic disorder: Clinical and preclinical mechanisms. *The Journal of Clinical Psychiatry, 59*(Suppl. 8), 24–28.

Nutt, D. J., Ballenger, J. C., Sheehan, D., & Wittchen, H. U. (2002). Generalized anxiety disorder: Comorbidity, comparative biology and treatment. *International Journal of Neuropsychopharmacology, 5*(4), 315–325.

Öhman, A. (2005). The role of the amygdala in human fear: Automatic detection of threat. *Psychoneuroendocrinology, 30*(10), 953–958.

Olthuis, J. V., Watt, M. C., Bailey, K., Hayden, J. A., & Stewart, S. H. (2016). Therapist-supported Internet cognitive behavioural therapy for anxiety disorders in adults. *Cochrane Database of Systematic Reviews, 3*, CD011565.

Palatnik, A., Frolov, K., Fux, M., & Benjamin, J. (2001). Double-blind, controlled, crossover trial of inositol versus fluvoxamine for the treatment of panic disorder. *Journal of Clinical Psychopharmacology, 21*(3), 335–339.

Patterson, E., Cryan, J. F., Fitzgerald, G. F., Ross, R. P., Dinan, T. G., & Stanton, C. (2014). Gut microbiota, the pharmabiotics they produce and host health. *The Proceedings of the Nutrition Society, 73*(4), 477–489.

Peck, K. J., Girard, T. A., Russo, F. A., & Fiocco, A. J. (2016). Music and memory in Alzheimer's disease and the potential underlying mechanisms. *Journal of Alzheimer's Disease, 51*(4), 949–959.

Peng, S., Koo, M., & Yu, Z. (2009). Effects of music and essential oil inhalation on cardiac autonomic balance in healthy individuals. *Journal of Alternative and Complementary Medicine, 15*(1), 53–57.

Pilkington, K., Kirkwood, G., Rampes, H., Cummings, M., & Richardson, J. (2007). Acupuncture for anxiety and anxiety disorders—a systematic literature review. *Acupuncture in Medicine, 25*(1–2), 1–10.

Pittler, M. H., & Ernst, E. (2003). Kava extract for treating anxiety. *Cochrane Database of Systematic Reviews, 1*, CD003383.

Qian, Y., Xia, X., Ochin, H., Huang, C., Gao, C., Gao, L., et al. (2017). Therapeutic effect of acupuncture on the outcomes of in vitro fertilization: A systematic review and meta-analysis. *Archives of Gynecology and Obstetrics, 295*(3), 543–558.

Raglio, A., Giovanazzi, E., Pain, D., Baiardi, P., Imbriani, C., Imbriani, M., & Mora, G. (2016). Active music therapy approach in amyotrophic lateral sclerosis: A randomized-controlled trial. *International Journal of Rehabilitation Research, 39*(4), 365–367.

Ramel, W., Goldin, P. R., Carmona, P. E., & McQuaid, J. R. (2004). The effects of mindfulness meditation on cognitive processes and affect in patients with past depression. *Cognitive Therapy and Research, 28*(4), 433–455.

Ravindran, L. N., & Stein, M. B. (2010). The pharmacologic treatment of anxiety disorders: A review of progress. *The Journal of Clinical Psychiatry, 71*(7), 839–854.

Rickels, K., Rynn, M., Iyengar, M., & Duff, D. (2006). Remission of generalized anxiety disorder: A review of the paroxetine clinical trials database. *The Journal of Clinical Psychiatry, 67*(1), 41–47.

Roemer, L., Orsillo, S. M., & Salters-Pedneault, K. (2008). Efficacy of an acceptance-based behavior therapy for generalized anxiety disorder: Evaluation in a randomized controlled trial. *Journal of Consulting and Clinical Psychology, 76*(6), 1083–1089.

Roest, A. M., de Jonge, P., Williams, C. D., de Vries, Y. A., Schoevers, R. A., & Turner, E. H. (2015). Reporting bias in clinical trials investigating the efficacy of second-generation antidepressants in the treatment of anxiety disorders: A report of 2 meta-analyses. *JAMA Psychiatry, 72*(5), 500–510.

Saitz, R. (1998). Introduction to alcohol withdrawal. *Alcohol Health and Research World, 22*(1), 5–12.

Salmon, P., Lush, E., Jablonski, M., & Sephton, S. E. (2009). Yoga and mindfulness: Clinical aspects of an ancient mind/body practice. *Cognitive and Behavioral Practice, 16*(1), 59–72.

Salzer, S., Winkelbach, C., Leweke, F., Leibing, E., & Leichsenring, F. (2011). Long-term effects of short-term psychodynamic psychotherapy and cognitive-behavioural therapy in generalized anxiety disorder: 12-month follow-up. *The Canadian Journal of Psychiatry, 56*(8), 503–508.

Sander, D., Grafman, J., & Zalla, T. (2003). The human amygdala: An evolved system for relevance detection. *Reviews in the Neurosciences, 14*(4), 303–316.

Sarris, J., LaPorte, E., & Schweitzer, I. (2011). Kava: A comprehensive review of efficacy, safety, and psychopharmacology. *Australian and New Zealand Journal of Psychiatry, 45*(1), 27–35.

Sarris, J., Moylan, S., Camfield, D. A., Pase, M. P., Mischoulon, D., Berk, M., Jacka, F. N., & Schweitzer, I. (2012). Complementary medicine, exercise, meditation, diet, and lifestyle modification for anxiety disorders: A review of current evidence. *Evidence-Based Complementary and Alternative Medicine, 2012*, 1–20.

Schellhammer, F., Ostermann, T., Krüger, G., Berger, B., & Heusser, P. (2013). Good scent in MRI: Can scent management optimize patient tolerance? *Acta Radiologica, 54*(7), 795–799.

Schweitzer, I., Maguire, K., & Ng, C. (2009). Sexual side-effects of contemporary antidepressants: Review. *Australian and New Zealand Journal of Psychiatry, 43*(9), 795–808.

Segal, Z. V., Williams, J. M. G., & Teasdale, J. D. (2002*). Mindfulness-based cognitive therapy for depression: A new approach to preventing relapse.* New York: Guilford Press.

Seitz, U., Schüle, A., & Gleitz, J. (1997). [3H]-monoamine uptake inhibition properties of kava pyrones. *Planta Medica, 63*(6), 548–549.

Shakeri, A., Sahebkar, A., & Javadi, B. (2016). Melissa officinalis L.—a review of its traditional uses, phytochemistry and pharmacology. *Journal of Ethnopharmacology, 188*, 204–228.

Silverstone, P. H. (2004). Qualitative review of SNRIs in anxiety. *The Journal of Clinical Psychiatry, 65*(Suppl. 17), 19–28.

Simon, N. M., Worthington, J. J., Moshier, S. J., Marks, E. H., Hoge, E. A., Brandes, M., et al. (2010). Duloxetine for the treatment of generalized social anxiety disorder: A preliminary randomized trial of increased dose to optimize response. *CNS Spectrums, 15*(7), 367–373.

Sovik, R. (2000). The science of breathing—the yogic view. *Progress in Brain Research, 122*, 491–505.

Steenen, S. A., van Wijk, A. J., van der Heijden, Geert, J. M. G., van Westrhenen, R., de Lange, J., & de Jongh, A. (2016). Propranolol for the treatment of anxiety disorders: Systematic review and meta-analysis. *Journal of Psychopharmacology, 30*(2), 128–139.

Steptoe, A. S., & Butler, N. (1996). Sports participation and emotional wellbeing in adolescents. *The Lancet, 347*(9018), 1789–1792.

Streeter, C. C., Whitfield, T. H., Owen, L., Rein, T., Karri, S. K., Yakhkind, A., Perlmutter, R., Prescot, A., Renshaw, P. F., Ciraulo, D. A., & Jensen, J. E. (2010). Effects of yoga versus walking on mood, anxiety, and brain GABA levels: a randomized controlled MRS study. *Journal of Alternative and Complementary Medicine, 16*(11), 1145–1152.

Sussman, N., & Ginsberg, D. (1998). Rethinking side effects of the selective serotonin reuptake inhibitors: Sexual dysfunction and weight gain. *Psychiatric Annals, 28*(2), 89–97.

Teasdale, J. D., Segal, Z. V., Williams, J. M. G., Ridgeway, V. A., Soulsby, J. M., & Lau, M. A. (2000). Prevention of relapse/recurrence in major depression by mindfulness-based cognitive therapy. *Journal of Consulting and Clinical Psychology, 68*(4), 615–623.

Treanor, M. (2011). The potential impact of mindfulness on exposure and extinction learning in anxiety disorders. *Clinical Psychology Review, 31*(4), 617–625.

Tyrer, P. (1988). Current status of beta-blocking drugs in the treatment of anxiety disorders. *Drugs, 36*(6), 773–783.

Volkow, N. D., Fowler, J. S., Wang, G. J., Baler, R., & Telang, F. (2009). Imaging dopamine's role in drug abuse and addiction. *Neuropharmacology, 56*, 3–8.

Warren, R., Smith, G., & Velten, E. (1984). Rational-emotive therapy and the reduction of interpersonal anxiety in junior high school students. *Adolescence, 19*(76), 893–902.

Weaver, L. L., & Darragh, A. R. (2015). Systematic review of yoga interventions for anxiety reduction among children and adolescents. *American Journal of Occupational Therapy, 69*(6), 6906180070p1.

Webster, C. S., Luo, A. Y., Krägeloh, C., Moir, F., & Henning, M. (2016). A systematic review of the health benefits of tai chi for students in higher education. *Preventive Medicine Reports, 3*, 103–112.

Wester, P. O. (1987). Magnesium. *The American Journal of Clinical Nutrition, 45*(5 Suppl), 1305–1312.

Wipfli, B. M., Rethorst, C. D., & Landers, D. M. (2008). The anxiolytic effects of exercise: A meta-analysis of randomized trials and dose-response analysis. *Journal of Sport & Exercise Psychology, 30*(4), 392–410.

Witte, S., Loew, D., & Gaus, W. (2005). Meta-analysis of the efficacy of the acetonic kava-kava extract WS1490 in patients with non-psychotic anxiety disorders. *Phytotherapy Research, 19*(3), 183–188.

Woelk, H., & Schläfke, S. (2010). A multi-center, double-blind, randomised study of the lavender oil preparation silexan in comparison to lorazepam for generalized anxiety disorder. *Phytomedicine, 17*(2), 94–99.

World Health Organization. (2004). The World Heath Report 2004—Changing history. Retrieved from http://www.who.int/whr/2004/en/

Yu, X., Fumoto, M., Nakatani, Y., Sekiyama, T., Kikuchi, H., Seki, Y., et al. (2011). Activation of the anterior prefrontal cortex and serotonergic system is associated with improvements in mood and EEG changes induced by Zen meditation practice in novices. *International Journal of Psychophysiology, 80*(2), 103–111.

Zhang, Y., Cai, J., An, L., Hui, F., Ren, T., Ma, H., & Zhao, Q. (2017). Does music therapy enhance behavioral and cognitive function in elderly dementia patients? A systematic review and meta-analysis. *Ageing Research Reviews*, 35, 1–11.

Zinbarg, R. E., Eun Lee, J., & Lira Yoon, K. (2007). Dyadic predictors of outcome in a cognitive-behavioral program for patients with generalized anxiety disorder in committed relationships: A "spoonful of sugar" and a dose of non-hostile criticism may help. *Behaviour Research and Therapy*, 45(4), 699–713.

20

Integrative Treatment of Emotional Traumas

ANNA TOBIA

Key Points

- Posttraumatic stress disorder (PTSD) is a multifaceted and multifactorial disorder often requiring complex integrated plans of therapy.
- Single therapies are often not successful in PTSD.
- Meditation programs such as mindfulness have been useful in PTSD patients.
- Acupuncture has been shown to be beneficial for reducing PTSD symptoms.
- The Neuro-Emotional Technique that combines cognitive restructuring, acupressure, and biofeedback has been shown to reduce the emotional response to traumatic memories.
- Biofeedback helps reduce the body's reactivity to traumatic stimuli.
- Eye movement desensitization and reprocessing has been particularly effective in PTSD patients.
- Various plant based compounds such as ashwagandha or chamomile can help reduce anxiety symptoms.
- Medical cannabis might be useful in selected PTSD patients.

Introduction to PTSD

Across cultures and generations, people have understood that traumatic events can alter human functioning and behavior. Kucmin, Kucmin, Nogalski, Sojezuk, and Jojezuk (2016) reviewed the history of trauma and posttraumatic disorders and found evidence dating back 4,000 years of symptoms similar to our modern day understanding of posttraumatic stress disorder (PTSD). Analysis of the descriptions revealed that the types of stressors have changed; however, the way people react to intensive distressing events is basically similar throughout time. Essentially, traumatic events create a stress reaction that decreases cognitive and emotional functioning in some manner. As our understanding of PTSD has evolved from the first edition of the *Diagnostic and Statistical Manual of Mental Disorders* (called "gross stress reaction") to the current *Diagnostic and Statistical Manual of Mental Disorders* (fifth edition [DSM-V]), what is clear is that there are many events that cause PTSD and the presentation of the disorder is highly individualized.

PTSD is a heterogeneous disorder in two ways. First, the type of trauma experienced differs from one individual to another and the exposure can include different types of traumatic events. Second, the clinical presentation varies between individuals in the symptoms experienced, the severity of those symptoms, and their duration. First we explore the controversy on what constitutes a traumatic event, and second we discuss the way the disorder presents itself.

Defining what constitutes a traumatic event can be challenging, and many people can experience a PTSD-like syndrome across a range of stressful events (Roberts et al., 2012). However, the DSM-V clearly limits the diagnosis of PTSD to those who have been exposed to actual or threatened death, serious injury, or sexual violence. Even within this narrow band, between individuals the type of trauma experienced differs from one to another. Exposure can include different traumatic life events such as military combat, a natural disaster, physical or sexual assault, life-threatening illness, a terrorist attack, or a severe motor vehicle accident, and these can be experienced directly or witnessed (e.g., watching a sibling or parent be physically abused or responding to a vehicle accident for an EMT).

Taken more broadly, traumatic events are highly stressful and consequential events in which the person feels overwhelmed by extreme negative emotions. There is debate about the core attributes of traumatic events, and it is arguable whether events that do not involve a threat to physical safety or bodily peril can be a traumatic experience. Although by no means an exhaustive list, divorce, significant employment difficulties, loss of a close friendship, sexual betrayal, alcoholic parents, and poverty can contribute to traumatic reactions. It is important to remain alert to possible PTSD symptoms that may develop from such atypical distressing events. Gold, Marx, Soler-Baillo, and Sloan (2005) studied 454 undergraduates and found that those students who experienced nontraumatic stressors such as divorce of parents, relationship problems, or imprisonment of someone close to them reported even higher rates of PTSD symptoms than students who had experienced classical trauma.

Another factor that can impact the development of PTSD is the degree of exposure to the traumatic event (Antai-Otong, 2002). Referred to as peritraumatic factors in the DSM-V, it is further noted that the greater the magnitude of the trauma, the greater the likelihood of PTSD and that personal injury and perceived life threat increase the likelihood of developing PTSD.

The variability in presentation of PTSD symptoms is influenced by several risk factors that contribute uniquely to an individual's vulnerability to trauma. Factors such as personal and family psychiatric history, cognitive deficits, emotional maturity, temperament, gender, hardiness, and social support create an increased vulnerability to developing PTSD (Antai-Otong, 2002; Brewin, Andres, & Valentine, 2000). The complex role social support plays demands further clarification.

Social support can be perceived as positive or negative. Positive support typically involves interactions where others take an interest and one feels cared for, whereas negative social support is characterized by friends and family making demands, criticizing, and creating arguments. Examining them separately revealed that positive social support is associated with better mental health outcomes while negative social support is linked to higher psychological distress in those with PTSD (Grills-Taquechel, Littleton, & Axsom, 2011). Another study found that PTSD symptoms are associated with a subsequent decrease in perceived positive social support (King, King, Taft, Hammond, & Stone, 2006). These researchers found that severe PTSD symptoms two-years' postcombat exposure were associated with lower perceived positive social support five years later.

The distress experienced and expressed by survivors of some traumas (including aggression, impulsiveness, irritability, and substance abuse) may lead others to withdraw thus reducing sources of support (Guay, Billette, & Marchand, 2006). Nickerson et al. (2017) conducted a longitudinal study of those with traumatic injury. Participants were interviewed at 3, 12, 24, and 72 months posttrauma. Findings suggested that high levels of PTSD symptoms were associated with decreases in perceived social support in the year after trauma exposure and greater increases in perceived negative social support over the six years following the traumatic event. High levels of perceived social support did not have a buffering or exacerbating effect on subsequent PTSD symptoms.

The specific diagnostic symptoms that develop are heterogeneous, but the DSM-V categorizes them in the following way. PTSD is characterized by four hallmark clusters of symptoms: re-experiencing, avoidance, negative cognitions or mood, and hyperarousal (American Psychiatric Association, 2013). Diagnostic criteria require that symptoms last for more than a month. The DSM-V indicates that patients may experience symptoms for extended periods or symptoms may come and go over time (American Psychiatric Association, 2013). One study found that a third of cases may persist for more than 60 months (Breslau et al., 1998).

There is a high level of comorbidity among those diagnosed with PTSD (Resnick, Kilpatrick, Dansky, & Saunders, 1993). Most commonly associated psychiatric disorders include major depression and anxiety disorders, but people with PTSD are more likely than the general population to use drugs and experience impairments in psychosocial functioning and to engage in suicidal behavior (Bailey, Cordell, Sobin, & Neumeister, 2013). Patients with PTSD are also at an increased risk for other diseases including cardiovascular disease, arthritis, hypertension, autoimmune diseases, fibromyalgia, irritable bowel disease, and chronic migraines (Dobie et al., 2004; Sherman, Turk, & Okifuji, 2000; Zarei et al., 2016).

General Integrative Therapeutic Approach to PTSD

As PTSD constitutes a complex and heterogeneous condition, therapeutic benefit can be achieved by modifying different aspects of its multifaceted presentation, preferably using an integrative psychiatric model. In other words, because the clinical picture can vary, treating and understanding the core mechanisms of the disease and not just the specific symptoms can be useful. To better understand the mechanisms of PTSD, Sripada, Rauch, and Liberzon (2016) explored the psychological mechanisms of PTSD to aid in recovery and treatment. Thorough understanding of the mechanisms that impact PTSD are important. Emotion processing theory posits that to recover from PTSD a patient must emotionally engage with the traumatic memory, organize and process the trauma, and modify the negative trauma-related beliefs about the world and him or herself. PTSD develops when one or more of these do not occur (Foa & Kozak, 1986). By activating the fear so that it can be available to be modified in the safe confines of therapy allows the individual to process and resolve the emotions. This further allows disconfirming information to be presented (e.g., "I am in control now") and integrated.

Another mechanism that impacts PTSD is contextualization, which means how one responds to cues, depending on the context in which the cues occur. A recent study suggests that an impaired ability to distinguish between safety and danger contexts is common in individuals with PTSD (Lissek & van Meurs, 2015). Functional magnetic resonance imaging (fMRI) data suggest that there is a failure to modulate fear response according to context in that those with PTSD showed exaggerated fear response in safety contexts and unaltered fear response in danger contexts, suggesting they are not optimally using danger contexts to enhance fear (Garfinkel et al., 2014). Hollifield (2011) theorized that PTSD patients get stuck in a freeze response and because they are unable to successfully process the event by fighting or fleeing danger, the perceived threat continues even when the acute danger has passed.

Sripada et al. (2016) emphasized the role of distress tolerance as critical to understanding PTSD in that those with PTSD have a diminished capacity to tolerate distressing negative states, including distressing emotions and physical discomfort. They report that distress tolerance is strongly associated with PTSD symptomology. For example, low distress tolerance is associated with higher PTSD reexperiencing and avoidance symptoms even after adjusting for number of traumas, time since trauma, and depressive symptoms. Moreover, low coping flexibility correlates with higher PTSD symptoms as the number of traumatic experiences increases. Those with greater coping flexibility had lower PTSD symptoms.

Finally, negative posttraumatic cognitions, including negative cognitions about the self and world, are a core component of PTSD and predict the course of the illness. One study found there is a bidirectional relationship between PTSD symptoms and negative cognitions. Baseline PTSD was prospectively associated with an increase in negative cognitions about the self and the world, and negative cognitions were associated with subsequent increases in PTSD symptoms (Shahar, Noyman, Schnidel-Allon, & Gilboa-Schechtman, 2013). Similarly, persistent PTSD was associated with initial negative cognitions that worsened over time, suggesting that the behavioral symptoms of PTSD and distorted appraisals of PTSD symptoms might themselves exacerbate posttrauma cognitions (Dekel, Peleg, & Solomon, 2013). Sripada et al. (2016) describe robust support for PTSD treatments that target negative posttraumatic cognitions as they effectively decrease PTSD symptomology.

Trauma-focused exposure and cognitive restructuring–based therapies, along with stress inoculation therapy, are some of the limited psychotherapeutic approaches that have the highest rating within the Department of Defense/Veterans Administration guidelines for the treatment of PTSD (Wynn, 2015). Trauma-focused exposure slowly exposes people to the psychological trauma by prompting them to reflect on various parts of their traumatic experiences so that they eventually are able to manage and react to it. Cognitive restructuring focuses psychotherapy on modifying the specific thoughts a patient has regarding traumatic events. Stress inoculation therapy is a psychotherapeutic intervention with the goal of teaching skills to help people react differently to stressful situations.

While each of these can be helpful, dropout rates can be high, and talking about the trauma may not be comfortable or preferred for some patients. A comprehensive literature review on the psychological therapies for chronic PTSD in adults found only low quality evidence that trauma-focused cognitive behavioral therapy (TFCBT) was better than waitlist/usual care in reducing traumatic symptoms and associated symptoms of depression and anxiety (Bisson, Roberts, Cooper, & Lewis, 2013). Although the evidence was of low quality, the review of 70 studies of 4,761 participants found that TFCBT did statically better than waitlist at reducing clinician-assessed PTSD symptoms. The Food and Drug Administration has approved only two medications in the treatment of PTSD, paroxetine and sertraline. However, a recent review of treatments for PTSD by the US Institute of Medicine concluded that the response rate rarely exceeds 60%, even fewer patients (20% to 30%) achieve clinical remission, and there was not sufficient evidence for any drug or class of drug for the treatment of PTSD (Bailey et al., 2013). Integrative medicine, which includes complementary and alternative medicine (CAM), can make an important contribution in the treatment of PTSD. There are many integrative medicine approaches that can address the aforementioned mechanisms for PTSD and be useful in relieving symptoms of PTSD. Many integrative medicine and CAM modalities do not focus on talking about the traumatic experience, which is appealing to some patients. As such, integrative medicine approaches provide additional treatment options available to clinicians and their patients to help with the various complex elements of PTSD.

Meditation in PTSD

Meditation is a mind–body technique that has the general goal of training the mind through regulation of attention and emotion to impact the way the body functions and responds. One form of meditation that has been well researched is mindfulness, which emphasizes attention to emotional and physical stimuli. It is intentional, present-focused, nonjudgmental awareness of experiences. Typically offered in a group format as the Mindfulness-Based Stress Reduction (MBSR) program, mindfulness training has been useful in reducing depression and anxiety. More specific to PTSD, a pilot study examining fMRI data before and after mindfulness-based exposure therapy in those with PTSD suggested that this treatment leads to changes in neural processing of social-emotional threat related to symptom reduction (King et al., 2016). More specifically, post-treatment there were significant changes observed in the medial frontal cortex and amygdala. The authors suggest that the increased amygdala activity participants experienced with longer processing of angry faces correlated to greater PTSD symptom reduction reflected greater engagement and less avoidance of threat-related cues and thus greater emotional processing of these cues. As discussed earlier with regard to contextualization, separating out a true threat and then responding more appropriately is beneficial in reducing PTSD symptoms. Mindfulness involves engaging and observing both what is happening and how one is reacting to it. This is in opposition to the distraction/avoidance or suppression of emotional responses that increases distress in those with PTSD. A systematic review and meta-analysis of meditation programs (Mindfulness-Based Stress Reduction, yoga, and the Mantram Repetition Programs) and posttraumatic stress (Hilton et al., 2017) found that meditation interventions performed along with treatment as usual (TAU) significantly reduced PTSD symptoms compared with TAU, education, or present-centered therapy, across all sources of trauma. However, the treatment effects were positive for but not statistically significant for quality of life and anxiety symptoms. There was no evidence of any adverse reactions as a result of the meditation interventions (Hilton et al., 2017).

In an effort to assess the specific aspects of mindfulness that have the greatest impact on PTSD symptoms, Stephenson, Simpson, Martinez, & Kearney (2017) explored the five facets of mindfulness (Acting With Awareness, Observing, Describing, Non-Reactivity, and Nonjudgement) and changes in four aspects of PTSD (Re-Experiencing, Avoidance, Emotional Numbing, and Hyperarousal symptoms) Increases in mindfulness were significantly associated with reduced PTSD symptoms. Specifically, Acting With Awareness and Non-Reactivity were the aspects most strongly and consistently associated with reduced PTSD symptoms. Increased mindfulness was related to decreased Hyperarousal and Emotional Numbing.

Using data from a multisite Veteran's Administration project, Heffner, Crean, and Kemp (2016) evaluated responses before and after a meditation program and TAU. The authors concluded that meditation programs show promise as effective interventions in reducing PTSD severity. More specifically, significant effect sizes were found for meditation programs versus TAU. Mindfulness and Non-Reactivity were factors that also had significant changes. Because mindfulness encourages the acceptance of thoughts and feelings, it is possible that the avoidance that leads to and perpetuates PTSD is reduced. Conversely, higher PTSD symptom severity predicted lower levels of mindfulness in a group of outpatients with PTSD and substance use problems (Bowen, De Boer, & Bergman, 2017). Moreover, the relationship between mindfulness and substance use was also significant. The authors explain that Acting With Awareness in the presence of symptoms and having a Nonjudgemental stance were critical factors in attenuating the relationship between trauma and substance dependence.

A comprehensive review of mindfulness meditation explored the mechanism by which mindfulness may act (Khusid & Vythilingam, 2016) The authors report that many PTSD symptoms result from decreased activation in the prefrontal cortex (PFC) and insufficient inhibition of the amygdala (leading to overactivity) and that mindfulness has the opposite effect on the PFC-amygdala neurocircuit by activating the PFC and reducing bilateral amygdala activity. They suggest that adjunctive MBSR be offered to combat veterans with PTSD interested in self-management to decrease PTSD symptoms and improve health-related quality of life and mindfulness skills. They conclude that mindfulness interventions are safe, portable, and cost-effective and can be recommended as an adjunct to standard care or self-management strategy.

Yoga

Many doctors will recommend physical activity and exercise to reduce stress and improve well-being. In a meta-analysis of studies on physical activity and PTSD, physical activity has been found to improve PTSD symptoms although the data is very limited given the number of studies (Rosenbaum et al., 2015). There has been extensive research on the impact of yoga on health and PTSD. Yoga is a physical practice that utilizes postures, poses, movements, and breathing to improve well-being and enhance mental health. There is a social element to yoga, which could be helpful to those with PTSD, as well the meditative aspect and sense of control, which can both be challenging following a trauma. Generally, yoga has been found to decrease stressful reactions (Ross & Thomas, 2010) among healthy people. In a study of women with chronic, treatment-resistant PTSD, those who participated in 10 weeks of yoga experienced a significant reduction in symptom severity compared to the control group who attended a seminar on women's health (van der Kolk et al., 2014). In a long-term follow-up of those who completed the yoga training, the majority continued to practice yoga, and the greater the frequency of yoga practice, the greater the decreases in PTSD symptom severity (Rhodes, Spinazzola, & van der Kolk, 2016). The authors note that the study group had reported persistent mental health problems related to trauma despite having been in trauma-focused psychotherapy for three years. Moreover, they found that more frequent yoga practice over extended periods helped to sustain decreases in both PTSD and depression; however, it did not significantly help with dissociation symptoms. For veterans with combat-related PTSD, a six-week trial of yoga showed significant improvements in hyperarousal and sleep-related symptoms (Staples, Hamilton, & Uddo, 2013).

Another study followed women with chronic treatment-resistant PTSD who were randomly assigned to 10 weeks of yoga or supportive health education as a one-hour-a-week intervention (van der Kolk et al., 2014). Yoga significantly reduced PTSD symptoms compared to the control group.

One form of yoga, Sudarshan Kriya Yoga, which has four breath techniques, is described in a review article on the clinical application of yoga as especially beneficial (Brown & Gerbarg, 2005). Ujjay, also called ocean breath because of the sound made, is a slow breath technique involving two to four breaths per minute. In contrast, during Bhastrika, air is rapidly inhaled and forcefully exhaled at a rate of 30 breaths per minute. The third breath technique is to chant "om" three times with very prolonged expiration. Finally, Sudarshan Kriya involves cyclical breathing at varying rates: slow, medium, and fast.

Traditional Chinese Medicine in PTSD

Traditional Chinese medicine (TCM) is a broad category that includes many different interventions such as Chinese herbal remedies and pills, cupping, and acupuncture. It is amongst the oldest of the healing arts. These interventions are used to treat a pattern of illness rather than specific symptoms. The Chinese medicine doctor would explore how symptoms come and go and how they cluster together. Given that PTSD is a heterogeneous disorder with a varied clinical presentation, TCM is an excellent treatment option. A basic understanding of TCM is that all living things are made up of five elements—water, wood, fire, earth, and metal—which are related to organ systems and corresponding seasons. The balance or imbalance in these systems can, over time, become hardwired into one's constitution. This constitution is what predisposes someone to certain illnesses. Interestingly, TCM does not make distinctions between the mind and body and therefore works on both the physical and emotional level. Comorbidity consequently is seen differently than in Western medicine. For example, having gastrointestinal problems and PTSD would be understood as having multiple patterns of disease based on imbalances.

In a pilot study of acupuncture (Hollifield, Sinclair-Lian, Warner, and Hammerschlag, 2007), a prominent component in TCM, PTSD symptoms declined significantly from pre- to posttreatment with acupuncture, and 63% of patients no longer met *Diagnostic and Statistical Manual of Mental Disorders* (fourth edition) criteria for PTSD posttreatment. These gains were maintained at three months posttreatment. In reviewing animal studies of acupuncture, Hollifield (2011) concluded that acupuncture has biological effects that are relevant to PTSD pathology in that acupuncture downregulates limbic functioning (Napadow et al., 2005).

In a review article of CAM in refugees and survivors of torture, Longacre, Silver-Highfield, Lama, and Grodin (2012) found high efficacy for acupuncture and commented that for some refugee groups it is similar to traditional medicine from their country of origin. The authors also reported that acupuncture has the potential to alleviate the chronic pain associated with torture. Finally, they reported evidence that acupuncture can treat isolated symptoms of PTSD.

A randomized controlled trial of subjects with PTSD was conducted comparing acupuncture and TAU to TAU alone and found encouraging results (Engel et al., 2014). A standardized acupuncture treatment was conducted over four weeks and for an additional four weeks the acupuncturist was allowed to adjust the treatment based on individual needs. Both groups were followed for 12 weeks. At the conclusion, the acupuncture group showed significantly greater improvements in PTSD symptoms as well as improvements on ratings of depression, pain, and physical and mental health functioning. A review article on CAM approaches in the treatment of PTSD recommended that clinicians strongly consider including acupuncture as part of a comprehensive treatment plan for those suffering from PTSD, especially because of the relatively rapid improvement that is seen (Wynn, 2015).

The Neuro-Emotional Technique

Another technique that combines TCM with principles of cognitive therapy is the Neuro-Emotional Technique (NET). In this approach, the treatment involves identifying the cognitions such as the nature of the thoughts and internal dialogue associated with the trauma, the emotions that recollecting the traumatic event elicits, and the behaviors that are impacted (e.g., how the recollections affect actions such as avoidance of accomplishing tasks). During the desensitization phase of treatment, while thinking about the traumatic event and the cognitions and emotions associated with it, patients stimulate acupressure points and do simple breathing exercises. Three to five sessions have been demonstrated to be efficient in resolving traumatic memories (Monti, Stoner, Zivin, & Schlesinger, 2007).

A more comprehensive study of NET analyzed fMRI results pre- and post-NET treatment in those with traumatic stress symptoms of at least six months' duration (Monti et al., 2017). The initial arterial spin labeling fMRI scans in the NET group and the waitlist control groups both showed significant increases in the bilateral parahippocampus and brainstem during recollection of the traumatic event (see Figure 20.1). These structures correspond with distress, emotional activation, and emotional memories. After an average of four sessions of NET, these structures had a significantly different activation pattern compared to controls. Specifically, the hippocampus no longer reacted to the traumatic stimulus, suggesting a "normalization" of the brain's response to the trauma. Those receiving the NET intervention also had significant reductions in distress as measured by the Brief Symptom Inventory-18

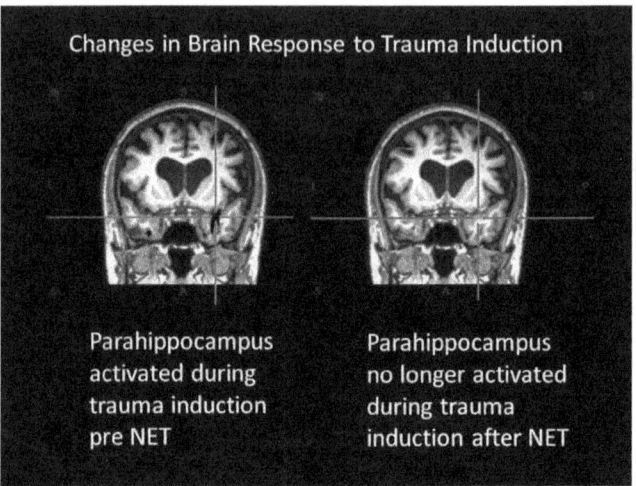

FIGURE 20.1. fMRI results of a representative subject showing difference between the pre- and post-NET scans in which subjects were exposed to the auditory presentation of their primary traumatic memory event. The scan shows activation in the parahippocampal region initially but no reactivity after undergoing the NET intervention. The implication is that the brain has "normalized" its reaction to the traumatic event.

global severity index, anxiety as measured by the State-Trait Anxiety Inventory (STAI) and traumatic stress as measured by the Impact of Events Scale (IES) and Posttraumatic Cognitions Inventory. This study showed that there were signature neurophysiological changes in brain function associated with clinical improvements after the treatment. Specifically, brain regions involved with traumatic memories and distress were markedly less responsive after the NET intervention.

Biofeedback in PTSD

Biofeedback teaches people to take control of their physiology like heart rate, respiratory rate, and muscle tension. Treatment involves training sessions during which one is connected to electrical sensors that give feedback about those areas of functioning. The goal is that one can learn to pace breathing and relax muscles to produce a reduction in distress and stress. Similarly, neurofeedback (also known as EEG biofeedback) seeks to alter patterns of brain activity associated with maladaptive cognitions and behaviors. This is done by giving an auditory or visual signal as a reward each time progress is made toward regulated neural activity. Because these techniques encourage one to actively control bodily functioning, they are particularly well suited for those with PTSD who often feel out of control and especially reactive. Moreover, research into brain functioning of those with PTSD revealed that there are altered patterns of brain functioning that can be corrected using feedback training (Johnson, Allana, Medlin, Harris, & Karl, 2013).

PTSD is associated with abnormal patterns of brain activity. Several brain regions have been found to be compromised in those with PTSD (Patel, Spreng, Shin, & Girard, 2012). More specifically, overengagement of the salience network, failure to properly recruit the central executive network and altered functional connectivity within the default mode network. Those with PTSD have also exhibited less activation of the medial PFC, which leads to a loss of top-down regulation of the emotional systems. This may contribute to amygdala hyperactivation, which has also been found in PTSD (Menon, 2011).

There is evidence that neurofeedback induces functionally and anatomically specific brain changes (Ros et al., 2013). In a review article on neurofeedback and PTSD, Reiter, Anderson, and Carlsson (2016) found a positive clinical effect and statistically significant reductions in targeted symptomology. Several of the studies included in the review found changes in brainwave activity and/or fMRI connectivity and a significant link between changes in network connectivity and calmness, particularly in the default mode network, central executive network, and salience network. Reiter et al. concluded that those with PTSD can have their brainwave activity and fMRI connectivity of core neurocognitive networks changed by neurofeedback training and that symptom resolution occurs.

Eye Movement Desensitization and Reprocessing

Another approach that is well researched and shows significant promise in PTSD is eye movement desensitization and reprocessing (EMDR; Shapiro 2001). It is a treatment for PTSD that is recommended by the Veterans Affairs and Department of Defense Clinical Practice Guidelines. The treatment involves inducing a series of rapid and rhythmic eye movements, sounds, or taps designed to facilitate cognitive changes and decrease anxiety. Patients bring the negative memories, emotions, and cognitions associated with the trauma to the forefront of their mind. One thought might be "I am powerless." Once the negative thoughts and feelings are processed, they can be replaced with positive cognitions such as "I am in control" or "I can handle it." The treatment continues until traumatic memories and emotions are significantly reduced (Wilson, Becker, & Tinker, 1995). One benefit to EMDR is that it works quickly to relieve symptoms. A meta-analysis of various treatments for PTSD found that EMDR tended to relieve symptoms more than behavior therapy and required fewer sessions (Van Etten & Taylor, 1998). A review study of EMDR compared the treatment to no treatment and other treatments (Shepherd, Stein, & Milne, 2000) and found that EMDR had a positive effect compared to no treatment and that it was as effective as exposure therapy and muscle relaxation and more effective than biofeedback-assisted relaxation and active listening therapy. The authors also found that the benefit was consistently attained after at least three sessions.

In a single-blind randomized controlled trial of outpatients in treatment for psychosis, those with PTSD were treated with either EMDR, prolonged exposure (PE), or a waitlist control (de Bont et al., 2016). Patients in the treatment group received eight weekly sessions, but all study participants were given medication, support of therapists, nursing care, and so on with the exclusion of trauma-focused treatment. The PTSD symptoms were successfully treated by both PE and EMDR. It is noteworthy in both groups that the severity of the paranoid thoughts decreased significantly and the rates of remission from psychotic disorders increased. It has previously been found that comorbid PTSD worsens the course and severity of psychotic disorders (Lysaker & Larocco, 2008). If comorbid PTSD can be diminished in those with psychosis, and that in turn leads to a reduction in psychotic symptoms, patients will be able to benefit twofold from a single approach. EMDR did not, however, reduce symptoms of depression in the de Bont et al. (2016) study.

A 2016 study utilized record review of active-duty military personnel. Personnel included in the study had visited mental health clinics where clinical outcomes had been monitored over a 10-week period using self-report measures of PTSD and disability (McLay et al., 2016). Service members who received EMDR were compared with those who had psychotherapy without EMDR. Results revealed that those receiving EMDR had significantly fewer therapy sessions over the 10 weeks but had significantly greater improvement on the PTSD Checklist.

There is some disagreement about the role of eye movements in the efficacy of EMDR, the mechanism of change, and if the eye movements are necessary (Davidson & Parker, 2001; MacCulloch, 2006). A meta-analysis by Lee and Cuijpers (2011) sought to clarify the importance of the effect of eye movements in EMDR treatment studies and to see if they significantly impact the processing of distressing memories. They included two groups of studies, those that used EMDR as treatment for anxiety disorders or in the treatment of a distressing memory and those in a laboratory format where participants thought of a distressing memory and were treated in a single session. The studies in the treatment group found a significant medium effect size advantage for eye movements over no eye movements. For those studies in the nontherapy contexts, a significant medium to large effect advantage was found for eye movements. The authors argue that focusing on an emotional memory and performing another task like eye movements disrupts the traumatic memory storage and that when these memories lose their vividness, trauma recovery can occur.

In as study comparing EMDR to a pill placebo or fluoxetine (a psychopharmacologic agent), EMDR was significantly superior to the placebo in terms of reducing PTSD symptoms and showed a greater percentage of loss of diagnostic status (van der Kolk et al., 2007). When compared to fluoxetine, EMDR was superior in attaining complete remission of symptoms at six months post treatment. Fifty-eight percent of the EMDR group were asymptomatic compared with none in the fluoxetine group, and self-reported depressive symptoms were significantly improved for the EMDR group.

Animal-Assisted Therapy

Some with PTSD can benefit from assistance from animals. Many individuals form strong bonds to their pets, companion dogs, and working animals. These bonds can have a significant positive psychological and physiological effect (Wynn, 2015). There are two means to incorporate animals into the care of those with PTSD, service dogs and animal-assisted therapy. Service animals are trained to perform tasks and assist people with disabilities. More than only a seeing-eye dog for those with visual impairments, dogs can be trained to remind people to take medication or can calm a person with PTSD. These animals undergo rigorous training to be able to assist with tasks the individual cannot perform.

Animal-assisted therapy is a structured therapy where the animal–human interaction facilitates progress toward specific therapeutic goals (Fine, 2000). Interactions with animals can decrease blood pressure and have a calming effect on those with dissociative disorder (Katcher, 1981) Wynn (2015) suggests that this model may be especially beneficial for those with PTSD who are experiencing issues of isolation and difficulty with social interactions. Animals have been demonstrated to facilitate social interactions and reduce loneliness, which may help people with PTSD connect to those around them (Wood, Giles-Corti, & Bulsara, 2005).

In a meta-analysis of animal-assisted interventions in those with trauma, there was a reduction in depression symptoms, PTSD symptoms, and anxiety (O'Haire, Guerin, & Kirkham, 2015). Several studies found improvements in social outcomes with one study finding an increase in involvement in helping others and feelings of social support, in addition to decease in frequency of nightmares. The authors concluded that the current data supports the short-term subjective benefits of animal-assisted interventions for trauma. However, intervention procedures varied greatly, making it difficult to recommend a specific treatment protocol.

A 2015 study explored the effectiveness of a specific form of equine therapy, Equine Partnering Naturally, which incorporates mindful observation (Earles, Vernon, & Yetz, 2015). Participants experienced a Criterion A traumatic even and had elevated scores on the PTSD Checklist. Six weekly, two-hour sessions focused on engaging with the horses while developing mindfulness skills. Participants' PTSD symptoms, emotional distress, anxiety symptoms, depression symptoms, and alcohol use decreased significantly by the completion of the study. Mindfulness increased following treatment.

Plant-Based Medicine

There has been a growing interest in herbal alternatives to traditional medications in the treatment of mental health disorders. Interventions that may improve anxiety disorders are classed as anxiolytics and typically impact the gamma-aminobutyric acid (GABA) system. A 2013 article reviewed clinical studies of plant-based medicines that were either anxiolytics with clinical evidence or psychotropic plant-based medicines with potential anxiolytic applications (Sarris, McIntyre, & Camfield, 2013). The results are summarized next.

Ashwagandha is an adaptogenic herb popular in Ayurvedic medicine. The name comes from Sanskrit and is a combination of *ashva* meaning "horse" and *ghadha* meaning "smell" because the root has a strong, horse-like smell. It has been found to produce an anxiolytic effect comparable to lorazepam in rats (20 and 50 mg/kg once daily for five days). A six-week study in humans diagnosed with anxiety disorders found that 500 mg twice a day resulted in 88% of patients meeting improvement on the Hamilton Anxiety Rating Scale to a score of 12 or below compared with 50% of the placebo (Sarris et al., 2013). However, clinician and patient ratings of improvement did not differ between the groups.

Preclinical research has found that brahmi, a leaf used throughout India for centuries, demonstrates antidepressant, anxiolytic, and antioxidant effects. A 12-week randomized controlled trial (RCT) involving elderly patients with mild cognitive impairment found that a brahmi extract of 300 mg/day significantly reduced anxiety scores on the STAI but the clinical effect was minor. A 12-week double-blind study using the same dose also found a significant reduction in STAI anxiety (Sarris et al., 2013).

Bitter orange, an oil from the bitter orange blossom, is purported to exert a psychologically calming effect. In a rat study, inhalation of the oil was compared to diazepam. Both effectively mitigated corticosterone response to the acute elevated plus-maze provoked stressor. Only one study was found using humans. In an acute double-blind placebo-controlled study of patients with preoperative anxiety, the bitter orange group had lower STAI-State and decreased scores on the Amsterdam Preoperative Anxiety and Information Scale compared to the placebo (Sarris et al., 2013).

Chamomile is commonly used in teas to produce a calming effect. It is a daisy-like plant used throughout Europe and was popular in the Middle Ages. Its flowers contain volatile oils and flavonoids. However, it is unclear if its effect is sedative or anxiolytic. One study concluded that the effect was not likely to be related to GABA-A receptor activation, and another showed chamomile inhibited both glutamic acid decarboxylase and GABA-transaminase. An eight-week double-blind RCT investigating chamomile extract found a significant reduction in anxiety symptoms compared to the placebo in patients with generalized anxiety disorder (GAD). This study used a dose ranging from 220 to 1,100 mg of an extract standardized to 1.2% apigenin varying according to response (Sarris et al., 2013).

Echinacea, an herb native to the western United States, Canada, and Europe, was used by Native Americans for a variety of ailments and may also have some anxiolytic effects. In a study of rats, there was a decrease in anxious behavior in the elevated plus maze test, social interaction, and social avoidance tests. In a healthy sample of adults given one to two tablets per day (20 or 40 mg concentrated echinacea extract) over one week, the higher dose significantly decreased STAI scores within three days until day 7 and for the two weeks of follow-up observation. The lower dose was not effective (Sarris et al., 2013).

Galphimia is traditionally used in Mexican and Central American cultures, and the leaves and stems are extracted from a small evergreen shrub. It has been shown to be effective in reducing anxiety. Using an aqueous extract of galphimia in a positive-controlled, double-blind RCT, patients with a Hamilton Anxiety Rating Scale (HAM-A) score over 19 were given either 1 mg of lorazepam twice daily or a 0.348 mg capsule of galphimine twice daily. Both treatments were effective, and there was no significant difference between groups (61.2% reduction for galphimia and 60.29% reduction for lorazepam), but whereas 21.33% of participants receiving lorazepam reported excessive sedation, no significant adverse effects were noted in the galphimine group. Another study reported in Sarris et al. (2013) found a greater reduction in HAM-A scores in the galphimia treatment group compared to lorazepam over 15 weeks.

Lemon balm is indigenous to southern Europe, Iran, and Central Asia and is in the mint family. Although it has not been as well studied, Sarris et al. (2013) suggest that it has does provide a clinically meaningful reduction in anxiety. In those with a diagnosis of anxiety disorder and sleep disturbance, lemon balm leaf extract was given at a dose of 300 mg twice daily for 15 days. There was a significant reduction in anxiety and associated symptoms from baseline, and insomnia was reduced significantly by 42%. Given that those with PTSD often struggle with insomnia, this may be an especially useful herb to consider.

Passionflower is a vine or shrub that is native to the southeastern United States from Virginia to Florida and as far west as Texas, Mexico, and Central and South America. It can be recommended for anxiety and sleep disorders, particularly the leaves, which have the greatest anxiolytic action. Several clinical trials described in Sarris et al. (2013) demonstrated significant reductions in anxiety symptoms. In a double-blind RCT with outpatients with GAD, a group taking passionflower extract at 45 drops plus a placebo tablet was compared with a group taking placebo drops and oxazepam at 30 mg per day. At the end of four weeks, both groups had a significant reduction in total mean HAM-A scores with no significant difference between groups.

Cannabinoids and Psilocybin

Given recent legal changes in the United States that make medical cannabinoids available, there have been more studies conducted on the effectiveness of psilocybin and cannabis. Psilocybe mushrooms contain the psychoactive compound psilocybin, which is a classical hallucinogen of the indoleamine class. Compared to lysergic acid diethylamide (LSD), the hallucinogenic experience associated with psilocybin has been described as more euphoric, less emotionally intense, as well as being associated with less panic and paranoia (Passie, Seifert, Schneider, & Emrich, 2002). In an effort to understand the impact of psilocybin on anxiety, Grob et al. (2011) gave 200 ug/kg of psilocybin or 250 mg of niacin to advanced-stage cancer patients. Measures were collected during the six-hour treatment period, as well as again two weeks later and at monthly follow-up visits for six months. During the acute treatment phase, a significant alteration in consciousness was found in the psilocybin group compared to the niacin, including a significant elevation in positive mood. At the two-week follow-up, there was a trend toward a greater reduction in the Profile of Mood States score in the psilocybin group compared to the niacin group. The longer term results were also positive. The psilocybin group had a significant reduction it STAI-Trait anxiety (at both one and three months), and there was a significant improvement in mood noted on the Beck

Depression Inventory (at six months). No significant adverse psychological effects were found to be associated with psilocybin.

There is clear evidence that the recreational or nonmedical use of cannabis (NMC) can increase mental health problems across a range of conditions from anxiety and depression to psychosis (Moore et al., 2007; Patton et al., 2002). NMC can lead to cannabis abuse or dependence, cognitive deficits, and impairment in attention and memory (Lundqvist, 2005). However, cannabis for therapeutic purposes (CTP) has shown benefit for physical health disorders and mental health concerns (Belendiuk et al., 2015). For anxiety generally, a review of the literature revealed that relaxation and relief of anxiety are the most widely reported motives for using CPT and NMC (Walsh et al., 2017). Among those with PTSD, 19% of CPT users report doing so to manage PTSD, and the use is associated with improved sleep and enhanced ability to cope with negative affect (Bonn-Miller, Boden, Bucossi, & Babson, 2014). A study of first-time CPT users seeking treatment for non-PTSD conditions found that 25% screened positive for a lifetime diagnosis for PTSD (Bohnert et al., 2014).

The question remains: Does CPT work for those with PTSD? Oral tetrahydrocannabinol (THC) and synthetic cannabinoids have demonstrated effectiveness for improving sleep duration and quality and reducing nightmares and daytime flashbacks in treatment-resistant patients with PTSD (Roitman, Mechoulam, Cooper-Kazaz, & Shalev, 2014). In a study on the efficacy of CPT on PTSD symptomology through analysis of data extracted from 46 articles, Yarnell (2015) found that taken together the studies suggest that there is a decrease in PTSD symptoms with marijuana use. Using a synthetic cannabinoid modulator, nabilone, Fraser (2009) gave 0.5 mg prior to bedtime. Participants had experienced PTSD-related nightmares for two years and had been unresponsive to conventional therapy. Seventy-two percent of the patients experienced total cessation or lessening of severity of the nightmares. These results were replicated in male military personnel with PTSD who had trauma-related nightmares that did not respond to standard treatment (Jetly, Heber, Fraser, & Boisvert, 2015).

Evidence suggests that patients with chronic PTSD already on stable medication may benefit from the addition of THC. Roitman et al. (2014) gave orally absorbable THC twice a day (5 mg) as an add-on treatment to stable psychotropic medication. Not only was it safe and well tolerated but more importantly it demonstrated a significant improvement in global symptom severity, sleep quality, frequency of nightmares, and PTSD hyperarousal symptoms.

In a review of the literature on cannabinoids and PTSD, Zer-Aviv, Segev, and Akirav (2016) concluded that animal studies suggest that administering cannabinoids following exposure to a traumatic event could prevent the development of dysfunctional stress-related processes and can prevent the effects of stress on emotional functioning and memory processes, facilitate fear extinction, and have an anti-anxiety effect in a variety of tasks. Moreover, they report that the studies they describe suggest that cannabinoids may offer therapeutic benefits for PTSD, especially for sleep quality, frequency of nightmares, and hyperarousal. They stress the need for a large-scale clinical trial examining the potential decrease in PTSD symptomology with the use of cannabis.

Conclusion

Several integrative medicine approaches can be incorporated into a comprehensive PTSD treatment program. When considering which approaches to bring together for a particular patient, there are several factors that the research has found to be important. In determining what works in the treatment of PTSD, Wampold et al. (2010) devised a table listing the elements of treatment that are effective in targeting PTSD (see Box 20.1).

Box 20.1 Elements of Effective Treatment

- Cogent psychological rationale that is acceptable to patient
- Systematic set of treatment actions consistent with the rationale
- Development and monitoring of a safe, respectful, and trusting therapeutic relationship
- Collaborative agreement about tasks and goals of therapy
- Nurturing hope and creating a sense of self-efficacy
- Psychoeducation about PTSD
- Opportunity to talk about trauma (i.e., tell their story)
- Ensuring the patient's safety, especially if the patient has been victimized as in the case of domestic violence, neighborhood violence, or abuse
- Helping patients learn how to avoid revictimization
- Identifying patient resources, strengths, survival skills, and intra- and interpersonal resources and building resilience
- Teaching coping skills
- Examination of behavioral chain of events
- Exposure (covert in session and in-vivo outside of session)
- Making sense of a traumatic event and patient's reaction to event
- Patient attribution of change to his or her own efforts
- Encouragement to generate and use social supports
- Relapse prevention

Wampold, B. E., Imel, Z. E., Laska, K. M., Benish, S., Miller, S. D., Fluckiger, C., et al. (2010). Determining what works in the treatment of PTSD. *Clinical Psychology Review, 30*, 923–933, Table 3. Reprinted with permission.

As this chapter explains, PTSD is a heterogeneous disease with varied causal events, clinical presentation, and comorbidity. There is no effective "one-size-fits-all" treatment for everyone. Many integrative medicine treatments reviewed are effective at quieting one's physiology and refocusing one's mind. As such, integrative medicine can play an important role in a comprehensive and successful treatment protocol for patients with PTSD.

REFERENCES

American Psychiatric Association. (2013). *Diagnostic and statistical manual of mental disorders: DSM-5(5th ed.)*. Arlington, VA: American Psychiatric Association.

Antai-Otong, D. (2002). Culture and traumatic events. *Journal of the American Psychiatric Nurses Association, 8*(6), 203–208.

Bailey, C. R., Cordell, E., Sobin, S., & Neumeister, A. (2013). Recent progress in understanding the pathophysiology of posttraumatic stress disorder: Implications for targeted pharmacological treatment. *CNS Drugs, 27*(3), 221–232.

Bisson, J. I., Roberts, N. P., Cooper, A. M., & Lewis, C. (2013). Psychological therapies for chronic post-traumatic stress disorder (PTSD) in adults. *Cochrane Database of Systematic Reviews, 2013*, 12.

Bohnert, K. M., Perron, B. E., Ashrafioun, L., Kleinberg, F., Jannausch, M., & Llgen, M. A. (2014). Positive posttraumatic stress disorder screens among first-time medical cannabis patients: Prevalence and association with other substance use. *Addictive Behaviors, 39*, 1414–1417.

Bonn-Miller, M. O., Boden, M. T., Bucossi, M. M., & Babson, K. A. (2014). Self-reported cannabis use characteristics, patterns and helpfulness among medical cannabis users. *The American Journal for Drug and Alcohol Abuse, 40*, 23–30.

Bowen, S., De Boer, D., & Bergman A. L. (2017). The role of mindfulness as approach-based coping in the PTSD-substance abuse cycle. *Addictive Behaviors, 64*, 212–216.

Breslau, N., Kessler, R. C., Chilcoat, H. D., Schultz, L. R., Davis, G. C., & Andreski, P. (1998). Trauma and posttraumatic stress disorder in the community: The 1996 Detroit Area Survey of Trauma. *Archives of General Psychiatry, 55*, 626–632.

Brewin, C. R., Andrews, B., & Valentine, J. D. (2000). Meta-analysis of risk factors for posttraumatic stress disorder in trauma-exposed adults. *Journal of Consulting and Clinical Psychology, 68*, 748–766.

Brown, R., & Gerbarg, P. (2005). Sudarshan Kriya yogic breathing in the treatment of stress, anxiety, and depression: Part II—clinical applications and guidelines. *Journal of Alternative and Complimentary Medicine, 11*(4), 711–717.

de Bont, P. A., van den Berg, D., van der Vleugel, B., de Roos, C., de Jongh, A., van der Gaag, M., & van Minnen, A. (2016). Psychosis, depression and social functioning in patients with chronic psychotic disorders. *Psychological Medicine, 46*, 2411–2421.

Dekel, S., Peleg, T., & Solomon, Z. (2013). The relationship of PTSD to negative cognitions: A 17-year longitudinal study. *Psychiatry, 76*, 241–55.

Dobie, D. J., Kiviahn, D. R., Maynard, C., Bush, K. R., Davis, T. M., & Bradley, K. A. (2004). Posttraumatic stress disorder in female veterans: Association with self-reported health problems and functional impairment. *Archives of Internal Medicine, 164*, 394–400.

Earles, J., Vernon, L., & Yetz, J. (2015). Equine-assisted therapy for anxiety and posttraumatic stress symptoms. *Journal of Traumatic Stress, 28*, 149–152.

Engel, C., Cordova, E., Benedek, D., Liu, X., Gore, K. L., Goertz, C., et al. (2014). Randomized effectiveness trial of a brief course of acupuncture for posttraumatic stress disorder. *Medical Care, 52*(12), S57–S64.

Fine, A. H. (Ed.). (2000). *Handbook on animal-assisted therapy: Theoretical foundations and guidelines for practice*. San Diego, CA: Academic Press.

Foa, E. B., & Kozak, M. J. (1986). Emotional processing of fear: Exposure to corrective information. *Psychological Bulletin, 99*, 20–35.

Fraser, G. A. (2009). The use of synthetic cannabinoid in the management of treatment-resistant nightmares in PTSD. *CNS Neuroscience & Therapeutics, 15*, 84–88.

Garfinkel, S. N., Abelson, J. L., King, A. P., Sripada, R. K., Wang, X., Gaines, L. M., & Liberzon, I. (2014). Impaired contextual modulation of memories in PTSD: An fMRI and psychophysiological study of extinction retention and fear renewal. *Journal of Neuroscience, 34*, 13435–13443.

Gold, S. D., Marx, B. P., Soler-Baillo, J. M., & Sloan, D. M. (2005). Is life stress more traumatic than traumatic stress? *Journal of Anxiety Disorders, 19*(6), 687–698

Grills-Taquechel, A. E., Littleton, H. L., & Axsom, D. (2011). Social support, world assumptions, and exposure as predictors of anxiety and quality of life following a mass trauma. *Journal of Anxiety Disorders, 25*, 498–506.

Grob, C. S., Danforth, A. L., Chopra, G. S., Hagerty, M., McKay, C. R., Halberstadt, A. L., & Greer, G. R. (2011). Pilot study of psilocybin treatment for anxiety in patients with advanced-stage cancer. *Archives of General Psychiatry, 68*(1), 71–78.

Guay, S., Billette, V., & Marchand, A. (2006). Exploring the links between posttraumatic stress disorder and social support: Processes and potential research avenues. *Journal of Traumatic Stress, 19*, 327–338.

Heffner, K. L., Crean, H. F., & Kemp, J. E. (2016). Meditation programs for veterans with posttraumatic stress disorder: Aggregate findings from a multi-site evaluations. *Psychological Trauma: Theory, Research, Practice, and Policy, 8*(3) 365–374.

Hilton, L., Maher, A. R., Colaiaco, B., Apaydin, E., Sorbero, M. E., Booth, M., et al. (2017). Meditation for posttraumatic stress: Systematic review and meta-analysis. *Psychological Trauma: Theory, Research, Practice, and Policy, 9*(4), 453–460.

Hollifield, M. (2011). Acupuncture for posttraumatic stress disorder: Conceptual, clinical and biological data support further research. *CNS Neuroscience and Therapeutics, 17*, 769–779.

Hollifield, M., Sinclair-Lian, N., Warner, T. D., & Hammerschlag, R. (2007). Acupuncture for posttraumatic stress disorder: A randomized controlled pilot train. *Journal of Nervous and Mental Disorders, 195*, 504–513.

Jetly, R., Heber, A., Fraser, G., & Boisvert, D. (2015). The efficacy of nabilone, a synthetic cannabinoid, in the treatment of PTSD-associated nightmares: A

preliminary randomized, double-blind, placebo-controlled cross-over design study. *Psychoneuroendocrinology, 51,* 585–588.
Johnson, J. D., Allana, T. N., Medlin, M. D., Harris, E. W., & Karl, A. (2013). Meta-analytic review of P3 components in posttraumatic stress disorder and their clinical utility. *Clinical EEG and Neuroscience, 44,* 112–134.
Katcher, A. H. (1981). Interactions between people and their pets: Form and function. In B. Fogle (Ed.), *Interrelations between people and pets* (pp. 41–67). Springfield, IL: C. C. Thomas.
Khusid, M. A., & Vythilingam, M. (2016). The emerging role of mindfulness meditation as effective self-management strategy, part 1: Clinical implications for depression, post-traumatic stress disorder, and anxiety. *Military Medicine, 181*(9), 961–968.
King, A. P., Block, S. R., Sripada, R. K., Rauch, S. A. M., Porter, K. E., Favorit, T. K., et al. (2016). A pilot study of mindfulness-based exposure therapy in OEF/OIF combat veterans with PTSD: Altered medial frontal cortex and amygdala responses in social-emotional processing. *Frontiers in Psychiatry, 7,* 154.
King, D. W., King, L. A., Taft, C. T., Hammond, C., & Stone, E. R. (2006). Directionality of the association between social support and post-traumatic stress disorder: A longitudinal investigation. *Journal of Applied Social Psychology, 36,* 2980–2992.
Kucmin, T., Kucmin, A., Nogalski, A., Sojezuk, S., & Jojezuk, M. (2016). History of trauma and posttraumatic disorders in literature. *Psychiatria Polska, 50*(1), 269–281.
Lee, C., & Cuijpers. P. (2011). A meta-analysis of the contribution of eye movements in processing emotional memories. *Journal of Behavior Therapy and Experimental Psychiatry, 3*(44), 231–239.
Lissek, S., & van Meurs, B. (2015). Learning models of PTSD: Theoretical accounts and psychobiological evidence. *International Journal of Psychophysiology, 98,* 594–605.
Longacre, M. M., Silver-Highfield, E., Lama, P., & Grodin, M. A. (2012). Complementary and alternative medicine in the treatment of refugees and survivors of torture: A review and proposal for action. *Torture, 22*(1), 38–57.
Lundqvist, T. (2005). Cognitive consequences of cannabis use: comparison with abuse of stimulants and heroin with regard to attention, memory and executive functions. *Pharmacology, Biochemistry and Behavior, 81*(2), 319–330.
Lysaker, P. H., & Larocco, V. A. (2008). The prevalence and correlates of trauma-related symptoms in schizophrenia spectrum disorder. *Comprehensive Psychiatry, 49,* 330–334.
MacCulloch, M. (2006). Effects of EMDR on previously abused child molesters: Theoretical reviews and preliminary findings from Ricci, Clayton, and Shapiro. *Journal of Forensic Psychiatry and Psychology, 17,* 531–537.
McLay, R. N., Webb-Murphy, J. A., Fesperman, S. F., Delany, E. M., Gerard, S. K., Roesch, S. C., et al. (2016). Outcomes from eye movement desensitization and reprocessing in active-duty service members with posttraumatic stress disorder. *Psychological Trauma, 8*(6), 702–708.
Menon, V. (2011). Large-scale brain networks and psychopathology: A unifying triple network model. *Trends in Cognitive Science, 15,* 483–506.

Monti, D. A., Stoner, M. E., Zivin, G., & Schlesinger, M. (2007). Short term correlates of the neuro-emotional technique for cancer-related traumatic stress symptoms: A pilot case series. *Journal of Cancer Survivorship, 1*, 161–166.

Monti, D. A., Tobia, A., Stoner, M., Wintering, N., Matthews, M., He, X. S., et al. (2017). Neuro-emotional technique effects on brain physiology in cancer patients with traumatic stress symptoms. *Journal of Cancer Survivorship: Research and Practice, 11*(4), 438–446.

Moore, T. H., Zammit, S., Lingford-Hughes, A., Barnes, T. R., Jones, P. B., Burke, M., & Lewis, G. (2007). Cannabis use and risk of psychotic or affective mental health outcomes: a systematic review. *Lancet, 370*(9584), 319–328.

Napadow, V., Makris, N., Liu, J., Kettner, N. W., Kwong, K. K., & Hui, K. K. (2005). Effects of electroacupuncture versus manual acupuncture on the human brain as measured by MRI. *Human Brain Mapping, 24*, 193–205.

Nickerson, A., Creamer, M., Forbes, D., McFarlane, A. C., O'Donnell, M. L., et al. (2017). The longitudinal relationship between post-traumatic stress disorder and perceived social support in survivors of traumatic injury. *Psychological Medicine 47*(1), 114–126.

O'Haire, M., Guerin, N., & Kirkham, A. (2015). Animal-assisted intervention for trauma: A systematic literature review. *Frontiers in Psychology, 6*, 1121.

Passie, T., Seifert, J., Schneider, U., & Emrich, H. M. (2002). The pharmacology of psilocybin. *Addiction Biology, 7*(4), 357–364.

Patel, R., Spreng, R. N., Shin, L. M., & Girard, T. A. (2012). Neurocircuitry models of posttraumatic stress disorder and beyond: A meta-analysis of functional neuroimaging studies. *Neuroscience & Biobehavioral Reviews, 36*, 2130–2142.

Patton, G. C., Coffey, C., Carlin, J. B., Degenhardt, L., Lynskey, M., & Hall, W. (2002). Cannabis use and mental health in young people: cohort study. *British Medical Journal, 325*(7374), 1195–1198.

Reiter, K., Anderson, S. B., & Carlsson, J. (2016). Neurofeedback treatment and post-traumatic stress disorder. *Journal of Nervous and Mental Disease, 204*(2), 69–77.

Resnick, H. S., Kilpatrick, D. G., Dansky, B. S., & Saunders, B. E. (1993). Prevalence of civilian trauma and posttraumatic stress disorder in a representative national sample of women. *Journal of Consulting and Clinical Psychology, 61*(6), 984–91.

Rhodes, A., Spinazzola, J., & van der Kolk, B. (2016). Yoga for adult women with chronic PTSD: A long-term follow-up study. *Journal of Alternative and Complementary Medicine, 22*(3), 189–196.

Roberts, A. L., Dohrenwend, B. P., Aiello, A. E., Wright, R. J., Maercker, A., Galea, S., & Koenen, K. C. (2012). The stressor criterion for posttraumatic stress disorder: does it matter? *Journal of Clinical Psychiatry, 73*(2), e264–270.

Roitman, P., Mechoulam, R., Cooper-Kazaz, R., & Shalev, A. (2014). Preliminary, open-label, pilot study of add-on oral 9-tetrahydrocannabinol in chronic post-traumatic stress disorder. *Clinical Drug Investigation, 34*, 587–591.

Rosenbaum, S., Vancampfort, D., Steel, Z., Newby, J., Ward, P., & Stubbs, B. (2015). Physical activity in the treatment of post-traumatic stress disorder: A systematic review ad meta-analysis. *Psychiatry Research, 230*, 130–136.

Ros, T., Yheberge, J., Frewen, P. A., Kluetsch, R., Densmore, M., Calhoun, V. D., & Lanius, R. A. (2013). Mind over clatter: Plastic up-regulation of the fMRI salience network directly after EEG neurofeedback. *Neuroimage, 65,* 324–335.

Ross, A., & Thomas, S. (2010). The health benefits of yoga and exercise: A review of comparison studies. *Journal of Alternative and Complementary Medicine, 16,* 3–12.

Sarris, J., McIntyre, E., & Camfield, D. A. (2013). Plant-based medicines for anxiety disorders, part 2: A review of clinical studies with supporting preclinical evidence. *CNS Drugs, 27,* 301–319.

Shahar, G., Noyman, G., Schnidel-Allon, I., & Gilboa-Schechtman, E. (2013). Do PTSD symptoms and trauma-related cognitions about the self-constitute a vicious cycle? Evidence for both cognitive vulnerability and scarring models. *Psychiatry Research, 205,* 79–84.

Shapiro, F. (2001). *Eye movement desensitization and reprocessing: Basic principles, protocols, and procedures* (2nd ed.). New York: Guilford Press.

Shepherd, J., Stein, K., & Milne, R. (2000). Eye movement desensitization and reprocessing in the treatment of post-traumatic stress disorder: A review of an emerging therapy. *Psychological Medicine, 30,* 863–871.

Sherman, J. J., Turk, D. C., & Okifuji, A. (2000). Prevalence and impact of post-traumatic stress disorder-like symptoms on patients with fibromyalgia syndrome. *Clinical Journal of Pain, 16,* 127–134.

Sripada, R. K., Rauch, S. A., & Liberzon, I. (2016). Psychological mechanisms of PTSD and its treatment. *Current Psychiatry Report, 18,* 99.

Staples, J. K., Hamilton, M. F., & Uddo, M. (2013). A yoga program for the symptoms of PTSD in veterans. *Military Medicine, 178*(8), 854–860.

Steenkamp, M. M., Litz, B. T., Hoge, C. W., & Marmar, C. R. (2015). Psychotherapy for military-related PTSD: A review of randomized clinical trials. *JAMA, 314,* 489–500.

Stephenson, K. R., Simpson, T. L., Martinez, M. E., & Kearney, D. J. (2017). Changes in mindfulness and posttraumatic stress disorder symptoms among veterans enrolled in Mindfulness Based Stress Reduction. *Journal of Clinical Psychology, 73*(3). 201–217.

Van der Kilk, B., Spinazzola, J., Blaustein, M., Hopper, J., Hopper, E., Korn, D., & Simpson, W. (2007). A randomized clinical trial of eye movement desensitization and reprocessing (EMDR), fluoxetine, and pill placebo in the treatment of post-traumatic stress disorder: Treatment effects and long-term maintenance. *Journal of Clinical Psychiatry, 68*(1), 37–46.

Van der Kolk, B. A., Stone, L., West, J, Rhodes, A., Emerson, D., Spinazzola, J., et al. (2014). Yoga as an adjunctive treatment for posttraumatic stress disorder: A randomized controlled trial. *Journal of Clinical Psychiatry, 75*(6), e559–565.

Van Etten, M., & Taylor, S. (1998). Comparative efficacy of treatments for post-traumatic stress disorder: A meta-analysis. *Clinical Psychology and Psychotherapy, 5,* 126–144.

Walsh, Z., Gonzalez, R., Crosby, K., Thiessen, M., Carrol, C., & Bonn-Miller, M. (2017). Medical cannabis and mental health: A guided systematic review. *Clinical Psychology Review, 51,* 15–29.

Wampold, B. E., Imel, Z. E., Laska, K. M., Benish, S., Miller, S. D., Fluckiger, C., et al. (2010). Determining what works in the treatment of PTSD. *Clinical Psychology Review, 30*, 923–933.

Wilson, S. A., Becker, L. A., & Tinker, R. H. (1995). Eye movement desensitization and reprocessing (EMDR) treatment for psychologically traumatized individuals. *Journal of Consulting and Clinical Psychology, 63*, 928–937.

Wood, L., Giles-Corti, B., & Bulsara, M. (2005). The pet connection: Pets as a conduit for social capital? *Social Science & Medicine, 61*, 1159–1173.

Wynn, G. H. (2015). Complementary and alternative medicine approaches in the treatment of PTSD. *Current Psychiatry Report, 17*, 62.

Yarnell, S. (2015). The use of medicinal marijuana for PTSD: A review of the current literature. *The Primary Care Companion for CNS Disorders, 17*(3).

Zarei, M. R., Shabani, M., Chamani, G., Abareghi, F., Razavinasab, M., & Nazeri, M. (2016). Migraine patients have a higher prevalence of PTSD symptoms in comparison to chronic tension-type headache and healthy subjects: A case-control study. *Acta Odontological Scandinavica, 74*(8), 633–635.

Zer-Aviv, T. M., Segev, A., & Akirav, I. (2016). Cannabinoids and post-traumatic stress disorder: Clinical and preclinical evidence for treatment and prevention. *Neurobehavioural Pharmacology, 27*, 561–569.

21

Addictions: Evidence for Integrative Treatment

MARY F. MORRISON, KAREN LIN, AND SUSAN GERSH

Key Points

- Substance use disorders are common among all demographics of the population.
- Many people with substance use disorders turn to integrative medicine approaches to help overcome this disorder.
- Conventional therapies such as pharmacological approaches are underutilized.
- Acupuncture may be helpful with substance use disorder, particularly with regard to ameliorating withdrawal symptoms.
- Yoga may be a helpful complementary therapy to tradition approaches for substance use disorder.
- Exercise appears to be an effective adjuvant to conventional smoking cessation treatment.
- Meditation approaches such as mindfulness may cause brain changes that reduce cravings and addictive behaviors.
- Mindfulness may help with relapse prevention after a person achieves abstinence.
- Biofeedback and neurofeedback may be useful for the treatment and prevention of various substance abuse disorders, but they require studies of longer duration with greater numbers of subjects.
- Herbal therapies have been suggested as possible complementary therapies in patients with substance abuse, but well-designed trials are required to determine their clinical use.

Introduction

This chapter focuses on integrative treatments for substance abuse disorder in which the use of substances leads to clinical and functional impairment or distress, specifically focusing on integrative therapies for alcoholism, drug abuse, and tobacco use disorder. Addiction is a common, chronic relapsing medical disorder with a neurobiological basis in the reward system in the brain and is categorized as either a substance addiction or a behavioral addiction. This chapter addresses only substance addictions, and nonsubstance-related behavioral addictions such as gambling, sex, and Internet addiction are not covered.

A substance use disorder is based on a problematic pattern of behaviors and feelings related to the use of the substance. Loss of control over the use of the substance is a key symptom in the transition from recreational use of the substance to a substance use disorder. The person may take more of the substance than he or she originally intended, use it more frequently, or take it instead of participating in social or professional activities. Craving is manifested by an intense desire to use the drug and signifies a transition from recreational use to a substance use disorder. A substance use disorder is evident when the substance use causes difficulty with work, relationships, or health and the person fails to cut down or abstain from the substance despite the difficulties that its use is causing. Initially, use of a substance is often associated with a rewarding feeling, such as euphoria, relaxation from stress, or a pleasant sense of omnipotence. Individuals who use substances chronically may undergo unpleasant withdrawal symptoms manifested by fatigue, irritability, anxiety, lack of motivation, and other physiologic symptoms caused by dependence on the specific substance withdrawn. For some people and for certain drugs, avoiding withdrawal symptoms is as important to ongoing addiction as drug craving and desire. The legal substance use disorders reviewed for the chapter include cigarette smoking, alcohol, marijuana (in some states), prescription opiates and benzodiazepines, as well as illegal substances such as cocaine, heroin, methamphetamine, and phencyclidine (PCP). However, the majority of studies regarding integrative treatments concentrate on cigarette smoking, alcohol, and opiate use disorders.

Can integrative medicine techniques help individuals with substance use disorders? The integrative approach combines mainstream medical therapies with complementary and alternative therapies for which there is some high-quality scientific evidence of safety and effectiveness. Many patients express interest in or are already using some form of these alternative therapies. A 2006 survey disclosed that 27% of smokers were using some form of complementary and alternative therapies (Sood, Ebbert, Sood, & Stevens, 2006). The same survey showed that 67% of smokers trying to quit were interested in using practices such as meditation, yoga, or massage to relieve stress and aid in cessation of tobacco use. Integrative therapies tend to be more acceptable to people and are perceived as more natural and health promoting. Integrative medicine therapies are common, with at least one-third of American adults using some form of complementary therapies. Another benefit of integrative practices is that they are often less expensive and may have fewer side effects compared with conventional therapies. The focus of integrated medicine practices on enriching health may enhance outcomes for addiction treatment, as well as attract vulnerable individuals who are desperate to reduce their harmful behavior. Substance abuse treatments should improve an individual's self-regulation of emotion, behavior, and cognition around substances. Integrative therapies can also target disorders that make recovery from addiction more difficult such as attention deficit disorder, since individuals with attention deficits and comorbid substance abuse have lower abstinence rates and are less likely to complete treatment programs. Despite an expanding number of scientific studies and clinical trials that suggest benefit of integrative practices in the treatment of addiction, the available studies are often limited by small sample sizes, lack of control groups, and widely varied outcome measures. More rigorous, evidence-based research is needed to further support and delineate the mechanisms for the therapeutic effects of these therapies as well as their efficacy and cost-effectiveness.

Magnitude of the Problem

Abuse and misuse of legal drugs, prescription drugs, and illicit drugs is a highly prevalent public health issue. Illicit drug use is a common disorder with 9.2% of the US population age 12 and older reporting having used illicit drugs (not including marijuana) in 2015 (Substance Abuse and Mental Health Services, 2016). Encouragingly, the 2015 numbers for tobacco and alcohol use represent a slight decline in use from 2014; however, the 2015 data also reveal that 7.1% of the adolescent/adult population reported misuse of prescription psychotherapeutics and 13.5% of the adolescent/adult population used marijuana. For legal drug use in adolescents/adults, the prevalence is even higher, with 29.2% using tobacco products and 65.7% using alcohol (Substance Abuse and Mental Health Services, 2016). Abuse of tobacco, alcohol, and illicit drugs is expensive, costing more than $700 billion annually in the United States including costs related to crime, lost work productivity, and healthcare, including more than

$165 billion in healthcare costs alone (National Institute of Drug Abuse, 2015). Globally, tobacco, alcohol, and illicit drugs are a substantial cause of mortality. In 2002, the World Health Organization estimated that 8.8% of deaths worldwide were related to tobacco use, 3.2% were related to alcohol use, and 0.4% were related to illicit drugs, with the majority of deaths in men.

Conventional Therapies

Conventional treatment for tobacco, alcohol, and illicit drug disorders consist of behavioral/psychotherapeutic approaches as well as pharmacologic approaches. Pharmacologic approaches tend to be underutilized by healthcare professionals, and even when they are utilized in ideal populations, such as clinical trials, they have limited efficacy (Lee, Kresina, Campopiano, Lubran, & Clark, 2015). Contingency management is based on the idea of rewarding individuals with addiction for a desired behavior, namely abstinence or substance reduction. Contingency management is effective in retaining patients in treatment and reducing substance use but can be costly. Other psychotherapeutic methods for substance use disorders include cognitive-behavioral therapy, family therapy, and motivation enhancement therapy. A complete review of conventional therapies for substance abuse treatment is beyond the scope of this chapter, which is focused on integrative therapies, but readers are referred to Galanter, Kleber, and Brady (2015) for conventional treatment approaches.

Integrative Therapies: Acupuncture

Acupuncture is the practice of inserting thin, solid needles into specific designated acupuncture points in the body. This therapeutic modality is part of traditional Chinese medicine and is based on the principle that there is a network of energy pathways called meridians in which the body's energy, qi, flows. The theory of Yin and Yang is a core concept of traditional Chinese medicine and maintains that all things in the universe may be categorized as either Yin or Yang. However, nothing is ever all Yin or all Yang but rather a balance between these two forces that are opposite but complementary and interdependent. Yin is generally associated with concepts and objects that are dark, cold, and still; examples include winter, death, female, night, and the body's solid organs. Yang is generally associated with ideas or items that are bright, warm, and in motion; examples include summer, birth, male, day, and the body's hollow organs. Additionally, any given frame of reference has a Yin and Yang aspect—for example, time can be divided into day (Yang) and night

(Yin). Bodily functions are optimal when there is a balance between the Yin and Yang in the body with smooth flow of qi in the meridians; however, when there are blockages in the flow of qi, symptoms emerge. Acupuncture can be used to relieve these blockages and restore balance, thereby alleviating symptoms. During acupuncture, needles are strategically placed subcutaneously and may be manipulated manually. Alternatively, an electrical stimulator is used on skin electrodes to deliver electric current or laser light is directed onto acupuncture points.

Acupuncture has been practiced in China since 2500 BC and has been gaining worldwide popularity as an alternative, complementary, and integrative therapeutic intervention for a multitude of medical conditions. Its use for substance abuse dates back to 1972 when Dr. Wen, a neurosurgeon in Hong Kong, observed that acupuncture used for preoperative anesthesia also decreased opiate withdrawal symptoms in patients with opiate addiction (Lin, Chan, & Chen, 2012). Anesthesia acupuncture points initially were the basis for treating drug abuse with acupuncture. The procedure was developed by Dr. M. Smith in 1985 and was known as the NADA (National Acupuncture Detoxification Association) protocol (Stuyt & Voyles, 2016). In 1996, the World Health Organization (WHO) specified 64 conditions for which acupuncture can be considered. Alcohol dependence and detoxification, cocaine, heroin, opium, and tobacco dependence were proposed as conditions for which a therapeutic effect has been shown but for which further proof is needed (WHO, 2003). In the same year, the Center for Substance Abuse Treatment of the National Institutes of Health (NIH) published a report, Treatment Improvement Protocol Series 19: "Detoxification from Alcohol and Other Drugs," that gave modest support for the use of acupuncture in opiate detoxification (Lin et al., 2012).

The following year, the NIH published the Acupuncture NIH Consensus statement, which concluded, "There are other situations such as addiction . . . for which acupuncture may be useful as an adjunct treatment or an acceptable alternative or be included in a comprehensive management program." Further developments in acupuncture treatment for opiate abuse were made by Dr. Han of Peking University in Beijing in 2005. His treatment modification used electrical stimulation of skin electrodes at acupuncture points (Lin et al., 2012).

The best-known and -understood mechanism of acupuncture in the treatment of drug abuse is its effects on the endogenous opiate system. Both manual acupuncture and electroacupuncture trigger a cascade of events that lead to the release of endogenous β-endorphin, enkephalin, and dynorphin in the central nervous system (Han, 2004). Further evidence that acupuncture exerts an effect on the opioid system is that the injection of naloxone, an opiate antagonist, can extinguish the opioid-induced analgesic effects of acupuncture. Other prominent effects of acupuncture include increases in epinephrine, serotonin, norepinephrine, and dopamine in the central nervous system and bloodstream, all of which might mediate effects on substance abuse (Motlagh, Ibrahim, Fashid, Seghatoleslam, & Habil, 2016).

The research supporting the effectiveness of acupuncture has been limited for various reasons. The gold standard Western approach to research and determining robust evidence-based therapies are randomized, double-blind, placebo-controlled trials. While it is possible to randomize acupuncture subjects, it is difficult to blind the recipient to acupuncture, and it is not at all possible to blind the acupuncturist performing the treatment. An appropriate placebo is also difficult to establish as significant evidence suggests that "sham" acupuncture (needle placement at nonacupuncture points) is not completely inert. In addition, acupuncture is often performed as a holistic therapy in which point selection may be individualized and unique to a patient's specific clinical presentation. Quality issues of existing studies include small sample size, lack of control arm, and lack of randomization. Other design issues to be considered are variability in outcome measures, point selection for similar disorders, and type of acupuncture (body, auricular, or other microsystem acupuncture, with or without electrical stimulation).

While acupuncture point selection for substance abuse has some variability, the NADA protocol utilizes five specific auricular points for the treatment of addiction. Needles are inserted, without electrical stimulation, into ear acupuncture points called sympathetic, shen men, kidney, lung, and liver. The NADA protocol aims to relieve withdrawal symptoms and alleviate or prevent symptoms of craving. Treatment is usually performed in a group setting and has been shown to increase patient participation rates in long-term treatment programs (Lin et al., 2012). There is growing evidence of the NADA protocol's positive effects, but large-scale studies are currently lacking (Han, 2004). Some advantages of the NADA protocol as an adjunct to comprehensive drug treatment programs are its easy administration, lack of adverse effects, and acceptability to patients (Motlagh et al., 2016).

As with much of acupuncture research, the heterogeneity of the acupuncture modalities and study designs makes it difficult to draw strong conclusions with regard to the effect of acupuncture on the treatment of alcohol addiction. There are two large randomized single-blind, placebo-controlled trials with conflicting results on the effects of acupuncture on reducing alcohol use. Other studies show no reduction in the duration and severity of alcohol withdrawal symptoms with auricular acupuncture or laser auricular acupuncture therapy. However, laser therapy utilized on body acupuncture points was shown to increase the release of endorphins and decrease symptoms of alcohol withdrawal (Motlagh et al., 2016). One study did show promising results of using acupuncture as an adjunctive treatment to carbamazepine (Karst, Passie, Friedrich, Wiese, & Schneider, 2002).

The most recent *Cochrane Database of Systemic Reviews* research on the use of acupuncture for nicotine dependence in 2014 included 38 trials. While firm conclusions could not be drawn due to research methodological problems and lack of evidence, the analysis did suggest that there are possible short-term effects of ameliorating nicotine withdrawal with acupuncture, acupressure, or acupuncture laser therapy. However, no conclusions could be made about long-term benefits. In a randomized, sham-controlled trial of the use of the NADA protocol for smoking cessation, the NADA protocol, when used along with education and counseling, was more effective at decreasing smoking (44%) than sham acupuncture with education and counseling (22%) or than the NADA protocol as a stand-alone treatment (10%; Bier, Wilson, Studt, & Shakleton, 2002). Again, the evidence points to the usage of the NADA protocol as an adjunctive therapy within a more comprehensive substance abuse treatment program. In addition, the results showed that the greater the estimated pack/year history before treatment, the greater the decrease in total number of cigarettes smoked per day following treatment.

As discussed earlier, acupuncture causes the release of endogenous opioids, and its analgesic effects can be reversed by naloxone, an opiate receptor antagonist. Many studies have been performed examining the reduction of opiate physical withdrawal symptoms, but the evidence has been inconclusive and difficult to interpret due to issues of methodology and study heterogeneity (Jordan, 2006; Lin et al., 2012). In contrast, a 2014 systematic review and meta-analysis indicated a statistically significant benefit of acupuncture for improving the psychological symptoms of depression and anxiety associated with opioid addiction (Boyuan, Yang, Ke, Xueyong, & Sheng, 2014). Functional magnetic resonance imaging (fMRI) has been utilized to examine the effect of acupuncture on specific brain areas related to craving and involved in reward, learning and memory, cognition, and emotion. Acupuncture at specific points can decrease activation of these craving-related brain regions and therefore may be helpful in the treatment of substance abuse (Lin et al., 2012).

Mind–Body Therapies

Mind–body therapies are a hallmark of integrative medicine practices and focus on the interaction between the brain, mind, body, and behavior. The mind–body practices that have received the most attention for addiction treatment include yoga, meditation/mindfulness practices, hypnosis, and exercise.

Many studies on the use of these therapies to treat addiction group these modalities together. The effect of integrative modalities for distinct types of addiction may be different, as the underlying pathophysiologic mechanisms for each addiction are somewhat dissimilar.

Yoga, which means "union" in Sanskrit, has its origins in ancient Indian philosophy. It is a mind–body therapy that incorporates physical postures (*asanas*), breath work, meditation, and relaxation. The yoga philosophy is to unite and align the mind, body, and spirit. There are numerous schools of yoga with Hatha yoga being the most commonly practiced in the United States and Europe, emphasizing postures *(asanas)* and breathing exercises *(pranayama)*.

Yoga has been shown to lower blood pressure and heart rate and to be effective in improving anxiety, stress, and depression. According to the 2007 National Health Interview Survey, which included a comprehensive survey on the use of complementary health approaches by Americans, yoga is the sixth most commonly used complementary health practice among adults. A network of yogis called "Yoga of Recovery" offers courses and retreats for recovering addicts at leading yoga centers all over the country.

What is the evidence for the use of yoga in treating opioid, alcohol, and tobacco abuse disorders? There are no studies that specifically address the role of yoga in the treatment of opioid addiction; however, there is evidence for the use of yoga in treating back pain and other musculoskeletal pain syndromes (Williams et al., 2009). Using yoga to treat painful musculoskeletal disorders may help prevent prescription opioid addiction by obviating the need for opioid medication in the first place. Regarding the use of yoga as a therapy for alcohol dependence, a small Swedish study (18 patients) examined yoga as an adjunct treatment for alcohol dependence and showed a nonsignificant reduction in alcohol consumption in the usual treatment plus yoga group (Hallgren, Romberg, Bakshi, & Andreasson, 2014).

Does yoga help with smoking cessation treatment? A 2012 study provided preliminary evidence that yoga may be an effective adjunctive treatment for smoking cessation in women (Bock et al., 2012). Women in the yoga group also experienced less anxiety and reported improved perceptions of health and well-being. There are only a few other nonrandomized studies on yoga, adjunctive to cognitive behavior therapy, for smoking cessation with the overall trend suggestive of a positive effect. However, there is not enough rigorous evidence to determine if these practices are as efficacious as the evidence-based modalities currently used in practice.

Other mind–body therapies may also be useful for smoking cessation. A large meta-analysis reviewed the effect of various mind-body therapies including mindfulness, breath work, and yoga on smoking cessation (Carim-Todd, Mitchell, & Oken, 2013). The meta-analysis included a total of 14 studies with 8 focusing on mindfulness, 3 on breath work, and 3 on yoga. The results showed five of the studies exhibiting smoking abstinence rates of 21% to 56% following treatment (range seven days to two years). Six of the studies found significant reductions in both cigarette cravings and desire to smoke. Two of the studies showed a 20% to 26% decrease in the number of cigarettes smoked in the treatment groups. The studies included in this large meta-analysis were of variable quality, with different outcome measures. The lack of robust study design prevented definite conclusions, but there was an overall suggestion that yoga and meditation-based therapies have the potential to reduce cigarette smoking and aid in smoking cessation. All 14 of the studies demonstrated some positive results.

Meditation and Hypnosis

Neuroimaging studies are bringing light to the profound brain changes that occur with engagement in regular mindfulness practices. Meditation affects activity in the amygdala, which is the part of the brain involved in processing emotions. Brain images of meditators show increased gyrification (more folds in the outer layer) of the brain suggesting more permanent effects over time (Luders et al., 2012).

What is the evidence regarding mindfulness and its role in treating addictions? "A Narrative Review of Yoga and Mindfulness as Complementary Therapies for Addiction" examines the theoretical basis for yoga and mindfulness as an integrative approach to treat the most common and costly addictions, namely smoking, alcohol dependence, and illicit substance use (Khanna & Greeson, 2013). Since these practices target multiple brain regions that play a role in the behavioral processes implicated in addiction and relapse, they have the potential to address the physical, psychological, and spiritual aspects pertinent to addiction. A small but growing number of well-designed clinical trials support the clinical effectiveness of these practices for treating addiction. Future studies are needed to better elucidate which specific practices work best for each type of addiction and then tailor them to individual patients to maximize efficacy.

Similar to the evidence regarding yoga for smoking cessation, the few randomized studies on mindfulness-based interventions for smoking cessation favor positive results, but the evidence is not rigorous enough to compare its efficacy to the conventional smoking cessation treatments currently in standard practice. A summary of the existing data on the use of mindfulness for smoking cessation can be found at the National Center for Complementary and Integrative Health, which is a center at the NIH, the federal focal point for medical research in the United States. In a 2011 study that compared two behavioral interventions, mindfulness training versus a standard behavioral smoking cessation treatment (the American Lung Association's Freedom From Smoking [FFS] treatment), individuals who received mindfulness training showed a greater rate of reduction in cigarette use immediately after treatment and at 17-week follow-up compared with the FFS intervention (Brewer et al., 2011). In a neuroimaging study, mindful attention reduced smoking associated craving and also decreased activity in a craving-related brain region of the brain (Westbrook et al., 2013). A 2015 review of 13 studies of mindfulness-based interventions for smoking cessation presented overall promising results regarding craving, smoking cessation, and relapse prevention (De Souza et al., 2015).

Data on the use of mindfulness-based practices in treating addictive disorders other than tobacco are suggestive of overall benefit. A French review of the literature from 1980 to 2009 on the use of mindfulness for the treatment of addictive disorders located six clinical trials (Skanavi, Laqueille, & Aubin, 2011). Of those, five discovered significant reductions in substance use and four showed mindfulness interventions more effective than control conditions. In another review of 24 studies in the English literature, the authors concluded that, overall, the evidence suggested that mindfulness-based interventions reduced the consumption of several substances including alcohol, cocaine, amphetamines, marijuana, cigarettes, and opiates to a significantly greater extent than control groups (waitlist controls, nonspecific educational support groups, and some specific control groups; Chiesa & Serretti, 2014).

Mindfulness-based therapies have been more studied with regard to relapse prevention. Mindfulness-Based Relapse Prevention (MBRP) is a technique modeled after Mindfulness-Based Stress Reduction (MBSR) developed by Jon Kabat-Zinn in the 1990s. MBRP integrates the techniques of mindfulness practices with cognitive-behavioral relapse prevention therapy. MBRP is designed to focus on experiences of craving and negative mood that play a role in relapse from addictions. The goal of MBRP, which is taught after stabilization from substance abuse, is to help patients tolerate uncomfortable states, like craving, and to experience difficult emotions, like anger or fear, without the automatic reaction of returning to the substance of abuse. In a large study, MBRP reduced both heavy drinking and drug use days (Bowen et al., 2014). At 12-month follow-up, MBRP was better at reducing heavy drinking and drug use days compared to both the relapse prevention intervention as well as treatment as usual. Several studies have looked at the feasibility, acceptability, and efficacy of MBRP methodology in ethnically diverse and challenging populations. One pilot study demonstrated that MBRP participants experienced fewer and shorter relapses compared to control patients (Witkiewitz,

Greenfield, & Bowen, 2013). Dialectical behavior therapy is also an evidence-based therapy for substance abuse that incorporates mindfulness. In a study of American native adolescents with substance use disorders, use of dialectical behavior therapy modified to incorporate native practices was associated with improvement in over 90% of adolescents, though there was no comparison group (Beckstead, Lambert, DuBose, & Linehan, 2015).

Hypnosis is a mind–body therapy that is exclusively therapeutic in orientation and not primarily a wellness and health modality. Hypnosis, which has been coupled with dissociation, has been considered an unconscious phenomenon, unlike mindfulness. Hypnosis has been used to enhance smoking cessation and prevent relapse for many years. In a study of veterans who wished to quit smoking with the aid of a nicotine patch, hypnosis was compared with standard behavioral counseling. The hypnosis intervention was designed to promote abstinence and the enhancement of self-regulatory coping responses (Carmody et al., 2008). Overall, the study demonstrated no treatment related differences in efficacy. However, in a subgroup analysis looking at abstinence in the groups with and without a history of depression, those with a history of depression had significantly improved abstinence with hypnosis compared with counseling. In a meta-analysis of gender differences in outcomes from hypnosis-based treatments for smoking cessation, men were more likely to be abstinent from hypnosis-based treatments compared with women (Green, Lynn, & Montgomery, 2008). Hypnosis responsive subgroups should be considered for further smoking cessation study.

Exercise

The health benefits of regular exercise include improvements in the function of the cardiovascular, pulmonary, and endocrine systems. Exercise also has cognitive benefits, with studies suggesting benefit in executive functions of learning, working memory, multitasking, and planning. There is some clinical evidence indicating that endurance aerobic exercise like marathon running can prevent the development of certain drug addictions. In addition, it is thought to be an effective adjunct treatment for drug addiction.

Just as with the other modalities discussed thus far, the data on exercise for alcohol addiction and substance use disorder is suggestive of benefit for the use of exercise as an adjunct therapy, but the studies are not rigorous enough to make definitive conclusions. For tobacco addiction, there is stronger evidence that exercise is an effective adjuvant treatment (Taylor, Ussher, & Faulkner, 2007). Exercise was found to be as effective as CBT and even more effective when combined with nicotine replacement therapy than CBT alone (Wang,

Wang, Wang, Li, & Zhou, 2014). Another study reported similar effects for moderate to vigorous exercise combined with nicotine replacement or bupropion treatment (Prochaska et al., 2008).

Biofeedback and Neurofeedback

While the conscious brain responses to drug and alcohol craving have been well studied, the response of the autonomic nervous system and its role in maintaining addiction has received little attention. The physiologic parameter of heart rate variability reflects the individual's autonomic system ability to respond to changing situational demands or stress. Chronic drug use disorders and alcohol dependence have been associated with lower heart rate variability (Eddie, Kim, Lehrer, Deneke, & Bates, 2014). In a pilot study of young men in treatment for alcohol or drug use disorders, the use of heart rate variability biofeedback was studied in addition to treatment as usual. Biofeedback was targeted at increasing heart rate variability by visualizing heart rate deviations on a computer screen. At baseline, high stress scores were associated with low heart rate variability (Eddie et al., 2014). After three weeks, the biofeedback group had reduced craving, but the effect was not significantly different compared with the usual treatment group. Learning to control one's autonomic nervous system after the loss of control associated with addiction is likely therapeutic. Biofeedback deserves studies of longer duration to investigate effects on addiction associated craving and associated symptoms of stress, anxiety, and depression.

Neurofeedback is a therapeutic method thought to target brain connectivity dysfunction. Neurofeedback is a biofeedback technique aimed at training patients to alter their brain function through conditioning to alter brain waveforms. The patient's electroencephalogram (EEG) is analyzed in real time using statistics to provide biofeedback to the patient. Three major neurofeedback methodologies exist: (a) real-time z-score surface neurofeedback, (b) low-resolution electromagnetic tomography (LORETA), and (c) fMRI neurofeedback (Simkin, Thatcher, & Lubar, 2014). LORETA neurofeedback provides estimates of deep brain structures like the anterior cingulate. Functional MRI neurofeedback can examine deep subcortical areas of the brain, but it is expensive and not portable (Simkin et al., 2014).

Focusing on changes in brainwave activity change with neurofeedback could be useful both to treat as well as prevent addiction. Substance abuse can have varied effects on a quantitative EEG depending on the substance, whether it is use or abuse, acute use, or chronic use (Simkin et al., 2014). For example, chronic cocaine and marijuana use has been associated with an increase in alpha brainwave activity, and chronic alcohol abuse has been associated with increased beta brainwave activity. Excessive fast beta brainwave activity has been associated with an increased risk of relapse in alcoholics. Relevant to prevention for the children of alcoholics, increased fast brainwave activity has also been associated with an increased risk of alcohol use disorder (Simkin et al., 2014). Other populations of children at risk for substance abuse disorders that could be identified with neurofeedback include children and adolescents with attention deficit disorder. Using neurofeedback for treatment, in a small study of alcoholics, adult subjects were treated with 20 sessions of eyes-closed alpha-theta neurofeedback. At the 21-month follow-up, there was only one relapse and depressive symptoms were significantly improved (Saxby & Peniston, 1991).

Real-time fMRI neurofeedback to strengthen craving related neural activation is considered promising though it is impractical for routine substance abuse treatment. The two substance abuse populations that are currently being studied: include nicotine cigarette smokers and alcohol-dependent adults (Hartwell et al., 2016; Karch et al., 2015). During fMRI sessions, subjects are exposed to stimuli associated with drug or alcohol use, which elicits craving. Concurrently, a neuronal network is activated by the drug-associated stimuli. In real time, brain region activation information is fed back to the individual so that control of the activated brain area can be trained and enhanced. After training, the individual should be able to regulate brain activity in critical brain areas such as the anterior cingulate and decrease craving. While intriguing, the stability of the neurofeedback effect, generalizability, and linkage to decreased substance use and relapse will need further study.

Music and Art Therapy

Both art therapy and music therapy are useful in addiction treatment to enhance self- expression through nonverbal, imaginative, meaningful, and enjoyable exercises. The use of art therapy for addiction treatment dates back to the 1950s (Aletraris, Paino, Edmond, Roman, & Bride, 2014). Art therapy includes a number of different exercises, such as an "incident exercise," which is used to explore an incident in which substances are used. Exploring the incident, the patient may express emotions and understand stressors related to continued substance use. Benefits that have been ascribed to art therapy include decreasing denial about substance use, improving communication, decreasing shame, and moving people from reflecting on their disorder to begin to change. Approximately 36.8% of substance abuse treatment programs reported providing art therapy (Aletraris et al., 2014). For adolescents in particular, art therapy is thought to be an excellent technique as the creative process can provide an opportunity to take an inner feeling to an outer depiction.

Music therapy has been perceived to enhance communication, decrease stress, and increase positive feelings. Approximately 14.7% of substance abuse treatment programs report providing music therapy (Aletraris et al., 2014). Adolescents are thought to be particularly interested in music therapy, given their use of music in daily life. Traditionally, music therapy has been provided by trained music therapists to groups or individuals. Examples of clinical music therapy include lyric analysis, musical games, songwriting, and musical improvisation based on emotions or another focus of treatment. Drumming has been associated with relaxation and may be useful for patients with multiple relapses who are trying to decrease stress and manage craving.

Music therapy has been related to a willingness to attend substance use treatment. One study found that music therapy was better than verbal therapy regarding readiness to change scores on substance abuse assessments (Silverman, 2011). A small study of men with substance use disorders demonstrated that depression scores, rated by a blinded observer, improved if improvisational music therapy sessions were added to the usual group addiction treatment (Albornoz, 2011). However, recent systematic reviews have concluded that most studies of music therapy for addictive disorders are descriptive, focused on positive feelings, not reduction of substance use, and music therapy cannot yet be considered an evidence-based practice (Silverman, 2011).

Nutrition, Vitamins, Herbal Therapies

Nutritional and vitamin deficiencies are common in substance use disorders. Illicit drug use has been associated with micronutrient deficiencies and is thought to cause cravings for low-nutrient calories (Schroeder & Higgins, 2017). In a large, population-based US study, dietary fat was positively associated with illicit drug use in women (Schroeder & Higgins, 2017). For men in the Multiple Risk Factor Intervention Trial (at baseline), smokers drank more alcoholic beverages and ate more meals away from home (Stamler, Rains-Clearman, Lenz-Litzow, Tillotson, & Grandits, 1997). The greater the number of cigarettes, the higher the intake of high-fat meats and the lower the consumption of fruits and vegetables. During the six years of follow-up, the early smoking quitters were able to make healthier dietary changes compared with the continuing smokers, suggesting that healthy nutritional changes may track with improvements in substance abuse. For alcohol, in a Finnish study, people with alcohol use disorders consumed a lower percentage of carbohydrates (8%; Rintamaki et al., 2014). The results are in agreement with other studies that have found that alcohol tends to replace healthier carbohydrates in the diet. In an Australian study of diet in addicted individuals admitted to the hospital for detoxification, the prevalence of mild-moderate malnutrition was 24% (Ross, Wilson, Banks, Rezannah, & Daglish, 2012). Fifty percent of subjects were deficient in at least one vitamin or in iron on testing. Low vitamin A levels were found in 18% of subjects tested, and low iron levels were found in 18%. Thiamine (vitamin B1) deficiency is commonly linked with alcohol use disorders and is also associated with disabling neurological problems such as Wernicke's encephalopathy (mental status changes, ataxia and ocular abnormalities) and Korsakoff's syndrome (severe amnestic disorder). Adequate nutrition is particularly critical during pregnancy. The role of nutrients to prevent or alleviate symptoms of fetal alcohol spectrum disorder has been recently reviewed, but there are few systematic human studies of dietary interventions during pregnancy in substance abusers (Young, Giesbrecht, Eskin, Aliani, & Suh, 2014). While marijuana is known to increase appetite, there is little study of marijuana abuse and diet. In a large US population-based study, caloric intake increased as marijuana use increased, with heaviest users consuming the most calories (Smit & Crespo. 2001). Heavy marijuana users consumed more of their calories as alcohol, though overall marijuana users did not appear to be malnourished. Intake of vitamin C and carotenes was lower in heavy marijuana users compared with nonusers. Not surprisingly, substance abuse has been associated with vitamin and nutritional deficiencies, and adequate treatment of substance use disorders requires enhancing patient health through improved diet.

In spite of these findings, limited studies have explored the potential use of nutritional supplementation as a way of helping with substance use disorders. There are a few studies that have reported some benefits of herbal supplements for reducing withdrawal symptoms. For example, one study of opiate withdrawal showed that the herbal extract Passionflower used in conjunction with a maximum daily dose of 0.8 mg of clonidine showed a significant superiority over clonidine alone in the management of mental symptoms associated with detoxification (Akhondzadeh et al., 2001). Other herbal preparations have also been suggested as possible therapies to treat substance use disorders for either reducing cravings or minimizing withdrawal symptoms, but well-designed, controlled trials will be required to determine whether they are useful clinically (Carai et al., 2000).

Conclusion

Addiction to and abuse of alcohol, nicotine, and illicit and prescription drugs is costly to our society, both financially and with regard to the health and well-being of addicted individuals. Conventional therapies and programs can be effective but are costly for some. Pharmacologic interventions are infrequently used outside of specialty substance abuse treatment providers. An integrative approach may offer a less stigmatized, more rewarding intervention in treating these disorders either alone or in combination with conventional therapies. In addition, many of these mind–body therapies have other effects that are beneficial to one's overall health and well-being.

Of the integrative therapies discussed, mindfulness-based therapies have both the greatest number of and most rigorous studies. The evidence favors overall benefit in treating tobacco, alcohol, and other substance use disorders, but more data with longer term outcomes are needed. For research in acupuncture, biofeedback and neurofeedback, nutritional and other supplements, art and music therapy, there is a lack of good-quality, well-powered research studies with valid, interpretable outcomes. Also, many studies lack the characteristics seen in clinical populations, including co-occurring medical illness, so generalizability of significant findings to more complicated patient populations with medical and psychiatric comorbidities is a challenge. When methodologically sound data is available then hopefully integrative therapies will be part of standard practice, either alone or in conjunction with traditional approaches and help to lessen the impact of addiction on patients and society.

REFERENCES

Akhondzadeh, S., Kashani, L., Mobaseri, M., Hosseini, S. H., Nikzad, S., & Khani, M. (2001). Passionflower in the treatment of opiates withdrawal: A double-blind randomized controlled trial. *Journal of Clinical Pharmacy & Therapeutics, 26*(5), 369–73.

Albornoz, Y. (2011). The effects of group improvisational music therapy on depression in adolescents and adults with substance abuse: A randomized controlled trial, *Nordic Journal of Music Therapy, 20*(3), 208–224.

Aletraris, L., Paino, M., Edmond, M. B., Roman, P. M., & Bride, B. E. (2014). The use of art and music therapy in substance abuse treatment programs. *Journal of Addictions Nursing, 25*(4), 190–196.

Beckstead, D. J., Lambert, M. J., DuBose, A. P., & Linehan, M. (2015). Dialectical behavior therapy with American Indian/Alaska native adolescents diagnosed with substance use disorders: Combining an evidence based treatment with cultural, traditional, and spiritual beliefs. *Addictive Behaviors, 51*, 84–87.

Bier, I. D., Wilson, J., Studt, P., & Shakleton, M. (2002). Auricular acupuncture, education and smoking cessation: A randomized, sham-controlled trial. *American Journal of Public Health*, 92(10), 1642–1647.

Bock, B. C., Fava, J. L., Gaskins, R., Morrow, K. M., Williams, D. M., Jennings, E., et al. (2012). Yoga as a complementary treatment for smoking cessation in women. *Journal of Women's Health*, 21(2), 240–248.

Bowen, S., Witkiewitz, K., Clifasefi, S. L., Grow, J., Chawla, N., Hsu, S. H., et al. (2014). Relative efficacy of mindfulness-based relapse prevention, standard relapse prevention, and treatment as usual for substance use disorders: A randomized clinical trial. *JAMA Psychiatry*, 71(5), 547–556.

Boyuan, Z., Yang, C., Ke, C., Xueyong, S., & Sheng, L. (2014). Efficacy of acupuncture for psychological symptoms associated with opioid addiction: A systematic review and meta-analysis. *Evidence-Based Complementary and Alternative Medicine*, 2014, 313549.

Brewer, J. A., Mallik, S., Babuscio, T. A., Nich, C., Johnson, H. E., Deleone, C. M., et al. (2011). Mindfulness training for smoking cessation: Results from a randomized controlled trial. *Drug & Alcohol Dependence*, 119(1–2), 72–80.

Carai, M. A., Agabio, R., Bombardelli, E., Bourov, I., Gessa, G. L., Lobina, C., et al. (2000). Potential use of medicinal plants in the treatment of alcoholism. *Fitoterapia*, 71(Suppl. 1), S38–S42.

Carim-Todd, L., Mitchell, S. H., & Oken, B. S. (2013). Mind-body practices: An alternative, drug-free treatment for smoking cessation? A systematic review of the literature. *Drug & Alcohol Dependence*, 132(3), 399–410.

Carmody, T. P., Duncan, C., Simon, J. A., Solkowitz, S., Huggins, J., Lee, S., & Delucchi, K. (2008). Hypnosis for smoking cessation: A randomized trial. *Nicotine & Tobacco Research*, 10(5), 811–818.

Chiesa, A., & Serretti, A. (2014). Are mindfulness-based interventions effective for substance use disorders? A systematic review of the evidence. *Substance Use & Misuse*, 49(5), 492–512.

De Souza, I. C., De Barros, V. V., Gomide, H. P., Miranda, T. C. M., de Paula Menezes, V., Kozasa, E. H., & Noto, A. R. (2015). Mindfulness-based interventions for the treatment of smoking: A systematic literature review. *Journal of Alternative and Complementary Medicine*, 21(3), 129–140.

Eddie, D., Kim, C., Lehrer, P., Deneke, E., & Bates, M. E. (2014). A pilot study of brief heart rate variability biofeedback to reduce craving in young adult men receiving inpatient treatment for substance use disorders. *Applied Psychophysiology & Biofeedback*, 39(3–4), 181–192.

Galanter, M., Kleber, H. D., & Brady, K. T. (2015). *The American Psychiatric Publishing textbook of substance abuse treatment* (5th ed.). Retrieved from http://psychiatryonline.org/doi/book/10.1176/appi.books.9781615370030

Green, J. P., Lynn, S. J., & Montgomery, G. H. (2008). Gender-related differences in hypnosis-based treatments for smoking: A follow-up meta-analysis. *American Journal of Clinical Hypnosis*, 50(3), 259–271.

Hallgren, M., Romberg, K., Bakshi, A., & Andreasson, S. (2014). Yoga as an adjunct treatment for alcohol dependence: A pilot study. *Complementary Therapies in Medicine*, 22(3), 441–445.

Han, J. S. (2004). Acupuncture and endorphins. *Neuroscience Letters, 361,* 258–261.

Hartwell, K. J., Hanlon, C. A., Li, X., et al. (2016). Individualized real-time fMRI neurofeedback to attenuate craving in nicotine-dependent smokers. *Journal of Psychiatry & Neuroscience, 41*(1), 48–55.

Jordan, J. B. (2006). Acupuncture treatment for opiate addiction: A systematic review. *Journal of Substance Abuse Treatment, 30*(4), 309–314.

Karch, S., Keeser, D., Hummer, S., Paolini, M., Kirsch, V., Karali, T., et al. (2015). Modulation of craving related brain responses using real-time fMRI in patients with alcohol use disorder. *PLoS One, 10*(7), e0133034.

Karst, M., Passie, T., Friedrich, S., Wiese, B., & Schneider, U. (2002). Acupuncture in the treatment of alcohol withdrawal symptoms: A randomized, placebo-controlled inpatient study. *Addiction Biology, 7,* 415–419.

Khanna, S., & Greeson, J. M. (2013). A narrative review of yoga and mindfulness as complementary therapies for addiction. *Complementary Therapies in Medicine, 21*(3), 244–252.

Lee, J., Kresina, T. F., Campopiano, M., Lubran, R., & Clark, H. W. (2015). Use of pharmacotherapies in the treatment of alcohol use disorders and opioid dependence in primary care. *BioMed Research International, 2015,* 137020. http://dx.doi.org/10.1155/2015/137020

Lin, J. G., Chan, Y. Y., & Chen, Y. H. (2012). Acupuncture for the treatment of opiate addiction. *Evidence-Based Complementary and Alternative Medicine, 2012,* 739045. doi:10.1155/2012/739045

Luders, E., Kurth, F., Mayer, E. A., Toga, A. W., Narr, K. L., & Gaser, C. (2012). The unique brain anatomy of meditation practitioners: Alterations in cortical gyrification. *Frontiers in Human Neuroscience, 6,* 1–9.

Motlagh, F. E., Ibrahim, F., Fashid, R. A., Seghatoleslam, T., & Habil, H. (2016). Acupuncture therapy for drug addiction. *Chinese Medicine, 11,* 16.

National Institute of Drug Abuse. (2015). Trends and statistics. Retrieved from https://www.drugabuse.gov/related-topics/trends-statistics#costs

Prochaska, J. J., Hall, S. M., Humfleet, G., Munoz, R. F., Reus, V., Gorecki;, J., & Hu, D. (2008). Physical activity as a strategy for maintaining tobacco abstinence: A randomized trial. *Preventive Medicine, 47*(2), 215–220.

Rintamaki, R., Kaplas, N., Mannisto. S., Montonen, J., Knekt, P., Lönnqvist, J., & Partonen, T. (2014). Difference in diet between a general population national representative sample and individuals with alcohol use disorders, but not individuals with depressive or anxiety disorders. *Nordic Journal of Psychiatry, 68*(6), 391–400.

Ross, L. J., Wilson, M., Banks, M., Rezannah, F., & Daglish, M. (2012). Prevalence of malnutrition and nutritional risk factors in patients undergoing alcohol and drug treatment. *Nutrition, 28*(7–8), 738–743.

Saxby, E., & Peniston, E. G. (1991). Alpha-theta brainwave neurofeedback training: An effective treatment for male and female alcoholics with depressive symptoms. *Journal of Clinical Psychology, 51*(5), 685–693.

Schroeder, R. D., & Higgins, G. E. (2017). You are what you eat: The impact of nutrition on alcohol and drug use. *Substance Use & Misuse, 52*(1), 10–24.

Silverman, M. J. (2011). Effects of music therapy on change readiness and craving in patients on a detoxification unit. *Journal of Music Therapy, 48*(4), 509–531.

Simkin, D. R., Thatcher, R. W., & Lubar, J. (2014). Quantitative EEG and neurofeedback in children and adolescents: Anxiety disorders, depressive disorders, comorbid addiction and attention-deficit/hyperactivity disorder, and brain injury. *Child & Adolescent Psychiatric Clinics of North America, 23*(3), 427–464.

Skanavi, S., Laqueille, X., & Aubin, H. (2011). [Mindfulness based interventions for addictive disorders: A review]. *Encephale, 37*(5), 379–387.

Smit, E., & Crespo, C. J. (2001). Dietary intake and nutritional status of US adult marijuana users: Results from the third national health and nutrition examination survey. *Public Health and Nutrition, 4*(3), 781–786.

Sood. A., Ebbert, J. O., Sood. R., & Stevens, S. R. (2006). Complementary treatments for tobacco cessation: A survey. *Nicotine & Tobacco Research, 8*(6), 767–771.

Stamler, J., Rains-Clearman, D., Lenz-Litzow, K., Tillotson, J. L., & Grandits, G. A. (1997). Relation of smoking at baseline and during trial years 1-6 to food and nutrient intakes and weight in the special intervention and usual care groups in the multiple risk factor intervention trial. *American Journal of Clinical Nutrition, 65*(1 Suppl.), 374S-402S.

Stuyt, E. B., & Voyles, C. A. (2016). The National Acupuncture Detoxification Association protocol, auricular acupuncture to support patients with substance abuse and behavioral health disorders: Current perspectives. *Substance Abuse and Rehabilitation, 7*, 169–180.

Substance Abuse and Mental Health Services Administration. (2016). 2015 National Survey on Drug Use and Health. Retrieved from https://www.samhsa.gov/data/sites/default/files/NSDUH-DetTabs-2015/NSDUH-DetTabs-2015/NSDUH-DetTabs-2015.pdf

Taylor, A. H., Ussher, M. H., & Faulkner, G. (2007). The acute effects of exercise on cigarette cravings, withdrawal symptoms, affect and smoking behavior: A systematic review. *Addiction, 102*(4), 534–543.

Wang, D., Wang, Y., Wang, Y., Li, R., & Zhou, C. (2014). Impact of physical exercise on substance use disorders: A meta-analysis. *PLoS One, 9*(10), e110728.

Westbrook, C., Creswell, J. D., Tabibnia, G., Julson, E., Kober, H., & Tindle, H. A. (2013). Mindful attention reduces neural and self-reported cue-induced craving in smokers. *Social Cognitive & Affective Neuroscience, 8*(1), 73–84.

Williams, K., Abildso, C., Steinberg, L., Cooper, L., Steinberg, L., Epstein, B., et al. (2009). Evaluation of the effectiveness and efficacy of Iyengar yoga therapy on chronic low back pain. *Spine, 34*(19), 2066–2076.

Witkiewitz, K., Greenfield, B. L., & Bowen, S. (2013). Mindfulness-based relapse prevention with racial and ethnic minority women. *Addictive Behavior, 38*(12), 2821–2824.

World Health Organization. (2002). Management of substance abuse. Retrieved from http://www.who.int/substance_abuse/facts/global_burden/en/

World Health Organization. (2003). Evidence based acupuncture. Retrieved from http://www.evidencebasedacupuncture.org/who-official-position/

Young, J. K., Giesbrecht, H. E., Eskin, M. N., Aliani, M., & Suh, M. (2014). Nutrition implications for fetal alcohol spectrum disorder. *Advances in Nutrition, 5*(6), 675–692.

INDEX

Tables, figures, and boxes are indicated by an italic *t*, *f*, and *b* following the page/paragraph number

Aboelsaad, F., 329
Acceptance and Commitment Therapy (ACT), 319–320, 322–323
acetylcholinesterase inhibitors, for cognitive decline, 432
acetyl-L-carnitine, 446
acoustic neuritis, vertigo from, 249
ACRM cognitive rehabilitation manual, 422–423
ACTIVE trial, 408, 412, 413–415
acupuncture, 205, 219–229. *See also* traditional Chinese medicine (TCM)
  for addiction, 228, 558–561
  for anxiety, 220–223, 513–514
  biomedicine and, 229–230
  for depression, 223–225, 354–355, 482–483
  efficacy, 220
  for insomnia, 226
  modern practice, 219–220
  on opiate system, 559–560
  for pain disorders, 226–227
  points
    artificial lines connecting, 211, 216*f*
    meridians, 219
  for PTSD, 538–539
  research difficulties, 220
  for schizophrenia, 225–226
  for smoking cessation, 228–229
  theory, 558–559
  treatments, 559
Adapt-232, 442
adaptogens, for cognitive decline, 442–446
  Adapt-232, 442
  Ginkgo biloba, 445–446
  huperzine A, 445
  other, 446
  polyphenols and pomegranate juice, 442–443
  probiotics, 443
  reservatrol, 443–444
  vitamin E, 444–445
addiction. *See also specific types*
  contingency management, 558
  conventional therapies, 558
  craving, 556
  fundamentals, 556–557
  prevalence, 557–558
  religion on, 129–130
  symptoms, 556
  withdrawal symptoms, avoiding, 556
addiction, integrative treatment, 558–570
  acupuncture, 228, 558–561
  art therapy, 567–568
  biofeedback, 566
  conventional therapies, 558
  exercise, 565–566
  herbal therapies, 569
  hypnosis, 565
  meditation, 563–565
  mind–body therapies, 561–563

576 Index

addiction, integrative treatment (*cont.*)
   Mindfulness-Based Relapse Prevention, 320, 323, 564
   music therapy, 568
   neurofeedback, 566–567
   nutrition, 568–569
   patient interest, 556–557
   vitamins, 568–569
   yoga, 562
Adey, Ross, 331, 338
Adrian, E. D., 330
Advanced Cognitive Training for Independent and Vital Elderly (ACTIVE), 408, 412, 413–415
aerobic exercise. *See also* exercise
   for brain health, 433–434
   on cerebral blood flow, 55–56
   on cognitive function, 58
   on mental health, 51 (*see also* exercise, on mental health)
   on neuroplasticity, 53
   on neurotrophic factors, 54
   on serotonin, 55
   on sympathovagal balance, 56
aging
   brain changes, 52–53
   cognitive, normal *vs.* pathological, 405
Akhondzadeh, S., 516
Akirav, I., 547–548
Akkermania muciniphila, 12
Alavia, A., 367
alcoholism
   functional neuroimaging, 365–366
   neurotransmitter studies, 365
   prevalence, 557–558
alcoholism, integrative treatment
   diet and nutrition, 568–569
   fMRI neurofeedback, 567
   homeopathy, 272–273
   Mindfulness-Based Relapse Prevention, 323
alcohol use
   on anxiety, 508
   for insomnia, 389
   religion on, 129–130
Alexander Technique, for anxiety, 511
Alladin, A., 302
alpha-tocopherol, 35–37, 444–445. *See also* Vitamin E
alpha waves, 331, 332
   in depression, 332–333
α-linoleic acid (ALA), 21–22

alternating attention, 425–426
Alzheimer's disease. *See also* cognitive decline
   glucose metabolism, 440
   integrative treatment
      transcranial direct current, 448
      transcranial magnetic stimulation, 448
   prevalence, 431
   rosacea, as risk factor, 439
Amen, D. G., 351
Amen database, 351
Ames, B. N., 23, 42
Amminger, G. P., 24
Amsterdam, J. D., 516–517
amygdala
   activation, 501
      meditation on, 105–106
   on hypothalamic-pituitary-adrenal axis, 356
Anderson, S. B., 541
animal-assisted therapy, for PTSD, 543–544
animal diet, on gut microbiome, 7–8
antioxidants. *see also specific types*
   fruit, 446
anxiety (disorders). *See also* stress
   alcohol, 508
   associations, 499
   caffeine, 507–508
   characteristics, 499
   with chronic disease, 500
   definition, 499
   DSM-V criteria, 499–500
   functional neuroimaging, 356–358
   generalized anxiety disorder, 499–500
   vs. health, 498–499
   health and, 500
   hypothalamic-pituitary-adrenal axis, 502
   inflammation, 507
   pathophysiology, 501
   prevalence, 499
   smoking, 508
anxiety (disorders) treatment
   exposure therapy, 505
   medical, 502–504
      adverse effects, 500, 502
   mind-based cognitive therapy, 322
   psychodynamic therapy, 505
   psychotherapeutic, 504–505
   rational emotive behavior therapy, 505
anxiety (disorders) treatment, integrative, 505–517
   acupuncture, 220–223, 513–514

Index

Alexander Technique, 511
aromatherapy, 512–513
art therapy, 512
Ayurveda, 514
biofeedback, 300–301, 301*t*
botanicals, 515–517
chamomile, 545
diet, 506–508
exercise, 64–67, 73*t*, 508–509
gut microbiome, 506–507
massage therapy, 513
mind-based cognitive therapy, 322
mind-based stress reduction, 321
mind–body modalities, 509–511
Mindfulness-Based Cognitive Therapy, 505
mindfulness-based interventions, 324
Mindfulness-Based Stress Reduction, 357, 509–510
music therapy, 512
omega-3 fatty acids, 506
supplements, 514–515
tai chi and chi gong, 511
tiers, 505
traditional Chinese medicine, 513
yoga, 511
apnea-hypopnea index (AHI), 391
Apter, A., 24
arginine vasopressin, meditation on, 103*t*, 107
Arns, M., 339
aromatherapy, for anxiety, 512–513
Artemesia absinthium (wormwood), 191–192
Artemesia vulgaris (mugwort), 192
arterial spin labeling, 349
art therapy
 for addiction, 567–568
 for anxiety, 512
 Mindfulness-Based Art Therapy, 320, 323
ashwagandha, 192–193
 for PTSD, 544
Asser, S. M., 135
atorvastatin, 437
atrial natriuretic peptide (ANP), exercise on, 57
Atropa belladonna (belladonna), 196–197
attention
 alternating, 425–426
 deficits, 425–426
 divided, 426
 focused, 425
 sustained, 425

attentional deployment, conscious, 160–163, 161*f*, 162*f*
attention deficit hyperactivity disorder (ADHD)
 causal theory, 337
 integrative therapy
  exercise, 71–72, 73*t*
  homeopathy, 265
  Mindfulness Awareness Program, 320
  neurofeedback, 337–341
 prevalence, 337
attention management, 161–163, 161*f*, 162*f*
 happiness focus, 163–166
Attention Process Training, 426
Au, T. K., 131
autism, homeopathy on, 273–274
autonomic balance, exercise on, 56
autonomic-cortical activity, meditation on, 108–109
autonomic nervous system (ANS)
 biofeedback, 292–293
 heart rate variability biofeedback, 299–300
 meditation on, 106–107
Ayele, H., 121
Ayurveda, for anxiety, 514

Bach, P., 323
Bachner-Melman, R., 291
Bacopa monnieri, 446
Bacteroidetes, 5, 7, 7*b*
Baill, 446
Baker, E. L., 303
Ballesteros, S., 410
Balvers, M. G. J., 30–31
Barabasz, A., 290
Barabasz, M., 302, 303
Barga, J., 303
Barker, A. T., 333
Bassuk, S. S., 132
Beauregard, M., 341
being on your case *vs.* being on your side, 167–168
being on your side, tools for, 168–170, 169*t*
belladonna, 196–197
Belmaker, R. H., 24
benign paroxysmal positional vertigo (BPPV), 249
 chiropractic on, 250–252
Benson, H., 510
benzodiazepines, for anxiety, 502, 503
Berbaum, D., 296

Berbaum, M., 296
Berger, Hans, 330
Berkman, L. F., 132
beta blockers, for anxiety, 503
beta waves, 331
β-endorphin, meditation on, 103t, 107–108
β-hydroxybuterate (BHB), 440
biofeedback
    for addiction, 566
    for ANS disorders, heart rate variability biofeedback, 299–300
    for anxiety disorders, 300–301, 301t
    fundamentals, 291–292
    goal, 541
    for headaches and migraine, 294, 295t
    heart rate variability
        for ANS disorders, 299–300
        for cognitive decline, 448
    for hypertension, 298–299, 299t
    for major depression, 301–302
    mechanisms, 292–293, 293t
    mind–body medicine, 287–288
    for pain, acute and chronic, 295–297
    in psychiatric populations, 300
    for PTSD, 540–541
    research, methodological limitations, 288
    treatment sessions, 541
biotin deficiency, 33
bipolar disorder
    functional neuroimaging, 355–356
    integrative approaches, 484–486
        exercise, 73t
        omega-3 fatty acids, 24, 25
        vitamin D_3, 29
Birbaumer, N., 297
bitter orange, for PTSD, 545
Blaccioniere, M. J., 128
Black, S., 513
Blanchard, E. B., 298
blood–brain barrier (BB), diet and microbiome on, 11
blood oxygen labeled dependent (BOLD), 349–350
blood pressure, 437
Blumenthal, J. A., 128
Bodman, F., 268
Boericke, W., 274
Boltz, O., 268–269
Boone, T. L., 131
botanicals, in psychiatry, 177–200
    for addiction, 569

    for anxiety, 514, 515–517
    clinical effectiveness not demonstrated or inadequate testing, 191–196
        Artemesia absinthium (wormwood), 191–192
        Artemesia vulgaris (mugwort), 192
        Eleutherococcus senticosus (Siberian ginseng), 193, 446
        Eschscholzia californica (California poppy), 195
        Leonurus cardiaca (motherwort), 193–194
        Melissa officinalis (lemon balm), 194–195
        Papaver rhoeas (corn poppy), 195
        Scutellaria (skullcap), 195–196
        Withania somnifera (ashwagandha), 192–193
    clinically effective, evidence of, 181–191
        Cannabis sativa (marijuana), 187–188, 200t
        Coffea arabica, Coffea robusta (coffee, caffeine), 181–182, 200t
        Ginkgo biloba (ginkgo), 182, 200t, 445–446
        Humulus lupulus (hops), 183, 200t
        Hypericum perforatum (St. John's wort), 183–184, 200t, 475–476, 486
        Lavender angustifolia (English lavender), 188–189
        Matricaria chamomilla, Matricaria recutita (chamomile), 190, 200t
        Panax ginseng, Panax cinquefolius (ginseng), 184–185, 200t
        Passiflora incarnata (passionflower), 189–190
        Piper methysticum (kava), 185–186
        Rauwolfia serpentina (snakeroot, reserpine), 186–187, 200t
        Rhodiola rosea (goldenroot), 190–191, 200t, 446, 478–479
        Valeriana officinalis (valerian), 187, 200t
    in current practice, 180–181
    evaluation, problems, 179
    history, 177–178
    illegal, toxic, or addictive, 196–199
        Atropa belladonna (belladonna), 196–197
        Catha edulis (khat), 197
        Ephedra sinica, Ephedra spp., 198
        Erythroxylum coca (cocaine), 198–199

psychoactive plant substances, 177
  for PTSD, 544–546
  regulations and control, 178–179
Bowen, S., 130
Bracha, Z., 24
Brady, K. T., 558
brahmi, for PTSD, 544
brain-derived neurotropic factor (BDNF)
  in depression, 335
  exercise on, 54
  transcranial magnetic stimulation on, 335
brain health pillars, 433–437
  aerobic exercise, 433–434
  cognitive engagement, 433, 435
  diet and nutrition, 433, 435–436
  sleep, 433, 436–437
  social engagement, 433, 434
BrainHQ, 412
brain mapping, qEEG, 330–331
brain plasticity, 406
BrainTrain®, 411–412
brain training. see cognitive interventions
Bresee, C., 25
Bretteler, M., 339
Brot, C., 27
bruxism, sleep, 399t
Bryant, R., 291
Buckler, R. E., 134
Burdette, A. M., 128
buspirone, for anxiety, 503–504
Butki, B., 131
B vitamins, 31–35. See also vitamin B
Byrd, R. C., 136

caffeine, 181–182, 200t
  on anxiety, 507–508
calcium, 41
California poppy, 195
Camellia assamica, 446
cannabinoid receptors, exercise on, 54–55
cannabinoids
  on dopamine, 188
  on PTSD, 547–548
Cannabis sativa (marijuana), 187–188, 200t
  on dopamine, 188
Cannon, W. B., 293
Captain's Log, 411–412
Carlsson, J., 541
Carpenter, T., 244
Carroll, D., 515

cataplexy, 395
Catha edulis (khat), 197
celiac disease, 8
central sleep apnea (CSA), 391–394, 392b
cerebral blood flow (CBF)
  aerobic exercise on, 55–56
  atorvastatin on, 437
  functional neuroimaging, 348, 349f
    fMRI, 349
    PET and SPECT, 348, 349f
cerebral metabolism, functional neuroimaging, 348, 349f
Ceretec, 348
Cerletti, Ugo, 333
chamomile, 190, 200t
  for anxiety, 545
  for depression, 478
  for PTSD, 545
chamomile, German, for anxiety, 516–517
Chan, Y. Y., 559–561
Chapman, E. H., 265
Cheal, K., 133
Chen, H., 133
Chen, Y. H., 559–561
Chi, 207–208
chi gong, for anxiety, 511
Chinese medicine. *see* acupuncture; traditional Chinese medicine (TCM)
chiropractic, 238–253
  innate wellness and recovery, mechanism, 242–243
  for neurologic conditions, 247–252
    benign paroxysmal positional vertigo, 250–252
    chronic pain, 247–248
    epilepsy, 252
    Meniere's disease, 250
    vertigo, 248–249
  practice and history, 239–241
  on psychiatric conditions, 245–247
  research, 243–245, 245t
  risk, 252–253
  scientific theories and principles, 238–239
cholesterol, blood, 437
choline, 41, 446
Chopra, D., 168–169
Choufani, D., 383, 383b
chronic fatigue syndrome, homeopathy on, 265

Cialdini, R., 160
Cicerone, K., 425
cingulate cortex
　in ADHD, 357
　chiropractic on, 245t
　dorsal anterior, self-criticism, 168
　meditation on, 101–102, 101f, 102f
　mindfulness-based interventions on, 322
　Mindfulness-Based Stress Reduction on, 357
　in obsessive compulsive disorder, 363
　in pain processing, 159
cingulate cortex, anterior
　acupuncture on, 225, 354
　biofeedback on, 297
　in depression, 332, 354
　in schizophrenia, 359
　in self-criticism, 168
cocaine, 198–199
Coffea arabica (coffee, caffeine), 181–182, 200t
Coffea robusta (coffee, caffeine), 181–182, 200t
coffee, 181–182, 200t
cognition. See also specific types
　gut, microbiome, and, 10–11
　insulin resistance, 13
cognitive aging, normal vs. pathological, 405
cognitive behavioral therapy (CBT), for anxiety, 502, 504
cognitive decline. See also specific types
　costs, estimated, 432
　physiology, 432
　prevalence, 431
　risk factor reduction, 432
cognitive decline, integrative approaches, 431–450. See also specific approaches
　brain health pillars, 433–437
　combination therapies, 432–433
　disease-halting therapies, 432
　fundamentals, 431–432
　integrating multiple approaches, 448–449
　neuromodulation, 446–448
　　heart rate variability, 447–448
　　meditation, 447
　　repetitive transcranial magnetic stimulation, 448
　　yoga, 446–447
　pharmacologic

　　acetylcholinesterase inhibitors, 432
　　memantine, 432
　　risk factor reduction, 432, 437–439
　supplements, 439–446
　　adaptogens, 442–446 (see also adaptogens, for cognitive decline)
　　combination formulations, 446, 447b
　　medium chain triglycerides, 440–441
　　omega-3 fatty acids, 441–442
　　over-the-counter, 439–440
cognitive engagement, for brain health, 433, 435
cognitive function, exercise on, 58, 60–61, 73t
cognitive hypnotherapy, 302–303
cognitive interventions, 404–427, 435
　benefits, 404
　cognitive skill acquisition, factors, 406–408
　　cognitive reserve, 406–407
　　cognitive resilience, 406–407
　　neuroplasticity, 406
　　transfer of learning and generalization, 407–408
　combined programs, 412–419
　　ACTIVE trial, 408, 412, 413–415
　　FINGER study, 416–418, 448–449
　　NeuroGrow Brain Fitness, 415–416, 449
　　research overview, 412–413
　　SMART trial, 418–419
　computerized cognitive training (CCT), 408–412
　　BrainTrain® and Captain's Log, 411–412
　　economics, 409
　　history and fundamentals, 408–409
　　LUMOSITY®, 409–411
　　Posit Science and BrainHQ, 412
　definition, 404
　with healthy cognitive function, 405
　remediation and rehabilitation, 405, 422–426 (see also cognitive remediation and rehabilitation)
　scientific consensus, on brain training industry, 419–421
　terminology, 404–405
cognitive remediation and rehabilitation, 405, 422–426
　ACRM cognitive rehabilitation manual, 422–423
　attention deficits, 425–426
　Attention Process Training, 426
　computer-based programs, early, 423

Index **581**

definitions and focus, 422
Ecologically Oriented Neurorehabilitation of Memory, 423
Goal-Plan-Do-Review, 425
of memory, 423
memory peg technique, 424
metacognitive strategy training, 425
Write-Organize-Picture-Rehearse strategy, 424–425
cognitive reserve, 406–407
cognitive resilience, 406–407
cognitive restructuring, for PTSD, 534
cognitive skill acquisition, factors, 406–408
    cognitive reserve, 406–407
    cognitive resilience, 406–407
    neuroplasticity, 406
    transfer of learning and generalization, 407–408
Cohen, J., 58, 59*f*
coherence, 339
Cojan, T., 291
complementary and alternative medicine (CAM), 206, 240. *See also specific practices*
    classification, 474
    history and documentation, 206
computerized cognitive training (CCT), 408–412
    BrainTrain® and Captain's Log, 411–412
    economics, 409
    history and fundamentals, 408–409
    LUMOSITY®, 409–411
    Posit Science and BrainHQ, 412
Comstock, G. W., 126
concussion, chronic, functional neuroimaging, 366–369, 368*f*
conscious attentional deployment, 160–163, 161*f*, 162*f*
conscious decisionmaking, 159
consciousness, EEG assessment, 331
constitution, 279
Constitutional Type Questionnaire (CTQ), 279–280
contextualization, in PTSD, 533
contingency management, 558
continuous positive airway pressure (CPAP), for obstructive sleep apnea, 393–394
Contrada, R. J., 127
Conwell, Y., 133
coping
    exercise on, 60

flexibility, in PTSD, 534
with medical problems, religion on, 134
corn poppy, 195
Coronado, R. A., 243–244
cortisol
    acupuncture on, 224, 514, 560
    in depression, 57
    exercise on, 57
    meditation on, 101*f*, 103*t*, 107, 108
    in panic disorder, 57
    Qi Gong Therapy on, 511
    in stress response, 357, 501
    yoga on, 57, 447, 481
Covey, S., 160–161
Coward, D. D., 134
craving, 556
Crawford, C., 266
Crawford, H. J., 291
Crean, H. F., 536
Cuijpers, P., 542
Cullen-Drill, M., 24
Cummings, M., 513
Curcuma longa, 446
Cutshall, C., 302
cystine, for cognitive decline, 441–442

Darroch, J. E., 131
Datscan (ioflupane), 348
Davidson, J., 266–267
Davidson, R. J., 332–333
Davies, M., 130
de Bont, P. A., 542
decisionmaking, conscious, 159
delirium tremens, homeopathy for, 272–273
delta waves, 331
dementia. *See also* Alzheimer's disease; cognitive decline
    cognitive interventions for, 406–407 (*see also* cognitive interventions)
    costs, estimated, 432
    prevalence, 432
depression. *See also* bipolar disorder; major depressive disorder (MDD)
    alpha asymmetry, frontal, 332–333
    brain changes, 53, 332
    brain-derived neurotropic factor, 335
    costs, morbidity, and mortality, 472
    diagnosis challenges, 331–332
    functional neuroimaging, 350–355, 350*f*
    hypothalamic-pituitary-adrenal axis, 502
    incidence, 472–473
    monoamine theory, 335

depression (*cont.*)
  neurotransmitter studies, 350
  qEEG and, 331–333
  treatment barriers, 473
depression, integrative approaches, 472–487
  acupuncture, 223–225, 354–355, 482–483
  biofeedback, 301–302
  bipolar disorder, 484–486
  CAM use, prevalence of, 473–475
  Chamomile, 478
  chiropractic, 246
  clinical trials, methodological issues, 475
  Dialectical Behavior Therapy, 322
  diet and nutrition, 483–484
  exercise, 73t, 483–484
  homeopathy, 267–268
  Hypericum perforatum (St. John's wort), 183–184, 200t, 475–476, 486
  magnesium, 37–38
  meditation, 355
  mind-based cognitive therapy, 322
  mind-based stress reduction, 321
  mindfulness-based interventions, 324, 479–480
  neuromodulation, 333–337
  omega-3 fatty acids, 24, 25, 477
  religion, 133–134
  Rhodiola rosea, 478–479
  S-adenosyl-methionine (SAMe), 476–477, 486
  spirituality, 133–134, 480–481
  transcranial magnetic stimulation, 333–337, 353, 448
  Trauma-Informed-MBSR, 323
  tryptophan and hydroxytryptophan, 479
  vitamin D and D$_3$, 10, 29–30
  yoga, 481
  zinc, 40–41
Detinis, L., 267–268
Dialectical Behavior Therapy (DBT), 319, 322
diet. *See also specific types and disorders*
  for addiction, 568–569
  for anxiety, 506–508
  for brain health, 433, 435–436
  cognition, gut, microbiome, and, 10–11
  for depression, 483–484
  religion on, 129
diet and gut, 3–13. *See also* microbiome, gut
  animal *vs.* plant diet, 7–8
  cognition, microbiome, and, 10–11
  gluten, 8
  gut microbiome, 4–8 (*see also* microbiome, gut)
  gut regulators, 8–9
  insulin, 12–13
  metagenomics, 6
  metascriptomics, 6
  neuroinflammatory markers, 12
  short-chain fatty acids, 5, 11–12
  vitamin D, 10
  Western diet
    on brain, 11–13
    inflammation and mood, 4
    risks, 3–4
  zonulin, 8–9
Dietary Approaches to Stop Hypertension (DASH), 435
diffusion tensor imaging (DTI), 350
  schizophrenia, 361
  traumatic brain injury, 369
direct current, transcranial, for cognitive decline, 448
diversity of style, embracing, 163
divided attention, 426
Dix-Hallpike maneuver, 251–252
Dobson-Stone, C., 291
docosahexaenoic acid (DHA), 21
  marine-derived, 441
  serotonin and, 22–23, 42
Doghramji, K., 383, 383b, 385, 391t, 394
Doghramji, P. P., 385, 391t
dopamine
  acupuncture on, 560
  in ADHD, 337
  in alcoholism, 366
  branched-chain amino acids on, 485
  caffeine on, 507
  cannabis on, 188
  cocaine on, 199
  in depression, 350
  exercise on, 55
  functions, 55
  hypnosis on, 291
  kava on, 185
  meditation on, 100f, 103–104, 358, 510
  monoamine theory, 330, 335
  nicotine on, 508
  in nucleus accumbens, 105
  in obsessive compulsive disorder, 363
  SAMe in synthesis of, 476
  serotonin and, 110
  stressors on, 358
  transcranial magnetic stimulation on, 335

in traumatic brain injury, 368
yoga nidra on, 103–104, 358
dopamine hypothesis, schizophrenia, 360
dopamine receptors, in restless legs syndrome and periodic limb movement disorder, 398
dopaminergic activity, PET and SPECT of, 98
dorsal anterior cingulate
  emotion processing in, 353
  pain in, 159
  in self-criticism, 168
dorsolateral prefrontal cortex (DLPFC), transcranial magnetic stimulation of, 334
dose-response phenomenon, 260
Downs, J. H., 291
Drescher, David, 409
drug abuse. *See* addiction
Duberstein, P. R., 133
Duncan, N. L., 422
dysbiosis, gut, 4–5. *See also* gut; microbiome, gut
  reversal, 6

eating disorders, Mindfulness-Based Eating Awareness Training on, 323
eating habits, 19–20
Ebstein, R. P., 291
Ebster, C., 411
echinacea, for PTSD, 545
Eck, J. C., 128
Eckroth-Bucher, M., 411
Ecologically Oriented Neurorehabilitation of Memory, 423
EEG
  consciousness level, 331
  definition, 331
  epilepsy assessment, 331
  waveforms, 331
EEG, quantitative (qEEG)
  brain mapping, 330–331
  cordance, 336
  depression, 331–333
  development, 331
eicosapentaenoic acid (EPA), 21–22
  serotonin and, 22–23, 42
Eisenberg, D. M., 136
Eisenberger, N. I., 159, 161
Eleutherococcus senticosus (Eleuthero, Siberian ginseng), 193, 446
Ellison, C. G., 128

emotional intelligence model, 171
emotional pain, reframing *vs.* avoiding, 162
emotional reactivity, Mindfulness-Based Stress Reduction on, 321–322
emotional trauma. *See also* posttraumatic stress disorder (PTSD)
  integrative treatment, 530–549
emotion processing theory, 533
endocannabinoids
  exercise on, 54–55
  placebos on, 278
endorphins, post-exercise, 54
Engel, G. L., 288
English lavender, 188–189
enzogenol, 446
Ephedra sinica, 198
Ephedra spp., 198
epilepsy
  chiropractic on, 252
  EEG assessment, 331
Epley, J. M., 251
Epley maneuver, 251
Epworth Sleepiness Scale, 384
Equine Partnering Naturally, 544
equine therapy, for PTSD, 544
Erickson, K. I., 53, 58, 59*f*
Erythroxylum coca (cocaine), 198–199. *See also* addiction
  Freud on, 329–330
Eschscholzia californica (California poppy), 195
excessive daytime somnolence (EDS), 383, 385
exercise
  for brain health, 433–434
  guidelines on, current, 76
  health benefits, 565
  religion on, 130
  for smoking cessation, 565–566
exercise, on mental health, 50–78
  addiction, 565–566
  anxiety, 508–509
  clinical effects
    on ADHD, 71–72, 74*t*
    on anxiety, 64–67, 73*t*
    on bipolar disorder, 73*t*
    on cognitive function, 60–61, 73*t*
    on depression, 73*t*, 483–484
    on mood, 61–64
    on obsessive compulsive disorder, 69, 74*t*
    on panic disorder, 73*t*

exercise, on mental health (cont.)
    on PTSD, 67–69, 74t
    on schizophrenia, 69–71, 74t
  clinical implications, 72–77
    clinical practice implementation, 75
    effectiveness, maximizing, 76
    implementation, 72
    motivating factors and barriers, 74–75
    personal program and capabilities, 77
    risk minimization, 76
  depression, 73t, 483–484
  psychological effect, mechanisms, 51–60, 52b
    autonomic balance, 56
    cerebral blood flow, 55–56
    cognitive function, 58
    conceptual model, 58, 59f
    coping, 60
    dopamine, 55
    endocannabinoids and cannabinoid receptors, 54–55
    heart rate variability, 56
    hypothalamic-pituitary-adrenal axis, 57
    inflammatory response and neuroinflammation, 57–58
    mind diversion and focus, 58–59
    mindfulness, 59–60
    muscular tension reduction, 60
    neuroplasticity and neuroplasticity, 52–53
    neurotrophic factors, 54
    norepinephrine, 55
    physical health, 58
    serotonin, 55
    sleep, 60
    social interactions, 60
    vagal tone, 56
  summary, 73t–74t
  types, 51
exposure therapy
  for anxiety, 505
  for PTSD
    Mindfulness-Based Exposure Therapy, 365
    trauma-focused exposure, 534
eye movement desensitization and reprocessing (EMDR), for PTSD, 541–543

faith healing, 139
Farah, A., 33–34
FDG PET. *See* PET

fear, defined, 499
feeling–thinking balance, 159–160
fibroblast growth factor (FGF-2), exercise on, 54
fibromyalgia, homeopathy on, 265
Figueredo, V. M., 51, 56
Fine, T. H., 298
Finnish Geriatric Intervention Study to Prevent Cognitive Impairment and Disability (FINGER), 416–418, 448–449
Firmicutes, 5, 7, 7b
Firmicutes/Bacteroidetes ratio
  gut microbiome, 5, 7, 7b
  obesity, 11
fish oils. *See also* omega-3 fatty acids
  contamination, 26
Fitzgerald, P. B., 336
five elements, 215–219
  balance, 218–219
  elements and properties, 217t
  meridians and, 215–216
  Shen and Ko cycles, 216–218, 218f
Flor, H., 297
fluorodeoxyglucose (FDG), 348. *See also* PET
fMRI, 331. *See also specific applications*
  alcoholism, 366
  applications, 349–350
  arterial spin labeling, 349
  bipolar disorder, 356
  blood oxygen labeled dependent, 349–350
  cerebral blood flow, 349
  depression treatment, 352–353
  diffusion tensor imaging, 350, 361, 369
  meditation, 97–98
  PTSD, 365, 533
  traumatic brain injury, 369
fMRI neurofeedback
  for alcoholism, 567
  for smoking cessation, 567
focused attention, 425
FokI polymorphism, 28
folate, on cognitive decline, 437–438
folate deficiency, 33
folic acid, vitamin B_{12} masking, 34–35
Fotuhi, M., 415
fractional anisotropy (FA)
  obsessive compulsive disorder, 363–364
  schizophrenia, 361–362
Fraser, G. A., 547

Frederick, C., 302
Freeman, D. H. Jr., 127
Freeston, I. L., 333
Frei, H., 266
Freud, S., 329–330
functional magnetic resonance imaging (fMRI). *See* fMRI
functional neuroimaging, 347–369. *See also specific types*
  alcoholism, 365–366
  anxiety, 356–358
  applications, 347–350
  bipolar disorder, 355–356
  cerebral metabolism and blood flow, 348, 349*f*
  concussion, chronic, 366–369, 368*f*
  depression, 350–355, 350*f*
  meditation, 97–98, 358, 358*f*
  obsessive compulsive disorder, 362–365, 362*f*
  PET, 348, 349*f*
  posttraumatic stress disorder, 364–365
  schizophrenia, 358–362, 359*f*
  SPECT, 348
  tracers, 348
functional somatic syndromes, homeopathy on, 266

Galanter, M., 558
Gallavardin, J., 272
galphimia, for PTSD, 545
gamma aminobutyric acid (GABA)
  in anxiety, 501
  meditation, 102–103, 103*t*
  transcranial magnetic stimulation on, 335
gamma waves, 331
Gay, C. W., 245
Gellhorn, E., 108–109
generalization, 407–408
generalized anxiety disorder (GAD). *See also* anxiety
  chamomile for, 545
  DSM-V criteria, 499–500
  Mindfulness-Based Stress Reduction for, 509–510
German chamomile, for anxiety, 516–517
Gertsik, L., 25
Giacino, J., 425
Gilbert, D., 164
Ginkgo biloba (ginkgo), 182, 200*t*
  for cognitive decline, 445–446

ginseng, 184–185, 200*t*
  Siberian, 193, 446
Glass, T. A., 132
gliadins, 8
glutamate
  meditation on, via prefrontal cortex, 108
  transcranial magnetic stimulation on, 335
gluten, 8
  gliadins and glutenins in, 8
  on zonulin, 8
glutenins, 8
Goal-Plan-Do-Review (G-P-D-R), 425
Gold, S. D., 531
goldenroot, 190–191, 200*t*
  for cognitive decline, 442, 446
Goleman, D., 159, 171
Gonsalkorale, W., 297
Gonsalves, A., 244
gratitude expressions, 164–165
Grazyna, M., 273
Greenaway, M. C., 422
Greenberg, C. L., 163, 165, 166
Greenberg-Walt, C. L., 163
Greenwald, S., 130
Gritsenko, I., 291
Grob, C. S., 546
Grodin, M. A., 538–539
Guernsey, H., 280
Gumpricht, E., 35–36
Gunkelman, J., 339
Gur, M., 131
gut. *See also* diet and gut
  bacterial mass, 5–6
gut-brain connection
  vitamin D, 10
  zonulin in dysfunction of, 9
gut dysbiosis, 4–5
  reversal, 6
gut microbiome. *See* microbiome, gut
gut regulators, 8–9

Hahnemann, Samuel, 259–260, 277, 279–280
Haidvogl, M., 273
hallucination, Acceptance and Commitment Therapy on, 323
Hampstead, B. M., 423
HAPIE model, 164
happiness
  focus, 163–166
  tips, 164
  traps, 164

happiness and satisfaction, behavioral
  strategies, 157–171
  being on your side, tools for,
    168–170, 169t
  being on your side vs. being on your
    case, 167–168
  conscious attentional deployment,
    160–163, 161f, 162f
  conscious decisionmaking, 159
  emotional pain, reframing vs.
    avoiding, 162
  feeling–thinking balance, 159–160
  further strategies, 170
  gratitude expressions, 164–165
  HAPIE model, 164
  happiness focus, 163–166
  interpersonal neurobiology, 160
  measures and quantification, 157–158
  models and self-leadership concepts, 159
  natural tendency, 158
  neural circuitry, for physical and
    emotional pain, 159
  neural circuitry, for physical and social
    pain, 161
  positive psychology, 158
  prosperity, 166
  return on investment, 166–167
  salience network, 160
  self-awareness, 159, 165–166
  self-criticism, 167–168
  self-evaluations, 167, 170
  Seligman's theory, 158
  set point, 164
  thought processes, ordinary vs.
    inspirited, 159
  well-being, sense of, 165
  wellness, sense of, 165
  whipping vs. redirecting, 168–169
Harmann, G. W., 246
Harrington, G., 291
Harris, W. S., 136
Harvard Hypnotic Susceptibility scale,
  289, 289b
hatha yoga. See yoga
Hatira, P., 296
Hayes, S. C., 323
headaches, biofeedback
  for, 294, 295t
health, defined, 498
heart rate variability (HRV), 299–300
  biofeedback on
    for ANS disorders, 299–300

for cognitive decline, 448
in cognitive decline, 447–448
definition, 447
exercise on, 56
mindfulness meditation on, 446
vagal tone, 447–448
Heckmann, R. C., 134
Heffner, K. L., 536
Heng, S., 356
Henriques, J. B., 332–333
herbal therapy. See botanicals; specific herbs
Hermann, D., 407–408
Herwig, U., 336
Hess, S. A., 120
Hilgarde, E. R., 289
Hill, T. D., 128
hippocampus
  gut microbiome, 11
  on hypothalamic-pituitary-adrenal
    axis, 356
  meditation on, 105–106
  in mental illness, 53
  neuroplasticity, 53
Hirshkowitz, M., 386t
Hodges, S. D., 128
Hoexter, M. Q., 364
Hollifield, M., 533–534, 538
homeopathy, 258–282
  constitution, 279
  Constitutional Type Questionnaire,
    279–280
  Flexner report, 259
  history, 258–261
  hormesis, 260–261, 274
  individualized homeopathic
    consultation, 277
  materia medica, 260
  philosophical concepts, 260–261
  placebo as therapy, 275–278
  potentization, 259–260
  proving, 259, 261
  psychiatry and, 264–275
    ADHD, 265
    alcoholism and delirium tremens,
      272–273
    autism, 273–274
    depression, 267–268
    functional somatic syndromes, 266
    homeopathic hospital for mentally ill,
      first, 264
    mild traumatic brain
      injury, 265

psychosis, 268–271
  research difficulties, 265–266
  selection bias, patient choice of
    intervention, 264
  studies, 264
 research, 261–263
 treatment process, 279–281, 281t
homeostasis, 239
homeostenosis, 239
homocysteine hypothesis, 32
hops, 183, 200t
hormesis, 260–261, 274
Horton, J. E., 291
HP gene, schizophrenia, 9
Hummel, T., 244
Humphreys, S. C., 128
Humulus lupulus (hops), 183, 200t
Hung, L., 291
huperzine A, 445
hydroxytryptophan, for depression, 479
hyperhomocysteinemia, 438
Hypericum perforatum (St. John's wort),
  183–184, 200t, 475–476, 486
hypertension, biofeedback on, 298–299, 299t
hypnagogic hallucinations, 395
hypnopompic hallucinations, 395
hypnosis, 287–290, 295–298
  for addiction, 565
  fundamentals, 289–290, 289b, 290t
  Harvard Hypnotic Susceptibility scale,
    289, 289b
  hypnotizability, 289–290, 290t
  mechanisms, 291
  mind–body medicine, 287–288
  research, evidence
    irritable bowel syndrome, 297, 298b
    pain, acute and chronic, 295–296
    psychiatric populations, 300–302
  research, methodological limitations, 288
  Stanford Hypnotic Susceptibility scale,
    289, 289b
hypnotherapy, cognitive, 302–303
hypnotizability, 289–290, 290t
hypocretins, in narcolepsy, 396
hypoglossal nerve stimulation therapy, for
  obstructive sleep apnea, 394
hypoglycemia, reactive, 506
hypothalamic-pituitary-adrenal (HPA)
  axis, 502
  in anxiety and depression, 501
  exercise on, 57
hypothalamus, meditation on, 106–107

immune system, gut microbiome and, 6
imposter syndrome, 167
inadequate sleep hygiene, 386, 387b
individualized homeopathic consultation
  (IHC), 277
inflammation
  in anxiety, 507
  chiropractic on, 244
  exercise on, 57–58
  Lactobacilli on, 12
  Mediterranean-type diet on, 4
  omega-3 fatty acids on, 22
  Western diet on, 4
insomnia disorder, 387–391. *See also* sleep
  disorders
  classification, 387
  treatment
    acupuncture, 226
    nonpharmacologic, 388–389, 389t
    pharmacologic, 390, 391t
    wake after sleep onset, 390
insufficient sleep syndrome, 385–386, 386t
insulin, 12–13
insulin-like growth factor, 54
insulin resistance, on cognition, 13
interpersonal neurobiology, 160
intestinal barrier, 8
  zonulin, 9
ioflupane, 348
iron, 38–40
  brain, gut metagenome and, 10
  deficiency, 38–39
  dosing and side effects, 39–40
  function and benefits, 39
irritable bowel syndrome, hypnosis on,
  297, 298b
Iverson, J., 101, 103, 104, 105, 133
Ives, J., 266

Jalinous, R., 333
Jerneren, F., 42
Johnson, L., 426
Jojezuk, M., 530
Jonas, W., 266
Jones, R. K., 131

Kabat-Zinn, J., 59, 99, 165, 321, 509–510
Kandola, A., 53
Kaplan, B. J., 37, 39, 40, 41
Kark, J. D., 126
kava kava, 185–186
  for anxiety, 517

Kearney, D. J., 533–536
Keck, M. E., 335
Kemp, J. E., 536
Kennedy, D. O., 31–32
Kessler, R., 300
ketogenic diet, 440
ketone bodies, 440
khat, 197
Kiely, W. F., 108–109
Kimmel, H., 292
Kirkwood, G., 513
Kirsch, I., 275
Kladder, V., 121
Kleber, H. D., 558
Ko cycle, 218, 218f
Krames, E., 329
Krause, N., 132
Kropotov, Y., 330, 332, 339, 340
Kryger, M., 399t
kucha tea, 446
Kucmin, A., 530
Kucmin, T., 530
Kuzma, J. W., 128

labyrinthitis, vertigo from, 249
Lactobacilli, 12
Lama, P., 538–539
Lamont, J., 265
Lampit, A., 411
Lang, E. V., 296
Lannin, D. R., 135
Lansdowne, A. T. G., 28–29
Lansky, A., 273
Larson, D. B., 127, 130, 134
lavender, English, 188–189
Lavender angustifolia (English lavender), 188–189
lavender oil, for anxiety, 515–516
Law of Effect, 337
Lazar, S. W., 106
learning, transfer of, 407–408
Lee, C., 542
Lee, M. S., 511
Lefkowitz, E. S., 131
Lehman, M. E., 58, 59f
Lehner, E., 273
Leibovici, L., 136
Leigh, J., 130
lemon balm, 194–195
 for anxiety, 516
 for PTSD, 546
Leonurus cardiaca (motherwort), 193–194

Levesque, J., 341
Levkoff, S. E, 133
Lewis, G., 133
Liberzon, I., 533, 534
Lichtenberg, P., 291
light therapy, 436–437
Lin, J. G., 559–561
Linde, K., 262
Linden, D., 301
Liossi, C., 290, 296
liver meridian, 209–211, 211t, 212f
Long, C. R., 243
Longacre, M. M., 538–539
Longe, O., 167
lovingkindness meditation, 99
Lox, C. L., 131
LPS, 12
Lubar, Joel, 338–339
LUMOSITY®, 409–411
lung meridian
 grief, 214
 Jia Bia of, 211, 214f
Luria, A. R., 425
Lyons, J. S., 127
Lyubomirsky, S., 160

Ma, C., 297
Maes, M., 9
magnesium, 37–38
 for anxiety, 514–515
magnetic resonance spectroscopy, 486, 514
 of meditation, 103
 of traumatic brain injury, 369
major depression
 biofeedback, 301–302
 Dialectical Behavior Therapy, 322
 incidence, 472–473
 mind-based cognitive therapy on, 322
 prevalence, 20
major depressive disorder (MDD). *See also* depression
 MTHFR and B vitamins, 33–34
 MTHFR variants, 33–34
 omega-3 fatty acids, 24, 25, 477
Malone, P. S., 411
Mannheimer, E. D., 127
marijuana, 187–188, 200t
 diet and abuse of, 569
Marlatt, G. A., 130
Martin, A., 294
Martinez, M. E., 533–536
Marx, B. P., 531

Maslow, A., 158
massage therapy
  for anxiety, 513
  aromatherapy with, 512
  for fibromyalgia, 248
Mateer, C., 425, 426
materia medica, 260
Mathews, H. F., 135
Matricaria chamomilla (chamomile), 190, 200*t*, 516–517
Matricaria recutita (chamomile), 190, 200*t*
Maxim, 446
Mayas, J., 410
McDonald, P. G., 120
McDonel Herr, E. C., 133
McGrady, A. V., 298
McLane, S., 131
Mech, A. W., 33–34
meditation
  for addiction, 563–565
  on anxiety, 358, 358*f*, 509–510
  for cognitive decline, 447
  depression, 355
  functional neuroimaging, 97–98, 358, 358*f*
  on health, 137–138
  for PTSD, 537
meditation and stress reduction, neurobiology, 97–111. *See also* religion and spirituality
  autonomic-cortical activity, 108–109
  cingulate cortex activation, 101–102, 101*f*, 102*f*
  focused attention, 99
  functional neuroimaging, 97–98
  hippocampal and amygdala activation, 105–106
  hypothalamic and autonomic nervous system changes, 106–107
  initial studies, 97
  lovingkindness meditation, 99
  mindfulness meditation, 99
  neurophysiological network, 100–101, 100*f*
  parietal lobe deafferentation, 104–105
  prefrontal cortex
    activation, 101–102, 101*f*, 102*f*
    on other neurochemical systems, 107
  serotonergic activity, 109–110
  taxonomic keys, 99–100
  thalamic activation, 102–104, 103*t*
  types of, 99–101

Mediterranean-type diet
  components, 21
  with exercise, on cognitive decline, 449
  on inflammation, 4
  on microbiome, 443
  in MIND diet, 435–436
  in NeuroGrow Brain Fitness, 415, 449
  nutrients, 21
medium chain triglycerides, for cognitive decline, 440–441
melatonin
  for brain health, 436
  for insomnia, 390
  meditation, 103*t*, 110
Melissa officinalis (lemon balm), 194–195
  for anxiety, 516
  for PTSD, 546
Melzack, R., 295
memantine, 432
memory
  cognitive remediation and rehabilitation, 423
  Ecologically Oriented Neurorehabilitation of Memory, 423
memory peg technique, 424
Meniere's disease
  chiropractic on, 250
  vertigo from, 249
Menninger, C., 264
Mensour, B., 341
mental illnesses. *See also specific types*
  neuroinflammation, 20–21
  prevalence
    U.S., 312–313
    worldwide, 312
  public health burden, 313
mental illnesses, integrative treatments
  biofeedback, 300
  chiropractic, 245–247
  homeopathy, 264–275 (*see also under* homeopathy)
  hypnosis, 300–302
  religion, 132–133
meridians, 209–214
  8 extra, 211, 213*t*
  12 principal, 209–211, 210*t*–211*t*
    functions, 212–214
  definition and function, 209
  five elements and, 215–216
  liver, 209–211, 211*t*, 212*f*
  lung, 211, 214, 214*f*
  Pi Bu, 211, 215*f*

Merill, R. M., 131
Merizalde, B., 260
Mesmer, Franz, 289
metacognition, 425
metacognitive strategy training, 425
metagenomics, 6, 10
metascriptomics, 6
methyl-cobalamin, on cognitive decline, 437–438
methylenetetrahydrofolate reductase (MTHFR) variants, in depression, 33–34
methyl-folate, on cognitive decline, 437–438
Micouland-Franchigh, J. A., 293
microbiome, gut, 4–8. *See also* diet and gut
  animal *vs.* plant diet on, 7–8
  in anxiety, 506–507
  bacterial mas, 5–6
  blood–brain barrier, 11
  brain and body health, 6
  cognition, 10–11
  definition, 6
  diet on, 5
  Firmicutes/Bacteroidetes ratio, 5, 7, 7b
  hippocampus, 11
  immune system, 6
  ion deposition and siderophores, 10
  Mediterranean-type diet on, 443
  metabolic activity and functions, 6
  neuroinflammatory marker levels, 12
  on neurotransmitters, 507
  obesity, 10
migraine
  biofeedback, 294, 295t
  vertigo from, 249
Milburn, M. A., 265
mild traumatic brain injury, homeopathy on, 265
Miller, L., 130, 131
Miller, N., 292
Miller, W. R., 130
Milling, L. S., 290
mind–body medicine, 287–288. *See also specific types*
  for addiction, 561–563
  for anxiety, 509–511
MIND diet, 435–436
  omega-3 fatty acids, 441
mindfulness, 59. *See also specific techniques*
  exercise on, 59
Mindfulness Awareness Program (MAP for ADHD), 320

Mindfulness-Based Art Therapy (MBAT), 320, 323
Mindfulness-Based Cognitive Therapy (MBCT), 315–318, 322
  for anxiety, 505
Mindfulness-Based Eating Awareness Training (MB-EAT), 320, 323
Mindfulness-Based Exposure Therapy (MBET), for PTSD, 365
mindfulness-based interventions (MBIs), 312–325. *See also specific types*
  Acceptance and Commitment Therapy, 319–320
  on brain, 322
  for depression, 479–480
  Dialectical Behavior Therapy, 319
  for PTSD, 535–537
  for smoking, 563–564
Mindfulness-Based Relapse Prevention (MBRP), 320, 323, 564
  for addiction, 323
Mindfulness-Based Stress Reduction (MBSR), 165, 313–315, 321–322
  for anxiety, 357, 509–510
  for PTSD, 535–536
mindfulness meditation, 99
  on heart rate variability, 446
minerals, 37–41
  iron, 38–40
  magnesium, 37–38
  zinc, 40–41
Mitchell, J., 135
Mohammadian, P., 244
Monastra, V. J., 293, 341
monoamine theory of depression, 335
Montgomery, G. H., 296
Monti, D., 110, 219, 221, 320, 323, 365, 442, 475, 512, 539
mood
  exercise, 61–64
  vitamin D_3, 28–29
  Western diet, 4
mood disorders. *See also specific types*
  costs, morbidity, and mortality, 472
  definition, 472
  integrative approaches, 473 (*see also* depression, integrative approaches)
  mindfulness-based interventions on, 324
  treatment barriers, 473
Moore, T., 275
Morgan, A. H., 291
Morgenthaler, T., 389t

motherwort, 193–194
movement therapy, for anxiety, 511
MTHFR gene, 33–34
mugwort, 192
Mulligan, T., 121
multiple sclerosis, vertigo from, 249
Murray, D. W., 411
muscular tension, exercise on, 60
Musick, M. A, 128
music therapy
  for addiction, 568
  for anxiety, 512
mu waves, 339
myoinositol, for anxiety, 515

N-acetyl-cysteine (NAC), on cognitive decline, 437–438, 441–442
Nadler, R. S., 167–168
narcolepsy, 395–397, 397t
Nash, M. R., 303
Neeleman, J., 133
negative cognitions, in PTSD, 534
negative self-beliefs, Mindfulness-Based Stress Reduction on, 321–322
Nemets, B., 24
Nemets, H., 24
Nestoriuc, Y., 294
networked approach, to leadership, 163
neural plasticity, 406
neurodegeneration. *See also* cognitive decline
  inflammatory process, 432
  memantine for, 432
  physiology, 432
  prevalence, 431–432
  therapeutic agents, for pathogenesis, 432
Neuro-Emotional Technique (NET), for PTSD, 365, 539–540, 540f
neurofeedback
  for addiction, 566–567
  for ADHD, 337–341
  definition, 338
  mechanism of action, 566
  for PTSD, 541–542
neurogenesis, 52
NeuroGrow Brain Fitness, 415–416, 449
neuroimaging, functional, 347–369. *See also* functional neuroimaging; specific types
neuroinflammation
  diet on, 12
  exercise on, 57–58

in mental illness, 20–21
nutrient deprivation and, 20
Neurolite, 348
neuromodulation, 329–341. *See also* specific types
  ADHD and neurofeedback, 337–341
  definition, 329
  depression and, 333–337
  qEEG
    brain mapping, 330–331
    depression and, 331–333
neuromodulation, for cognitive decline, 446–448
  heart rate variability, 447–448
  meditation, 447
  repetitive transcranial magnetic stimulation, 448
  yoga, 446–447
neuroplasticity, 52–53, 406
neurotransmitters. *See also specific types*
  in alcoholism, 365
  in depression, 350
  gut microbiome on, 507
  in obsessive compulsive disorder, 363
  in panic disorder and social anxiety disorder, 357
  in PTSD, 357
  tracers for, 348
  in traumatic brain injury, 368, 369
neurotrophic factors. *See also specific types*
  exercise on, 54
Newberg, A. B., 51, 56, 98, 99, 101, 103, 104, 105, 133, 351, 510
Ngandu, T., 417
niacin deficiency, 33
Nickerson, A., 532
nightmare disorder, 399t
Nisbet, P. A., 133
N-methyl d-aspartate receptors (NMDAr), meditation on, 108
Nogalski, A., 530
norepinephrine
  acupuncture on, 514, 560
  exercise on, 55
  functions, 55
  meditation on, 103t, 106
  SAMe in synthesis of, 476
nutraceuticals, 446
nutrient pharmaceuticals, 446
nutrients, for brain health, 19–43. *See also specific nutrients*
  calcium, 41

nutrients, for brain health (*cont.*)
  choline, 41
  EPA and DHA–serotonin
      connection, 22–23
  minerals, 37–41
    iron, 38–40
    magnesium, 37–38
    zinc, 40–41
  neuroinflammation and mental
      illnesses, 20–21
  nutrient deprivation, 20
  omega-3 fatty acids, 21–26
  selenium, 41
  Standard American Diet, 19–20
  synergies, 42
  vitamins, 26–37
nutrition. *See also* diet; *specific topics*
  for addiction, 568–569
  for brain health, 433, 435–436
  for depression, 483–484
  religion on, 129

obesity
  Firmicutes/Bacteroidetes ratio, 11
  gut microbiome, 10
  short-chain fatty acids, 11
observant-self theory, 168
obsessive compulsive disorder (OCD)
  Acceptance and Commitment Therapy
      on, 323
  exercise on, 69, 73*t*
  functional neuroimaging, 362–365, 362*f*
  neurotransmitter studies, 363
obstructive sleep apnea (OSA), 391–394, 392*b*
  predisposing factors, 392, 392*b*
  snoring, 392
  treatment options, 393–394
occludin, 9, 10
Oleckno, W. A., 128
Olex, S., 51, 56
omega-3 fatty acids, 21–26
  for anxiety, 506
  with aspirin, 26
  for brain health, 21–22
    ALA, 21–22
    serotonin connection, 22–23
  with B vitamins, 42
  cautions, fish oil contamination, 26
  for cognitive decline, 441–442
  for depression, 24, 25, 477
  docosahexaenoic acid,
      marine-derived, 441
  dosing, 25–26
  EPA and DHA–serotonin
      connection, 22–23
  N-acetyl-cysteine, 441–442
  overview, 21–22
  phosphatidyl serine, 441
  for psychiatric illness, 23–25
    adjuvant, 24–25
    prevention, 23–24
  serotonin, 42
  side effects, potential, 26
omega-6 fatty acids, 22
operant conditioning punishment
    contingent relationships, 337
Oxford Happiness Inventory, 157, 170
Oxman, T. E., 127

Padberg, F., 336
pain. *See also specific types*
  acupuncture for, 226–227
  avoiding, natural tendency, 158
  chiropractic on, 243, 247–248
  diminished, as increased happiness, 158
  emotional, reframing *vs.* avoiding, 162
  spiritual, 136
pain, acute and chronic
  biofeedback on, 295–297
  hypnosis on, 295–296
pain neural circuitry
  emotional pain, 159
  physical pain, 159, 161
  social pain, 161
pain processing network (PPN), 245
Palmer, D. D., 239–240
Palmer, Joshua Bartlett, 240
Palsson, O., 297
Panax cinquefolius (ginseng),
    184–185, 200*t*
Panax ginseng (ginseng), 184–185, 200*t*
panic disorder
  exercise on, 73*t*
  mind-based stress reduction on, 321
  neurotransmitter studies, 357
pantothenic acid deficiency, 33
Papaver rhoeas (corn poppy), 195
Papp, K. V., 409
parasomnias, 399*t*, 400
Parenté, R., 407–408
parietal lobe
  acetylcholine on, 110
  acupuncture on, 225
  in Alzheimer's disease, 440

meditation on, 102, 102f, 103–105, 110
  in obsessive compulsive disorder, 362
Parkinson's disease, 431. *See also* cognitive decline
Partridge, K. B., 126
passionflower *(Passiflora incarnata)*, 189–190
  for addiction, 569
  for anxiety, 516
  for PTSD, 546
Patrick, R. P., 23, 42
Paule, L., 426
Peckham, P. H., 329
Pendleton, B., 136
Perez, N., 290
periodic limb movement disorder (PLMD), 397–398
personal mastery, 163–164
PET, 331
  alcoholism, 365–366
  anxiety and stress, 356–358, 358f
  applications, 348
  bipolar disorder, 355–356
  cerebral metabolism and blood flow, 348, 349f
  depression, 350–354, 350f
  meditation, 98
  neuroimaging, 348, 349f
  obsessive compulsive disorder, 362–363, 362f
  PTSD, 364–365
  schizophrenia, 358–360, 359f
  tracers, 348, 349f
  traumatic brain injury, 367–368, 368f
Phillips, R. L., 128
phosphatidyl serine, for cognitive decline, 441
physical exercise (activity). *See* exercise
physical health. *See also specific types*
  exercise on, 58
physical pain, neural circuitry for, 161
Pi Bu, 211, 215f
Pickar, J. G., 243
Piguet, C., 291
Pilkington, K., 513
Pinus pinaster, 446
Pinus radiata, 446
Piper methysticum (kava), 185–186
  for anxiety, 517
Pirozzi, T. O., 265
placebo
  antidepressants, 275

endocannabinoids, 278
  on rheumatoid arthritis, 276–277
  selection bias, patient choice of intervention, 264
  as therapy, 275–278
plant-based diet
  on gut microbiome, 7
  short-chain fatty acids, 5, 12
Poland, R. E., 25
Poloma, M., 136
polyphenols, for cognitive decline, 442–443
polysomnography, 385, 385b
pomegranate juice, for cognitive decline, 442–443
Pop-Jordanova, N., 303
poppy
  California, 195
  corn, 195
Positive and Negative Affect Scale (PANAS), 157, 170
positive psychology, 158
positron emission tomography (PET). *See* PET
Posit Science, 412
posttraumatic stress disorder (PTSD)
  comorbidity, 533
  contextualization, 533
  coping flexibility, 534
  development, 531–532
  distress tolerance, 534
  DSM-V diagnosis, 531, 532
  effective treatment, elements of, 548b
  emotion processing theory, 533
  functional neuroimaging, 364–365
  heterogeneity, 531
  history, 530
  meta-analyses, 323–324
  negative cognitions, 534
  neurotransmitter studies, 357
  peritraumatic factors, 531–532
  psychological mechanisms, 533
  psychotherapeutic approaches
    cognitive restructuring, 534
    stress inoculation therapy, 534
    trauma-focused cognitive behavioral therapy, 534–535
    trauma-focused exposure, 534
  social support, 532
  symptom presentation and risk factors, 532
  traumatic events, 531

posttraumatic stress disorder (PTSD),
    integrative treatment, 533–549
  animal-assisted therapy, 543–544
  biofeedback, 540–541
  cannabinoids, 547–548
  efficacy research, 321–324
    Acceptance and Commitment
      Therapy, 322–323
    Dialectical Behavior Therapy, 322
    mindfulness-based interventions,
      321–323
  exercise, 67–69, 73t
  eye movement desensitization and
    reprocessing, 541–543
  general approach, 533–535
  meditation, 535–537
  mind-based stress reduction, 321
  mindfulness-based interventions, 320
  Neuro-Emotional Technique, 365,
    539–540, 540f
  plant-based medicine, 544–546
    ashwagandha, 544
    bitter orange, 545
    brahmi, 544
    chamomile, 545
    echinacea, 545
    galphimia, 545
    lemon balm, 546
  psilocybin, 546–547
  traditional Chinese medicine, 538–539
  Trauma-Informed MBSR, 323
  yoga, 537–538
potentization, 259–260
Potie, A., 296
prayer, 136
prefrontal cortex
  acupuncture on, 225
  aging on, 53
  in alcoholism, 366
  in bipolar disorder, 356
  in depression, 53, 332
  exercise on, 53
  hypnosis on, 291
  on hypothalamic-pituitary-adrenal
    axis, 356
  meditation on, 101–102, 101f, 102f, 107
  mindfulness-based interventions on, 322
  in obsessive compulsive disorder,
    363–364
  paroxetine on, 351–352
  in PTSD, 364, 365, 536
  in schizophrenia, 360

  in self-criticism, 168
  stress on, psychosocial, 357
  transcranial magnetic stimulation on,
    334, 353, 448
Pressman, P., 127
probiotics, for cognitive decline, 443
prosperity, 166
proving, 259, 261
Provost, S. C., 28–29
pseudodementia, 439
psilocybin
  for anxiety, 504
  on PTSD, 546–547
psychoactive plant substances, 177. See also
  botanicals
psychodynamic therapy, for anxiety, 505
psychopharmacology
  effectiveness, limited, 330
  history, 329–330
  theory, 330
psychotic disorders. See also specific types
  homeopathy for, 268–271
  omega-3 fatty acids on, 24, 25
pycnogenol, 446
Pyle, C. M., 134
pyridoxine
  deficiency, 33
  upper limit, 35

qEEG, 331
  brain mapping, 330–331
  cordance, 336
  depression and, 331–333
Qi (Chi), 207–208
  cognitive and emotional
    expressions, 214

Rabiner, D. L., 411
Rajalakshmi, M. A., 273–274
Rampes, H., 513
Rapaport, M. H., 25
Raskin, S., 426
rational emotive behavior therapy, for
  anxiety, 505
Rauch, S. A., 533, 534
Rauwolfia serpentina (snakeroot,
  reserpine), 186–187, 200t
Raz, A., 291
reactive hypoglycemia, 506
Reales, J. M., 410
Reed, W. R., 243, 244
reframing, 162

rehabilitation, cognitive, 405, 422–426.
    See also cognitive remediation and rehabilitation
Reibel, D., 314
reinforcer, 337
Reiter, K., 541
relaxation response, 510
religion and spirituality, 118–140
    clinical studies, methodological issues, 121–126
        causality, direction of, 124
        compliance, 122
        correlational studies and confounding variables, 121
        cultural context, 125
        definitions, 122
        hierarchical social aspects, 125
        measures, 122–123
        measures, accuracy, 123–124
        multidisciplinary research/clinical teams, 126
        positive externalities, 124
        randomized controlled trials, 121
        subjects, recruiting and retaining, 122
        time frame, study, 125
        variability, affiliations and denominations, 124–125
        well-designed, challenges, 121
    for depression, 133–134, 480–481
    faith healing, 139
    future directions, 139–140
    in healthcare, 120–121
    history, 118–119
    importance, to patients and physicians, 119
    medical and scientific interest, 119
    meditation, 137–138
    negative effects, 134–135
    positive effects, 126–134
        access to healthcare resources, 132
        alcohol, tobacco, and drug abuse, 129–130
        behavior and lifestyles, 128–129
        coping with medical problems, 134
        depression, 133–134, 480–481
        diet and nutrition, 129
        disease incidence and prevalence, 126–127
        exercise, 130
        mental health, 132–133
        mortality and morbidity, 126–127
        outcomes, disease and surgical, 127–128
        sexual behavior, 130
        prayer, 136
        professional education on, 120
        on risky sexual behavior, 130
        spiritual pain and abuse, 136
        yoga, 138–139
remediation and rehabilitation, cognitive, 405, 422–426
    ACRM cognitive rehabilitation manual, 422–423
    attention deficits, 425–426
    Attention Process Training, 426
    computer-based programs, early, 423
    definitions and focus, 422
    Ecologically Oriented Neurorehabilitation of Memory, 423
    Goal-Plan-Do-Review, 425
    of memory, 423
    memory peg technique, 424
    metacognitive strategy training, 425
    Write-Organize-Picture-Rehearse strategy, 424–425
REM sleep behavior disorder, 399t
repetitive transcranial magnetic stimulation (rTMS)
    for cognitive decline, 448
    on depression, 353
Resch, D., 273
reserpine, 186–187, 200t
reservatrol, 443–444
resistance exercise. *See also* exercise
    on mental health, 51
    on neurotrophic factors, 54
restless legs syndrome (RLS), 397–398
return on investment, 166–167
reward, 337
Rezai, A., 329
rheumatoid arthritis, placebo on, 276–277
Rhodiola rosea (goldenroot), 190–191, 200t
    for cognitive decline, 442, 446
    for depression, 478–479
Richardson, J., 513
Rief, W., 294
Ring, C., 515
Robertson, A. G., 163
Rockway, S., 35–36
rosacea, 439

S-adenosyl-methionine (SAMe), for depression, 476–477, 486
Saine, A., 269–270

salience network, 160
  in PTSD, 541
Saperstein, G., 275
Sarkar, Kunal, 409
Sarris, J., 545–546
Satisfaction with Life Scale, 158, 170
Scanlon, Michael, 409
Schermer, C., 130
Schisandra chinensis, 446
schizophrenia
  acupuncture for, 225–226
  dopamine hypothesis, 360
  exercise on, 69–71, 73t
  functional neuroimaging, 358–362, 359f
  HP gene and plasma proteins, 9
Schofield, P., 291
Schonfeldt-Lecuona, C., 336
Schupp, C., 296
Schwartz, H. S., 246
Scoboria, A. N., 275
Scutellaria (skullcap), 195–196
sedentary habits, 433
Segev, A., 547–548
Seidlitz, L., 133
selection bias, patient choice of intervention, 264
selective serotonin and noradrenaline reuptake inhibitors (SNRIs), 502–503
selective serotonin reuptake inhibitors (SSRIs), 502
selenium, 41
self-awareness, 159, 165–166
self-beliefs, negative, Mindfulness-Based Stress Reduction on, 321–322
self-criticism, 167–168
self-evaluations, 167, 170
self-understanding, 163
Seligman, M., 158
sensori-motor rhythm (SMR), 338
Serefko, A., 37, 38
serotonergic activity
  meditation on, 103t, 109–110
  PET and SPECT of, 98
serotonin
  acupuncture on, 514, 560
  in alcoholism, 366
  in anxiety, 501–503
  in depression, 335, 350, 353–354
  EPA, DHA, and, 22–23, 42
  exercise on, 55
  functions, 55
  iron and, 39
  kava on, 185
  magnesium on, 37
  meditation on, 103t, 109–110, 510
  monoamine theory, 330
  MTHFR, 33
  omega-3 fatty acids, 42
  in panic disorder and social anxiety disorder, 357
  SAMe in synthesis of, 476
  in traumatic brain injury, 368
  tryptophan and, 55, 479
  vitamin D, 28, 42
serotonin receptors, in obsessive compulsive disorder, 363
serotonin syndrome, 476
set point, happiness, 164
Shen cycle, 216–218, 218f
Shevin, W., 271–272
short-chain fatty acids (SCFAs), 5, 11–12
Shusta, S. R., 302
Siberian ginseng, 193, 446
Siberski, J., 411
siderophores, 10
Sigman, M., 131
Sikoglu, E. M., 29
Silver-Highfield, E., 538–539
Sim, K., 356
Simons, D. J., 409
Simpson, T. L., 533–536
Singh, S., 131
single nucleotide polymorphisms (SNPs), vitamin D receptor, 28
single photon emission computed tomography (SPECT). *See* SPECT
Skinner, A. T., 411
Skinner, B. F., 337
skullcap, 195–196
sleep
  for brain health, 433, 436–437
  exercise on, 60
sleep apnea, 391–394, 392b
sleep bruxism, 399t
sleep disorders, 382–400
  acupuncture for, 226
  cataplexy, 395
  clinical approach, 382–384
    diagnostic process, 382–384, 383b
    physical examination, 384
    referral criteria, 384, 385b
  Epworth Sleepiness Scale, 384
  excessive daytime somnolence, 383, 385

hypnagogic hallucinations, 395
inadequate sleep hygiene, 386, 387b
insomnia disorder, 387–391
insufficient sleep syndrome,
    385–386, 386t
naps, 384
narcolepsy, 395–397, 397t
parasomnias, 399t, 400
periodic limb movement disorder,
    397–398
polysomnography, 385, 385b
restless legs syndrome, 397–398
sleep apnea, 391–394, 392b
sleep paralysis, 395
snoring, 392
sleep duration guidelines, 385, 386t
sleep hygiene measures, 386, 387b
sleepiness, 382–383
sleep paralysis, 395
sleep terrors, 399t
sleep walking, 399t
Sloan, D. M., 531
Smaldone, A., 24
SMART trial, 418–419
Smith, G. E., 422
smoking
    on anxiety, 508
    prevalence, 557–558
    religion on, 129–130
smoking cessation, integrative treatment.
    See also addiction
    acupuncture, 228–229
    diet and nutrition, 568–569
    exercise, 565–566
    fMRI neurofeedback, 567
    mindfulness-based interventions,
        563–564
    mind-therapies, 562–563
    patient interest, 556–557
    yoga, 562
snakeroot, 186–187, 200t
Snyder, P. J., 409
social anxiety disorder, neurotransmitter
    studies, 357
social engagement, for brain health,
    433, 434
social interactions, from exercise, 60
social pain, 161
social support, 532
sodium butyrate, 12
Sohlberg, M., 425, 426
Sojezuk, S., 530

Soler-Baillo, J. M., 531
Song, A. W., 356
Sozio, R. S., 243
SPECT
    Amen database, 351
    applications, 348
    cerebral metabolism and blood flow, 348
    of depression, 350–351, 353–354
    functional neuroimaging, 348
    of meditation, 98
    of obsessive compulsive disorder, 362
    tracers in, 348
    of traumatic brain injury, 367–368
spinal manipulative therapy or chiropractic
    adjustment (SMT), 243. See also
    chiropractic
spin labeling, arterial, 349
spiritual abuse, 136
spirituality. See religion and spirituality
spiritual pain, 136
Spitzer, M., 336
Spronk, D., 339
Sripada, R. K., 533, 534
Standard American Diet (SAD), 19–20. See
    also diet; Western diet
    anxiety, 506
    chronic diseases, 20
    components, 19
    eating habits, 19–20
    omega-6 fatty acids, 22
Stanford Hypnotic Susceptibility scale,
    289, 289b
Stefanek, M., 120
Stephenson, K. R., 533–536
Sterman, M. B., 338
Stern, L., 131
Stillman, C. M., 58, 59f
St. John's wort, 183–184, 200t
    for depression, 475–476, 486
Stoll, A. L., 25
Strafella, A. P., 334, 335
Strain, J. J., 127
Strehl, U., 341
stress. See also anxiety
    with cancer, Mindfulness-Based Art
        Therapy on, 323
    pathophysiology, 501
    tolerance, in PTSD, 534
stress inoculation therapy, for PTSD, 534
Stringer, A. Y., 423
stroke. See also cognitive decline
    prevalence, 431

Study of Mental Activity and Resistance Training (SMART), 418–419
Subjective Happiness Scale, 157–158, 170
subluxation, 242
substance use disorders. *See also* addiction; *specific types*
  contingency management, 558
  conventional therapies, 558
  craving, 556
  prevalence, 557–558
  symptoms, 556
  withdrawal symptoms, avoiding, 556
Sudarshan Kriya Yoga, for PTSD, 538
suicide, religiosity and, 133
supplements, for anxiety, 514–517
  fundamentals, 514–515
  German chamomile, 516–517
  kava kava, 517
  lavender oil, 515–516
  lemon balm, 516
  passionflower, 516
  valerian, 516
supplements, for cognitive decline, 439–446
  adaptogens, 442–446
  combination formulations, 446, 447b
  medium chain triglycerides, 440–441
  omega-3 fatty acids, 441–442
  over-the-counter, 439–440
sustained attention, 425
Suter, M., 515
Swan, R., 135
Swanson, M. S., 135
Swirsky-Sacchetti, T., 407
sympathovagal balance, exercise on, 56
synergies, nutrient, 42
Szeszko, P. R., 363

tai chi
  on anxiety, 511
  on autonomic nervous system, 56
  on executive function, 58
  on mental health, 51
  on mindfulness, 59–60
Tan, S. Y., 298
Tanzi, R. E., 168–169
Tartagni, M., 29
technological savvy, 163
terminology, 404–405
testosterone replacement, 439
thalamus
  chiropractic on, 244
  meditation on, 102–104, 103t
theacrine, 446
theoretical framework
  Qi (Chi), 207–208
  Yin and Yang, 208–209
theta waves, 331
Thorndike, E. L., 337
thought processes, ordinary *vs.* inspirited, 159
Thygerson, A. L., 131
Tibetan Buddhism, 99. *See also* meditation and stress reduction, neurobiology
tight junctions, 8, 9
tobacco. *See* smoking
tocotrienols, 35, 36
Tonigan, J. S., 130
Toril, P., 410
Townsend, M., 121
tracers, 348
traditional Chinese medicine (TCM), 206. *See also* acupuncture
  for anxiety, 513
  biomedicine and, 229–230
  clinical reports and literature reviews, 206–207
  efficacy, 220
  five elements, 215–219, 217t (*see also* five elements)
  fundamental principles, 538
  interventions, 538
  origins and creators, 206
  for PTSD, 538–539
  textual challenges, 206
  theoretical framework, 207–212
    meridians, 209–214 (*see also* meridians)
    Qi (Chi), 207–208
    Yin and Yang, 208–209
  Yellow Emperor's Internal Classics, 206
transactional symbol, 277
transcranial direct current, for cognitive decline, 448
transcranial magnetic stimulation (TMS). *See also* neuromodulation
  for alcoholism, 366
  on brain-derived neurotropic factor, 335
  on brain regional blood flow, 334
  for cognitive decline, 448
  for depression, 333–337, 353
  mechanisms of action, 333–334
  on neurotransmitters, 335
  pulse train stimulation, 334

transfer of learning, 407–408
trauma, emotional. *See also* posttraumatic stress disorder (PTSD)
    integrative treatment, 530–549
trauma-focused cognitive behavioral therapy (TFCBT), 534–535
trauma-focused exposure, for PTSD, 534
Trauma-Informed MBSR, 320, 323
traumatic brain injury (TBI)
    functional neuroimaging, 366–369, 368*f*
    mild, homeopathy on, 265
    neurotransmitter studies, 368, 369
    prevalence, 366
tryptophan, 55
    for depression, 479
    serotonin and, 55, 479
    vitamin D receptor, 28
tryptophan hydroxylase-2 enzyme (TPH2), vitamin D receptor, 28
Trzebiatowska-Trzeciak, O., 273
Tsai, C., 244
Turnbull, T., 24

Unger, J., 336
unhappiness. *See also* happiness and satisfaction, behavioral strategies
    study of, 158
upper airway stimulation therapy, for obstructive sleep apnea, 393–394
uvulopalatopharyngoplasty, 394

vagal tone
    definition, 447–448
    exercise on, 56
    heart rate variability, 447–448
Valenzuela, M., 411
Valeriana officinalis (valerian), 187, 200*t*, 516
van Groningen, L., 30
vascular risk factors. *See also specific types*
    brain health and, 437
vegetarian diet
    on gut microbiome, 7
    short-chain fatty acids, 5, 12
vertigo, chiropractic on, 248–249
vitamin B, 31–35
    coenzyme functions, 31–32
    deficiencies, brain-specific symptoms, 32–33
    dosing and side effects, 34
    folic acid masking, 34–35
    homocysteine hypothesis, 32
    MTHFR gene and variants, 33–34
    niacin and, 35
    with omega-3 fatty acids, 42
    upper limit, 35
vitamin B6
    deficiency, 33
    upper limit, 35
vitamin B_{12}
    for brain health, 437–438
    deficiency, 34
    folic acid masking, 34–35
vitamin D, 27–31
    gut–brain connection, 10
    serotonin and, 28, 42
    side effects, 31
    synthesis and metabolism, 27
vitamin D_3, 27–31
    for bipolar spectrum disorder, 29
    for brain health, 438–439
    for depression, 29–30
    dosing, 30–31
    on mood, primary prevention, 28–29
    side effects, 31
    synthesis and metabolism, 27
    therapeutic benefits, 29
vitamin D receptor, 27–28
    tryptophan hydroxylase-2 enzyme and tryptophans, 28
vitamin E, 35–37
    alpha-tocopherols, 35–37
    benefits, 35–36
    for cognitive decline, 444–445
    dosing, 36–37
    side effects, potential, 37
    tocotrienols, 35, 36
vitamins, 26–37. *See also specific vitamins*
    for addiction, 568–569
    for anxiety, 515
    definition and function, 26
    requirements, 26–27
voxel based morphometry (VBM), of schizophrenia, 360–361
Vuilleumier, P., 291

wake after sleep onset (WASO), 390
Wal, P. D., 295
Walsh, S. J., 409
Wampold, B. E., 548, 548*b*
Watson, D., 302
Weintraub, R. J., 265
Weitzenhofer, A. M., 289
well, sense of being, 165

well-being, on happiness, 165
wellness, sense of, on happiness, 165
Wen, Dr., 559
Wentink, M., 410–411
Wernicke-Korsakoff syndrome, 32
Western diet. *See also* diet; Standard American Diet (SAD)
   on brain, 11–13
   gut bacteria distribution, 8
   inflammation and mood, 4
   Lactobacilli, 12
   neuroinflammatory marker levels, 12
   risks, 3–4
   short-chain fatty acids, 5, 11–12
whipping *vs.* redirecting, 168–169
Willemsen, G., 515
Williams, D. R., 134
Willis-Ekbom's disease, 397–398
Wilson, B. A., 424
Wilson, W. P., 130
Withania somnifera (ashwagandha), 192–193, 446
withdrawal symptoms, avoiding, 556
Woerner, M., 298
Woo, E, 265
wormwood, 191–192
Write-Organize-Picture-Rehearse (W-O-P-R) strategy, 424–425
Wu, K., 302
Wynn, G. H., 543

Yaden, D. B., 105, 133
Yamagiwa, D., 330
Yang, 208–209, 558–559
Yang, J. D., 219
Yarnell, S., 547
Yellow Emperor's Internal Classics, 206
Yin and Yang, 208–209, 558–559
yoga. *See also* religion and spirituality
   for addiction, 562
   on anxiety, 511
   on autonomic nervous system, 56
   for cognitive decline, 446–447
   on cortisol, 57
   for depression, 481
   on dopamine, 55
   on executive function, 58
   on health, 138–139
   on mental health, 51
   on mindfulness, 59
   popularity of, 119
   for PTSD, 537–538
   on serotonin, 55
   for smoking cessation, 562
Yonker, R., 298
Young, K., 302
Yuan, H., 301–302
Yukimasa, T., 335

Zen Buddhism, 99. *See also* meditation and stress reduction, neurobiology
Zer-Aviv, T. M., 547–548
zinc, 40–41
Zollinger, T. W., 128
zonulin, 8–9
zonulin occludin, 9
Zubritsky, C., 133